Health

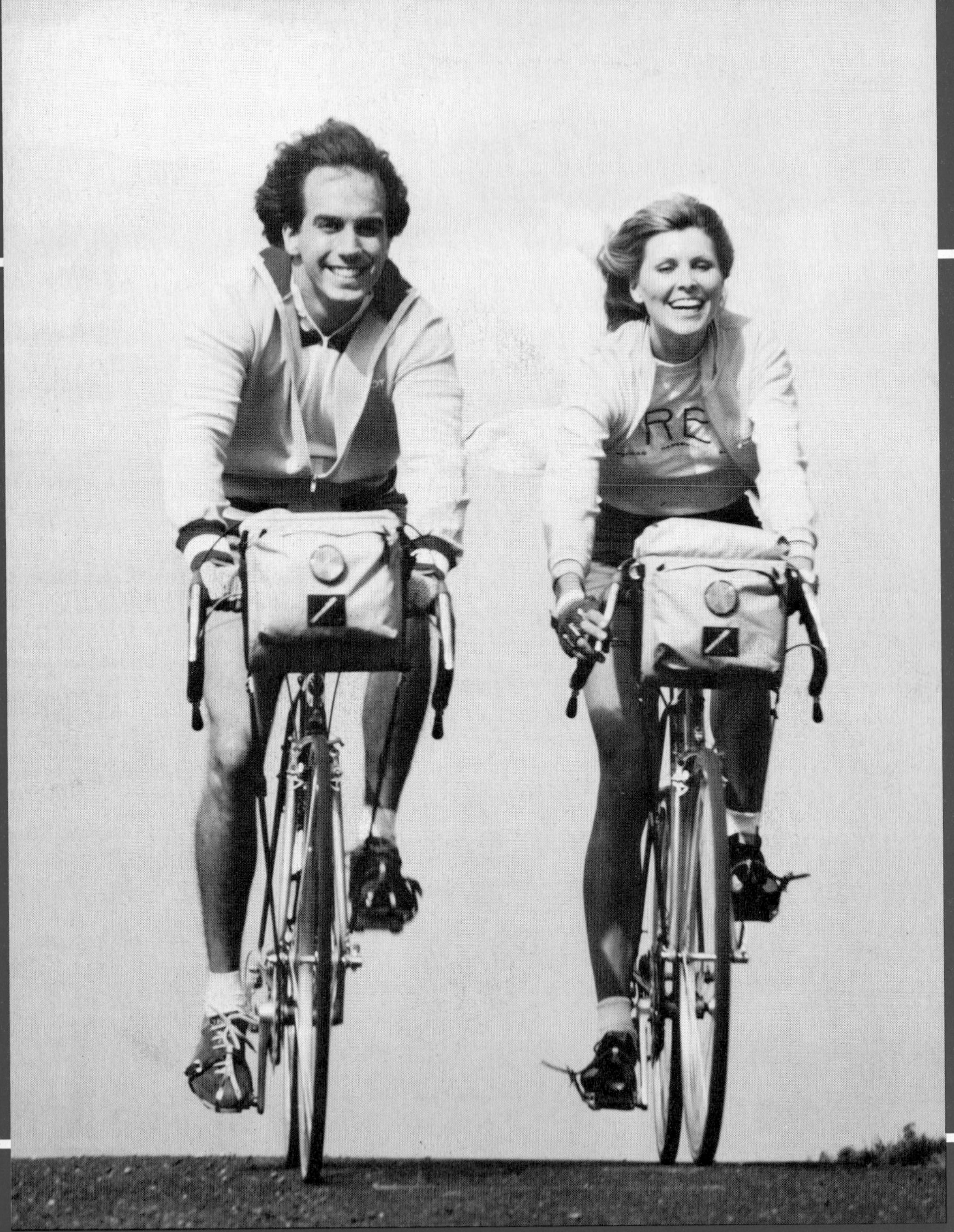

FIFTH EDITION

Health

John La Place, Ph.D.

Prentice-Hall, Inc., Englewood Cliffs, New Jersey 07632

Library of Congress Cataloging-in-Publication Data

LaPlace, John.
Health.

Bibliography: p.
Includes index.
1. Health. 2. Public health. I. Title.
[DNLM: 1. Health. 2. Public Health. WA 4 L312h]
RA776.L348 1987 613 86-25194
ISBN 0-13-384587-7

Editorial/production supervision: Joseph X. O'Donnell Jr.
Cover and interior design: Anne T. Bonanno
Photo editor: Lorinda Morris
Photo research: Ilene Cherna
Cover photo: The Stock Shop
Manufacturing buyer: Harry P. Baisley

Printed in the United States of America

10 9 8 7 6 5 4 3

ISBN 0-13-384587-7 01

Prentice-Hall International (UK) Limited, *London*
Prentice-Hall of Australia Pty. Limited, *Sydney*
Prentice-Hall Canada Inc., *Toronto*
Prentice-Hall Hispanoamericana, S.A., *Mexico*
Prentice-Hall of India Private Limited, *New Delhi*
Prentice-Hall of Japan, Inc., *Tokyo*
Prentice-Hall of Southeast Asia Pte. Ltd., *Singapore*
Editora Prentice-Hall do Brasil, Ltda., *Rio de Janeiro*

(Acknowledgments appear on pp. 539–540, which constitute
a continuation of the copyright page.)

Brief Contents

Contents

Boxes

1 *Mental Health*

2 *Stress*

3 *Accidents and Safety*

4 *Physical Fitness*

5 *Nutrition*

6 *Weight Control*

7 *Reproduction and Birth Control*

8 *Sexual Behavior*

9 *Life Styles*

10 *Aging, Dying, and Death*

11 *Alcohol*

12 *Tobacco*

13 *Drugs*

14 *Cardiovascular Diseases and Cancer*

15 *Communicable Diseases*

16 *Consumer Health*

17 *Environmental Health*

Preface

Today more than ever, we enjoy the benefits of modern medical science. We also receive more and more information related to health issues. Unfortunately, much of what is brought to our attention comes through the publications and advertisements of faddists and hucksters. The need to be able to distinguish between what is valid information and what is false, between what is fact and what is fabrication, is greater than ever. The fifth edition of *Health* is designed to help readers distinguish between information that could be beneficial and that which is worthless. *Health* gives its readers the opportunity to study and evaluate the full spectrum of health-related issues and to establish guidelines tailored to their own needs, values, and interests.

We take pride in our effort in this edition of *Health* to continue to present a text that is current in its issues; accurate in its information; free from bias in its reporting; and clear and concise in its writing. The success of *Health* in maintaining these standards through the first four editions is attested to by its wide acceptance in the field of health education. The fifth edition retains the acclaimed features of the past editions, supplementing them with a variety of new features.

Guides to Behavior Change

Advances in the medical sciences enable more people to overcome conditions that were once disabling or to survive disorders ordinarily fatal. Infants as well as adults benefit from new medical techniques that permit survival in situations once considered hopeless. And with a greater number of us responding more to medical advice by being more careful about our weight and diet, discontinuing smoking, drinking less alcohol, and exercising more, we find ourselves enjoying longer and more fruitful lives. Throughout *Health,* self-scoring inventories permit readers to assess their health habits and knowledge, so that they can judge for themselves the degree to which they incorporate healthful ways into their life styles. The first and most fundamental of these inventories appears in the Introduction. It provides the reader with the opportunity for an overall appraisal of fundamental health habits. It also suggests critical health areas that the reader may wish to pursue in the text for further information.

Problems and Controversies

Like the earlier editions, the fifth edition of *Health* presents the full range of health issues, including the controversial topics. In fact, the fifth edition features controversial issues in a special section of each chapter bearing the title "Problems and Controversies." A major purpose of a health course should be to sharpen decision-making skills, and we believe there is no better way to do this than through a lively debate over a controversial issue.

Boxes There are inevitably sidelights to every topic of discussion. They may reflect a unique point of view, point out something that may warrant being highlighted, or simply present another fact. These sidelights appear as boxed-off sections in each chapter of the text and are a source of supplementary information. They are listed on a separate page following the table of contents.

Where to Go for Help As a further aid in resolving possible personal problems, there is a new feature in most chapters—a listing of national agencies that provide assistance in dealing with specific health problems.

Consumer Concerns As the values of the marketplace invade the field of health, we find fashion and faddism rather than knowledge and judgment influencing our health decisions. Instead of questioning the validity of the latest health craze, many of us commit ourselves to ill-chosen food regimens and exercise programs, employ unqualified therapists, or indulge in psychic experiences that, too often, are psychologically damaging. As opportunists increasingly find the health field a lucrative area in which to operate, we are obliged to become more and more skeptical and also more capable of defending ourselves from maltreatment, unwise expenditures, or blatant fraud. Additionally, there is the inescapable fact that health expenditures continue to become an ever larger part of our total budget. How well we can manage the costs of health insurance, pharmaceuticals, medical fees, and, perhaps, nursing care is a problem each of us must face. Therefore, each chapter of *Health* concludes with a section labeled "Consumer Concerns" that is designed to give readers the opportunity to test their consumer skills.

Accidents and Safety Accidents are the fourth leading cause of death in the United States, following heart disorders, cancer, and stroke. But accidents are the principal cause of death for all of us until the age of thirty-seven. Because of the particular significance of accidents to those of college age, the fifth edition includes a separate chapter on accidents and safety. Related material on first aid has been included in a special appendix so that it may be treated as an optional topic.

Flexible Topic Sequence The fifth edition of *Health* presents topics in a logical sequence that is outlined in the Introduction, but the chapters are self-contained and so may be used in any order. Where information pertinent to one chapter is included in another (such as the influence of drug or alcohol abuse on prenatal development, or sexuality and fitness as applied to old age), cross-references are provided.

Other Features To make facts and figures easy to grasp, many are presented in the form of tables, charts, and graphs. Each chapter ends with a concise numbered summary. A glossary for the entire text follows the last chapter. Words that are glossed are defined in the text as they first appear and are printed in boldface type to indicate their presence in the glossary. A select bibliography keyed by chapter precedes the index.

SUPPLEMENTS

Classroom instructors will find the **Instructor's Resource Guide** that accompanies *Health* an excellent source of supplementary information. Prepared by Patrick Moffit of the University of Northern Iowa, it is coordinated with the Consumer

Concerns unit of each chapter and provides many other suggestions for classroom discussion as well. An excellent *Test Item File* prepared by Peter Koehneke of Canisius College is bound in with the Resource Guide.

The test file is also available in two other formats. It is a part of Prentice-Hall's Computerized Testing Service, whereby instructors can order customized tests direct from the publisher. For those who have access to an Apple II™ or IBM® PC, floppy disks containing the test questions are also available. This service allows users to add, change, or delete questions at their discretion.

Also available, on a separate floppy disk, is the Grade Book Program, which helps instructors maintain student grades, compute class statistics, print graphs, and sort by student name or grade.

Qualified adopters are eligible to receive free videotapes. Details on these and all of the supplements are available from local Prentice-Hall representatives.

The most frequent comment that we have received from students who have used earlier editions of *Health* is that they have enjoyed reading it. We trust that readers of the fifth edition will feel the same.

ACKNOWLEDGMENTS

I will always be indebted to my friend Saul Ostrow for his counsel in the writing of *Health* and to my friend Tonnes Vetland for the encouragement he provided. Many thanks to my daughter, Ellen, for her perspectives as my current "in-house reader" and to my wife, Olaug, for her role in keeping everything together.

I am grateful also for the advice of reviewers of the fourth edition and of the manuscript of the fifth, many of whose suggestions I have adopted:

Ruth Ann Althaus
Illinois Benedictine College

Ken Becker
University of Wisconsin, La Crosse

Andrew J. J. Brennan
Metropolitan Life Insurance Company

Lee N. Burkett
Arizona State University

Randall R. Cottrell
University of Oregon

Joyce E. Miller
Indiana University

Patrick Moffit
University of Northern Iowa

Larry K. Olsen
Penn State University

Frank Schabel
Iowa State University

Richard G. Schlaadt
University of Oregon

Mary H. Slaughter
University of Illinois at Urbana-Champaign

Sherman K. Sowby
California State University, Fresno

Harold E. Wingard
Indiana University of Pennsylvania

Thanks are owed, too, to Laurie Beck, who did the research for this edition; to Robert Mony, whose writing skills improved it; and to Ronald S. Csuha, who prepared the select bibliography.

I am also grateful for the help I have received from the members of the Prentice-Hall staff. I express my deepest appreciation and thanks for their contributions toward the preparation of this new edition.

John La Place

Introduction: Your Health Decisions

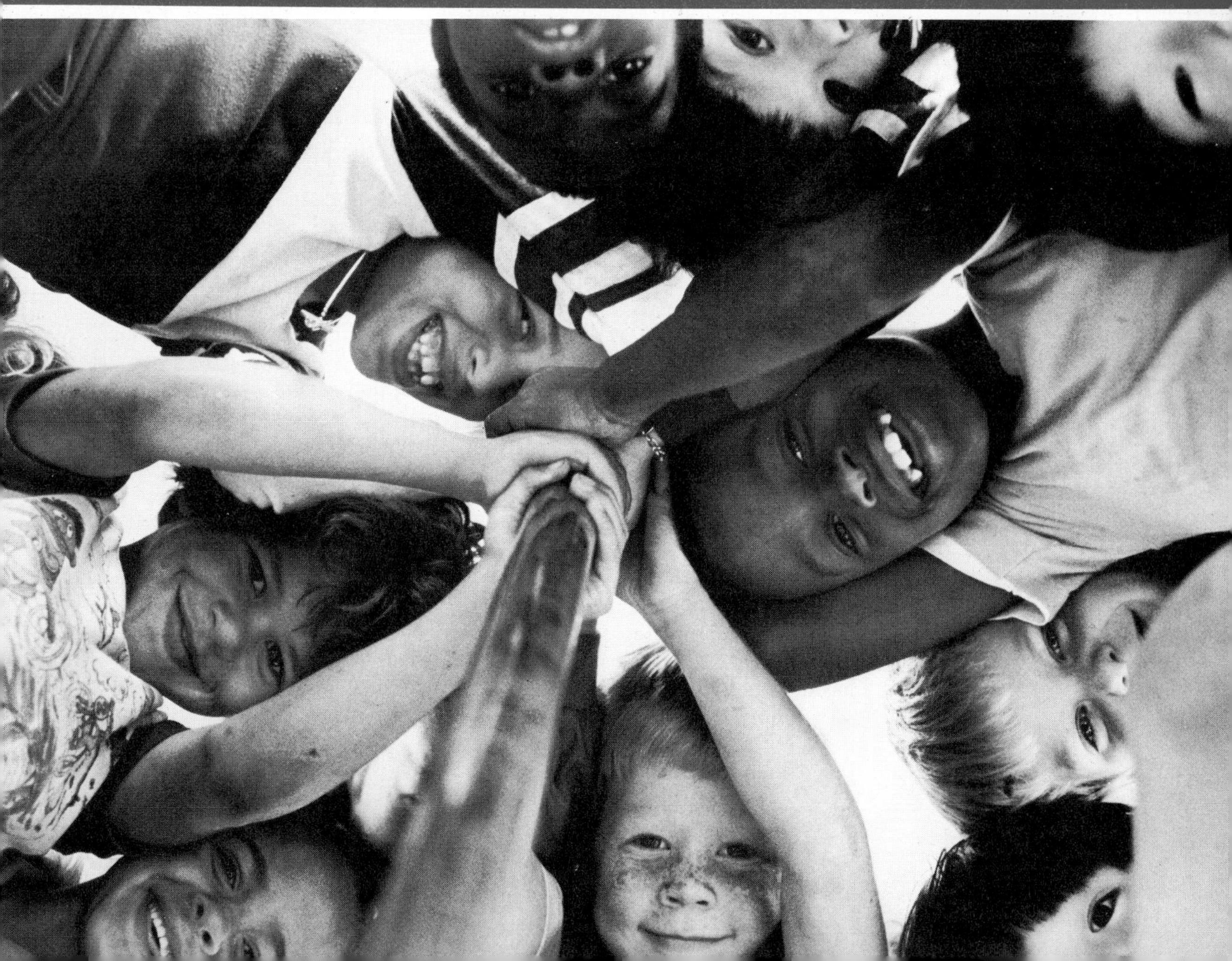

Health is more than the absence of injury or disease. If poor health is accompanied by lethargy and a reduced ability to function, then the reverse must be true of good health, and healthiness must elevate our level of energy and our capacity to perform, mentally as well as physically. This positive concept of health as an ever increasing level of well-being is gradually replacing the somewhat negative definition of merely avoiding illness. Those who have accepted the challenge of maximizing their well-being have made significant changes in their life styles as they have established new goals for themselves. They have committed themselves to programs of physical activity selected to improve their vital capacity. They have become more cautious in their choice of food, selecting their diet with greater purpose. And they have decided to avoid or limit their use of substances known to detract from well-being. Those who are in this group maintain that they benefit not only in improved mental and physical capacity but, just as important, in their attitudes toward themselves.

Each chapter of *Health* is designed to provide you with information essential to making decisions in an area of health critical to your well-being. Only if you have accurate information, validated by scientific study, will you have a legitimate basis upon which to exercise your judgment. Ultimately, it is your own personal values that will determine what options you choose in matters affecting your life style in such areas as diet, physical activity, rest, sexuality, abusable substances, safety, and stress. Understanding the future consequences of your present actions will enable you to make decisions in the interest of your future well-being and can give you the satisfaction of knowing that you are in control of your own life.

It would be wrong, however, to think that life style alone determines well-being. Each of us is born with a prospective life span determined in part by our genetic inheritance. We should make ourselves aware of any conditions or predispositions we have inherited that may impose limitations on our lives, for many diseases begin in a very subtle fashion. It is quite common for people to have disorders such as diabetes or glaucoma, both of which run in families, and not be aware of them. And cardiovascular impairment and cancer, our leading causes of death, can exist with little or no outward sign.

We all tend to be complacent about our health when we feel well. But periodic medical examinations by a qualified physician are essential for a complete and reliable assessment of our true physical condition. Such an assessment can help to prevent future illnesses as well as discover existing conditions while they are in an early stage and generally more amenable to treatment. It can also provide much vital information that may affect our health behavior. Knowing the level of cholesterol or sodium in our blood, for example, can influence our dietary choices. And it is essential to know our state of cardiovascular health before beginning any vigorous exercise program.

Such a medical examination requires qualified medical personnel. And other health counseling, in areas such as nutrition, mental health, and marital or sexual problems, requires equally competent and honest practitioners. Today's health complex is so vast an industry that it is difficult for us to evaluate its programs, products, and people. But doing so is important to our well-being. *Health* provides you with help in becoming a knowledgeable consumer.

Health is structured in units of related chapters. In the first unit, composed of chapters on mental health, stress, and accidents and safety, the common bond is the psychological—your frame of mind, your thinking, your attitudes. The chapter on mental health presents positive strategies directed toward maintaining psychological well-being. The chapter on stress shows you what factors cause stress and presents ways of handling what has become virtually the earmark of our society. Accidents are the leading cause of death among young people, and they are preventable. The chapter on accidents and safety presents considerations that can help you reduce the possibility of such mishaps in your life.

Physical fitness, nutrition, and weight control are at the core of our concept of well-being. These are areas over which you have considerable control. They are also areas where misinformation is rampant and exploitation of the public is commonplace. The chapters on these topics urge you to be particularly discerning in making decisions and give you specific advice on how to do so.

The next unit is composed of chapters on reproduction and birth control, sexual behavior, and life styles. No other material in the text brings forth feelings as intense as the personal and social issues discussed in this section. Clarifying facts, nevertheless, is a significant aspect of these subjects.

Our lives continue to lengthen, and the percentage of our population that we consider elderly continues to grow; therefore the phenomenon of aging becomes increasingly important to all of us, individually as well as collectively. How you adjust to life as you grow older, the care you may have to provide for others as they grow older, the provisions that exist for the elderly in our society, and our ability to deal with dying and death are discussed in this next chapter of the text.

Those of you who have opted for a healthier life style have probably made a very definite decision in respect to alcohol, tobacco, and other abusable substances. Among a considerable portion of the population the use of these substances has declined considerably. But, as we are all well aware, the problem of abuse has not disappeared. Use, sometimes leading to abuse, of potentially addictive substances is still too common in our society. The dimensions of this problem are discussed in the chapters on alcohol, tobacco, and drugs.

The cardiovascular diseases and cancer are our primary causes of death. Of special significance is the fact that signs of these diseases can often be detected early in life. Such early detection is of the utmost importance if the direction of the disease is to be altered. This chapter discusses the factors that contribute to the development of these diseases and presents the advice of authorities to guide you in avoiding them.

The chapter on communicable diseases describes the manner in which your immune system functions; brings to your attention the importance of our immunization programs; and discusses a variety of transmittable diseases that remain prevalent in our society. Of special concern is the fact that the sexually transmitted diseases are occurring with such frequency and that with the appearance of AIDS we are faced with a form that, so far, remains fatal.

One of the major concerns we all face in life is financing our well-being. It is essential that you learn to understand health insurance with its variety of options, the costs as well as the benefits. It is also important that you develop a skeptical attitude about health-promoting offers. The chapter on consumer health points out various debatable and fraudulent approaches to health care.

U.S. Life Expectancy at Various Ages, 1984

Age in 1984	Average years Life Remaining
At birth	74.7
1	74.5
5	70.7
10	65.8
15	60.8
20	56.1
25	51.4
30	46.7
35	42.0
40	37.3
45	32.7
50	28.4
55	24.2
60	20.4
65	16.8
70	13.6
75	10.7
80	8.2
85	6.2

Source: National Center for Health Statistics, 1985.

The magnitude of the problems affecting our environment is tremendous. Dealing with such problems as chemical wastes, sludge, acid rain, auto emissions, and radioactive wastes, all of which pose a threat to our health and well-being, requires concerted effort and legislative action. There is a role for all of us in this effort because social pressure is a tremendous force, and if we want a healthier environment, we must fight for it. This final chapter of the book presents you with the significant issues in environmental health.

Each of us, it is true, is born with a prospective life span that is determined by our genetic inheritance. But advancing medical knowledge and a corresponding adoption of sound health practices are enabling us to live out our potential lifespan to a constantly increasing extent, so that the child born in the United States today can anticipate living some seventy-five years. What is of special interest is to note how we benefit by remaining healthy and well: for each year of life that we survive, our potential moves forward. This can best be seen by looking at the life expectancy figures for those who have today reached the age of seventy-five—an age, by the way, already far beyond the average lifespan at the time of their birth. From the table at the left, we can see that those who are presently seventy-five can still expect over ten more years of life. So the rewards of making wise health decisions continue to accumulate.

Because your well-being is influenced considerably by your knowledge of health and the degree to which you put this knowledge to practice in your daily life, you may wish to respond to the following questions about your health habits and determine for yourself whether your life style is healthful.

Your Life Style

_________ 1. Have you had a physical examination conducted by a medical doctor within the past few years that provided you with the opportunity to discuss your medical and family history, your life style, and your feelings in general, as well as the test results?

_________ 2. Do you understand and follow medically recognized guidelines for proper nutrition in your daily intake of food?

_________ 3. Remaining mindful of these same nutritional guidelines, do you endeavor to control your consumption of calories?

_________ 4. Do you include at least three half-hour sessions of genuinely aerobic activity in your weekly routine?

_________ 5. Do you get enough rest?

_________ 6. Are you aware of the inherent hazard, and do you exercise appropriate caution, in respect to the following: caffeine, tobacco, alcohol, health foods, legal drugs, illegal drugs?

_________ 7. Is your sexual life guided by good judgment?

_________ 8. In your present mode of family living, do you fulfill your role, and do you find your role to be fulfilling?

_________ 9. In general, is your life wholesome and rewarding? For example, do you derive satisfaction from your work or your life as a student? Do you have interests that occupy your spare time? Are you happy with the state of your friendships?

1

Mental Health

Determinants of Personality
The Life Cycle
Defining Mental Health
Defense Mechanisms
Neuroses
Psychoses
Treatment Strategies
Mental Illness and Society
Therapists

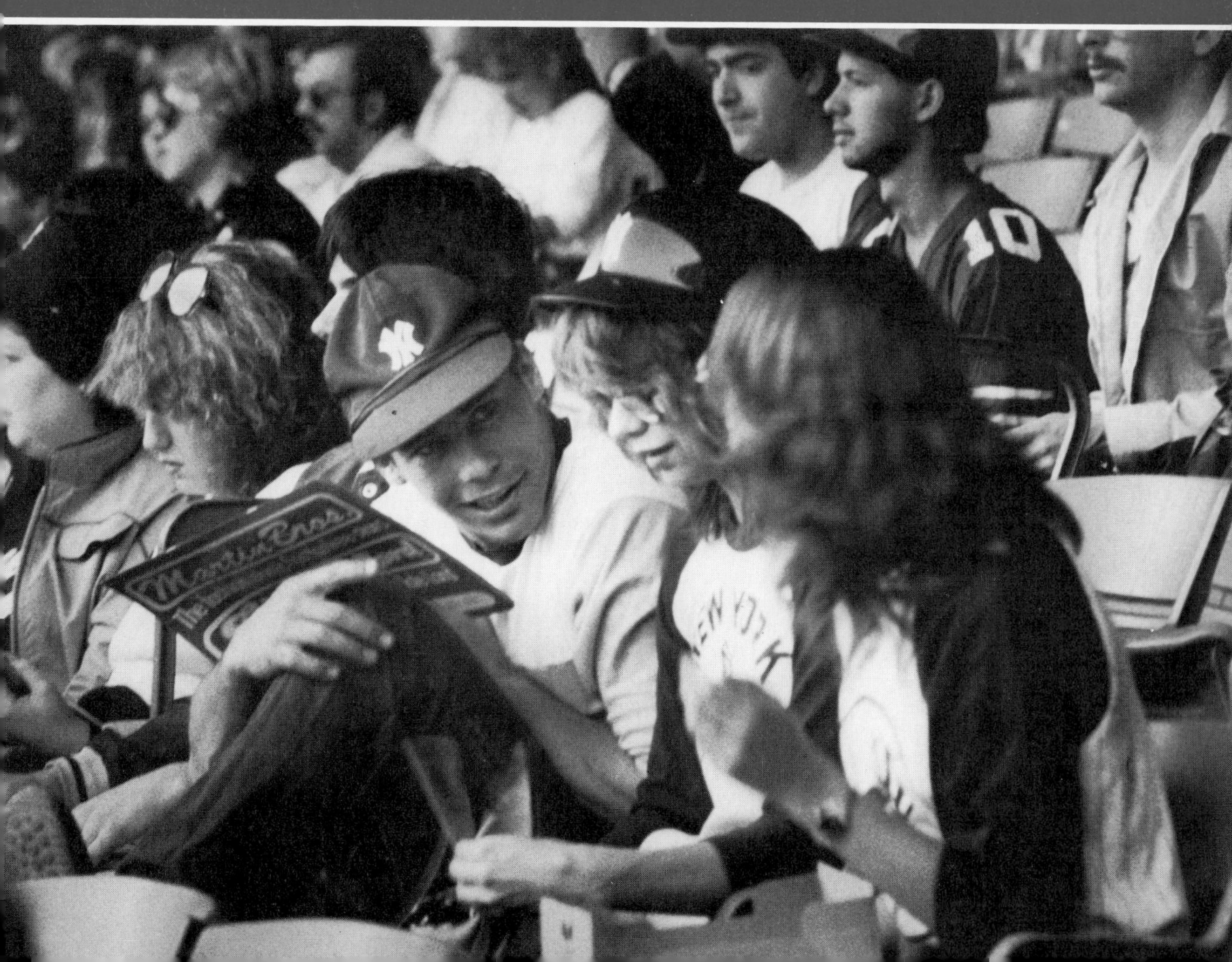

It has been estimated that one out of five Americans is suffering from some form of mental illness. If you do not have any psychological difficulties yourself, you probably know someone—either a family member or friend—who does. Mental illness is one of our gravest national health problems, but our country seems unwilling to do much to alleviate it. Of all the money spent on health by both federal and state governments, the least is given over to mental health. The major reason for this is society's attitude toward mental illness. Many people consider emotional disturbance to be a sign of character weakness. Many others have an irrational fear of mental patients and ex-patients and want them kept out of sight as much as possible. Still others recognize the signs of mental illness in themselves but are terrified of being labeled "crazy" and refuse to seek help.

People who have no symptoms of mental illness are not necessarily mentally healthy, however—just at people who have no symptoms of disease are not necessarily physically healthy. While inactive and overweight people may feel fine, they do not have the physical capacities of those who are fit and active. By the same token, those who are functioning from day to day with no signs of emotional disturbance may still lack certain positive definable characteristics that truly well-adjusted people possess.

What, then, constitutes mental well-being and mental illness? In this chapter we shall discuss some factors that influence personality makeup and review the major formative experiences of the life-cycle stages. Next, we will consider the defensive strategies people use in coping with emotional conflicts and follow this with a brief overview of the major types of neurotic and psychotic disorders. A variety of treatment strategies, ranging from psychoanalysis to drug therapy, will then be discussed. Toward the end of the chapter we shall return to society's attitudes toward mental disorders and finish by describing the training and capabilities of mental health professionals.

DETERMINANTS OF PERSONALITY

Personality is the totality of traits, attitudes, and ways of behaving that make each person unique. Despite lifelong growth, adjustment, and developmental change, personality tends to remain fairly stable.

It is generally accepted that heredity and environment interact to influence the development of our personality and behavior patterns. Experience and culture are both part of environment. Our inherited traits may be allowed their full expression or be modified by our life experiences. The culture in which we are raised determines, to a great extent, the nature of the experiences we are likely to have. Heredity and environment interact, as we shall see, throughout the life cycle.

Heredity

Heredity is the process by which certain characteristics are biologically transmitted from parent to child. We know that physical characteristics are inherited—for example, most of us resemble our parents in some way. (The process of genetic transmission is discussed in Chapter 7.) It is more difficult to determine whether personality traits are inherited as well. Environmental factors such as education, family upbringing, and social mores contribute greatly to the formation of personality. Identifying those characteristics that are specifically a function of heredity is therefore complicated.

Nevertheless, extensive research suggests that we inherit certain tendencies and potentialities. For example, babies display different temperaments almost from the moment of birth. There is a highly significant correlation between the intelligence of parents and the intelligence of their children. Identical twins, who are the same genetically, have been found to share a great number of personality traits—including certain mental disorders. Even identical twins who have been reared separately (and thus did not have the same environment) display many intellectual, emotional, and psychological similarities. Heredity also appears to influence the development of artistic, mathematical, and linguistic ability, although here environment as well plays a large role.

Environment: Experience and Culture

A child may inherit a tendency toward certain personality traits—introversion or extroversion, superior intelligence or average intelligence, and so on. But the way in which the tendency is developed depends to a large degree on the environment. Life experiences and culture can determine whether and how inherited potentials are expressed.

Experience. A lively and loving family, for example, can make a child with an inborn tendency toward introversion much more outgoing. On the other hand, an early environment of emotional deprivation can inhibit a child. Children raised in institutions from birth tend to be more withdrawn and less affectionate and intelligent than children raised in a warm and secure home environment.

Similarly, the experiences people have throughout their lives can affect their personality development. The possibility of personality change—for better or for worse—exists as long as a person is alive. Generally, the nature, intensity, and duration of a particular experience determine its effect. Momentary nontraumatic experiences usually have little effect on a person's normal development. A more prolonged or intense experience may inhibit a person's innate capacities or, conversely, reinforce them so they will be expressed more fully.

Culture. Cultural attitudes and expectations are another major influence on personality formation. By imitating the behavior of those around them, a process that is generally encouraged and reinforced, individuals incorporate into their own personalities the values of their country, community, and economic class.

Parents begin the process of **socialization** almost as soon as their child is born. Initial training usually involves the development of the child's gender identity—a young boy's aggressiveness, for example, might be greeted with approval, while a young girl's aggressiveness might be met with dismay. Studies have shown that many sex differences that were presumed to be hereditary are really the products of socialization. Parents also transmit to their child their speech accents, manners, social prejudices, and attitudes—all of which are absorbed by the child and become a part of his or her identity.

Many fundamental attitudes that we take for granted are really the product of our own time and place. The idea of the individual self, for example, which is so much a part of our cultural tradition, is a comparatively recent development

TABLE 1-1
Erikson's Stages of Psychosocial Development

Stage	Approximate Age	Challenges and Outcomes
1	Birth to 1 year	*Trust vs. Mistrust* Infants learn about the basic trustworthiness of the environment. If their needs for nourishment, attention, and affection are met, they will perceive the world as trustworthy and secure. If these needs are not met, they will come to view the world as inconsistent, stressful, and threatening.
2	1–3 years	*Autonomy vs. Shame and Doubt* Children learn about their own bodies and how to control them. Feeding, dressing, toileting, and walking all involve experimentation. When successful at these things, children gain a sense of self-confidence and self-control. When they fail continually and are labeled messy, inadequate, or bad, they learn to feel shame and self-doubt.
3	3–6 years	*Initiative vs. Guilt* Children begin to explore the world; they discover how it works and how they can affect it. If their activities are successful, they learn to deal with the world in a constructive way and gain a sense of initiative. If they are criticized and punished, they learn to feel guilty for many of their own actions.
4	6–11 years	*Industry vs. Inferiority* Children develop many skills and competencies in school, at home, and in the outside world of their peers. Comparison with peers becomes increasingly important. They can gain a sense of inferiority if negatively evaluated compared to others at this time.
5	Adolescence	*Ego Identity vs. Ego Diffusion* The adolescent must sort out and integrate various roles—such as older sister, student, friend, Christian—into one consistent identity. Adolescents also seek out basic values that cut across these roles. If an adolescent fails to integrate a central identity and cannot resolve major value conflicts, the result is ego diffusion.
6	Early Adulthood	*Intimacy vs. Isolation* Young adults seek not only sexual intimacy but also social intimacy in which they can share themselves with another person without fear of losing their own identity. Success at this task depends on how well the person has solved the five earlier conflicts.
7	Middle Adulthood	*Generativity vs. Self-Absorption* Having solved their earlier conflicts, adults can now attend more fully to assisting others. Parents find themselves by helping their children. Others may help solve social issues or do other constructive work. Failure to solve earlier conflicts results in self-preoccupation with health, psychological needs, comfort, and so on.
8	Late Adulthood	*Integrity vs. Despair* People look back over their lives and judge them. If they are satisfied that their life has had meaning and involvement, then they have a sense of integrity. If they see their life as a series of misdirected energies and lost chances, they have a sense of despair.

Source: Adapted from Grace J. Craig, *Human Development,* 4th ed. (Englewood Cliffs, N.J.: Prentice-Hall, 1986), pp. 44–46.

in human history. People in "primitive" societies often had no sense of self as we know it; instead, they felt themselves to be totally identified with their communities. Attitudes of aggression or cooperation, conformity or individuality, rationality or spirituality, and countless other attitudes are conveyed to us by our culture and form the basis of many of our beliefs and actions.

THE LIFE CYCLE

Theorists give varying degrees of importance to heredity, experience, and culture in personality development. In recent years they have stressed the importance of experience over heredity and culture. Experience is the element over which we can exercise the most control. We cannot choose our ancestors, nor can we change our culture. We can, however, learn which experiences affect us positively and negatively, develop ways of preparing for them, and let this knowledge guide our behavior toward others.

Although each individual has unique experiences, all human beings pass through fairly predictable stages of development. According to the psychologist Erik Erikson, knowledge and experience build from one stage to the next, so that the different needs and challenges of early stages must be met before a person can cope with problems at later stages. Erikson's eight-stage theory of psychosocial development explains how each stage of life presents a person with certain critical conflicts and challenges (see Table 1-1). The healthy person meets each challenge or resolves each conflict successfully. Although each of Erikson's stages poses two extreme resolutions—for example, initiative and guilt in stage 3—a wide range of other resolutions is possible. On balance, most people steer a middle course in which the experiences that give them a sense of initiative probably outnumber those that result in feelings of guilt.

Erikson's stages are called psychosocial because they indicate relationships between the personality and the expanding social world. The following sections describe experiences typically encountered over the life cycle. It will be useful to consult Table 1-1 as you read these sections.

Infancy

The interplay of heredity and environment affects human potential from the moment of conception. Genetic abnormalities in the embryo, for example, may cause the mother to miscarry. During pregnancy maternal nutrition, as the source of embryonic and fetal nutrition, directly affects the child's physical and mental development. It has long been known that inadequate maternal nutrition stunts the growth of brain cells in the fetus. The harmful effects of other substances have only recently been verified: Any but minimal amounts of alcohol consumed by the expectant mother can damage the fetus. The use of tobacco and hard drugs also retards fetal growth and intelligence. Likewise, the abuse of vitamin D during pregnancy can result in mental retardation; and one can only guess what fetal damage is being caused by a variety of chemical substances that enter the food chain either unintentionally, as pesticides, or during food processing. Even the act of birth itself can be harmful to the child. A mother's structural or physical abnormalities may deprive the child of sufficient oxygen during birth and cause severe brain damage and functional disability.

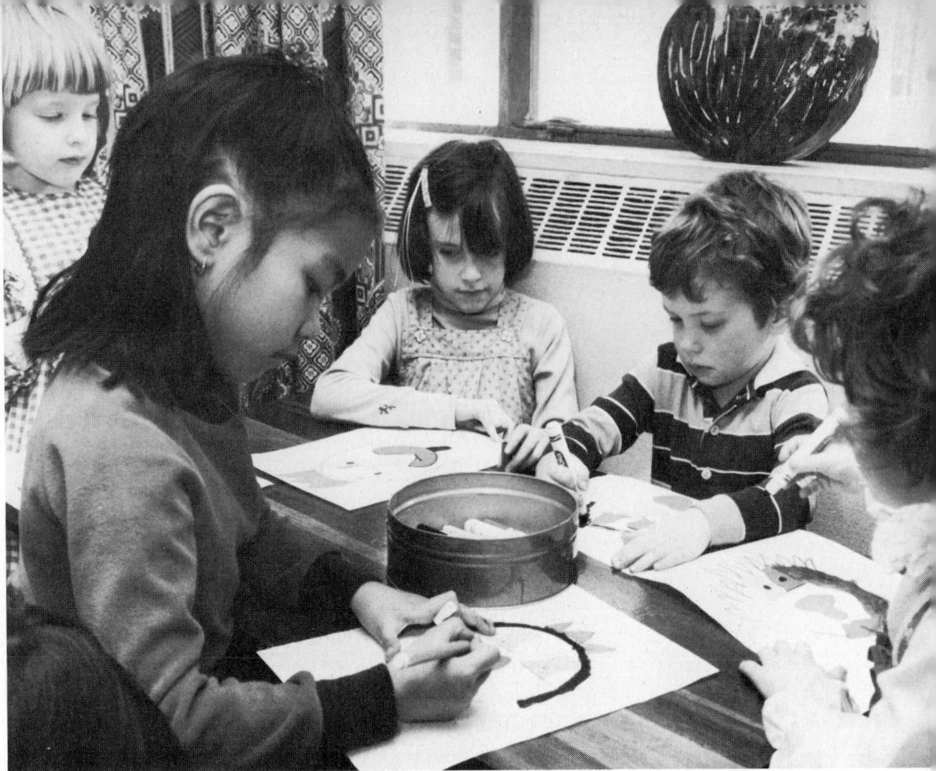

From the moment of birth, tender loving care becomes a necessity. The infant who is held securely and affectionately; who is touched and allowed to touch; who is fed, washed, and permitted to sleep undisturbed according to his or her needs; and who receives verbal attention by being spoken to is the infant who will begin to develop basic feelings of trust (Erikson's stage 1).

The opposite type of care—neglecting the infant's comfort and needs—creates a disturbing environment that hinders emotional development. Children raised in institutions are very likely to become mistrustful and emotionally disturbed, a direct consequence of emotional deprivation during the early years.

During their first years, children learn about themselves and their environment. They begin to recognize the sights and sounds of people and things around them, and they begin the process of self-exploration and identification. Providing young children with things to touch and moving objects (such as mobiles) to watch facilitates this development.

Released from the confinement of the crib and allowed to crawl, the infant begins to explore a totally new world. Progress may be slow, or occur in spurts, but the rewards, nevertheless, are gratifying. There are new things to see and to feel; there is the satisfaction of being able to touch and grasp desired objects. Thus the crawling stage provides the emotional reward of achievement, the mental stimulation that occurs with exploration, and the physical benefit derived from crawling itself.

As children grow less dependent upon others to bring things to them and begin to determine their own course of action, they start to become autonomous individuals (Erikson's stage 2). Legitimate concerns of the parents for the safety of their children or the preservation of the home may require them to warn their children and restrict their movements. If such situations are handled in a neutral, unthreatening manner, children will understand the limits that are being imposed.

Physical dexterity and independence of action are developed at this stage, as children begin to handle spoons, for example, and hold and use cups or glasses. That everything does not reach its mark is incidental. Criticism or comment will only destroy a child's confidence. Toys that provide opportunity for movement, such as inserting, pouring, lifting, rolling, stacking, and selecting, all help to develop coordination and dexterity. Parental encouragement and patience are important. A display of disappointment or excessively high expectations can create feelings of shame and self-doubt in children. During this period a child must be assured of being a person, of having a role, of being wanted and loved. A show of affection says much to a child.

Childhood

A child's unique individuality begins to emerge early in life. Perceptive parents recognize the particular characteristics of their child, acknowledge the fact that each human being is different and has a right to be so, and behave toward the child as befits his or her specific personality pattern. Acceptance of children as they are enhances their self-image and reduces parent-child tension. Children should not feel coerced or limited in their options by the threat of losing love or respect. They should be allowed to select interests and pursuits that satisfy them, not their parents; in other words, they should be encouraged to develop initiative (Erikson's stage 3). Receiving this respect and consideration will, in turn, encourage them to respect the rights and needs of others and to develop a sense of social concern. Parents should try neither to relive their own lives nor live the life they never lived through their children.

Many abilities that affect the child's self-esteem are developed during this period. All children want to feel that they are not only a part of the family but a contributing member as well. Their contribution to the family consists at first of merely being able to take care of themselves, to put away their clothes or their toys, and eventually to make their own beds. As they grow older, they will have opportunities to assume greater responsibilities—to run errands, take messages, and so on.

Decision making is another important skill that children must learn. Letting a child decide such things as what to wear on a particular day, what new clothes to buy, or what to have for lunch develops abilities that can be put to good use when larger decisions in life must be made. Teaching the child that there are consequences to each decision—that money spent on one item will leave nothing for another, for example—facilitates the maturation process.

When children begin school, it is important that parents talk with them, encourage their inquisitiveness, and help them to develop a feeling of competence (Erikson's stage 4) through industriousness. Parents should make every possible effort to increase their children's vocabulary skills. Reading stories to smaller children and making reading material available to older children are essential. The development of verbal and reading abilities, a sense of curiosity, and a feeling that the complex world can indeed be understood is the most important prerequisite for scholastic success and a resulting feeling of competence in the child.

A crucial factor in the child's development is the impact of the total community environment. If the net effect of the vital forces in a child's life—family, neighborhood, school, country—is one of caring and concern for the child's

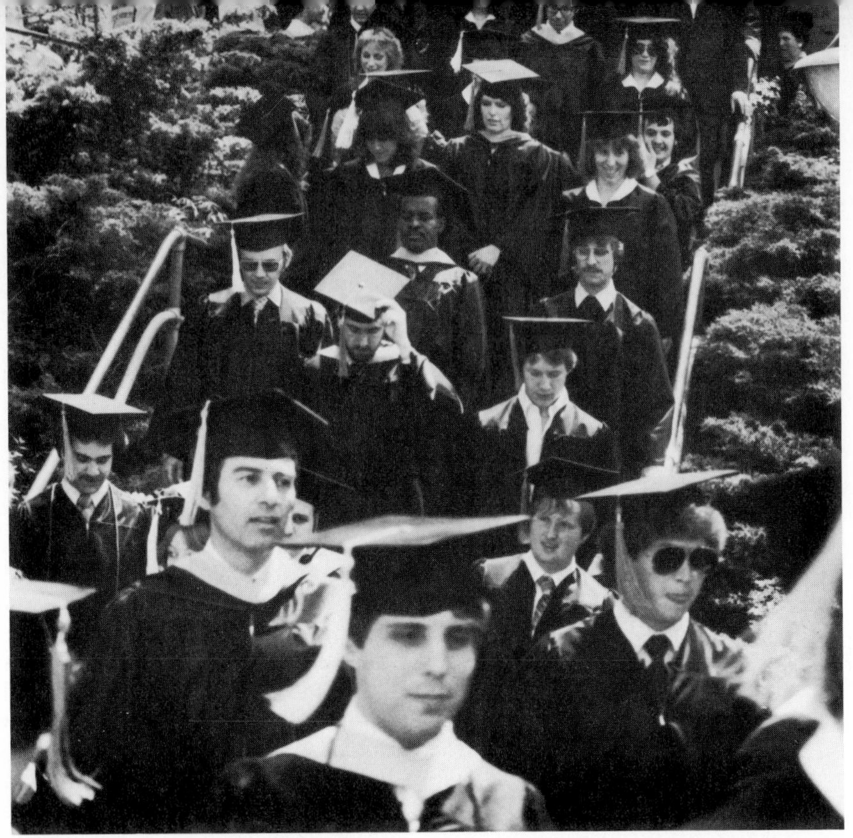

well-being and future, then a sense of acceptance, worth, and security will be engendered. Discrimination, poverty, poor housing, and inadequate social services foster feelings of inferiority and helplessness in a child.

Adolescence

Adolescence is a time of uncertainty. Conflicts between strongly held beliefs and newly acquired knowledge and experience can create tensions that must be resolved. The basic task of adolescence is putting together a coherent identity (Erikson's stage 5). At this stage a person asks, "Who am I?" "Where am I going?" "What do I believe in?" For an unfortunate number, these questions are never resolved, and ego diffusion results. The search for answers involves much exploration, experimentation, questioning, challenging, mood fluctuations, and seeking of supportive figures. Peers are most likely to provide this support, because they are the ones with whom lines of communication are most open, the ones who are least critical, and the ones who, because they are undergoing similar experiences, are most empathetic. For these reasons, peer influence is particularly strong during adolescent years.

Parents' efforts to impose standards often breed alienation and create resentment in adolescents because they feel they are being denied the right to make their own decisions. Consequently, adolescents may totally reject any rules or standards that are set. Furthermore, because adolescents are often offered little information for establishing a standard of behavior, they may follow the very course of action that their parents want them to avoid.

Parental influence, therefore, may seem to be minimal, because parents either abdicate their role or attempt to impose their standards and concepts upon their children instead of helping their children arrive at their own conclusions.

But parents' fears that their children's answers will not be the "right" ones (meaning in conformity with their own) are unwarranted. Whatever significance it may have, most children adopt their parents' opinions. In one study 85 percent of graduating high-school seniors said that in general they agreed with their parents' ideas and shared their values.

The process of maturation implies, among other things, the development of independent individuals, secure within themselves, capable of making decisions, and able to impose self-discipline when necessary. It follows that these traits can emerge only when individuals are given the opportunity to exercise independence during these formative years. Parents who maintain contact with their children by being interested in their activities and welfare; who schedule events that the entire family can enjoy together; who show their affection for their children by expressing their satisfaction, their trust, and their concern; and who are available to provide assistance and information when it is needed will probably find that their children, in turn, will have confidence in them, will seek their advice, and will share their concerns.

The community should provide constructive services to assist adolescents in their decisions and adjustments. The school and other community agencies should be able to complement the efforts of parents under ordinary circumstances and compensate, to whatever extent possible, for inadequate parental care and guidance.

Early Adulthood

In adulthood a person acquires legal independence and, more important, responsibility for his or her own life. The readiness for this period of self-determination is a measure of a person's emotional maturity. Many at this stage of life are not prepared to take responsibility for themselves or to become self-supporting. This could reflect emotional immaturity; an unwise life decision, such as marrying despite financial insecurity; or an educational involvement that preempts employment possibilities. The resulting dependence-independence conflict can often engender emotional stress.

In early adulthood (Erikson's stage 6) friends replace family as the source of an individual's most important relationships. People in this age group seek intimate relationships but may find it difficult to make emotional commitments until they become more sure of themselves. Relationships may dissolve as soon as they are formed, while the individual attempts to carve out an identity.

Gaining self-confidence and self-knowledge permits an increased commitment to others. Marriage may occur at this stage, as well as a resolution to master one's fate and achieve success in one's work. Individuals may acquire an older mentor to help them make critical decisions at this stage of life. Delay in achieving a sense of self-worth may lead to self-preoccupation and isolation and render a person unable to become deeply involved in a relationship or activity.

Far from being a final plateau, adulthood continues to present new challenges, new opportunities, and new responsibilities that change at each decade of life. Self-assessments and decisions are required all along the way.

Middle Adulthood

The thirties represent one of the most critical life stages. The individual at this point has had experience in coping with the real world of job, family, and friends. He or she must reassess preconceptions and hopes in the light of

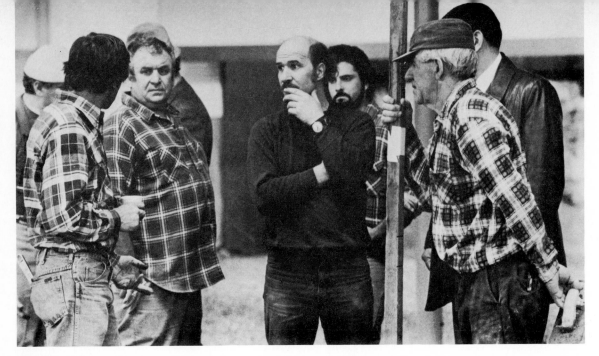

For many, middle adulthood is a time when self-image is dependent upon job satisfaction.

this reality. New questions may arise, such as "Where am I going?" "What is life all about?" "Why aren't other people more sympathetic to my problems?"

The individual may become preoccupied with obstacles that stand in the way of success. Work may be assessed not in terms of the satisfactions it provides but in terms of the status or financial rewards it offers. Friends and even family may be seen as hindrances rather than helpers. For the many whose employment opportunities are severely limited, this can be a particularly depressing time. Lack of opportunity, minimal job satisfaction, and the absence of any feeling of achievement—all have adverse effects on one's self-image and sense of satisfaction. Job changing, infidelity, and divorce are common during this stage of life.

The process of adjusting one's life goals and standards in the light of reality need not be a bitter or depressing experience, however. Many individuals evaluate themselves and those around them with a more benevolent eye. If a job is not proving to be as rewarding as expected, they renew attempts to achieve greater satisfaction. They may, for example, refocus their energies toward constructive, attainable goals. On the other hand, they may open up other areas of their lives—such as leisure-time pursuits—if they find it necessary to compensate for shortcomings in their jobs. They may also create new lines of communication with friends and family. This process of settling down and forming a realistic, satisfying life structure is an important step toward greater self-realization and fulfillment.

Late Adulthood

Late adulthood is characterized by a growing awareness that one's own death is inevitable and that the promise and hopes of one's youth may not have been completely fulfilled. For those who are overly self-involved, who have not achieved a sense of intimacy with others and a sense of mastery over their own destinies, this can be an extremely depressing time.

For others, however, this period may be marked by contentment. The strivings and conflicts of one's youth are viewed with nostalgia, amusement, and self-understanding. There is satisfaction with past accomplishments and a desire to enjoy the present. Individuals may experience what Erikson in his stage 7 calls *generativity*—the desire to advise, teach, and nurture others. Minor failures, faults, and conflicts lose their ability to disturb; there is a greater emphasis on a simpler, more intimate way of life. These are the most stable years of the life cycle.

Individuals who chose to raise a family rather than pursue a career expressed their generativity much earlier. For them, this period of life can offer new obstacles or new opportunities, depending on their point of view. The parental role has been sharply diminished, because by this time children are fully grown and independent. Those who have too closely identified their personalities with family life may have difficulty in adjusting to this new situation. For others, however, this period represents not purposelessness but rather freedom. There is a fresh opportunity to be oneself, to pursue one's own interests, and to act on one's own desires. The long-deferred education, job, or hobby can at last be pursued and enjoyed. (See also the discussion of the male and female climacteric in Chapter 8.)

The Later Years

Today most of us, including the elderly themselves, hold traditional, stereotyped concepts of the aging process that are inaccurate. Before 1950 very little research on the aging process existed. The few studies that had been done were virtually all confined to the elderly in institutions, who make up a very small percentage of those over 65.

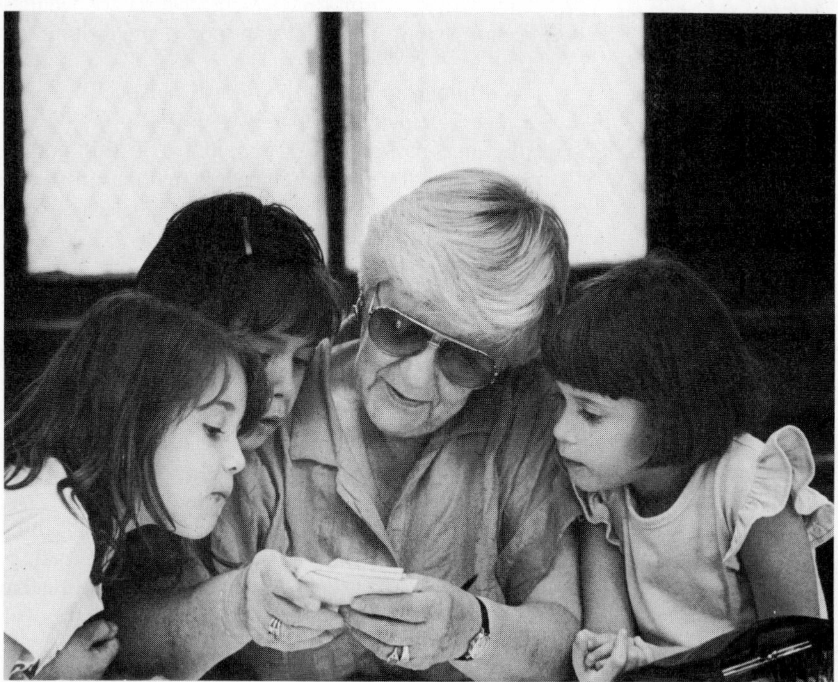

A growing body of research reveals some unexpected information about people in their later years. A leading example is the twenty-year study of 200 elderly people conducted at the Duke University Medical Center. This study showed that the vast majority of old people are in good health, are socially and sexually active, enjoy reasonable financial security, and are mentally alert until the final weeks of their life. Furthermore, the study revealed that far from lacking individuality, which is how the elderly are often depicted, old people maintain their uniqueness and a remarkable continuity of character. For many, old age is a time of peaceful reflection (Erikson's stage 8).

Not all elderly people are as fortunate as the Duke study might suggest, however. Many find that inflation has dissipated their savings, that private pensions are inadequate, or that it is extremely difficult, if not impossible, to survive on Social Security benefits. Child abuse and spouse abuse are much in the news; rarely do we hear of parent abuse, where resentful offspring who must provide lodging or financial support for indigent parents vent their feelings in the form of mental or even physical aggression.

Perhaps more commonly known are the scandalous conditions under which many of the elderly are forced to live in nursing homes or other residential situations. The lack of supervision of these facilities has permitted the exploiters to abuse the elderly while profiting greedily from funding systems such as Medicaid. Chapter 10 discusses the problems of aging in greater detail.

DEFINING MENTAL HEALTH

A good definition of mental health has to consider both the person and the larger society. For the person, criteria for wellness include both behavior and feeling. From the social standpoint, the welfare of other people is equally important.

Although different theoretical perspectives on mental health have put forth a range of ideas on what is essential to mental health, most prescriptions have the same basic theme: A mentally healthy person is able to meet the lifelong challenges of development while maintaining a satisfying sense of personal identity. Put another way, healthy individuals are able to adjust to their environment while maintaining their individuality.

The Personal and Social Perspectives

Whatever criteria we select as essential for wellness, they should include both external *behavior* and inner *feeling*. Many theorists would add the *consequences of behavior* for others and for society as a third consideration. Adjusting satisfactorily to the demands of life through *adaptive behavior*, for example, is insufficient if you nevertheless feel personal distress—depression, anxiety, unhappiness, or the sense that your identity is fragmented. Personal satisfaction or a feeling of elation is also an incomplete criterion for mental health, and could even be delusional in someone unable to cope with the demands of living.

The consequences of behavior from the standpoint of other people and society also deserve consideration. It is possible, taking into account only behavior and feelings, to imagine a successful computer bandit, dishonest political boss, or rich drug dealer who has met the criterion of adaptive behavior and who also enjoys feelings of happiness and self-integration. Are these people mentally healthy? They are clearly deviating from social norms and have broken the law. The legal definition of insanity, in fact, is the only one that introduces the concept of right and wrong. Legal and medical views of mental health have been historically at odds.

Perhaps we have two standards of mental health that need to be integrated. According to Erich Fromm, both social and individual welfare criteria have to be satisfied in a definition of mental health. From society's standpoint, a healthy individual adjusts to life by performing a socially productive role. From the individual's standpoint, mental health means optimal growth and happiness. A satisfactory definition of mental health would seem to require, *for* the individual, positive feelings and successful adjustment, and *from* the individual, behavior that is desirable.

Different Theories, Different Definitions

Individual mental health has never been defined by a list of fixed traits or characteristics. People like catchwords, however, and some concepts of mental health are even summarized in single words or phrases. For Erik Erikson, wellness is *integrity*, which is variously defined as wholeness, unity, or integration of the self. It is the goal of development over the stages of life. Humanistic psychologists, on the other hand, believe that the hallmark of mental health is the full development of one's potential as a unique human being.

Humanistic psychology is only one of three major schools of thought concerning mental health. The other two approaches, psychoanalysis and behaviorism, have different theories about psychological disorders and therefore different criteria for mental health and different recommendations for treatment.

The psychoanalytical school, founded by Sigmund Freud, holds that psychological problems are caused by inner conflicts. One central concept of psychoanalysis is the **unconscious,** a vast submerged area of the mind containing the basic drives that motivate our behavior. It also contains painful experiences and unacceptable desires that we have pushed into "forgetfulness," or **repressed,** but have not entirely eliminated. These repressed memories and feelings are the cause of our present emotional distress; and they reappear with all their original intensity in disguised forms—that is, as symptoms whose meaning and significance trained psychonalysts can recognize (see the section Defense Mechanisms, below). For psychoanalytical theorists, then, mental health means the absence of symptoms that indicate disorder, including anxiety and depression.

Behavioral psychologists, or **behaviorists,** including B. F. Skinner, have very different ideas about mental health. Behaviorists dismiss the unconscious and all internal mental and emotional states because these are unobservable events. Behaviorists study only observable behavior (responses) and treat psychological disturbances as problems in learning. Whereas psychoanalysts consider any problems in behavior to be symptoms of some underlying disorder, behaviorists treat the problem behavior directly. Behaviorists believe that faulty learning is the cause of disorder and therefore define mental health as the learning, or relearning, of effective responses to the problems we encounter in the environment.

The concept of mental health includes ideas from several other disciplines. It involves developmental change, learning, and states of consciousness. Biochemists studying the brain might say that mental health depends on how well the electrochemical activity in the brain cells and nervous system is balanced and regulated. Nutritionists and physical fitness researchers have also discovered important facts about mental health. Both groups have found clear correlations between mental health and the quality of diet and amount of exercise (see Chapters 4 and 5). While no line of research has all the answers, each theoretical school and profession has contributed significant pieces that help solve the puzzle of mental health.

Components of Mental Health

Though it is difficult to define good mental health explicitly, certain characteristics seem to typify healthy emotional attitudes and behavior. According to the National Association for Mental Health, people with good mental health tend to exhibit the following traits:

1. *They feel comfortable about themselves*. Mentally healthy individuals tend to accept themselves for what they are. They enjoy their own capabilities and make the most of them. Conversely, they are tolerant of their own flaws and inabilities and do not worry over them. They have a realistic view of themselves and can take life's disappointments in stride. They spend little time being worried, fearful, anxious, or jealous. Instead, they are usually calm, open to new ideas, spontaneous, humorous, and self-confident. Though they enjoy the company of others, they do not mind being alone. Perhaps

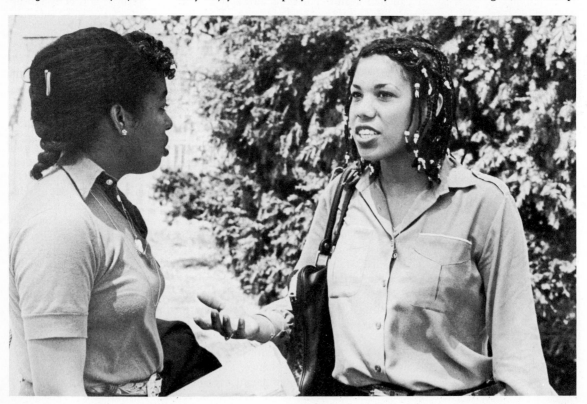

Mentally healthy people feel comfortable about themselves and right about other people.

most important, they have a value system derived from their own experiences—a personal sense of right and wrong.

2. *They feel right about other people*. Mentally healthy people tend to like and trust others, and take it for granted that other people will like and trust them. They are able to form warm and lasting relationships, and they consider and respect the interests of others. They do not allow themselves to be pushed around, nor do they try to dominate others. They have a sense of identification with humanity and feel a sense of responsibility toward others.
3. *They are able to meet the demands of life*. Mentally healthy individuals generally assume responsibility for their own actions and deal with their problems as they arise. They have realistic ideas about what they can and cannot do; thus they shape their environment whenever possible and adjust to it whenever necessary. They enjoy the basic experiences of life, but are not self-preoccupied. Instead, they seek experiences and challenges outside themselves. Persons with good mental health are unlikely to say, "I do the minimum amount of work I need to do to get by." Rather, they put their best effort into what they do and get satisfaction out of doing it.

Few people can always conform to these high standards of effective functioning. Everyone must contend with a number of frustrations and conflicts in his or her lifetime. Sometimes these conflicts are compounded by personal limitations—for example, one may wish to do something one is really incapable of doing, and the reality may be very hard to accept. Or an individual may be torn between several equally desirable but irreconcilable goals—such as going to summer school for extra credit or taking a summer job. These conflicts and frustrations can produce stress, which is the subject of Chapter 2. Often frustrations are a natural result of living in a society. The demands or expectations of society sometimes run counter to the individual's personal code of behavior. They may also be inherently contradictory—for example, it is hard to be selfless and success-oriented at the same time.

Ideally, the best way to handle almost all of these frustrations would be first to achieve an objective understanding of the situation and the alternatives it offers, and then to act on the basis of what will bring the most personal satisfaction and the greatest realization of one's potential. But almost everyone finds it impossible to adjust to every pressure and demand; and almost everyone is sometimes frustrated in his or her goals or occasionally experiences an emotional disturbance. The traits that characterize the mentally healthy individual, however desirable, are difficult to maintain in every situation. Ultimately, all individuals must determine for themselves the level of adjustment at which they can function comfortably and successfully.

DEFENSE MECHANISMS

Most of us are brought up to view certain feelings as undesirable or unacceptable, including envy, jealousy, anger, and other "selfish" emotions. When such feelings arise, they come into conflict with our ideas about how we ought to feel and what we ought to do. Such conflict is expressed as psychological stress—anxiety, guilt, and fear of disapproval or loss of love. Solving the conflict—that is, eliminating the anxiety—means either squashing the unacceptable feelings or making them acceptable. For most people, the first alternative is impossible; socialization is simply too strong. From time to time, we all use **defense mechanisms** to deny feelings that we know will meet with social disapproval. Basically, defense mechanisms are ways of deceiving ourselves (and others) about our real but unconscious desires, reactions, and emotions. Although defense mechanisms are part of Freudian theory, they are constructive strategies rather than symptoms of emotional disorder. An excessive reliance on any one defense might indicate a problem, but the use of defense mechanisms is considered necessary and normal.

Rationalization

Rationalization is the process by which a person justifies an action or event by distorting the real reasons for its occurrence. If a student has neglected to clean his room, he might explain this neglect by avowing that he didn't have time—that he had to study for exams. If a woman isn't dated again by a man she likes, she might rationalize that he was not intellectual enough for her. Rationalization can be a good way to maintain self-esteem in a world in which at least some failure is inevitable. But used to excess, rationalization keeps us from being in touch with reality and inhibits effective functioning. In the long run, it might be better if the student who does not straighten out his room simply admits that he does not want to bother with the task of cleaning. Similarly, rather than rationalizing a rejection, the woman might improve her social life if she tries to determine why the rejection occurred.

Sublimation

Sublimation is the replacement of a socially unacceptable goal with one that meets with society's approval. In terms of benefit to society, sublimation probably ranks highest among the defense mechanisms. It is diversion of an internal energy that the individual recognizes as "antisocial" into an external channel that is constructive and socially acceptable. For example, a man might divert the physical aggressiveness he feels but knows is unwelcome into a highly aggressive business career, such as sales.

Regression

When a person escapes an anxiety-producing conflict by retreating to an earlier and less mature form of behavior, he is **regressing.** For example, a person might cry or show anger when he has done something he is ashamed of, or when he simply wants attention. Sometimes illness is a regressive form of behavior in that the patient uses the illness as a way of getting the constant attention he or she received as a child.

An individual who consciously acknowledges to himself that he needs additional attention from friends or family might be able to achieve it in more mature ways. He could invite the others out to dinner more often, or simply visit them more frequently. Whether or not these methods achieve their goal, the person would at least be behaving in a more honest and direct manner.

Projection

People very much dislike admitting failure or experiencing guilt. Through **projection** they can avoid feelings of anxiety by attributing to others the motives or qualities of which they disapprove in themselves. For example, a person who habitually refuses to give to charities may claim that charities keep most of the money for themselves instead of distributing it to the needy. Rather than experience anxiety over his own selfishness, he attributes this quality to the charitable organizations. In the same way, a person filled with suppressed hostility sees hostility wherever he looks. "He doesn't like me" seems more acceptable than "I don't like him." A man who drives aggressively might constantly criticize other drivers; a woman feeling cranky and out of sorts might ask her husband why he is so grumpy.

Isolated instances of projection are fairly harmless. However, when a person habitually projects his negative personality traits onto others, he is using the mental mechanism of projection to avoid facing his own hostilities.

Repression

A person may blot out the memory of a painful feeling, event, or action from her conscious mind. In this way, she does not have to deal consciously with the anxiety caused by the memory. Such **repression** can be as harmless as forgetting an interview one fears or the room number of an exam for which one has not studied. However, severe repression can also result in distortion of or removal from reality. An extreme form is *psychological* (as opposed to physiological) *amnesia*, which involves the repression of something so painful to a person that it causes her memory to fail partially or totally.

When repression allows a person temporary relief from unpleasant or socially unacceptable feelings and desires, it can be beneficial. However, when repression is consistently used to deny reality, it can prevent self-fulfillment. For example, when a young woman applying to graduate school misses the deadline for each application, it would be well for her to analyze her true feelings. She may really prefer to go to work and may be suppressing her own desires in order to please her parents.

Identification

The extension of one's ego to include those outside oneself is called **identification.** A child will first identify with his parents and siblings, and later with members of his peer group, race, religion, and nationality. An adult may identify with the corporation for which she works or the branch of the armed forces in which she serves. Some individuals identify with an athlete or a movie star. Identification works as a defense mechanism by enabling a person to compensate for feelings of inadequacy by vicariously experiencing the achievements of others.

Fantasy and Daydreaming

An individual may escape from a frustrating or painful circumstance by creating a make-believe situation or a **fantasy** world that is more pleasurable to him than the real world. The most common form of fantasy is **daydreaming.** Everyone, at one time or another, engages in this delightful activity in which all dreams temporarily come true. A lonely person may daydream about what it would be like to be popular and surrounded by friends; a poor person might imagine herself enormously wealthy. Daydreams are harmless, although perhaps disappointing. Fantasy can, however, be a symptom of severe pathological disturbance when it becomes a way of life and causes the person to lose touch with reality.

Idealization

We are engaging in **idealization** when we see or interpret something according to our own desires rather than as it actually is. Thus someone might live in a shabby apartment but view it as beautiful and luxurious. Or a person with average children might see them as exceptionally smart or talented.

Idealization is often nothing more than one person's overvaluing the aptitudes or abilities of another person. It may also be a kind of request for similar appreciation of one's own potential. In other cases, idealization is a way of protecting one's own self-image by glorifying something or someone with whom one is associated.

Reaction Formation

Sometimes people are so successful in repressing their impulses that they outwardly express attitudes that are diametrically opposed to their true feelings. This is known as **reaction formation.** For example, a person who is ashamed of his sexual desires may become interested in organizations established to suppress vice and pornography. Or a mother who harbors repressed hostility toward her child might become excessively anxious and overprotective toward him.

Compensation

Made anxious by some personal inadequacy, people will often **compensate** or make up for their feelings of inferiority in one area by striving to succeed in other areas. For example, an individual who feels physically weak might devote a great deal of time to learning and playing chess. Sometimes people try to compensate in an area where they feel weakest. A timid individual, for example, may take lessons in self-defense. Compensation differs from sublimation in that with compensation, a real inadequacy or failure is experienced and offset.

NEUROSES

Unlike the defense mechanisms just discussed, neurotic disorders greatly impair an individual's ability to function effectively and realistically. **Neurosis** is characterized by inappropriate emotions and behavior that the individual is unable to explain or control.

Neurotic Reactions to Frustration

Occasionally, a normal individual may develop a *neurotic reaction* to a situation that is at least temporarily overwhelming. This type of reaction is characterized by inappropriate and self-defeating behavior and is often accompanied by anxiety.

The neurotic reaction worsens rather than alleviates a frustration: Individuals who experience such a reaction cannot work realistically toward a reasonable solution of their problem. For example, a student may become frustrated by the difficulty he is having in studying for an examination. To handle the situation realistically, he would probably seek help from a professor or a friend and devote extra time to studying the particular subject so that he would be assured of doing his best on the exam. A neurotic reaction, however, would be one in which worry over his exams prevents the student from utilizing even the least of his capabilities. The more worried he becomes, the less he can concentrate on his books; and the less he can concentrate, the more worried he becomes. Unable to avoid the frustrating situation or to deal with it effectively, the student responds neurotically and will usually experience feelings of anxiety.

Most people suffer from neurotic reactions of this type at some time in their lives. Some experience neurotic reactions more frequently than others, or they have more severe reactions. This does not necessarily mean that they are neurotic, but that a particular situation is too complex and painful for them to handle easily. Once this frustrating situation passes, normal individuals recover their emotional balance and perspective. And if they do need professional help to resolve a particular frustration or conflict, short-term treatment is all that is required.

Neurotic Individuals

Neurotic individuals, on the other hand, are not just temporarily unable to cope with specific difficulties or conflicts; their reactions are consistently inappropriate or excessive, even in situations with which normal individuals would find it comparatively easy to cope. For instance, normal people occasionally experience difficulty in making a decision, especially when faced with equally desirable or undesirable alternatives. But neurotic individuals often find it very difficult to make decisions even in situations that present little conflict. Part of the reason for this is that neurotic people are not merely dealing with objective problems; they are also dealing with the associations that each situation arouses. The actual situation is therefore distorted by their subjective interpretation of it. In other words, a neurotic's difficulties are compounded by problems and conflicts within his or her own personality.

Most neurotics have been chronically unable since childhood to deal effectively with the frustrations that are often part of life. Because neurotics do not feel they are in control of their own lives, they are overly sensitive to the approval or disapproval of others. Moreover, their anxiety levels are so high that even if others do approve of them, neurotics mistrust the approval they receive. Thus they lose the ability to assert themselves and become locked into their frustrations.

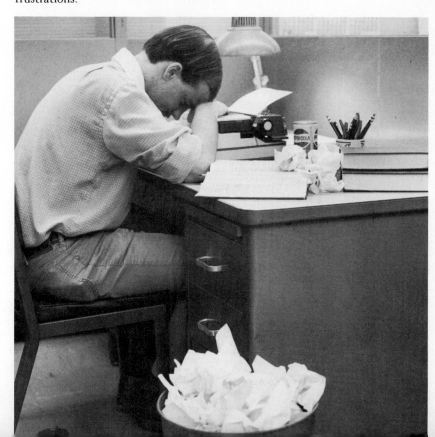

Frustration at a difficult task can be temporarily incapacitating, but most people recover quickly.

Anxiety Neurosis. A neurotic's reaction to frustration and conflict also usually differs in quality and degree from that of a normal person in a comparable situation. A normal person may feel anxious when in a specific uncomfortable situation. But the **anxiety** of neurotics is pervasive and free-floating—that is, capable of attaching itself to all their actions and thoughts. And the stronger this anxiety becomes, the more helpless the neurotic feels in dealing with a conflict.

For example, anyone might feel anxious about the approach of a difficult examination. But a neurotic's examination anxiety may trigger further anxieties concerning every detail of the academic program—every assignment, every paper, every meeting with the professor becomes the subject of free-floating anxiety. Neurotic individuals may respond to the situation by feeling that they are the only ones who are having difficulty as students, and they may begin to believe that they are intellectually inferior. Thus a gap develops between what they are potentially capable of doing and what they actually achieve. The ironic result is that neurotics may actually seem inferior to others because their internal conflicts (rather than external circumstances) have consistently defeated all their endeavors.

Neurotic Depression. Depression, like anxiety, is a debilitating state that most people have suffered at some point in their lives. **Neurotic depression,** however, is characterized by extreme hopelessness that lasts long after a precipitating event has passed, or is an extreme response to a relatively minor event—a slight by a friend or stranger, for example. In short, the sense of defeat seems excessive, given the nature of the event.

Anxiety and depression, because they are common reactions to stress even in the absence of neurosis, are discussed in Chapter 2. The relationship between anxiety and depression is not fully understood. Some psychologists believe that depression may be a response to extreme anxiety, a way of slowing down oneself and the world until one feels stronger or until a perceived or real emergency is over. Others see the two as distinct psychological and physiological states. Many forms of depression can be treated with drug therapy. There is no safe drug therapy for anxiety, however, as we shall see.

Other Neurotic Symptoms

In addition to the general personality and behavior distinctions that characterize neurotic individuals, certain specific symptoms may be manifested. However, these symptoms cannot be used as the basis for determining whether an individual is neurotic. Even if a person is severely neurotic, he or she may still appear to function harmoniously within society and may not show any of the symptoms discussed below. Furthermore, the average healthy individual may also exhibit these symptoms, though they are usually less elaborate and intense than in the neurotic person.

Phobias. As many as one in ten Americans suffers from some sort of **phobia.** A phobia is an irrational fear of an object or situation that usually has its origin in some event or experience long out of the person's memory. These fears can be of almost anything: flying, heights, dirt, elevators, trains, bridges, rats or snakes, closed places or open places, crowds, strangers, or the dark.

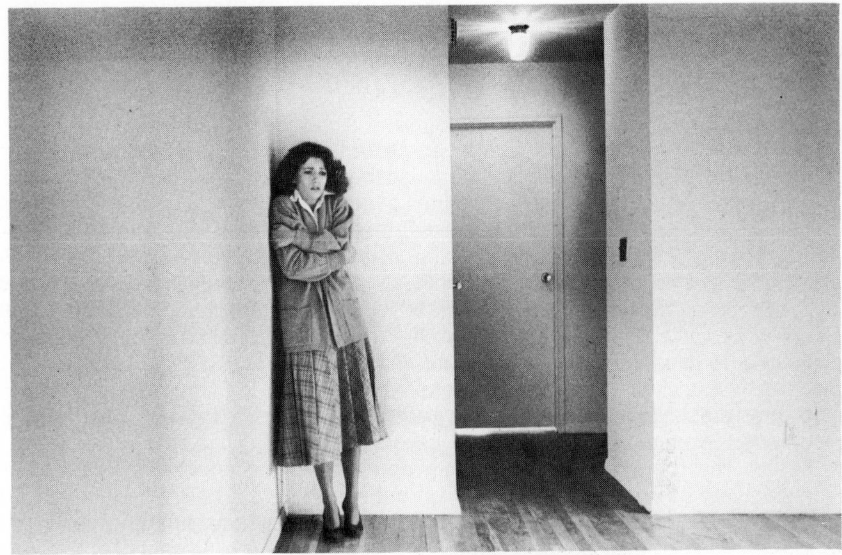

An irrational fear of open spaces is known as agoraphobia. Like other phobias, it is most successfully treated with behavioral techniques.

Behavioral treatment has proven remarkably successful with phobias, particularly in cases where the anxiety is centered on only one object or situation (see the section Behavioral Techniques, below).

Obsessions. When people's thoughts or fantasies become irrationally fixated on particular ideas or images, they are said to have an **obsession.** People with obsessions have no control over these particular thoughts; they constantly and persistently recur without conscious volition. For example, in one study, an individual reported that obsessions concerning the death or injury of others attached themselves to even his simplest actions. When he bought new shirts, for example, he believed that it was somehow a prelude to the murder of his two children. Even though he realized how irrational his fears were, he could not erase the idea from his mind until he finally returned the shirts. Such obsessions may be an unconscious attempt by the individual to control unacceptable urges. By focusing on one act or thought, the individual avoids dealing with more threatening emotions.

Compulsive Habits. Compulsive habits, such as washing one's hands dozens of times a day or methodically avoiding the cracks on the sidewalk, are ritualistic practices over which neurotics have little control. They may feel fearful or anxious if they do not complete the ritual. They may also believe that these particular practices protect them from harm or disaster of an undefined nature, and that if they break these compulsive habits, something terrible will occur. They would therefore prefer to follow their compulsions rather than confront their fears and suffer from anxiety.

Phobias and obsessive-compulsive disorders can be treated by psychotherapy and behavioral techniques discussed later in the chapter.

The Borderline Personality

Since 1980, psychiatrists have recognized a new category of mental disorder: the *borderline syndrome*, or *borderline personality*. Because the category is new and controversial, estimates of its prevalence vary. Some psychiatrists believe that up to 10 percent of Americans and perhaps 25 percent of those seeking therapy are borderlines.

The borderline personality is marked by impulsiveness, instability and unpredictability, and difficulty in forming intimate relationships. Borderlines often have a vague or inadequate sense of identity, a poor employment record, and a history of mild or short-lived delusional or other psychotic episodes. They become angry frequently and tend to manipulate others. They exhibit a high but superficial degree of sociability, and cannot tolerate being alone. Much of their behavior tends to be self-destructive and includes self-mutilation, drug abuse or drinking, and promiscuity.

Most psychiatrists trace the borderline's problems to infancy and to the unsolved developmental task of integrating clashing experiences (the mother who hugs and the mother who punishes, for example). The borderline's failure to accept both the positive and negative traits of the same person produces a defense mechanism called *splitting*. As adults, borderlines lack a sense of unity in their own personalities as well as others and therefore experience the world and themselves as fragmentary and contradictory. Borderline personalities are thought to seek states of consciousness that are similar to infantile states before the painful task of separating the self from the world. They seek a sense of oneness with the world and other people through sensuality and ectasy. They may therefore be drawn to drugs and nightlife and may be unable to find satisfaction in the world of work. Being alone gives borderlines a feeling of total isolation.

The fragmentation of modern society and rapid social change itself—in families and in role and career expectations, for example—may be especially hard for borderlines to cope with because of difficulties they already have in structuring experience and coping with contradictions.

Source: Louis Sass, "The Borderline Personality," *The New York Times Magazine* (August 22, 1982), pp. 12–15, 66–67.

Psychosomatic Disorders. The term **psychosomatic** is derived from two Greek words, *psyche* ("the soul") and *soma* ("the body"). It is used to describe physical disorders in which there is an intimate connection between physical symptoms and emotional states.

The operation of the brain is strongly influenced by the state of our emotions. The brain, in turn, controls most of our body functions. Therefore our emotions can influence the behavior of our body in a great many ways. Though anyone is potentially vulnerable to physical ailments when under great emotional stress, severely neurotic people are more apt to suffer from the physical manifestations of tension and anxiety than the average person. Psychosomatic disorders are often a means of evading a disagreeable situation. A common example is the person who gets a headache whenever an unpleasant appointment comes up. The person is usually unconscious of the connection between the physical discomfort and the feared appointment. But the headache, though psychosomatic in origin, *is* an actual headache.

Sometimes the tendency to develop psychosomatic illnesses is initiated by childhood experiences and is therefore very difficult to resolve. When a child is ill, for example, the mother is likely to display more concern and affection than at other times. When the child grows up, tension and stress are likely to bring unconscious recall of the security of the parent's presence during childhood illnesses. The symptoms of illness may then reappear, as much for the remembered security as from the bodily weakness resulting from tension.

PSYCHOSES

The **psychoses** are serious mental disorders in which a person is disabled owing to a breakdown in thinking ability or mood or both. Whereas neurotics are aware of their problems and in touch with reality, psychotics have lost contact with reality. They may withdraw completely from any interchange with the environment and other people or may respond with high emotional intensity.

The most common psychoses are schizophrenia and the affective, or mood, disorders, which include mania and psychotic depression, singly or in swing patterns.

Schizophrenia

There are several types of schizophrenia, but we do not have the space to cover them here. Most schizophrenics associate ideas and images, or ideas and feelings, not according to logic, but according to some arbitrary system or cue, such as rhyming or other linguistic devices. The inability to associate ideas meaningfully produces a host of irrational beliefs such as delusions of grandeur or superiority, of persecution, of control by interstellar radio waves, or of unredeemable fault or sin. Hallucinations, especially auditory ones, may accompany delusions. Emotional responses are disturbed and highly inappropriate—for example, a schizophrenic may become angry over an act of kindness or laugh at someone's misfortune. Emotional dullness is also typical. Most experts agree that biological factors and heredity play a significant role in schizophrenia; many of its symptoms can be treated by various drugs.

Affective Disorders

The affective disorders are depression, mania, or cyclic patterns of the two states. **Psychotic depression** is a crippling state of sadness in which a person can perform few, if any, ordinary functions. Symptoms include loss of appetite, loss of sexual interest, and severe sleep disturbances. The possibility of suicide is very real during periods of psychotic depression. (See the section Stress and Suicide in Chapter 2.)

Mania, extreme exuberance, is nearly the opposite of depression. In episodes of mania an individual may go without sleep for days, spend money lavishly or hatch grandiose plans, and jump from one activity to another, perhaps starting to paint the house at midnight and then two hours later telephoning acquaintances around the country. The manic person is impossible for family members to control and is a nuisance to others during the manic episode. The episode is usually followed by a crash into psychotic depression. Most manics can be treated with lithium, a drug that prevents attacks.

TREATMENT STRATEGIES

People who feel that their emotional problems or extreme anxieties are seriously interfering with their lives may want to seek some form of therapy or treatment. Others with less severe problems may seek therapy in order to improve their lives and develop their potential as fully as possible. Whatever the reasons for seeking professional help, there is a host of therapies to choose from. In this

Testing Your Assertiveness

How often do you get your own way? Do you often deny your own wishes in order to accommodate those of others? Assertive behavior is expressing our own needs and desires and standing up for them without hurting other people. Nonassertive behavior is sacrificing our own needs in order to satisfy others. Here is a test of assertive behavior.

Directions:

Indicate how characteristic or descriptive each of the following statements is of you by using the code given below.

+3 = very characteristic of me, extremely descriptive
+2 = rather characteristic of me, quite descriptive
+1 = somewhat characteristic of me, slightly descriptive
–1 = somewhat uncharacteristic of me, slightly nondescriptive
–2 = rather uncharacteristic of me, quite nondescriptive
–3 = very uncharacteristic of me, extremely nondescriptive

______ 1. Most people seem to be more aggressive and assertive than I am.
______ 2. I have hesitated to make or accept dates because of "shyness."
______ 3. When the food served at a restaurant is not done to my satisfaction, I complain about it to the waiter or waitress.
______ 4. I am careful to avoid hurting other people's feelings, even when I feel that I have been injured.
______ 5. If a salesperson has gone to considerable trouble to show me merchandise that is not quite suitable, I have a difficult time in saying no.
______ 6. When I am asked to do something, I insist upon knowing why.
______ 7. There are times when I look for a good, vigorous argument.
______ 8. I strive to get ahead as well as most people in my position.
______ 9. To be honest, people often take advantage of me.
______ 10. I enjoy starting conversations with new acquaintances and strangers,
______ 11. I often don't know what to say to attractive persons of the opposite sex.
______ 12. I will hesitate to make phone calls to business establishments and institutions.
______ 13. I would rather apply for a job or for admission to a college by writing letters than by going through with personal interviews.
______ 14. I find it embarrassing to return merchandise.
______ 15. If a close and respected relative were annoying me, I would smother my feelings rather than express my annoyance.
______ 16. I have avoided asking questions for fear of sounding stupid.

section we shall discuss briefly the most common forms of therapy, including traditional psychoanalysis, various psychotherapies, behavioral techniques, humanistic therapy, group therapy, and drug therapy.

The therapeutic techniques discussed here grew out of the theoretical schools

______17. During an argument I am sometimes afraid that I will get so upset that I will shake all over.
______18. If a famed and respected lecturer makes a statement that I think is incorrect, I will have the audience hear my point of view as well.
______19. I avoid arguing over prices with clerks and salespeople.
______20. When I have done something important or worthwhile, I manage to let others know about it.
______21. I am open and frank about my feelings.
______22. If someone has been spreading false and bad stories about me, I see him (her) as soon as possible to "have a talk" about it.
______23. I often have a hard time saying no.
______24. I tend to bottle up my emotions rather than make a scene.
______25. I complain about poor service in a restaurant and elsewhere.
______26. When I am given a compliment, I sometimes just don't know what to say.
______27. If a couple near me in a theater or at a lecture were conversing rather loudly, I would ask them to be quiet or to take their conversation elsewhere.
______28. Anyone attempting to push ahead of me in a line is in for a good battle.
______29. I am quick to express an opinion.
______30. There are times when I just can't say anything.

Scoring:

First, reverse the plus or minus signs you used for items 1, 2, 4, 5, 9, 11, 12, 13, 14, 15, 16, 17, 19, 23, 24, 26, and 30. Then add up your score. Scores can range from +90 to –90, with a plus score indicating assertive behavior and a minus score nonassertive behavior. The closer your score is to +90, the more assertively you usually act.

A pattern of nonassertive behavior can lead to problems in daily living. Nonassertive people who bottle up their feelings often become angry with others for using them and angry with themselves for not having stood up for their rights. Becoming more assertive is not easy, but can be done with practice. There are courses in assertiveness training and books about it. One such book is *When I Say No, I Feel Guilty*, by Manuel J. Smith (New York: Dial Press, 1975). Trying out assertive behavior in casual situations with friends can be a good first step.

Source: Spencer A. Rathus, "A 30-Item Schedule for Assessing Assertive Behavior," *Behavior Therapy*, IV (1973), pp. 398–406. Reprinted by permission of Academic Press.

discussed earlier in the chapter. As we shall see, some lend themselves better to certain problems than others. Moreover, some practitioners may subscribe to more than one school of thought. The best therapists are able to assess a person's problem and apply whichever therapy is likely to work best.

Psychoanalysis

As we saw earlier, Freudian psychoanalysts hold that people's conflicts and emotional problems are the result of painful memories and unacceptable feelings that have been pushed into the unconscious, or repressed. These conflicts may rise to the surface again in disguised forms, such as the symbolism of dreams or the outward symptoms of the various anxiety neuroses just discussed.

Traditional *psychoanalysis* is protracted and expensive. It is protracted because it takes a long time—usually several years—for a person to work back to the unconscious sources of conflict. It is expensive because psychoanalysts must undergo a long, rigorous training. The patient is thought to make best contact with the unconscious by free-associating ideas (Freud called his technique the "talking cure") while lying on a couch facing away from the analyst. Eventually the patient **transfers** his or her unresolved conflicts onto the person of the analyst, who remains silent and neutral throughout most of the treatment. For example, if a patient's suppressed hatred of her mother surfaced from the unconscious during treatment, that feeling would be transferred to the analyst. The analyst is specially trained to manipulate the transference situation so that the patient resolves the conflict. If the analysis is successful, the symptoms of inner conflict—anxiety or depression, for example—disappear, and the personality is effectively restored as a functioning, integrated whole.

Psychotherapy

The more modern version of psychoanalysis is called *psychotherapy*. That term, however, is often used to describe many methods of treating emotional problems, some of which are not based on psychoanalysis. Traditional psychotherapists, like psychoanalysts, believe that unconscious conflict is at the root of most emotional problems. However, psychotherapy is more directive than psychoanalysis and emphasizes meeting daily challenges and practical concerns. The therapist usually sits in a chair facing the patient and deals directly with the patient's conscious problems and concerns. Most psychotherapists today recognize that the people they treat hold jobs, live in families, or have other daily obligations that require fairly rapid improvement in their ability to cope or just get by, even if the real cause of their disorder takes longer to uncover and treat. For this reason, short-term psychotherapy has become increasingly popular (see box: New Trends in Therapy).

Psychoanalysis and psychotherapy are most effective for treating crippling anxiety or depression for which there are no clear causes or precipitating events, and for some severe neurotic disorders.

Behavioral Techniques

Behaviorists, as we have seen, dismiss all notions of internal mental states and unconscious processes. Instead, they believe most maladaptive behaviors, such as phobias and various compulsions, are learned in the same way all behavior is learned—through **reinforcement.** People tend to repeat behavior that has been rewarded (reinforced) in the past—that is, associated with pleasure. By the same token, behavior associated with pain is not likely to be repeated. A simple example of how behavior is reinforced is an infant's crying from hunger and getting fed as a consequence. Crying is then repeated as a successful behavior for getting food. When the child reaches the age of 7 or 8, crying is no longer rewarded as an appropriate signal for getting fed. According to behavioral theory, crying is slowly **extinguished** by parental disapproval, and the child learns new, approved strategies, such as pacing near the kitchen before the dinner hour.

Behavior therapists use a variety of techniques to change maladaptive behavior. For example, a student who has learned to be extremely timid, perhaps because shyness and dependence were rewarded by her parents, may now be having problems coping in college, where some degree of assertiveness is necessary just to survive. Behavioral therapy for such a person might involve **assertiveness training,** a method in which the therapist rewards assertive responses from the patient and gives no approval for passive behavior. Once the patient has increased her assertive behavior, perhaps over several sessions, the therapist may present her with situations that caused anxiety before therapy began: for example, asking someone out for dinner, insisting on help from the reference librarian, or saying no to a roommate. Therapist and patient work through these events until the patient feels comfortable with them. (See box: Testing Your Assertiveness.)

Another method used by behavior therapists is **systematic desensitization,** wherein patients are first taught relaxation techniques and then taught to approach the object or situation that causes intense fear or anxiety. For example, if a student had a fear of snakes, therapy would be directed at weakening this response. The patient might make a list of frightening events regarding snakes, from the least threatening (just thinking about a snake) to the most unbearable (being trapped in a room with a large snake). The therapist works through each situation while the patient is relaxed. Therapy may mean simply imagining the event or actually coming into contact with the feared object. In both assertiveness training and desensitization, the patient learns responses that effectively kill anxiety. Assertive responses tend to alleviate anxiety, and relaxation is the absence of anxiety.

Humanistic Approaches

Humanistic psychologists such as Abraham Maslow and Carl Rogers believe that mental health means developing one's potential to the fullest. To pursue this life goal, people have to feel up to the task. Humanistic therapy therefore focuses on restoring or developing feelings of self-worth in the patient. Whereas

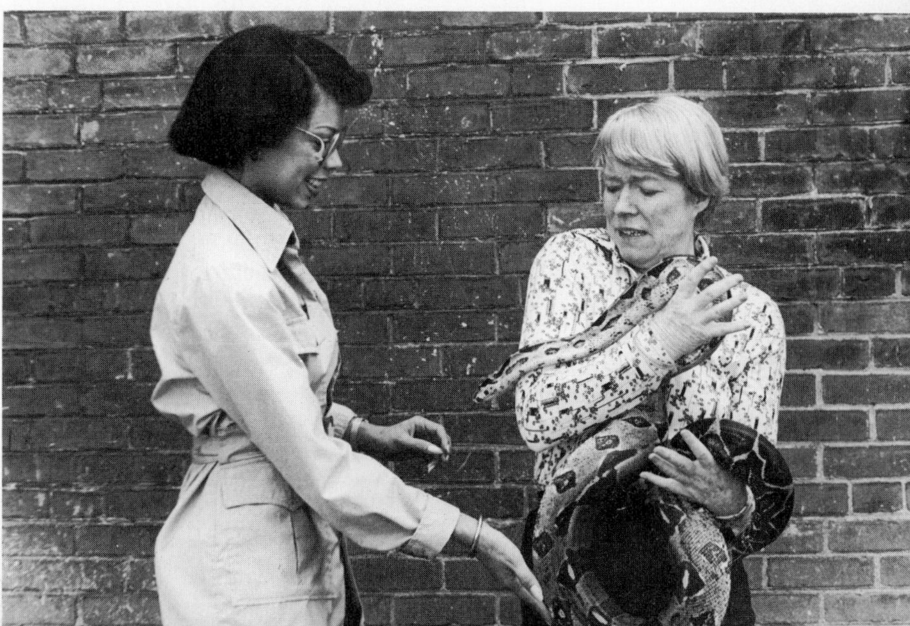

Systematic desensitization is often successful in curing phobias such as fear of snakes.

New Trends in Therapy

There was a time not so long ago when psychotherapy was limited mainly to treating the deep-seated problems of neurotics and psychotics. Such therapy was expected to last for years and cost many thousands of dollars; consequently, it was given only to the severely disturbed in institutions—or to the wealthy.

Now, however, many middle- and low-income "normal" adults are turning to a new type of psychotherapy for help with specific life problems such as depression, phobias, job anxieties, grief, and health worries. Many teenagers and young adults are also looking for help in arriving at a better understanding of themselves and what they want to do with their lives. Troubles like these can be overcome or at least greatly reduced in a relatively short time—say, twenty to forty hours of therapy.

The results of short-term therapy have been positive in two-thirds of the people treated, and most people have shown marked improvement in less than a year. To produce such results, the therapeutic profession has had to use a combination of several different theories and techniques such as behavior modification, cognitive therapy, and client-centered therapy. Furthermore, it has had to widen its ranks to include social workers, pastoral counselors, and psychiatric nurses, and broaden its field of operations to settings like corporation headquarters.

Many short-term therapists are considered by their patients to be intimate friends who help them express deep feelings and find ways of working out their personal problems. A word of caution is in order, however: Because some therapists are not well trained or well qualified, those seeking short-term help should carefully check the credentials of any prospective therapist.

Source: Adapted from Bryce Nelson, "Despite a Blur of Change, Clear Trends Are Emerging in Therapy," *The New York Times*, March 1, 1983, pp. C1, C6.

psychoanalysis explores the meaning of behavior and behavior therapy works to change behavior, humanistic therapy provides a setting in which the patient—often called the *client* by humanists—works out his or her own solutions to problems.

Client-centered therapy views behavior problems not as illness but as coping mechanisms the person chose in the past. The client is seen as a unique individual who is free to form new attitudes and behave differently. For this reason, the therapist neither approves nor disapproves of the client's feelings or behavior, but instead helps the client clarify his or her true feelings. Clients usually begin therapy with feelings of worthlessness, doubt, and confusion. By giving the client *unconditional positive regard* as a unique person, the therapist provides an atmosphere in which feelings of self-worth slowly emerge and the client finally creates solutions for problems.

Humanistic approaches may sound simple, but they take a great deal of skill, patience, and empathy on the part of the therapist. Such therapy works only if the therapist's regard for the client is believable. He or she has to be convincing to the client for progress to take place. Client-centered therapy works best for people who are motivated to improve their lives and take responsibility for their future.

Group Therapy

Group therapy can apply techniques from any of the theoretical schools we have discussed or can focus on special skills such as effective verbal communication or emotional expressiveness. Most people enter group therapy because they have problems interacting with others and forming relationships.

Participants in group therapy are given the opportunity to practice interacting with others in a supportive atmosphere and to see how others cope with communication problems, criticism or praise, and feelings of rejection. It is the therapist's job to make sure that group members do not "gang up" on any individual and to defuse potentially harmful situations.

Group therapy became popular in the 1960s and is now used in several institutional settings, including prisons, and for work groups as well as families.

Drug Therapy

The symptoms of serious mental illnesses such as the psychoses and the affective disorders have been successfully treated by a variety of drugs. The reason for this is that several of them seem to involve malfunctions in brain chemistry, although the precise mechanisms are not known. What is known is that certain drugs significantly alter behavior, in some cases eliminating the behavioral symptoms of disorder. Future research into brain chemistry may uncover causes of disorders that now remain a mystery.

The effectiveness of drug therapy in treating various disorders does not mean biochemical problems are the primary cause, only that they contribute to the problem. The causes of schizophrenia, as was pointed out earlier, are thought to be biologically based, and heredity is known to play a significant role. Certain drugs called **major tranquilizers** are effective in treating symptoms of schizophrenia but not in curing the disease. Many types of depression can also be treated with drugs. A class of antidepressant drugs called the **tricyclics** is usually effective and produces few side effects. One drug therapy that no one seems to argue about is the use of **lithium** to treat manic-depressive psychosis. Although how it works is only partially understood, it has been called a miracle drug. Many

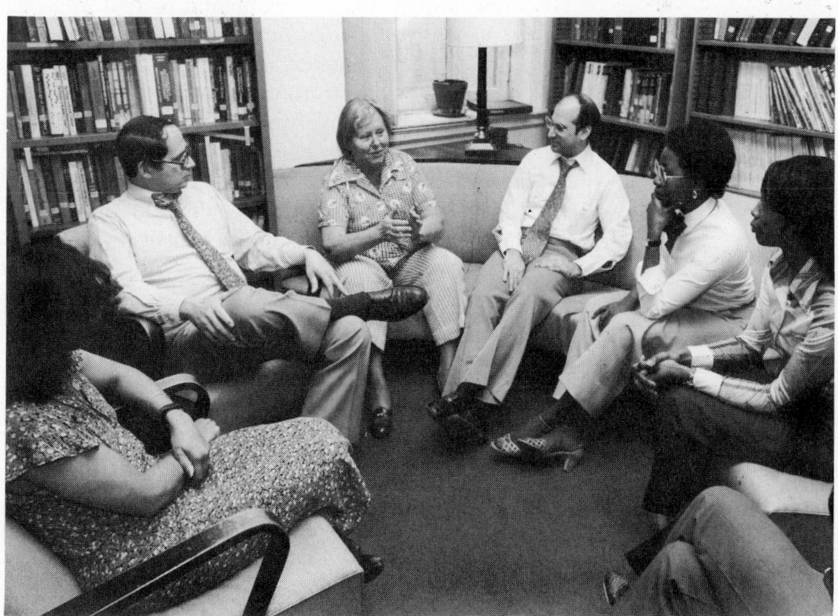

Group therapy is sometimes used to open up lines of communication in work groups.

thousands of patients who formerly experienced acute episodes of mania and were hospitalized are now maintained on lithium and lead normal lives.

The drug therapies discussed so far are primarily for serious illnesses, with the exception of the tricyclic antidepressants, which are commonly prescribed for depression that seems to be biologically caused. For all these drugs, the question of abuse generally does not apply. The drugs do not produce "highs," and may even produce unpleasant feelings in people who have no symptoms of disorder.

The **minor tranquilizers,** however, are frequently abused. These include the antianxiety drugs such as Librium and Valium, which are discussed at length in Chapter 13. Antianxiety drugs, most authorities now agree, should not be taken longer than two weeks at a time. They are highly addictive and frequently abused. Any person being maintained on a minor tranquilizer as a treatment for anxiety neurosis should get a second opinion. Unlike depression, which in many cases can be treated with relatively safe drug therapy, anxiety cannot yet be treated with safe, long-term drug therapy. This is not to say that the minor tranquilizers are not necessary medications for acute episodes or panic attacks. They are. But as yet, there is no safe maintenance medication for chronic anxiety.

MENTAL ILLNESS AND SOCIETY

Social attitudes about mental disorders may lead to abuses in our treatment of the mentally ill. It is no longer legal to discriminate against the ex-mental patient in housing or employment, and it is not socially acceptable openly to admit one's prejudice against the mentally ill or retarded. But the problem has not been solved: Studies show that most people would rather have an ex-prison inmate than an ex-mental patient as a neighbor.

One formerly widespread problem—the incarceration of eccentric or troublesome people in mental institutions on flimsily contrived evidence of their incompetence—has fortunately lessened. Indeed, **deinstitutionalization**—the policy of releasing nonviolent inmates from state hospitals because of overcrowding and insufficient funds—has come to replace it as a social problem. In urban areas homeless former inmates are adding to the numbers of vagrants and "shopping-bag ladies," people who live on the streets and are barely able to take care of themselves (see box: Deinstitutionalization).

Whatever one's opinion of institutional care, it is clear that the prevention of mental illness has been virtually ignored by our public and private health services. In most of the advanced countries of the world, mental health services are an integral part of health and welfare programs. Child and adolescent mental health facilities are available and widely used. This is in sharp contrast to the United States, where mental health facilities for children and youth are almost nonexistent.

The seriousness of this omission cannot be overstated. Childhood is the most crucial period of an individual's life in terms of emotional development. Adolescence is for many a period of conflict and anxiety for which they are unprepared. Our failure to seek out, detect, and treat the early signs of mental illness means

PROBLEMS AND CONTROVERSIES: *Deinstitutionalization*

No one living in a large city can have failed to notice the large number of shabby, troubled people aimlessly wandering the streets, hallucinating and muttering to themselves.

They are there because of the well-intended efforts of many psychiatrists and lawyers. During the 1950s mental health experts decided that most mental institutions were no more than warehouses for social outcasts, including the seriously disturbed. They felt that most of the mentally ill would be better served and treated at local community clinics and residential facilities. Accordingly, under a reform called *deinstitutionalization*, they released hundreds of thousands of mental patients over the next three decades. As a result, the mental hospital population declined by three-quarters, and the number of ex-patients swelled to almost 1.5 million. Many are in halfway houses and private homes, but most are on the street by themselves.

They wander the streets because very few community treatment facilities for them exist. The problem has grown worse because most of the federal funding for such services has been cut from the budget over the last five years. Even when funds have been available, many communities have fiercely resisted all attempts to locate group homes and treatment centers in neighborhoods.

One obvious solution is to reinstitutionalize many of these people, particularly the ones who have proved dangerous or unable to care for themselves. However, our legal system, which puts the highest value on personal freedom, makes it almost impossible to commit patients without their consent unless they pose a danger to themselves or others. Mental health experts feel that this policy does serious harm to both the mentally ill and society. They claim that under the present laws dangerously unbalanced people often deny that they are disturbed and refuse any form of counseling or treatment; the experts also point to the growing number of innocent people murdered by prematurely discharged mental patients.

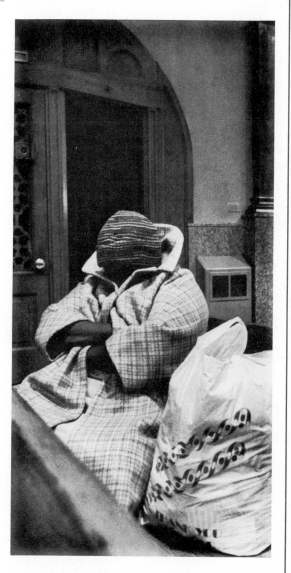

There are signs that society is beginning to realize that the deinstitutionalization movement has gone too far. The American Psychiatric Association has proposed laws that would allow dangerous hardcore cases to be recommitted. Legal authorities are trying to change the wording of state laws so that the "obviously mentally ill" or the "gravely impaired" can be reinstitutionalized.

that, as a society, we will be confronted with far more serious adult problems.

While some of our mental health facilities for adults are among the finest in the world, all too often the most competent therapists and the most effective treatment centers are inaccessible to many because they cannot afford them. Public welfare programs rarely include stipends for psychotherapy, and treatment for emotional illness is inadequately covered by our public and private medical insurance programs. This situation is disturbing, since the poor are particularly susceptible to mental health problems because of the severe stresses and strains of their lives.

One out of every five American adults suffers from some form of psychiatric disorder, according to a 1984 survey conducted by the National Institute of Mental Health. In decreasing order, the most frequently reported problems and the number of people affected are:

- Anxiety disorders (phobias, obsessive-compulsive behavior, panic attacks) 13,100,000
- Substance abuse (alcohol and drugs) 10,000,000
- Affective disorders (depression and manic depression) 9,400,000
- Cognitive impairment (disordered thinking) 1,600,000
- Schizophrenia 1,500,000
- Antisocial personality (low tolerance for frustration, violent and criminal behavior) 1,400,000

A significant finding of the study was that men and women are equally likely to be mentally disturbed (it had been assumed that women were more prone to mental illness). However, the kind of disturbance varies between the sexes: Women are more likely to suffer from depression and anxiety, while men have a higher incidence of substance-abuse and antisocial-personality disorders. Another interesting finding was that people over 45 are half as likely as younger people to experience any form of mental disturbance, while those over 65 are the least likely of all. Regardless of gender and age, there are 37 million severely disturbed Americans, a staggering number that should convince anyone of the need for increased federal and state funding for mental health.

Cultural attitudes toward mental health also need close examination. Many Americans hold contradictory views on mental illness and substance abuse. We abuse socially acceptable drugs but quickly label "street-drug" addiction a social problem. We agree that something should be done to improve the conditions in backward psychiatric institutions, but we tend to view a neighbor's acute depression as a character fault. If we find out that the neighbor is undergoing drug therapy, we might label the person weak, someone who has to rely on a chemical crutch to solve life problems we ourselves manage to cope with through courage and inner strength. Our enormous ignorance of therapy methods and substance abuse and our misplaced moralizing about mental illness are no doubt due to the stigma we attach to psychological disorders. If we changed our attitudes toward mental illness, we probably *would* get increased government budgets for research on the biological basis of mental disorders and for more help for people who do not belong in hospitals but are nevertheless ill.

One unfortunately ineffective program in recent years has been the **community psychology** approach to mental health and illness. Predicated upon the idea that an individual's problems do not develop in isolation, this approach was supposed to use the resources of a community both to prevent and to treat emotional illnesses. Emotionally disturbed children were to be identified early (usually in school) and referred to appropriate social agencies for counseling and treatment. The many thousands of severely disturbed people who were being released from state and mental hospitals into local communities were to be cared for and treated in group homes and neighborhood residential centers. However, the national government drastically reduced federal funding for these programs and shifted the responsibility to state and local governments. These governments have not been willing to take up the burden of preventing emotional illness in the young or caring for deinstitutionalized adults; at the most, some cities have provided shelter for the homeless.

THERAPISTS

Many students find their college years a time of severe stress and anxiety. Work pressures, competition for grades, the tensions of relating to people from very different backgrounds—all these factors can cause serious emotional and physical stress. From the discussion in this chapter it should be obvious that emotional and mental problems are nothing to be ashamed of, and that seeking

Mental Health: Where to Go for Help

Here is a list of resources for those seeking professional help for emotional problems and mental disorders. These services will provide you with the addresses of local branches and the names of the appropriate people to contact in your area.

- American Mental Health Foundation
  2 East 86th Street
  New York, N.Y. 10028
  (212) 737-9027

- National Association for Mental Health
  1800 North Kent Street
  Arlington, Va. 20006
  (703) 528-6408

- National Clearinghouse for Mental Health Information
  Public Inquiries Section
  Room 11A-21
  5600 Fishers Lane
  Rockville, Md. 20857
  (301) 443-4513

help for them is not a sign of weakness; quite the contrary, in fact. However, just as there are many types of therapy available, so are there many kinds of therapists who vary greatly in the amount and type of training they have had. Let us review some of the various kinds of professionals in the mental health field.

Psychiatrists are physicians who have received specialized medical training in mental illness and disease. Like all physicians, they are licensed by the state to practice medicine, treat patients, prescribe drugs, perform surgical operations, and institutionalize disturbed individuals.

Clinical psychologists who are qualified to practice psychotherapy usually have earned a Ph.D. degree and have received training in methods of treating mental illness. But since they do not have medical degrees, they cannot administer drugs (such as tranquilizers) to their patients. Clinical psychologists with an M.A. degree in their field may be trained in administering and evaluating psychological tests and often work in hospitals, schools, or clinics. In some states psychologists are regulated by a department of the state government, and they must meet specified educational standards before they can practice professionally as psychologists. Other states do not regulate psychologists at all. In general, any psychologist who is on the staff of a reputable clinic or social service agency, or who is recommended by a reputable agency, can be assumed to meet the standards of that organization.

Psychoanalysts are psychotherapists who have undergone specialized training in psychoanalysis. They must also be members of the American Psychoanalytic Association, the professional society of psychoanalysts in the United States, before being allowed to undertake the psychoanalysis of patients. Psychoanalysis may be practiced by some psychiatrists, clinical psychologists, and *lay analysts*, who, like psychologists, do not have a medical degree.

Psychiatric social workers, *occupational therapists*, and similar aides often have a college degree in their specialty. They are usually employed by a clinic or social service agency to administer tests, work up a case history, or provide limited treatment under the supervision of a psychiatrist or clinical psychologist. In many clinics a psychiatric social worker may also offer a limited amount of counseling.

In addition to these legitimate professionals, there are a great many nonprofessional, unlicensed therapists in practice. While some of them may offer sound, helpful therapy, many others are not only quacks but public menaces. They divert people who are in serious need of help from professional therapists and therapy programs, thereby delaying treatment and complicating existing problems. Some may suggest that a person is ill when he or she is not; others may actually induce emotional illness or even a breakdown in a particularly vulnerable individual. Many would-be therapists who use hypnosis techniques or encounter-group procedures are neither capable nor qualified to administer them, and again, may do lasting harm to susceptible clients.

People who seek treatment for emotional problems should make sure that any therapist they deal with is affiliated with a *recognized* professional organization. They would also be wise to examine any therapist's professional credentials and inform themselves beforehand about what educational and certification requirements the therapist has had to meet.

SUMMARY

1. *Personality* is the sum total of an individual's characteristics. *Heredity*, *experience*, and *culture* are the major factors influencing personality formation.

2. All human beings pass through certain stages of development. In *infancy* healthy emotional development is promoted by good care, affection, and encouragement of individuality and curiosity. In *childhood* a specific personality pattern emerges and the total community environment becomes significant. During *adolescence* the task is to put together a coherent identity. Peer influence becomes more important, and parental influence declines. During *early adulthood* a dependence-independence conflict often occurs. Resolution of this conflict is an important step in the maturation process and enables the individual to form intimate relationships. During *middle adulthood* individuals must adjust their goals and standards in the light of experience. Often greater self-realization results. During *late adulthood* self-indulgence may occur among those who have not resolved previous life conflicts. For others, feelings of contentment and generativity are common at this stage. During the *later years* individuals must deal with societal expectations and inadequate care for the elderly. However, a sense of satisfaction with one's life and experiences, and a feeling that one has participated fully in life, help to maintain one's personality and sense of well-being.

3. According to the National Association for Mental Health, mentally healthy people feel comfortable about themselves, feel right about other people, and are able to meet the demands of life.

4. According to Freudian theory, we all use *defense mechanisms* to deny feelings that will meet with social disapproval. The most frequently used defense mechanisms are *rationalization*, *sublimation*, *regression*, *projection*, *repression*, *identification*, *fantasy and daydreaming*, *idealization*, *reaction formation*, and *compensation*. All of these defenses help us cope with everyday problems.

5. *Neuroses* occur when people's emotions are consistently inappropriate to a situation; because of their self-defeating behavior, neurotics are unable to cope with the frustrations of daily life. *Anxiety neurosis* arises when anxiety pervades thoughts and actions, producing a feeling of helplessness in dealing with daily conflicts. *Neurotic depression* occurs when people feel a sense of extreme hopelessness, even in response to trivial events. Neurotics may also suffer from *phobias* (irrational fears of objects or situations), *obsessions* (fixations on particular ideas and images), *compulsive habits* (uncontrollable ritualistic behavior), and *psychosomatic disorders* (physical ailments caused by emotional distress). However, even though they are plagued by anxiety and depression and other specific symptoms, neurotics are in touch with reality.

6. *Psychoses* are much more severe mental disorders that involve a breakdown in thinking and mood and a loss of touch with reality. The most common kinds of psychosis are *schizophrenia*, *psychotic depression*, and *mania*.

7. Treatment strategies for emotional problems include *psychoanalysis*, *psychotherapy*, *behavioral techniques*, *client-centered therapy*, *group therapy*, and *drug therapy*.

8. The number of emotionally disturbed Americans is staggering. *Deinstitutionalization*, the policy of releasing inmates from state hospitals to save money, has resulted in a large number of "street people" who are barely able to care for themselves. Unlike other advanced countries, the United States has few mental health facilities for children and adolescents. While government spending on mental health is

grossly inadequate to the need, our own attitudes are also at fault. We tend to stigmatize people with emotional problems.

9. The *community psychology* approach to mental health offered the hope that community resources could be used to detect and treat emotional disturbances at an early age. Unfortunately, federal funding for community programs has been drastically cut back in recent years and state and local governments have not taken over the burden.

10. Mental health professionals include *psychiatrists*, *clinical psychologists*, *psychoanalysts*, *lay analysts*, *psychiatric social workers*, and *occupational therapists*. Besides these, a great many unlicensed therapists are in practice, some of whom can do lasting harm to susceptible persons. People seeking therapy should be careful to thoroughly check a therapist's credentials and educational background.

CONSUMER CONCERNS

1. Personal problems are often resolved through a discussion with someone in whom you have confidence. The person need not be an accredited counselor or therapist. In addition to a good friend, a family member, or a member of the school staff, what other persons might prove to be good listeners?
2. Before assigning yourself to a professional therapist, what credentials would you look for?
3. How would you judge the effectiveness of a specific group employing some form of group therapy? Is it necessary to go beyond satisfaction as the measure of the adequacy of a program?
4. If you believe you need psychological assistance, how should you begin to look for it?

2

Stress

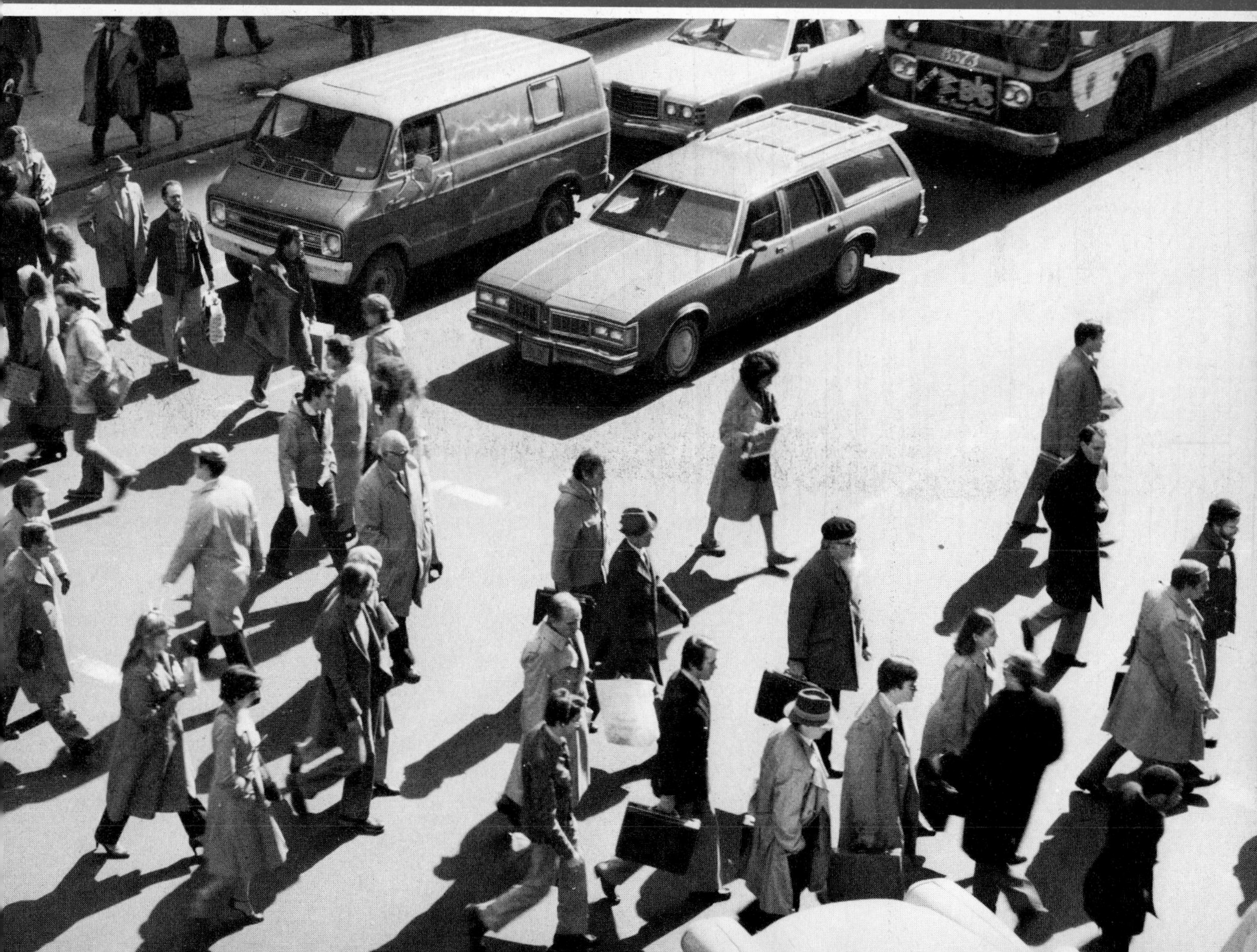

A concert pianist stepping onto the stage to perform; a construction worker inching his way over a girder high above the city; a college student jumping up and down in the stands, urging the college team to fight harder—all are under stress. At one time, stress was defined simply as body or mental tension caused by some physical, chemical, or emotional factor. It seemed an obvious and easily discernible condition. Students, for example, who stayed up all night studying for a final exam had no difficulty recognizing stress.

The concept of stress has been broadened over the past fifty years, however. Research has shown that the consequences of stress in our lives are much more far-reaching than was originally thought. It is now accepted, for example, that we are all under stress of one sort or another most of the time; to be alive is to be under stress. Also, stress is not necessarily a negative influence on our minds and bodies; it can be motivating psychologically as well as physically in a very positive way. In the broadest sense, stress of one sort or another can be thought of as having been responsible for most of mankind's achievements, since it is discomfort or dissatisfaction that spurs us out of the status quo.

So stress, as defined by modern scientists and medical experts, has implications much more complex than a simple dictionary definition of the word would indicate.

In this chapter we shall first see that the body responds to all forms of stress, both helpful and harmful, in the same way. Complex chemical responses evoke in us the fight-or-flight reaction, preparing us to cope with life events. We shall see that some persons are more prone than others to the stress of life events; that accidents, heart disease, ulcers, and even cancer have been related to stress proneness; and that the college years are a time of particular stress for many people. In the long run, however, it is not so much stress per se that is important, but rather our ability or inability to cope with it.

THE DEFINITION OF STRESS

A leading researcher in the field of stress, and a man who to a great degree enlarged our view of the subject, was Dr. Hans Selye. Selye defined **stress** as *the nonspecific response of the body to any demand*. In other words, stress demands that the body adapt to some factor—whether pleasant or unpleasant. All causes of stress produce the same biochemical changes in the body.

In a series of tests on laboratory animals, Selye observed that their response to injections of poisons and nonpoisons, as well as to cold, heat, and other stimuli, was usually the same. He called this response the **General Adaptation Syndrome (G.A.S).**

The G.A.S. has three stages. First is the alarm reaction, a generalized call to arms of the body's defenses when it is confronted with a **stressor**—that is, with any factor that causes stress. Second is the stage of resistance, a form of adaptation to the threat, for no organism can live in a perpetual state of alarm. Third is the stage of exhaustion, the symptoms of which are a wearing down of the organism, a premature aging due to wear and tear. Selye called the syndrome *general* "because it is produced by agents which have a general effect upon large portions of the body." He called it *adaptive* because it stimulates bodily defenses and thereby helps the organism to cope with stress. He called it a *syndrome* "because its individual manifestations are coordinated and even partly dependent upon each other."

Eustress and Distress

Stress evokes the G.A.S. whether it is caused by pleasant or unpleasant conditions. Stress, Selye said, "is all-inclusive," embodying both the positive and the negative, "just as cold and heat are specific variants of temperature changes." But Selye distinguished two varieties of stress: **distress,** the negative, or harmful, response; and **eustress** (from the Greek *eu*, "good"), the positive, or constructive, response. The G.A.S. is the same for both eustress and distress.

The stressor excites or agitates. Though it cannot be predicted whether a stressor will produce eustress or distress, individuals tend to follow a pattern of response. For example, in a clutch situation one baseball player more often gets the needed hit, while another is more apt to strike out. In the stress of final exams one student's powers of recall function, while another's fail. Different people cope with stress in different ways and with different degrees of success.

STRESS AND HEALTH

The most important application of the stress concept to general health is the discovery that the body meets all demands with the same basic adaptive defense mechanism. An understanding of this mechanism will teach us how to combat disease by strengthening the body's own defenses against stress. Research has shown that bodily changes during stress act upon our mental outlook—and vice versa. We must learn how to recognize the symptoms of stress and how to control our reactions when they become overwrought and threaten our well-being.

The Physiology of Stress

When we are faced with a threat—whether real or imagined—the body responds in what is called the **fight-or-flight reaction.** That is, it actively prepares to fight the threat or, alternatively, to escape it. Virtually every organ and every chemical constituent of the human body is involved in this reaction. The thyroid releases hormones that stimulate metabolism. The liver provides energy-yielding material to satisfy the body's increased demands and regulates the concentration of sugar, protein, and other elements in the blood. The white blood cells regulate the immune reaction to various foreign substances. The hypothalamus stimulates the pituitary gland, which secretes hormones into the blood. Blood flows away from the skin and digestive organs and to the brain and muscles, and this leads to those manifestations of stress that we can readily observe: agitation, loss of appetite, accelerated pulse, dry mouth, dilated pupils, increased blood pressure (which is evident by the thumping of the heart), sweat secretion, and a feeling of tension, excitement, and anxiety.

All of these physiological responses prepare us to act. But the responses are very strong indeed and can result in damage to the body if they are summoned too often or last too long. It is as though we had been given a hand grenade to dispose of a mosquito. The danger is compounded because we are not always aware that we have triggered these intense reactions when we are undergoing stress. Hans Selye prepared a list of manifestations of stress, particularly of the more dangerous distress, that can help us determine when we are overreacting (see box: Signs of Distress).

Signs of Distress

Hans Selye, in his book *The Stress of Life*, listed a number of stress signs that we can usefully monitor in our everyday lives. "Depending upon our conditioning," he wrote, "we all respond differently to general demands. But on the whole, I think that each of us tends to respond particularly with one set of signs, caused by the malfunction of whatever happens to be the most vulnerable part in our machinery, and when they appear, it's time to stop or change our activity—that is, find a diversion." Ask yourself whether you associate any of these symptoms with stressful events in your own life. Whenever you recognize them, prepare to take action.

_______ 1. General irritability, hyperexcitation, or depression.
_______ 2. Pounding of the heart (an indicator of high blood pressure often caused by stress)
_______ 3. Dryness of the throat and mouth
_______ 4. Impulsive behavior, emotional instability
_______ 5. The overpowering urge to cry or run and hide
_______ 6. Inability to concentrate
_______ 7. Feelings of unreality, weakness, or dizziness
_______ 8. Fatigue, loss of joie de vivre
_______ 9. Free-floating anxiety (feeling fear without knowing the cause)
_______ 10. Emotional tension and alertness, being keyed up
_______ 11. Trembling, nervous tics
_______ 12. Tendency to be easily startled by small sounds
_______ 13. High-pitched, nervous laughter
_______ 14. Stuttering and other speech difficulties
_______ 15. Grinding of the teeth
_______ 16. Insomnia
_______ 17. Hypermotility (inability to keep still)
_______ 18. Sweating
_______ 19. Frequent need to urinate
_______ 20. Diarrhea, indigestion, queasiness in the stomach, and sometimes vomiting (signs of disturbed gastrointestinal function that can lead to peptic ulcers and ulcerative colitis)
_______ 21. Migraine headaches
_______ 22. Premenstrual tension or missed menstrual cycles
_______ 23. Pain in the neck or lower back
_______ 24. Loss of or excessive appetitie
_______ 25. Increased smoking
_______ 26. Increased use of legally prescribed drugs, such as tranquilizers
_______ 27. Nightmares
_______ 28. Accident proneness

Source: Adapted from Hans Selye, *The Stress of Life*, rev. ed. (New York: McGraw Hill Book Company, 1978), pp. 174–177. Used by permission. Copyright © 1956, 1976 by Hans Selye. Reprinted by permission of Paul R. Reynolds, Inc., New York, N.Y.

STRESS-PRONE PERSONALITIES

Researchers are becoming convinced that certain personalities are more prone to what many consider stress-related diseases than others. According to one school of thought, definite personality profiles are connected with such illnesses as heart disease, asthma, arthritis, colitis, migraine, and even cancer. One such model has been constructed to identify those who have a high risk of heart disease.

Type A and Type B Behavior Patterns

Two physicians, Meyer Friedman and Ray H. Rosenman, have developed a profile of people whose behavior may encourage stress-induced medical problems such as heart disease. They call this the Type A behavior pattern.

Type A people are constantly involved in a struggle to do more and more in less and less time. They are intensely competitive, often hostile, aggressive, impatient, anxious, and eager for praise.

Type B behavior is the opposite of Type A. People with this pattern are rarely harried by a desire to crowd a great deal of achievement into a small segment of time. They may have a considerable amount of drive, but its character gives confidence and steadies, rather than goads, irritates, and infuriates, as it does with Type A people.

Recent research tends to show that not all Type A behavior is necessarily bad for everyone. Some people thrive on a fast-paced schedule, while others suffer from it. Researcher Redford Williams has hypothesized that of all Type A traits, it is hostility that is most related to disease.

Friedman and Rosenman estimate that roughly 90 percent of the population is easily identifiable as Type A or Type B (see box: Are You Type A or Type B?). Their experience in working with patients has shown them that the Type A personality can be modified into practicing behavior that is more healthful. We discuss some of these methods later in the chapter in the section Coping with Stress.

Cancer Personality

Many researchers now think that the way some people react to stress makes them more likely to develop cancer. People with the cancer personality have trouble dealing with stress, studies indicate. They are quiet, placid, emotionally repressed people. In fact, they have trouble expressing any feelings at all. When something bad happens to them, they do not blow up or fight back. Instead they withdraw into helplessness and despair. They simply give up. The theory is that a lifetime of pent-up emotion causes the release of a variety of hormones

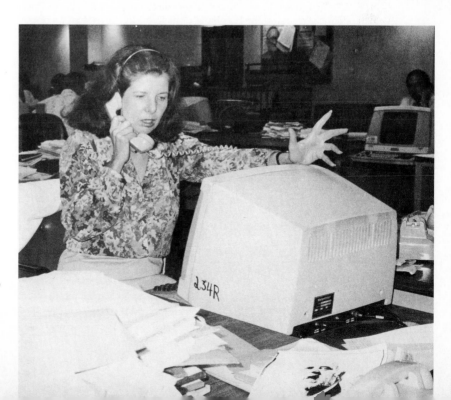

Type A people typically try to crowd more and more work into less and less time.

Are You Type A or Type B?

DO YOU:

_______ 1. Have (a) a habit of explosively accentuating various key words in your ordinary speech even when there is no real need to do so, and (b) a tendency to utter the last few words of your sentences far more rapidly than the opening words?

_______ 2. *Always* move, walk, and eat rapidly?

_______ 3. Feel (particularly if you openly exhibit to others) an impatience with the rate at which most events take place?

_______ 4. Frequently strive to think of or do two or more things simultaneously?

_______ 5. Find it *always* difficult to refrain from talking about or bringing the theme of any conversation around to those subjects that especially interest and intrigue you, and, when unable to accomplish this maneuver, pretend to listen but really remain preoccupied with your own thoughts?

_______ 6. Almost always feel vaguely guilty when you relax and do absolutely nothing for several hours to several days?

_______ 7. No longer observe the more important or interesting or lovely objects that you encounter in your milieu? For example, are you unable to recall what was in a strange office, store, or home after you have left?

_______ 8. Have no time to spare to become a person worth *being* because you are so preoccupied with getting the things worth *having*?

_______ 9. Attempt to schedule more and more in less and less time, and in doing so make fewer and fewer allowances for unforeseen contingencies?

_______ 10. On meeting another severely afflicted Type A person, instead of feeling compassion for his affliction, find yourself compelled to "challenge" him?

_______ 11. Resort to certain characteristic gestures or nervous tics? For example, in conversation frequently clench your fist, bang your hand upon a table, or pound one fist into the palm of your other hand in order to emphasize a point?

_______ 12. Believe that whatever success you have enjoyed has been due in good part to your ability to get things done faster than others? Are you afraid of what might happen if you slowed down a little?

_______ 13. Find yourself increasingly and unavoidably committed to translating and evaluating not only your own but also the activities of others in terms of "numbers"?

These are Type A behavior patterns. The following are Type B:

_______ 1. Are you completely free of *all* the habits and do you exhibit none of the traits listed above that harass the severely afflicted Type A person?

_______ 2. Do you never suffer from a sense of time urgency with its accompanying impatience?

_______ 3. Do you harbor no free-floating hostility, and do you feel no need to display or discuss either your achievements or accomplishments unless such exposure is demanded by the situation?

_______ 4. When you play, do you do so for fun and relaxation, not for exhibiting your superiority at any cost?

_______ 5. Can you relax without guilt, just as you can work without agitation?

Source: Meyer Friedman and Ray H. Rosenman, *Type A Behavior and Your Heart* (New York: Alfred A. Knopf, Inc., 1974), pp. 100–103. © 1974 by Meyer Friedman. Adapted by permission.

that weaken the body's immune system. Two specific hormones are thought to be responsible: corticosteroids and catecholamines, both of which are known to inhibit the white blood cells that patrol the body in search of cancer. Instead of seeking out tiny cancers and killing them, they let them get away, and the cancers grow and spread. One long-term study—stretching over seventeen years—found that men who were prone to depression were twice as likely to have died from cancer as others. In still another study doctors found a higher incidence of breast cancer among women who, in tests, proved to be suppressing their anger.

Not only do people with this personality pattern develop cancer more often, but they seem to be more likely to die quickly from the disease once it strikes. Several studies have shown that patients who keep fighting, hope for a turnaround, and express their emotions live longer. Recurrence-free survival is significantly more common among patients who initially react to cancer by denial, or who fight, than among those who respond with stoic acceptance or feelings of helplessness and hopelessness. Cancer survivors, in fact, are often feisty complainers.

THE STRESS OF LIFE EVENTS

In our society a premium is put upon achievement and competition, and this creates a climate that is conducive to stress. Most of us will have no trouble recognizing the probability of higher stress inherent in crowded urban settings, in difficult job situations, and in strained personal relationships. What is less obvious, however, and consequently more insidious, is that many events in our lives that we take for granted may well induce stress without our being aware of it until we are suffering the consequences.

Even such common events as going to college, changing jobs, getting married, or moving to another community can provoke stress. The stress will be even greater if several of these events occur at the same time. (see box: Life Events Stress Test). We often perceive any kind of change—even a beneficial one—as threatening. This is because we are put in a position of having to adapt, to learn how to cope, and this causes stress.

Anything that challenges our values and beliefs is a source of stress. The social tumult of the 1960s, for example, which brought about a reassessment

Promptness in American Society

Promptness is . . . valued highly in American life. If people are not prompt, it is often taken either as an insult or as an indication that they are not quite responsible. There are those, of a psychological bent, who would say that we are obsessed with time. They can point to individuals in American culture who are literally time-ridden. And even the rest of us feel very strongly about time because we have been taught to take it so seriously. We have stressed this aspect of culture and developed it to a point unequaled anywhere in the world, except, perhaps, in Switzerland and north Germany. Many people criticize our obsessional handling of time. They attribute ulcers and hypertension to the pressure engendered by such a system. Perhaps they are right.

Source: Edward T. Hall, *The Silent Language* (New York: Doubleday-Anchor, 1973), p. 9.

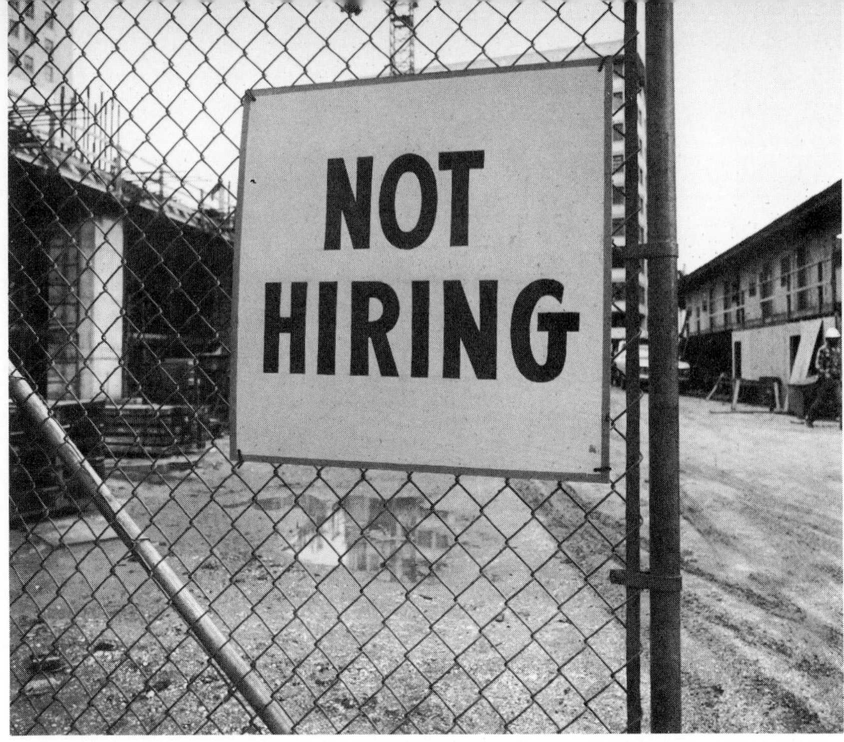

Holmes and Rahe found losing one's job to be a major source of stress; see the Life Events Stress Test on pages 50–51.

of so many beliefs, generated stress. A prime instance has been the women's movement, which has forced both sexes to reinterpret their roles and has placed a burden of coping with change on each.

More and more of us are living in urban areas where we are forced to cope with noise, air pollution (see the sections Noise Pollution and Air Pollution in Chapter 17), and frequent indifference or outright hostility on the part of our fellow citizens. Many people work in jobs that they do not like. This leads to feelings of being trapped, bored, and powerless—which create a prime climate for stress. It has been shown that people who spend a good part of their lives

The Hardy Personality

Recently, investigators have found that some people do not react to stressful events by suffering and becoming ill; some people seem to respond to stress more effectively than others. Psychologist Suzanne C. Kobasa studied executives and found that while some experienced illness due to high stress, it did not have this effect on others. She identified a personality—*the hardy personality*—that characterized those who did not experience illness. This personality has three dimensions involving *control*, *commitment*, and *challenge*. Hardy personality types tend to feel that life events can be controlled and influenced; this belief enables them to avoid feeling helpless when difficult situations arise. The commitment component is reflected in a tendency to become actively involved in events, rather than to be passively influenced by them. Hardy personality types show a sense of purpose and meaning in their lives. Finally, these people view life events as a challenge and an opportunity to develop rather than as a painful ordeal to be endured. They transform threat into a challenge. It seems that hardy people experience stress, but their response to stress diminishes its negative effects.

Source: Stephen Worchel and Wayne Shebilske, *Psychology: Principles and Applications*, 2nd ed. (Prentice-Hall, 1986), p. 358. Reprinted by permission.

doing something that matters to them can withstand a great deal more stress than those whose job means nothing more than killing time.

Different people react differently to the stress of life events, and the way in which they react is an important factor in whether the stress will cause them physical or emotional harm. One researcher has identified three characteristics of people who respond positively to the stress of life events—people she has described as having a *hardy personality*. These characteristics are summarized in the accompanying box The Hardy Personality.

THE HASSLES OF DAILY LIFE

It is easy to see how certain major life events can induce stress and cause illness. But what about all the little annoyances of daily life that make our hearts pound and our blood boil? Do they have a significant effect on our health?

Two kinds of stressful change in daily life—called hassles and uplifts—have been identified in a recent study. *Hassles* are the small, irritating events that come up unexpectedly in the course of a day; they include misplacing things, overscheduling, and becoming angry at other people's behavior. You arrive at the gym, for example, and discover that you left your membership card at home. After a tiring day, you force yourself to go out to a concert when you would much rather spend a quiet evening at home. The person in front of you in the supermarket checkout line waits until the total flashes on the cash register to open her purse and dig into it for her checkbook. What makes these little occasions stressful is that they disrupt the predictable flow of daily events. They are evidence that we do not have complete control over our lives.

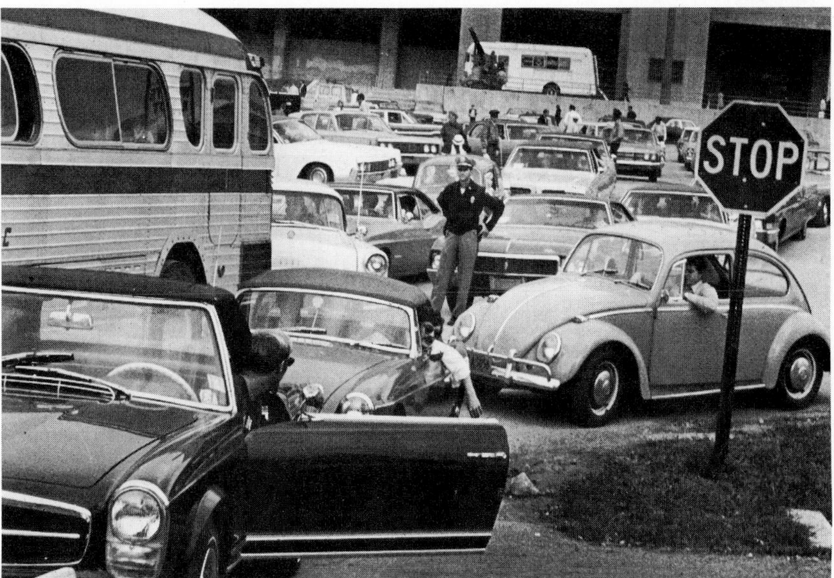

Daily hassles can cumulatively do us as much harm as major life events.

Life Events Stress Test

The death of Paul ("Bear") Bryant, one of the most famous of all American coaches, shortly after his announced retirement from football in 1982 was not surprising to those who have studied life events and their cumulative effect on health. As early as 1967, Holmes and Rahe conducted a scientific survey to test the effects of a number of life events on the health status of a large number of subjects. Their data revealed that the more stressful events one encountered, the more likely one was to begin to show symptoms of disease. The following suggestions are for using Holmes and Rahe's Social Readjustment Rating Scale for the maintenance of your health and prevention of illness:

1. Become familiar with the life events and the amount of change they require.
2. Put the scale where you and the family can see it easily several times a day.
3. With practice you can recognize when a life event happens.
4. Think about the meaning of the event for you and try to identify some of the feelings you experience.
5. Think about the different ways you might best adjust to the event.
6. Take your time in arriving at decisions.
7. If possible, anticipate life changes and plan for them well in advance.
8. Pace yourself. It can be done even if you are in a hurry.
9. Look at the accomplishment of a task as a part of daily living and avoid looking at such an achievement as a "stopping point" or a "time for letting down."
10. Remember, the more change you have, the more likely you are to get sick. Of those people with 300 or more Life Change Units for the past year, almost 80% get sick in the near future; with 150 to 299 Life Change Units, about 50% get sick in the near future; and with less than 150 Life Change Units, only about 30% get sick in the near future.

    So, the higher your Life Change Score, the harder you should work to stay well.

Life Event	Mean Value	Score
1. Death of spouse	100	____
2. Divorce	73	____
3. Marital separation from mate	65	____
4. Detention in jail or other institution	63	____
5. Death of a close family member	63	____
6. Major personal injury or illness	53	____
7. Marriage	50	____
8. Being fired at work	47	____
9. Marital reconciliation with mate	45	____
10. Retirement from work	45	____
11. Major change in the health or behavior of a family member	44	____
12. Pregnancy	40	____
13. Sexual difficulties	39	____
14. Gaining a new family member (e.g., through birth, adoption, oldster moving in, etc.)	39	____
15. Major business readjustment (e.g., merger, reorganization, bankruptcy, etc.)	39	____

Uplifts, on the other hand, are the small, radiant moments in the day when you feel that all's right with the world. You have finished a term paper ahead of time and can now take the weekend off and go to the beach with friends.

Life Event	Mean Value	Score
16. Major change in financial state (e.g., a lot worse off or a lot better off than usual)	38	____
17. Death of a close friend	37	____
18. Changing to a different line of work	36	____
19. Major change in the number of arguments with spouse (e.g., either a lot more or a lot less than usual regarding child rearing, personal habits, etc.)	35	____
20. Taking out a mortgage or loan for a major purchase (e.g., for a home, business, etc.)	31	____
21. Foreclosure on a mortgage or loan	30	____
22. Major change in responsibilities at work (e.g., promotion, demotion, lateral transfer)	29	____
23. Son or daughter leaving home (e.g., marriage, attending college, etc.)	29	____
24. Trouble with in-laws	29	____
25. Outstanding personal achievement	28	____
26. Wife beginning or ceasing work outside the home	26	____
27. Beginning or ceasing formal schooling	26	____
28. Major change in living conditions (e.g., building a new home remodeling, deterioration of home or neighborhood)	25	____
29. Revision of personal habits (dress, manners, association, etc.)	24	____
30. Troubles with the boss	23	____
31. Major change in working hours or conditions	20	____
32. Change in residence	20	____
33. Changing to a new school	20	____
34. Major change in usual type and/or amount of recreation	19	____
35. Major change in church activities (e.g., a lot more or a lot less than usual)	19	____
36. Major change in social activities (e.g., clubs, dancing, movies, visiting, etc.)	18	____
37. Taking out a mortgage or loan for a lesser purchase (e.g., for a car, TV, freezer, etc.)	17	____
38. Major change in sleeping habits (a lot more or a lot less sleep, or change in part of day when asleep)	16	____
39. Major change in number of family get-togethers (e.g., a lot more or a lot less than usual)	15	____
40. Major change in eating habits (a lot more or a lot less food intake, or very different meal hours or surroundings)	15	____
41. Vacation	13	____
42. Christmas	12	____
43. Minor violations of the law (e.g., traffic tickets, jaywalking, disturbing the peace, etc.)	11	____
Your Score	**Total**	________

Source: T. H. Holmes, and R. H. Rahe, "The Social Readjustment Rating Scale," *Journal of Psychosomatic Research*, 11 (1967), pp. 213–218, Pergamon Press, Ltd. Reprinted with permission.

An old friend whom you have been missing calls out of the blue to say that she's arriving next month. You feel a glowing exhilaration after a thirty-mile bike ride.

Thus change of any kind—large or small, good or bad—causes the body to activate the stress response. In fact, hassles and uplifts may have a stronger effect on mood and health than more dramatic life events do. According to a year-long study of 100 middle-aged, middle-class people done in 1983, the more daily hassles we experience, the poorer our overall health. This holds true even if we have also had an unusual number of uplifts. In fact, uplifts seem to have a temporary adverse effect on some women's emotional state and mental health.

Boredom. While the small, unexpected changes of daily life can impair mental and physical health, so, too, can the lack of change. Monotony and boredom—the lack of stimulation—can create stress just as major and minor life events can. For this reason, many people must learn techniques for creating change in their lives. We can break the monotony of a daily routine by varying the route of our homeward journey. Or we can accept a small challenge, a calculated risk, by opening a conversation with a stranger in class. These techniques, though trivial, can reduce the stress of boredom and add spice to our lives.

STRESS IN COLLEGE

Certainly no period is more rife with stress than the college years. In addition to the normal adolescent and early adulthood conflicts, the college student experiences many special stresses and anxieties. The following discussion describes some of the pressures that are characteristic of college life and offers some ways of coping with them.

Doubts About the College Experience. For most of us, the process of education follows a set pattern: Eight years of elementary school are followed by four years of high school and two to four years of college. Unfortunately, our personality or psychological development often does not fit conveniently into this pattern. We may not always be ready to meet the new demands of each stage in the educational process.

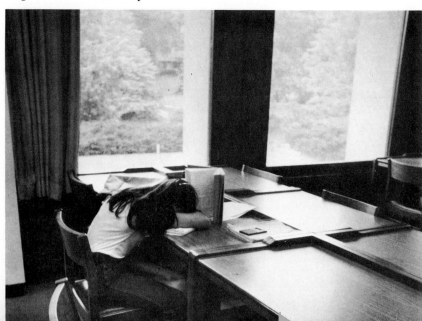

This may be particularly true of the transition from high school to college. Many people go to college for reasons other than acquiring an advanced education. Parental pressure, the influence of friends, or simply an unwillingness to start working for a living may be the motivation. These motives, however, may not be enough to enable the individual to deal with the pressures of college life.

The independence expected of the college student may also cause adjustment problems. During the high school years most students are protected by their families from taking any real responsibility for themselves. The home environment is often a comforting one, and many students hold on to the last vestiges of childhood dependence. When they enter college, however, they are expected to assume more responsibility. There is no one to monitor them periodically and make sure they are keeping up with their assignments, as there was in their earlier school days.

Academic Pressures. The freedom to create their own work schedule and to integrate the various aspects of their lives is a mixed blessing for college students. If they are unable to exercise self-discipline within the new scope of freedom, they will be considerably more vulnerable to the pressures placed on them by professors and administrators.

How well a student does in college can have enormous lifetime consequences. For this reason, college students experience an inordinate amount of stress over grades. While from an educational standpoint this might be desirable, it often has negative psychological consequences. Students become preoccupied with how they are judged rather than with the learning process itself. Rather than attempting to master the subjects they are studying—which requires a regular, daily commitment to course work—they concentrate on doing well on tests. The often impersonal nature of the classroom contributes to this attitude. In any case, the learning process and peace of mind both suffer. A grade becomes transformed from a judgment of work to a judgment of self-worth.

Social Pressures. The new and more complex interactions of the college years can be another source of stress for the student. The security of family and neighborhood relationships may be supplanted by the new and perhaps alien social community of college. Making friends and establishing satisfactory relationships may be more difficult than they were in high school. And yet, because the student is often removed from familiar surroundings, the need to form such relationships will be greater.

There may also be stresses in the area of sexuality. Many students come to college expecting to lead an unrestricted sexual life. Often they find that intimate relationships are difficult to form. The difference between expectation and reality may lead to frustration, anger, and diminished self-esteem. Conversely, other students find college too permissive. Coed dormitories, unrestricted visitation rights, and the generally more liberal atmosphere of a college may create strain for individuals who prefer to follow traditional patterns of sexual behavior. Peer-group pressure to conform to more permissive standards can create troubling inner conflicts.

PROBLEMS AND CONTROVERSIES: Cramming and the Use of Stimulants

Students who lack the self-discipline to devote sufficient time each day to course work pay a heavy price in stress when exam time rolls around. They have to cram a month's or a semester's worth of studying into the space of a few hours the night before. While it is no doubt better to cram than not to study at all, staying up all night, perhaps with the help of stimulants, takes its toll on mental efficiency, as *Newsweek* writer Keith Ablow points out:

For some people, disruptions in the regular sleep cycle can cause temporary intellectual lapses—and stimulants can set off severe side effects. Thus, for every student who manages to memorize the chemical synthesis of buna-S-rubber at 5 A.M. *and then triumphantly finds that precise question on his test at 9, there are more than a few who lament the "obvious" answers they blew on a multiple-choice exam because they "just couldn't focus.". . .*

Heavy use of stimulants can compound the problem. Many students assume that large quantities of coffee or a few amphetamines will increase alertness; they don't. In fact, stimulants merely disguise—briefly—a reduced capacity to grasp, retain, and retrieve information. [According to David Buchholtz, a neurologist and sleep therapist at The Johns Hopkins Hospital in Baltimore], "Caffeine does not correct the cognitive impairment caused by lost sleep. A person may be awake, but he'll have to deal with an intellectual deficit, and his concentration won't be there. He can actually have 'microsleeps' and stare at the same word for five minutes.". . .

In the end, the best formula to follow when finals arrive is one that students have been taught for years—moderation. There will surely be times when excelling, or perhaps just passing, requires pushing bedtime back, but any major changes in sleep patterns should be made cautiously. As Buchholtz suggests, "The key is keeping perspective and not ever overdoing it."

Source: Keith Ablow, "The Dangers of Cramming," *Newsweek on Campus*, May 1985, p. 25.

Pressures Concerning the Future. College students are generally in the process of maturation. They are in a period of life characterized by uncertainty and indecisiveness. Yet they are expected to make decisions of frightening importance. The student is under pressure from family and friends to make plans for the future and to choose an occupation. Although many students will have formulated their goals by the end of their freshman or sophomore year, some postpone their career decisions until much later. Anxiety concerning these decisions is often quite severe.

Help for Problems. One way to avoid these difficulties is to postpone going to college until ready for it. Readiness includes not only preparation for and awareness of the demands of college, but also enthusiasm for the learning process itself—an enthusiasm people find difficult to develop unless they are sure that a college education is really what they desire.

For students already in college who are undergoing stress, perhaps the first thing to do is to try to determine whether they belong in college in the first place. If their intellectual capabilities, educational background, interests, or temperaments are unsuited for college—and if they do not have a strong desire to be in college and to try to compensate for their inadequacies—they should see an adviser and explore their motives for remaining in school. Are they staying in school to please their parents? Would they be embarrassed to leave?

Would they really be happier doing something else? Do they simply need a year off to marshal their resources? An adviser can help them decide what course of action would be best.

Those who are experiencing stress in college but who feel they belong in school and should be doing better have a more complex problem to contend with. The first thing to do is to try actively to counteract the feeling of hopelessness that problems engender. Everyone experiences emotional difficulties to some degree. The decision to cope with these difficulties is the first step toward resolving them.

Students can solve many problems themselves. A tough required course is best dealt with through extra study—ineffectual worrying is of no help at all. Perhaps a professor or friend can be approached for guidance. Feelings of isolation are not overcome by sulking but by making efforts to meet other people. Most people respond to a friendly, honest approach, particularly when circumstances are appropriate, such as at a party or student center. The important thing is not to be defeated before one begins or even after failing in the first few attempts; an attitude that one is in control of one's destiny—that one's actions can have an impact—will ultimately bring about solutions.

Some problems, of course, are of a more severe nature and require outside help. Here, too, a determination to solve one's problems will provide momentum toward solutions. Students often fail to take advantage of the aid of faculty members or advisers, even in small colleges where students and faculty may know each other quite well. Yet even the process of explaining one's problems to someone else helps crystallize one's thoughts and allows useful ideas to emerge. And competent, sympathetic advisers, once located, can offer useful suggestions.

When problems are really severe—when deep feelings of depression, inadequacy, and helplessness take hold—professional assistance should be sought immediately. Waiting for emotional problems to solve themselves generally exacerbates them and makes them more difficult to handle.

EFFECTS OF STRESS

Most researchers agree that stress contributes to the incidence and deadliness of disease. A source of confusion is why some people become ill under stress and others remain healthy. One theory is that we have only so much energy to devote to our well-being, and when we channel large portions of it into coping with reactions of our body—such as the stress reaction—it leaves only a small margin to defend ourselves against the onslaught of disease. In other words, a too-frequent summoning of the stress reaction described above seriously depletes our ability to cope with our environment.

What is clear is that many people do become ill when they have to cope with crises or, in some cases, even when they have to deal with a series of ordinary life events.

It is still being debated whether some specific diseases are actually *caused* by stress. Peptic ulcers have long been associated with stress in the popular mind and in much research literature. Many hold that hypertension, or high blood pressure, is stress-induced. Others dispute this. What has been clearly demonstrated, however, is that stress has an extremely harmful effect on the course of hypertension when someone is already suffering from it. (Hypertension is discussed in Chapter 14.) Migraine headache and depression have also been widely associated with stress.

Suicide Prevention

Do you know what to do if someone threatens suicide? First, you are not responsible if he or she follows through with threats and makes an attempt. But you should observe the following guidelines if you are forced to react:

- *Don't* make light of the issue or say "That's crazy" or "You can't be serious." (The person wants you to listen.)
- *Don't* challenge the person by disguising your concern in an attempt at "reverse psychology." (This can backfire.)
- *Don't* play psychiatrist by trying to analyze the person's problems. (Depression is unresponsive to digressive, speculative chitchat.)
- *Do* listen attentively and communicate to the best of your ability that you really care about the person.
- *Do* remind the person of choices other than death. Death is always available, so it can be put off while other avenues are explored. Death is also irreversible, whereas other options can be tried and then canceled.
- *Do* try to reassure the person that depression passes no matter how permanent it may feel.

It is frightening to react to a suicide threat. Try not to let your fear push you toward either of two extremes: a panicky, emotional reaction or a too-cool, intellectual lecture. Be totally there for the person, communicate empathy, and follow the list of do's and don'ts.

A **migraine headache** is a severe, throbbing pain in the head caused by a constriction of the arteries supplying blood to a part of the head. This constriction of the arteries may be the result of tension in a person undergoing stress. Migraine is often accompanied by other symptoms—distorted vision, nausea, vomiting—all indications that the constriction is interfering with the normal functioning of the brain. The constriction results in the dilation of other arteries as the nervous system attempts to compensate for the decreased blood flow.

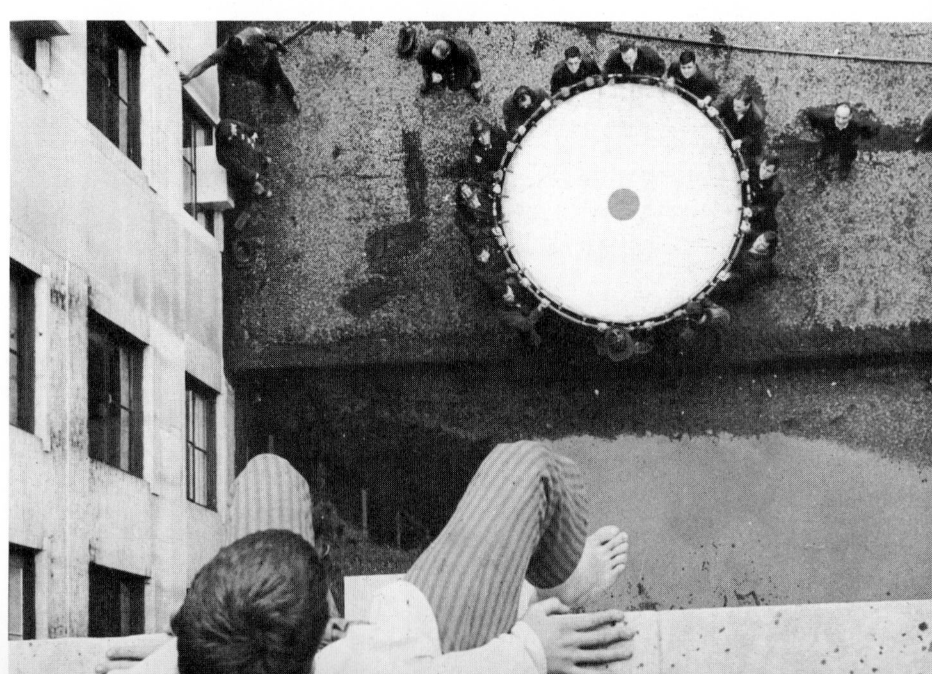

The pressure exerted by the dilated arteries upon the nerve endings embedded in the walls of the arteries causes the severe pain of a migraine headache. The headache throbs because the dilated arteries pulsate along with the blood as it is pumped through them by the heart. Headaches are usually treated with painkillers such as aspirin or codeine, depending upon their severity. Recurring headaches should be checked by a physician. Those that are not a symptom of a physical illness may require psychotherapy as treatment.

Depression is an example of a passive response to stress, the symptoms of which include sadness, hopelessness, withdrawal, isolation, feelings of worthlessness, and apathy. Physical symptoms may include insomnia and loss of appetite.

Everybody feels depressed sometimes. In fact, depression can be beneficial in helping a person adjust to new circumstances. But a depression that lasts a long time or that has no immediate realistic cause can be a serious problem. It is a symptom that something is wrong in the affected person's life, something that demands a solution.

People who periodically suffer from depression have been found to share certain personality traits. They are usually overly conscientious, idealistic, serious-minded, and unrealistic in the standards and goals they set for themselves and others. Ironically, depressed people are likely to suffer from impaired judgment, which may lead them to commit errors that only add to their depression. One of the most pervasive symptoms of depression is a feeling of helplessness and immobilization. A breaking of this vicious cycle is often a part of successful therapy.

Stress and Suicide

A great many people who see no way out of their depression and feelings of hopelessness look for some means to end it all. Depression is thought to play a major role in some four out of every five suicide attempts, and, as we have seen, depression is a frequent response to stress.

While suicide occurs more often among older people (see Chapter 10), in the last few years it has reached almost epidemic proportions among young Americans aged 10 to 20. Half a million teenagers, 90 percent of them girls, try to kill themselves each year. (Of the 5,000 who succeed, however, 75 percent are boys.)

Several social factors are responsible for this phenomenon. One major factor is family breakdown. Many older children and teenagers feel estranged from their families and report a lack of love and affection, particularly from their fathers. Others feel that they have failed to live up to their parents' high expectations of them. Still others hold themselves responsible for the disharmony and violence in their families and therefore decide to put themselves out of the way so that the rest of the family can live more happily.

The casual violence that pervades so much of American society is another major factor in suicide among the young. Too much exposure to meaningless violence on television and in motion pictures has a numbing effect. Also, the ready availability of handguns makes suicide all the easier; handguns were used in 62 percent of all youth suicides in 1986. (See box: Gun Control in Chapter 3.)

Suicide Among College Students. The suicide rate is particularly high among college students—50 percent higher than among same-aged persons not in college. Surveys have found that 30 percent of all college students think occasionally of suicide, and 10 percent consider it seriously. Of the 10,000 who attempt it each year, 1,000 succeed—again, the great majority of them male.

The most frequent causes of suicide among this group are academic failure and troubled personal relationships—or the lack of personal relationships. College students rely on grades for a feeling of security and self-worth; and they rely on personal relationships for a sense of identity. (It is interesting that during the 1960s protest movements the student suicide rate dropped sharply; the protest movements created a sense of intimacy and identity among students that counteracted feelings of alienation.) Equally important, many young men are under enormous pressures from their families to succeed and achieve a high standard of living. When they get low grades, they see it as mortifying evidence that they do not have what it takes to succeed. Instead of asking for help, as many women do, they resort to suicide.

Failure in personal relationships is also a potent source of suicidal feelings. The end of a love affair or the inability to make friends can bring on feelings of rejection and abandonment. It is in this context that most of the unsuccessful suicides occur. Many a failed suicide is often a disguised cry for help; it may also be an attempt to manipulate others: to instill feelings of guilt in friends or parents, to win an argument, or to call attention to oneself.

Evaluating a Suicide Risk. There are a number of signs and symptoms that should alert you to the possibility that a person may be about to attempt suicide. First, those who are chronically depressed or alcoholic are always potentially suicidal. So also are many loners who have no supportive family network or circle of friends, or who are alienated from others for various reasons. Likewise, those who are facing a specific stressful life event such as the loss of a means of livelihood or a serious illness may be considering suicide.

People who are about to attempt suicide will often discuss their plans in detail—for example, the advantages and disadvantages of certain methods, what should be done with their property after they die, and the setting in which they intend to die. They should be taken seriously, especially if they are male, and listened to (see box: Suicide Prevention).

COPING WITH STRESS

The human body has to adapt continually to an ever-changing world—to physical aspects such as temperature, humidity, and noise, and to social factors such as tight work schedules and troubled personal relationships. It makes these adaptations to keep working in a balanced way—that is, to maintain **homeostasis.** The act of making such adjustments is called **coping.**

Much of our physical coping with stress is automatic. When, for example, humid weather stresses our bodies, we sweat; we do not have to will our sweat glands to give up moisture to cool us off, nor is there much we can do to stop them. When we have just missed the bus and are going to be late for class, we respond automatically by gritting our teeth and getting a tight stomach. We can either let ourselves continue to fume and worry, or we can decide to

Twelve Tips on How to Cope with Stress

- *Try physical activity*. Exercising vigorously, mowing the lawn, or washing the car will relieve the "uptight" feeling, relax you, and turn frowns into smiles.
- *Talk out your worries*. Don't hesitate to ask for help when you feel you need it. If your problem is really serious, seek professional help from a psychologist, psychiatrist, or social worker.
- *Know your limits*. Learn to accept what you cannot change. If things are beyond your control, don't fight the situation.
- *Don't mask your problems with hard drugs and alcohol*. Although drugs and alcohol relieve stress temporarily, they do nothing to alleviate the conditions that caused the stress in the first place.
- *Take care of your health*. Make sure to eat well and get enough rest every day. Neglecting your diet and losing sleep will make you less able to deal with stressful situations.
- *Make time for fun*. Play is just as important to your well-being as work. It is essential to allow time for amusement and recreation.
- *Get involved with others*. If you are bored, sad, and lonely, get out and go where it's all happening. Offer your services to neighborhood and volunteer organizations. Help yourself by helping others.
- *Organize your time*. Don't try to do everything at once. Rank your tasks in order of importance and concentrate on the essential ones first.
- *Give in once in a while*. You don't always have to be right. Don't let other people upset you because they don't do things your way.
- *Realize that it's all right to cry.* Relieve your anxiety with a good cry; it may prevent a headache and other physical symptoms.
- *Create your own peace and quiet*. If you can't get away from your problems, try imagining a quiet country scene or a deserted beach. Escape into the pages of a good book or play some music you enjoy. Any one of these activities can induce a sense of peace and tranquility.
- *Learn how to relax*. The next time you feel tight and tense, take ten deep breaths. It works wonders in reducing tension. The relaxation techniques listed in the box The Relaxation Response, below, can relieve most symptoms of stress and can be used anywhere any time.

Source: Adapted from Louis E. Kopolow, M.D., "Plain Talk About Handling Stress," DHHS Publication No. (ADM) 83-502, National Institute of Mental Health, Division of Scientific and Public Information; Plain Talk Series, ed. Ruth Kay.

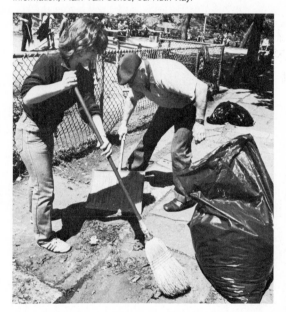

take advantage of the extra time and get out the morning newspaper. Thus by our own choices and actions, we can reduce the stress of many everyday situations.

In this section we shall discuss a number of ways by which you can reduce the amount of stress in your life and become a happier, more contented person. Some involve a fundamental change in mental habits, others a change in life style.

Manage Your Time

A major cause of stress is time pressure. Many people feel victimized by the strict time schedules, constant interruptions, and difficult deadlines that prevail in most schools and offices. That such stressful conditions take their toll on health is shown by the fact that people who are constantly battling to meet deadlines in their work suffer high rates of heart disease. Jane Brody and Donald Norfolk suggest a number of ways to cope with time pressure.* These include setting priorities, working at your own pace, formulating realistic goals, and keeping a flexible schedule.

Set Your Priorities. Rank your tasks in order of importance and save your energy for the essential ones. Delegate the less important tasks to others and put all the rest out of your mind. Next, identify what time of day you do your best work and reserve it for the most important projects. Eliminate activities that waste time. You may find, for example, that you can do with a lot less television watching.

Work at Your Own Pace. The next step is to find the rate at which you work most comfortably and keep to it. Concentrate on one thing at a time and don't watch the clock. Clock watchers just create more stress for themselves, and their performance often suffers from it. As Norfolk advises, you will find you get the most done at a "steady, comfortable pace. Try to follow the Taoist maxim: 'Don't push the river, let it flow.' "

Formulate Realistic Goals. Resist, if you can, the impulse to accommodate others and take on more than you can comfortably handle. Furthermore, accept the fact that you will not be able to do your very best in every situation; instead, be satisfied with what you can accomplish.

Keep Your Schedule Flexible. You may find that you need to work longer on some days and less on others; try not to let yourself be confined by rigid working hours. You should also try to carve out some breathing space during the day. Schedule in some extra time between tasks to take care of unforeseen emergencies. Try also to take the long view of things and anticipate stressful situations that may come up in the next few months. If you think several are going to occur at the same time, try to reschedule them in order to give yourself a break.

Have Fun

One of the most effective ways of coping with stress is to divert your mind from work concerns and emotional problems. A diversion such as doing a crossword puzzle, reading an interesting book, or even taking a walk around the block is often more effective for relieving the symptoms of stress than mere resting. As mentioned earlier, however, many competitive Type A personalities find it difficult to really relax. If you tend to be one of these, learn to enjoy an amusement or game simply for the fun of it instead of focusing on how well you are doing or on what you are ultimately going to get out of it. If you still find yourself preoccupied with troubles at work or feel your anger

*Jane Brody, *Jane Brody's The New York Times Guide to Personal Health* (New York: Avon, 1983); Donald Norfolk, *The Stress Factor* (New York: Simon and Schuster, 1979).

building up over trivial things, then use your powers of fantasy. Imagine yourself standing in a field of wildflowers, or in a quiet forest, or by a waterfall. After five or ten minutes of this you should be able to view your troubles from a more positive perspective.

Express Your Feelings

On the other hand, no host of golden daffodils is going to help you come to terms with real anger, anxiety, tension, or sadness. Holding in such feelings produces more stress than expressing them; in fact, it can lead to high blood pressure, ulcers, heart disease, and—as we have seen—cancer. (See box: Testing Your Assertiveness, in Chapter 1.)

The important considerations in dealing with emotions are, first, allowing yourself to express them, and second, expressing them over the right things. Much anxiety, tension, and depression, for example, can be relieved by a good, old-fashioned cry, as many women are well aware. But most men are taught from childhood to think of crying as a sign of weakness and effeminacy and therefore never permit themselves to do it except on the most extreme occasions. Women, on the other hand, emerge from emotional crises far stronger because as children they learn that crying is an acceptable response to overwhelming problems.

The second consideration is to conserve your emotional resources for the appropriate times. For example, let your anger or sadness flood out when the occasion truly warrants it and not over every minor setback. You can also avoid a lot of unnecessary anger by not insisting on being right all the time. Learn to give in once in a while; you'll feel much better for it.

Learn to Live in the Present. Don't worry too much about what is going to happen tomorrow. One of the greatest sources of stress is anticipation. As Mark Twain once said, "I'm an old man, and I have known troubles in my life, most of which never happened." In almost every case, the fear of the event is worse than the actual event itself. Learn to quell your worry about future and uncontrollable events.

Similarly, don't waste energy regretting past failures. The past no longer exists, and tomorrow will take care of itself. Keep the Zen motto in mind: "The present moment is all there is."

Seek Help When You Need It. One of the most effective stress-reducing measures is to talk things over with a close friend or family member. If you are having severe emotional problems, however, you should seek out some form of counseling or other professional assistance.

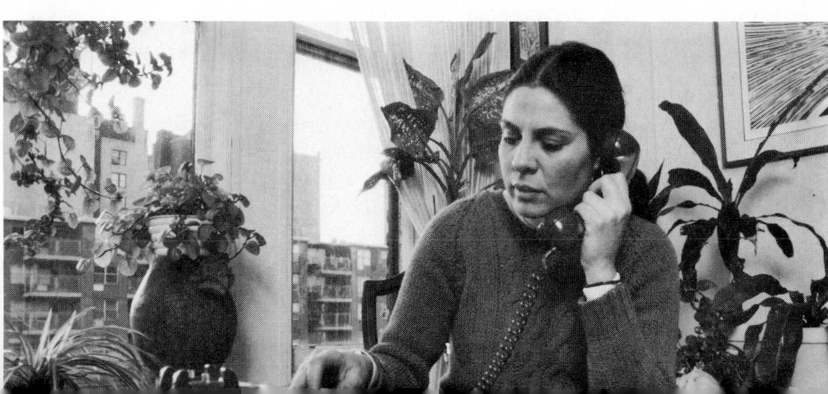

Getting involved with other people is a good way to reduce stress.

Get Involved with Others

People under stress often spend far too much time and mental energy on themselves and their problems. As a result, they are lonely, bored, frustrated, and depressed. As we pointed out earlier, the answer is to get involved with other people. Join a neighborhood organization or volunteer your services for a worthwhile cause. By getting more involved in the outside world and less wrapped up in yourself, you will become more attractive to others. You will thus expand your circle of friends and acquaintances and broaden your scope of activities.

Change Your Life Style

The efficient use of time and the appropriate expression of feelings are two fundamental ways of coping with stress, but these are basically mental procedures. Let us take a look now at some of the physical ways in which you can help your body cope with stress.

Watch Your Body Symptoms. Stress is such a constant background presence in our lives that we have become desensitized to it. Many of us feel that physical discomfort, anxiety, and tension are a normal part of life. For this reason, it is essential to stay alert to the signals the body gives off as it copes with these conditions (see the box Signs of Distress, page 44). Watch especially for tightness in the stomach, headaches, and back pain; when these appear, take a little fantasy vacation as suggested above. Again, it is men who have the most difficult time recognizing dangerous body symptoms because they are conditioned from childhood to ignore pain.

Drugs, Including Alcohol. Many people rely on drugs—stimulants, sedatives, and alcohol—to temporarily relieve the effects of stress but do nothing about the conditions that cause it. Instead of apportioning their time rationally and giving themselves a few needed breaks in the course of the day, they take stimulants to get work done, alcohol to relax, and sedatives to induce sleep. By their very nature, however, such drugs are habit-forming and thus compound the stress they were meant to alleviate.

The Relaxation Response

1. *Sit quietly in a comfortable position.*
2. *Close your eyes.*
3. *Deeply relax all your muscles, beginning at your feet and progressing up to your face. Keep them relaxed.*
4. *Breathe through your nose. Become aware of your breathing. As you breathe out, say the word "ONE," silently to yourself. For example, breathe IN . . . OUT, "ONE"; IN . . . OUT, "ONE"; etc. Breathe easily and naturally.*
5. *Continue for 10 to 20 minutes. You may open your eyes to check the time, but do not use an alarm. When you finish, sit quietly for several minutes, at first with your eyes closed and later with your eyes opened. Do not stand up for a few minutes.*
6. *Do not worry about whether you are successful in achieving a deep level of relaxation. Maintain a passive attitude and permit relaxation to occur at its own pace. When distracting thoughts occur, try to ignore them by not dwelling upon them and return to repeating "ONE." With practice, the response should come with little effort. Practice the technique once or twice daily, but not within two hours after any meal, since the digestive processes seem to interfere with the elicitation of the Relaxation Response.*

Source: Herbert Benson, M.D., with Miriam Z. Klipper, *The Relaxation Response* (New York: William Morrow and Company, 1975), pp. 114–115. Reprinted by permission.

Nutrition. You cannot handle stress unless you are in good health, and to be in good health, you must eat sensibly (see Chapter 5 for recommendations on diet and nutrition). To provide extra energy when you need it, you should make sure to take in enough complex carbohydrates. For more stamina in the daytime and a sounder sleep at night, eat a healthy breakfast, an adequate lunch, and a light dinner.

Relaxation Techniques. Many symptoms of stress can be controlled by a number of relaxation techniques. Meditation practices such as Zen, Yoga, and transcendental meditation are rooted in ancient Eastern traditions and have been proven effective at regulating the autonomic nervous system. (The autonomic nervous system controls and regulates the internal organs automatically.) Modern adaptations of these methods include autogenic training, biofeedback, progressive relaxation of muscle groups, imagery, and behavior modification. Dr. Herbert Benson's relaxation response (see box: The Relaxation Response), for example, borrows from ancient Zen techniques. Several temporary relaxation techniques will also quickly relieve the pressures of a heavy schedule—for instance, taking ten deep breaths, stretching, and walking around for a few minutes. Any of the deep relaxation techniques, practiced regularly, will release muscle tension, lower blood pressure, and slow the heartbeat and breath rates. Recent research shows that they can also lower cholesterol levels and strengthen the immune system, thereby reducing susceptibility to viral infection.

Exercise. Finally, one of the best ways to reduce tension is regular, vigorous exercise. When performed at least three times a week, exercise gives you the physical stamina to withstand stress. It not only relaxes the body, but enhances well-being in many other ways. Compared to sedentary people, regular exercisers have less trouble coping with frustration, boredom, and feelings of anger and hostility. In addition, exercise has been shown to relieve the symptoms of depression as effectively as psychotherapy.

SUMMARY

1. Stress is unavoidable, but it is not always harmful. Stress can be beneficial; the positive response to stress is termed *eustress*. *Distress* refers to negative tensions that have been aroused in our bodies by some environmental, social, or chemical factor. According to Selye, stress is the nonspecific response of the body to any demand—that is, the body makes the same response to any kind of stress. Selye labeled this response the *General Adaptation Syndrome* (G.A.S.). The G.A.S. has three stages: alarm reaction, resistance, and exhaustion.

2. When under stress our body undergoes a complex series of chemical reactions that are holdovers from a more primitive and physically active time. Any kind of threat—real or imagined—sets off a *flight-or-fight reaction* that equips us, in almost every case, for physical action. When this reaction is evoked too often, our body can actually be damaged and worn down and our resistance to disease weakened.

3. According to some researchers, certain personalities are more prone to certain stress-related diseases than others. One example is the *Type A personality*, which runs a higher risk than average of acquiring heart disease. Also, researchers have found common responses to stress among certain cancer patients, sug-

gesting that there may be such a thing as a cancer-prone personality.

4. In our society the social causes of stress are numerous and not always obvious; most people would recognize a crowded, noisy, polluted city as a possible source of stress, but might not realize that a job promotion or marriage can also summon a stress reaction.

5. The little hassles and uplifts of daily life, however, often have a stronger effect on our moods and health than major life events. The more minor annoyances we experience from day to day, the poorer our overall health. Boredom and monotony likewise take their toll on mental and physical health, and we must learn ways to break out of them.

6. Stress is particularly severe during the college years because of the vast changes most people must make in their lives when leaving home and confronting academic and social pressures, as well as concern for the future. When stress for college students becomes incapacitating—that is, when it causes deep depressions or feelings of inadequacy and helplessness—it is important to seek professional help.

7. Though the causal connection between stress and disease has not been fully established, there is a consensus that stress undoubtedly aggravates a disease once it is present. Also, few would dispute that stress can be responsible for such disorders as *migraine headaches* and *depression*.

8. Stress is also responsible for the high suicide rate among teenagers and young adults. Social factors such as the breakdown of the family and the casual violence and availability of guns in American society have been blamed for the phenomenon. Academic failure and troubled personal relationships are the primary causes of suicide among college students. Those who are chronically depressed, alcoholic, and loners are the most likely to attempt suicide; they often signal their intentions by discussing plans for suicide in detail. They should be taken seriously.

9. *Homeostasis* refers to the adjustments the body makes to keep itself balanced. Stress threatens homeostasis; the effort to bring the body back into balance is called *coping*. By our own choices and actions, we can prevent many of the harmful effects of everyday stress. A major way to reduce stress is to manage our time more efficiently by setting priorities, working at our own pace, formulating realistic goals, keeping a flexible schedule, and establishing regular habits. Another effective way to reduce stress is to divert ourselves frequently from work concerns and emotional problems by engaging in amusing activities for the fun of it or escaping into momentary fantasy. Suppressed emotions are a prime source of stress-induced illness; we must allow ourselves to express our feelings freely, and learn to express them over the right things. We must also learn not to worry too much about the future or waste time regretting past mistakes and failures. Talking problems over with a friend, relative, or counselor is one of the most effective ways of reducing stress. Getting involved with others and participating in outside activities is an effective cure for boredom and loneliness.

10. Several life-style changes can help the body cope with stress. We should learn what the body symptoms of stress are and stay alert to them. Relying on drugs and alcohol to work, sleep, and relax only increases stress because drugs are habit-forming. Following a sound diet will maintain physical stamina, and learning relaxation techniques will control the symptoms of stress. Exercising vigorously three times a week not only relaxes the body but also enables us to cope with anxiety and depression.

CONSUMER CONCERNS

1. Before paying good money to learn a "relaxation technique," do a little library research or ask a local health counselor for information related to the offered technique.
2. Check with your school health service to see what sort of services it provides for stress management.
3. When is the last time you had a physical checkup?
4. Does one of your school's academic departments offer a course on stress management? If not, perhaps your local division of continuing education provides such a course for the general public.

3

Accidents and Safety

Accident Patterns   Causes of Accidents   Accident Prevention

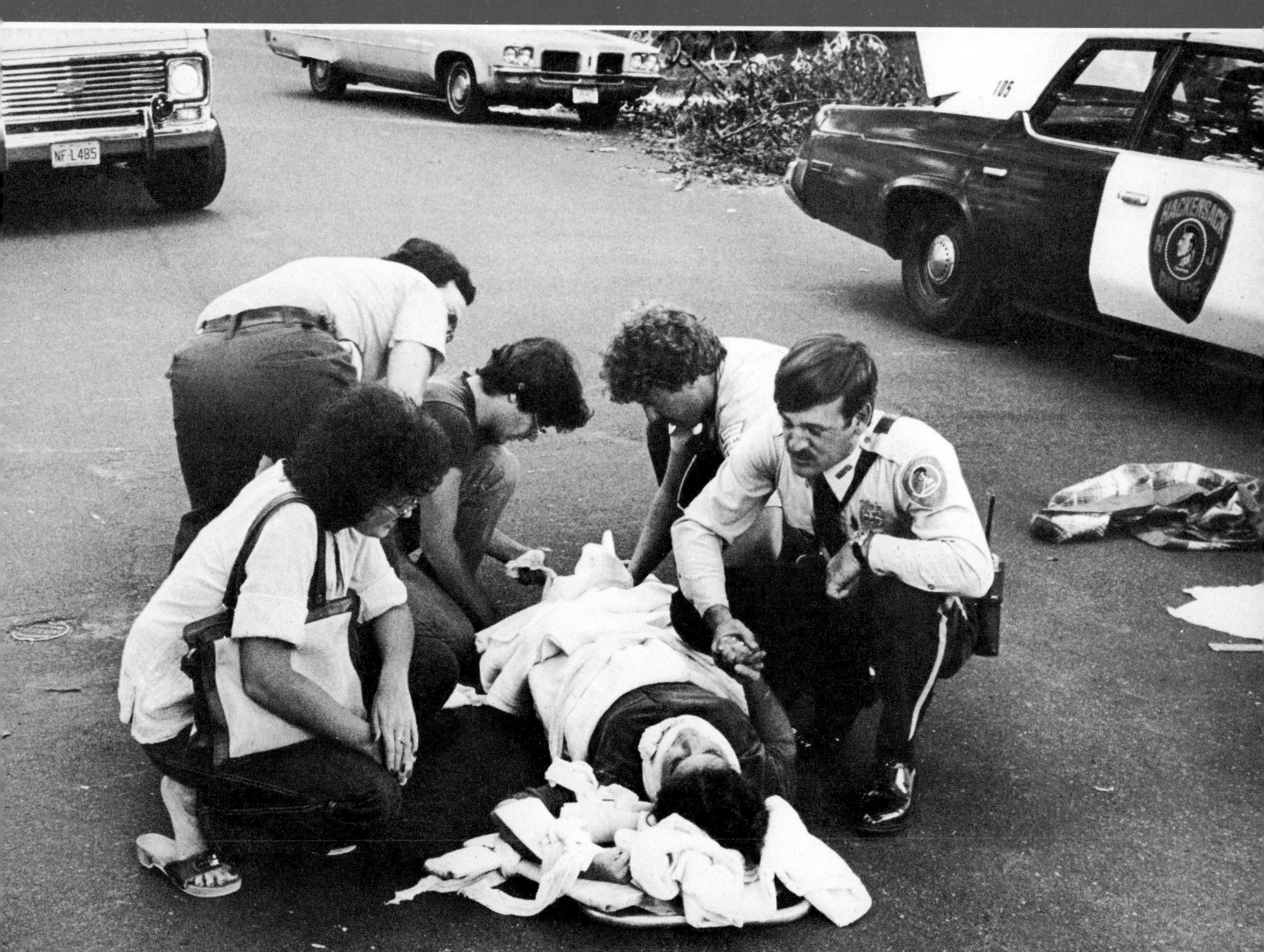

Accidents are the fourth leading cause of death in the United States, after heart disease, cancer, and stroke. Even though there has been an encouraging drop in the accident rate through the years, accidents are clearly a major contemporary health concern. They are the cause of almost 100,000 deaths each year and some 8.7 million disabling injuries. Whereas the major chronic diseases have their greatest impact on the elderly, accidents affect most severely the young and middle-aged, who ordinarily have many healthy and productive years ahead of them. In the 1- to 37-year age group accidents are the leading cause of death; among persons 15 to 24 years of age accidents are responsible for more deaths than all other causes combined.

We shall see that psychological factors, and stress in particular, are at the root of many accidents. Hans Seyle, in fact, estimated that more accidents have occurred under the influence of stress than under the influence of alcohol. In this chapter we shall discuss the scope of the accident problem, describe the major factors that lead to accidents, and suggest ways accidents can be avoided and their harmful effects minimized. Accidents are by far the most preventable of the major causes of death and disability. Individuals who learn to recognize and deal with hazardous situations can enormously increase their chances of living full, productive lives.

ACCIDENT PATTERNS

Accidents cause one death every six minutes and one injury every four seconds. The cost in lives and injuries is enormous, and the cost in dollars—$97 billion a year—is staggering. This figure includes wage losses, medical fees, insurance costs, motor vehicle damage, fire loss, and the money value of time lost by those who were not injured but who were involved in accidents.

The overall death rate from accidents in 1984 was 39 per 100,000 population. There are interesting and significant variations, however, among the major categories of accidents—work, home, public, and motor vehicle. Rates also differ for the two sexes, for various age groups, and by geographical location.

By far the greatest number of deaths occur in motor vehicle accidents; home accidents, however, account for the greatest number of injuries (see Table 3-1). In all age groups men are involved in about 70 percent of total accidental deaths, and are particularly overrepresented in deaths from motor vehicle, drown-

TABLE 3-1

Accidental Injuries by Severity of Injury, 1984

Severity of Injury	Total*	Motor Vehicle	Work	Home	Public Non-motor Vehicle
Deaths	92,000	46,200	11,500	20,000	18,500
Nonfatal disabling injuries	8,700,000	1,700,000	1,900,000	3,000,000	2,300,000
Permanent impairments	330,000	140,000	70,000	80,000	50,000
Temporary total disabilities	8,400,000	1,600,000	1,800,000	2,900,000	2,300,000

* Figures for the four separate classes add up to more than the total because of rounding of numbers and duplication between classes.

Source: National Safety Council, *Accident Facts, 1985 Edition*.

TABLE 3-2
Accidental Deaths by Age, Sex, and Type, 1982[a]

Age and Sex	All Types[b]	Motor Vehicle	Falls	Drowning[c]	Fires, Burns[d]	Ingestion of Food, Object	Firearms	Poison (solid, liquid)	Poison by Gas	% Male All Types
All ages	94,082	45,779	12,077	6,351	5,210	3,254	1,756	3,474	1,259	70%
Under 5	4,108	1,300	137	752	778	341	44	67	37	60%
5–14	4,504	2,301	103	715	482	59	235	16	31	68%
15–24	21,306	15,324	453	1,742	466	125	543	514	272	79%
25–44	25,135	14,469	976	1,772	941	358	588	1,765	404	79%
45–64	15,907	6,879	1,779	834	1,030	664	227	679	294	72%
65–74	8,224	2,825	1,635	287	648	581	84	212	115	61%
75+	14,898	2,681	6,994	249	865	1,126	35	221	106	46%
Male	65,754	33,191	6,354	5,294	3,180	1,859	1,524	2,311	914	
Female	28,328	12,588	5,723	1,057	2,030	1,395	232	1,163	345	
Percent male	70%	73%	53%	83%	61%	57%	87%	67%	73%	

[a] Latest official figures. [b] Includes some deaths not shown separately. [c] Includes drowning in water transport accidents. [d] Includes deaths resulting from conflagration regardless of nature of injury.
Source: National Safety Council, *Accident Facts, 1985 Edition*.

ing, and firearm accidents (Table 3-2). Overall, the male accident death rate is about 58 per 100,000 and the female death rate is about 24.

The highest rates of accidental deaths occur among those between the ages of 15 and 24, with deaths caused primarily by motor vehicle accidents, and among those 65 and over, with deaths due principally to falls and motor vehicle accidents. The lowest accidental death rate is found among those between the ages of 5 and 14. In analyzing the statistics for the different cases of accidental death among the various age groups, a pattern emerges that suggests there is a certain predictability to accidents—a fact to be kept in mind when we discuss accident prevention later in this chapter.

Geographically, death rates from all accidents combined are highest in the mountain and south-central areas of the country and lowest in the northeastern region. Alaska has the highest death rate from accidents in the United States, probably because of its large number of accidents involving air and water transport. New Jersey has the lowest rate. As might be expected, pedestrian deaths (those resulting from an individual's being struck by a motor vehicle) are highest in areas of high population density. Surprisingly, though, motor vehicle fatalities tend to be *lower* in the northeastern states, where there are large numbers of motor vehicles, and highest in the mountain states, where traffic is generally less congested. One explanation is that the lack of congestion makes high-speed driving—and thus accident fatalities—much more likely. Interesting patterns are also seen with regard to specific types of accidents. Deaths by fire, for example, are highest in southern states, where there are large numbers of flammable dwellings; deaths from falls tend to be highest where there are large numbers of older people, such as in New England; and deaths from drowning are highest in two states with extensive coastlines—Alaska and Florida.

CAUSES OF ACCIDENTS

The accident patterns we have described make it apparent that there are certain calculable causes of accidents, at least on a large scale. It is reasonable to assume, for example, that a rigid enforcement of lower speed limits (we have general proof of this since the 55-mile-per-hour limit was imposed) in the mountain states and the use of nonflammable materials in housing construction in the South would do much to lower the accident rates in those areas. It is more difficult to see that many accidents can be avoided on an individual basis—that there are many attitudes, behaviors, and conditions that contribute to accidents, and that these can be recognized and dealt with by the individual to minimize the likelihood of an accident.

Attitudinal Factors

Most people do not view accidents as having specific causes, as do diseases, or indeed, most other events. The occurrence or avoidance of accidents is attributed to "luck," "chance," or "God's will." Folklore holds that accidents are fated to happen when they do, or that, even after an exceptionally good record of safety, "one's number comes up."

In fact, only a minority of accidents can be attributed entirely to chance. People who are "too busy" to have their car brakes adjusted even though they are defective are clearly more likely to have an auto accident than those who keep their cars in perfect working order. The innocent victim of an accident—

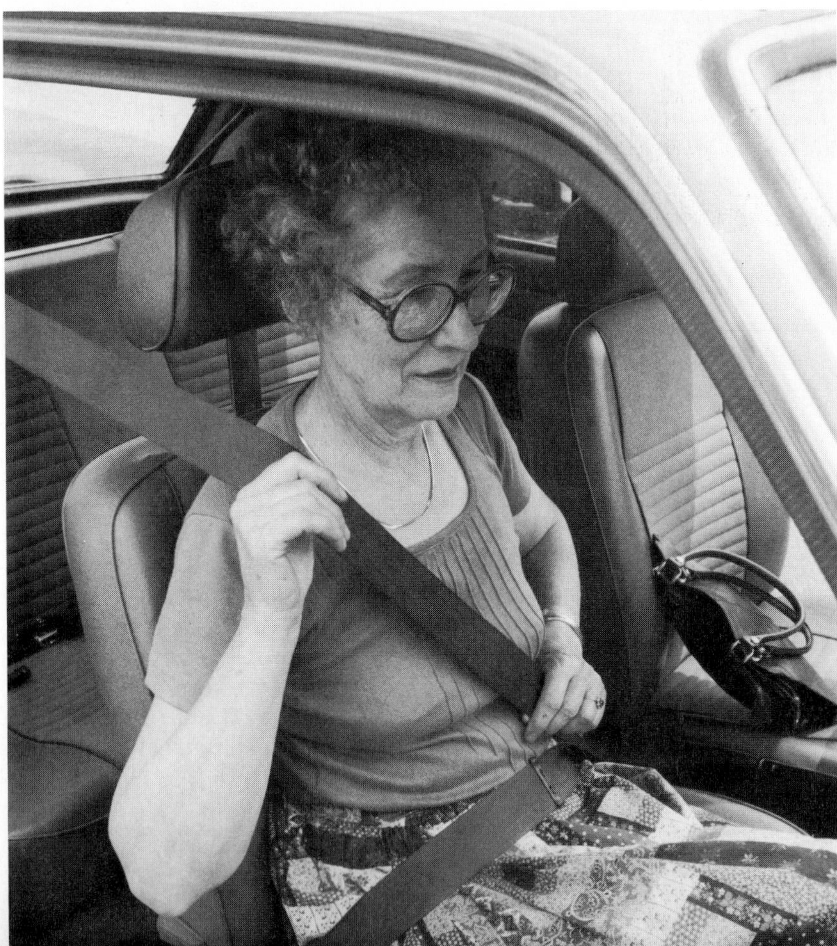

a pedestrian struck by a car whose driver is intoxicated, for example—suffers because of negligence in many areas: the driver's drinking, perhaps the bartender's lack of foresight, and society's unwillingness to keep irresponsible drivers off the road. In short, when we say events are due to luck or chance, it really means we have failed to identify their causes. An accident might be unintentional or unexplained, but it is generally preventable.

The consequence of viewing accidents as spontaneous events is a lack of concern for accident prevention on both the individual and the societal level. Though the lifesaving benefits of seat belts, for example, have been highly publicized, a great many Americans still do not use them. Society is not much better than individuals when it comes to accident prevention. A tragedy or a highly publicized disaster is invariably required to make society realize the importance of safety factors. Only after repeated incidents of children dying in abandoned refrigerators, for example, was legislation passed requiring that the doors be removed from large discarded appliances. Hotel and factory fires in which many people died occurred before laws were passed regarding fire alarms, fire escapes, sprinklers, and the like. The reluctance to spend money or take commonsense precautions to prevent accidents comes from viewing accidents as something that cannot be controlled.

Psychological Factors

At one time or another, most of us have seen an exceptionally angry looking man storm into his car and race off with tires squealing. It may have occurred to us that this man was under great stress and that he was very likely headed for an accident. Perhaps on the other side of town he crashed into a utility pole at high speed. Onlookers and police would attribute the accident to excessive speed with consequent loss of vehicle control. But the real source of this accident was the man's psychological state.

A variety of personality traits can make an individual more likely to have an accident. Overestimating one's abilities—by swimming past the point of fatigue, for example—can lead to trouble. Selfishness and self-centeredness might cause an accident, especially if one is reckless and ignores the presence of others—such as other cars on the road. Feelings of alienation might lead to an accident if they cause one to ignore laws designed to minimize accidents (such as traffic regulations and laws against driving while intoxicated). A highly aggressive person might get into hazardous situations a more mild-mannered individual would avoid. Finally, any one of a number of emotional problems might cause an individual to behave in an irrational manner or to become mentally distracted so that he or she is less able to avoid an accident.

Accident Proneness and Stress

All of us have periods when nothing seems to go right. We might have an absentminded spell of losing and forgetting things. Similarly, we might have an accident-filled day. We might begin by tripping over a pair of slippers as we get out of bed, then bang our head on the door of the medicine cabinet and burn our fingers on the toaster. While we may perceive a connection between all these episodes, we are all too likely to ascribe them to a "bad day." But spells such as these are more than a chain of unpleasantnesses. They may reflect our temporary inability to cope with stress—caused, perhaps, by a death in the family, anxiety over money, uncertainty over career decisions, or the end of a relationship. Generally, when the particular problem of stress is resolved, the period of accident proneness ends.

Some people, however, seem to suffer chronic accident proneness. They may have chronic personality disorders that make them particularly vulnerable to accidents. They possess traits such as selfishness, hostility, aggressiveness, improper judgment, poor self-image, and general feelings of insecurity. Unable to cope with stress, these people compensate for their inadequacies by thwarting authority and its symbols through attention-getting ploys. They might drive through red lights, ignore traffic policemen, disregard or challenge other drivers, or otherwise act like menaces on the road. Such individuals will continue in their accident-prone behavior until they seek out methods to quell or control the stress in their lives. (See the section Coping with Stress in Chapter 2.)

Personal Factors

Other personal factors influence the individual's likelihood of having an accident. For example, a person who is either very young or very old is more likely to perish or be seriously injured in a fire than someone in the middle years. This is because young children and the elderly have less mobility and physical skill, a reduced sense of danger, and slower reaction times than other people. Both groups require—but do not always get—special attention to prevent accidents. Age-related physiological impairments are sometimes compounded by the fact that many older people refuse to acknowledge symptoms of deterioration, either to themselves or to others. Hence, they may not ask for assistance when they

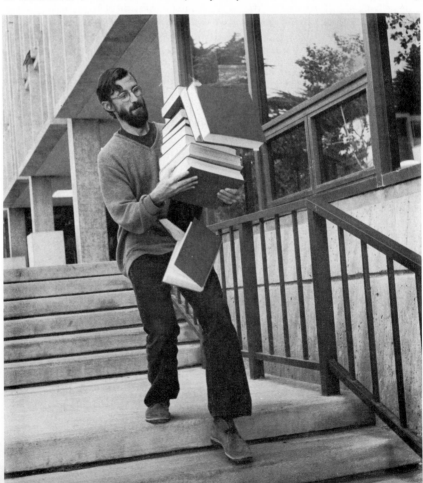

Accident proneness may reflect our temporary inability to cope with stress.

need it. The children of the elderly may also be to blame if an accident occurs. Accustomed to viewing their parents as independent, self-reliant adults, they are frequently reluctant to reverse roles and assume responsibility for their parents when it becomes necessary to do so. (See Chapter 10, Aging, Dying, and Death.)

An otherwise logical and safety-oriented person may become more accident prone after taking a substance that distorts normal perceptual abilities. Alcohol, marijuana, tranquilizers, and amphetamines, for instance, affect a person's ability to react effectively. Fatigue or excitement may cause a usually steady individual to have an accident, because he or she is too tired or disturbed to notice a hazard.

Cultural Factors

Cultural beliefs and attitudes also contribute significantly to the occurrence of accidents. It is not surprising that a country like ours, which has always placed an enormous premium on such values as technology, conspicuous consumption, risk taking, individualism, mobility, and masculinity, has a high accident toll.

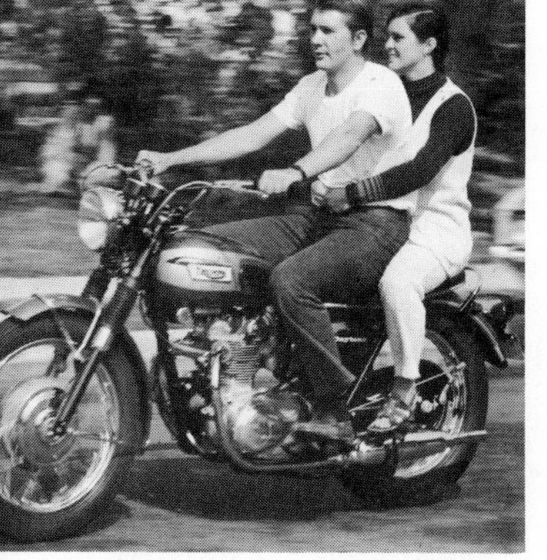

We are taught early in life that our environment is to be manipulated and exploited (from the "winning of the West" to the "conquest of space") rather than adjusted to. We tend to emphasize individual effort over group endeavors and to equate masculinity with daring and forcefulness. We encourage activities that are challenging, especially if they have an exciting element of danger. Regulations aimed at reducing the risk of some of our more hazardous activities—such as requiring the wearing of helmets when riding a motorcycle—are seen as infringements of our freedom. In short, many attitudes in our culture predispose us to risk-filled behavior.

One reason teenage drivers have the highest motor vehicle accident and death rates is that they adopt many of these cultural values before they have the experience to handle them. In addition, they are permitted few outlets for their energy and are at a time of life characterized by many anxieties. It is not hard to see how driving a car dangerously might be an attractive activity for many in this age group.

Equipment Factors

The kind and quality of equipment in use today influence overall accident rates. A power saw, for example, can do more damage more quickly than a handsaw. Similarly, an automobile capable of high speeds can cause more damage to its occupants on impact with another object than an automobile with a moderate top speed.

Breakdown in equipment and defective parts can also cause accidents—brakes that do not hold at the critical moment, for example. Poor equipment design can also be a factor in accidents—for instance, sharp edges in a car interior or ineffective highway barriers can turn a potentially minor mishap into a fatal accident.

Environmental Factors

There are many natural disasters over which we have no direct control. Hurricanes, tornadoes, floods, and earthquakes take many lives each year because we can neither prevent these events nor, as yet, predict them accurately. Nevertheless, we can prepare ourselves for such occurrences by keeping necessary equipment in readiness and having a systematic plan that will minimize the danger to people and property.

Environmental factors of a less destructive nature—such as snow, fog, or rain—may also cause accidents. We can minimize the hazards of these conditions by either avoiding or preparing for them. For example, we may wisely determine that it is better not to drive through a severe rainstorm or snowstorm. But we should also ensure that windshield wipers are functioning and, in snowy areas, that snow tires are mounted routinely for the winter season.

Human enterprise creates environmental hazards. The accumulation of smog (which reduces visibility), the proliferation of toxic substances, the contamination of food, air, and water, and so on, all increase the likelihood of accidents.

ACCIDENT PREVENTION

We have described the major factors affecting the incidence of accidents. In this section we will discuss in greater detail the kinds of accidents that occur in each of the major accident categories. We will also suggest ways to improve conditions and attitudes so that the likelihood of accidents will be minimized.

Work Accidents

Although the number of workers has more than doubled since 1912, reaching over 104 million, the on-the-job accident rate has decreased 76 percent, from 21 to 5 per 100,000, and the actual number of accidental deaths has dropped from about 19,000 to 11,500 annually. The total number of disabling injuries

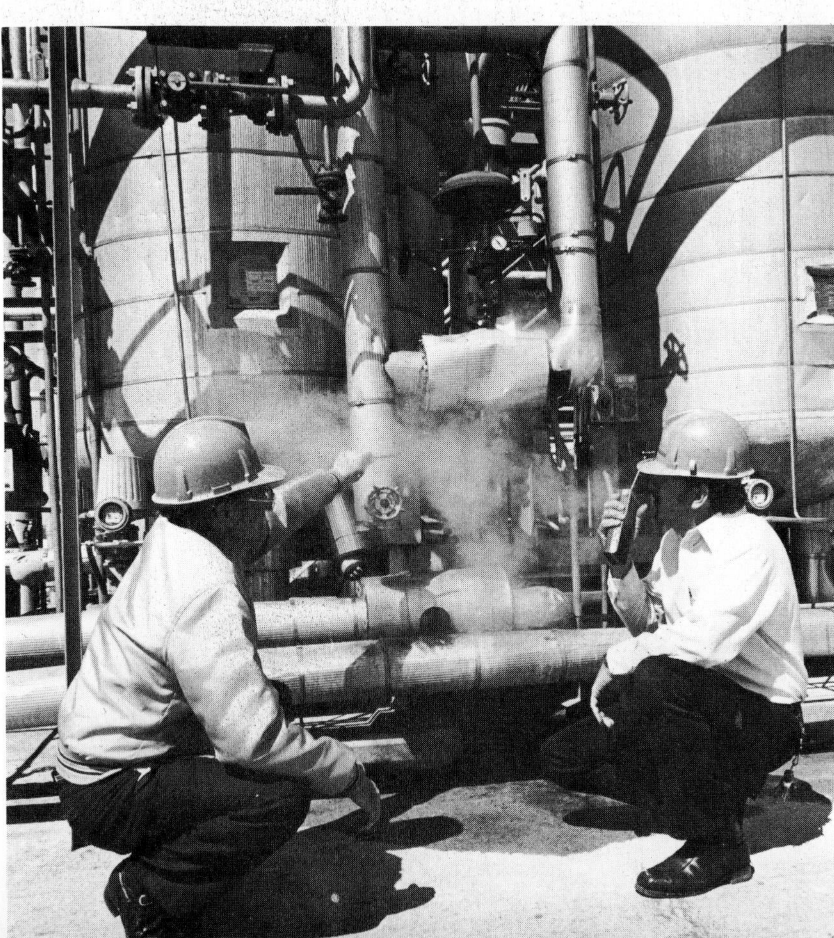

Work accidents can be reduced by the wearing of protective equipment such as hard hats in potentially dangerous areas.

resulting from work accidents was 1.9 million in 1984; the total cost of work-related accidents was $33 billion. Even though these figures are high, workers today actually have more accidents off the job than on the job: Three out of every four accidental deaths and more than half of all accidents involving workers take place outside the work environment.

The largest number of disabling accidental injuries occur in industries with the largest work force: service, 410,000 injuries; trade, 330,000; and manufacturing, 300,000. The highest death rate, however, is found in the mining industry (60 per 100,000 in 1984).

The **Occupational Safety and Health Act,** passed in 1971, established mandatory safety and health standards for virtually all industries. These standards are enforced by Labor Department inspectors, who have the power to issue citations and recommend penalties. The act also established a National Institute for Occupational Safety and Health to conduct research into work-related hazards and threats to health. Though there has been progress in improving working conditions, this law has come under criticism. Budgetary support for it has been inconsistent, and employers have not been adequately advised of its regulations. Perhaps most important, it has been ineffective in reducing the most significant occupational hazards, particularly the presence of toxic or carcinogenic (cancer-causing) substances, in many industries. (More than 100,000 workers, for example, were diagnosed as having an occupational disease in 1983.)

Prevention of Work Accidents. An important first step toward minimizing occupational hazards would be to improve the effectiveness of the Occupational Safety and Health Act. Any program of prevention, however, must involve three things: (1) improvement of the working environment; (2) elimination or modification of hazardous conditions; and (3) training and supervision of workers.

The physical conditions in which workers operate must be designed and maintained to keep accidents at a minimum. A safe work environment requires adequate space to guarantee freedom of movement, good lighting to ensure accuracy, noise reduction to decreasing hearing loss, proper ventilation, and efficient sanitation facilities to counteract exposure to irritants and contaminants. Potentially dangerous pieces of machinery should be equipped with safety and warning devices. Operators should be required to wear whatever protective apparel—such as goggles, gloves, helmets, lead aprons—might be warranted. New equipment should be tested before it is put into normal use.

Personal factors also play an important part in work accidents. Workers may operate a piece of equipment without permission or adequate instruction. They may fail to alert others, neglect to activate safety devices, or forget to wear protective attire. They may also display behavior that is incompatible with the operation of precision equipment. Workers who play pranks or otherwise distract fellow workers may provoke an accident that involves many others besides themselves. For this reason, it is important that only responsible people be permitted to work in areas of potential hazard.

Home Accidents

Because of the private nature of the home, statistics regarding home accidents are perhaps the most difficult to obtain. Nevertheless, it is estimated that in

1984 there were over 3 million home accidents resulting in disabling injuries—more than in any other accident category. It is estimated that an additional 21 million less serious home accidents occur each year. The total annual cost of these accidents is about $10.8 billion, excluding property damage.

Home accident deaths number about 20,000 annually; the most frequent cause of such deaths is falls, followed by fires and burns, poisoning, suffocation, and firearm accidents (see box: Gun Control).

Home Accident Prevention. Infants may fall when left unattended in high places or near stairs. Keeping watch over young children is therefore the best way to prevent this type of home accident. For the safety of individuals of all age groups, but particularly the elderly, floors should be left uncluttered, rugs should always be anchored, and stairways should be well lit, sturdy, and unobstructed. Stairs should also be equipped with handrails, and rubber treads should be used where necessary. Rubber mats should be used to prevent slipping in the bathtub. Ladders should be steady, strong, and correctly placed.

Among the major causes of fire in the home are carelessness in smoking, poor wiring, fuel explosions, and storage of matches where children can reach them. Thus the first step in accident prevention is to exercise elementary precaution in where one smokes—smoking in bed or near highly flammable materials creates a serious hazard. Fire prevention also requires that proper attention be paid to electrical equipment—unplugging appliances when they are not in use, checking for frayed wires, avoiding overloaded sockets, grounding appliances, and using proper fuses. The Underwriters' Laboratory, a private agency, monitors electrical appliances for compliance with established industry standards.

If at all possible, flammable liquids such as paint or fuel should not be kept in the home. If their presence is unavoidable, they should be stored in a cool area. Grease spills should be wiped up immediately, as grease accumulation is a common fire hazard.

A plan of action should be developed in case a fire does start. Every house should be equipped with a fire extinguisher, and the emergency telephone number of the local fire department should be immediately accessible. In addition, some convenient means of exit should be provided, such as an alternate doorway, a rope ladder, or the like.

We commonly think of poisoning as a child-related accident, but most cases of fatal poisoning occur among individuals between 25 and 44 years of age. The most common causes of poisoning are the ingestion of unlabeled or mislabeled substances, food poisoning (discussed in Chapter 15), overdoses of medication, and the use of outdated medications. For adults, how to prevent poisoning accidents is self-evident: proper labeling of all dangerous materials and proper use of all medications. The Appendix of this book contains a section on first aid for poisoning.

The 1970 **Poison Prevention Packaging Act** required that hazardous substances be packaged in child-resistant containers. Over 500 national poison control centers were also established in an attempt to save lives. Ultimately, however, responsibility for children's safety lies with their parents. Parents must never underestimate their child's ability to reach things; nor should they assume that because a substance smells bad the child will not eat or drink it. Medicines should never be referred to as "candy." Household chemicals and medications

Where to Go for Help

Several of the federal agencies described in the section Federal Sources of Consumer Aid and Information in Chapter 16, Consumer Health, provide information about such things as product safety.

should be kept out of children's reach. Parents should also immediately repaint objects or surfaces that have peeling lead-based paint, since eating lead paint has been a cause of poisoning among children.

Suffocation is another type of home accident common among children. Infants who cannot lift their heads should not sleep on pillows. Thin plastic, such as that protecting dry-cleaned goods, should never be used as a crib cover nor given to an infant to play with. As the infant inhales, the filmy material can cling to his nose and mouth, sealing off air. Abandoned refrigerators and old trunks also present the danger of suffocation. Doors or lids on all such objects

PROBLEMS AND CONTROVERSIES: *Gun Control*

Privately owned firearms cause an alarming number of accidental deaths in the United States each year. Gun owners are killed while cleaning their own firearms. Hunters are often mistakenly shot by other hunters. The ordinary citizen who buys a pistol to protect himself from intruders has been known to kill a family member with that same pistol, believing him or her to be an intruder. But the number of persons killed in incidents such as these pales in comparison to the number killed by handguns in the heat of an argument, either at home or in a public place.

The United States has the highest rate of homicide by handgun of any industrialized country. Within the last decade the number of deaths by handgun has risen 61 percent. In addition, the number of suicides committed using firearms has almost doubled in the last twenty years. Much of this violence is related to stress and occurs within families. Almost 20 percent of all murderers are close relatives of their victims, and half of these cases involve husbands or wives killing spouses. Violent behavior in these situations has been shown to escalate to the point of murder if there is a weapon nearby, especially if that weapon is a handgun.

These incidents, and the use of guns in attacks upon many prominent public figures and public officials, have prompted many groups to demand more stringent laws governing the sale of firearms and a more effective system for registering the ownership of firearms. People concerned with public safety generally support two related legislative solutions to the problem: (1) requiring registration of all firearms, so that records would exist as to the ownership and sale of guns, and (2) requiring that those who wish to own firearms pass strict proficiency and qualification standards. Additional recommendations include much stricter control over the manufacture and distribution of firearms and stiffer, mandatory penalties for their misuse. Some people also feel that private ownership of handguns should be sharply curbed or outlawed, as these are the weapons employed in most crimes involving guns and are rarely used by licensed hunters.

Polls of the public indicate a high degree of popular support (over 80 percent) for at least some of these measures. But the powerful National Rifle Association (NRA) in concert with other groups has conducted a well-organized and well-financed battle against any form of effective firearms legislation. The NRA makes the false claim that gun legislation would violate the constitutional right to bear arms. (In the first place, the Constitution actually grants the right to bear arms only in military service. In the second place, most gun-control advocates do not want to outlaw private gun ownership, but to regulate it.) The NRA and its supporters also claim that weapons other than guns are also used to kill, but the facts reveal that guns are the weapon used in more than half of all murders.

The gun lobby is so effective in controlling the votes of our national legislators that no public opinion poll has mattered, no assassination or attempted assassination of a President or high official has made a difference. The only major gun legislation passed in recent years, in fact, was a 1986 law that *eased* controls over the interstate shipment of long guns and reduced many violations of gun laws to lesser criminal offenses.

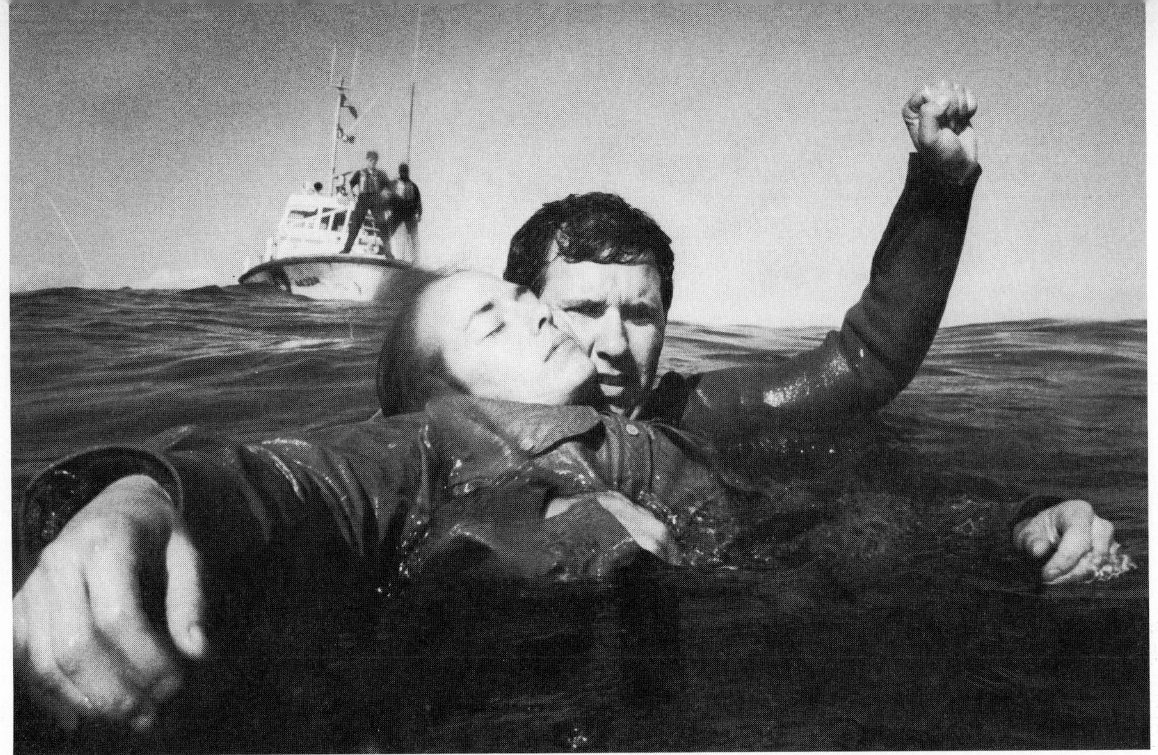

Rescue training by the U.S. Coast Guard. Before going into the water after a drowning person, one should attempt to throw her a lifeline or life preserver.

should be removed to prevent accidents. Very small toys, playthings with leaking stuffing, dolls with loose eyes, and other such objects should be kept away from young children, as small objects might be swallowed and cause the child to suffocate.

The **Consumer Product Safety Commission** was formed in 1973. It is a federal regulatory agency intended to remove hazardous consumer items from the marketplace. The commission has, for example, issued regulations regarding the packaging of drugs and the flammability of children's sleepwear. It has also banned hazardous toys, appliances, and other products until their safety defects are corrected.

Public Accidents

In 1984, there were 18,500 deaths from public accidents. Public accidents are deaths or injuries in public places such as beaches, parks, stadiums, and other public facilities. They do not include motor vehicle or work accidents.

The single largest cause of public accident deaths is falls. Drowning, the next largest cause, accounted for 3,500 deaths in 1984. This number, however, does not include drownings involving boats. When those deaths are added in, the total number of drowning deaths in 1984 was 5,700. Drownings involving boats are often caused by inattention to weather advisories, improper loading of the boat, and use of the boat in water inappropriate for small craft. Other types of public accidents include railroad and air transport injuries and fire injuries in public places. Public accidents involving firearms account for about 1,800 deaths each year, and there are about 50,000 reported cases annually of family violence involving handguns. Thus firearms have become a public safety problem of increasing magnitude and concern. In the accompanying box we discuss the problem of firearm accidents and the related issue of gun control; in the following section we examine ways in which death by drowning can be prevented.

Drowning Prevention. Drowning accidents occur at the rate of 2.4 per 100,000 people. Only about 2,100 of the 5,700 drowning deaths in 1984 involved individuals who were swimming or playing in the water. The rest were nonswimming fatalities—that is, they involved people who fell into the water accidentally from boats, docks, bridges, or shores. It is therefore essential that everyone planning to be in or even near water know how to swim. Swimmers should follow water safety practices, such as never swimming alone in unattended areas. Passengers in small vessels should be equipped with life jackets. If a boat capsizes, passengers should cling to it rather than attempt to swim to shore. People should try to aid a swimmer in trouble without endangering themselves. Going into the water after a swimmer in trouble is a last resort; attempts should first be made to throw the victim a life preserver or another object (such as a lifeline) to effect rescue. Infants and young children should never be left unsupervised in water, no matter how shallow.

Although the National Safety Council, Red Cross, scouting groups, and other organizations all provide water safety programs, deaths from accidental drowning have been steadily rising in the past ten years. Americans enjoy seashores and lakesides as vacation spots, but not enough of them have been properly trained in swimming or water safety, and thus are too lax about the potential hazards.

Motor Vehicle Accidents

Motor vehicle accidents are the single largest cause of accidental deaths in this country. Almost half are caused by collision with other motor vehicles; over one-quarter are noncollision accidents, such as overturning; about 18 percent involve pedestrians. In 1984 there were 46,200 deaths and 1.7 million disabling injuries involving motor vehicles. Accidents that did not result in disabling injuries totaled 31 million. Thus almost one out of every five licensed drivers—nearly 33 million out of 157 million—was involved in a reported accident. The total financial cost of these accidents is over $47.6 billion, including lost wages, medical and insurance costs, and property damage. In the discussion that follows, we will describe separately three elements that play a part in the occurrence of motor vehicle accidents: road conditions, the car, and the driver.

Road Conditions. The condition of the road has been implicated as a causative factor in many accidents. Though speeds are higher on interstate highways, for example, the number of deaths per million miles traveled is lower on them than on other roads. Fatal accidents happen mostly on rural roads, while nonfatal injuries and property damage occur mostly in accidents in urban areas.

Important road hazards include exits at poorly chosen locations (where visibility is poor, for example) and exit turns that are too sharp or poorly marked;

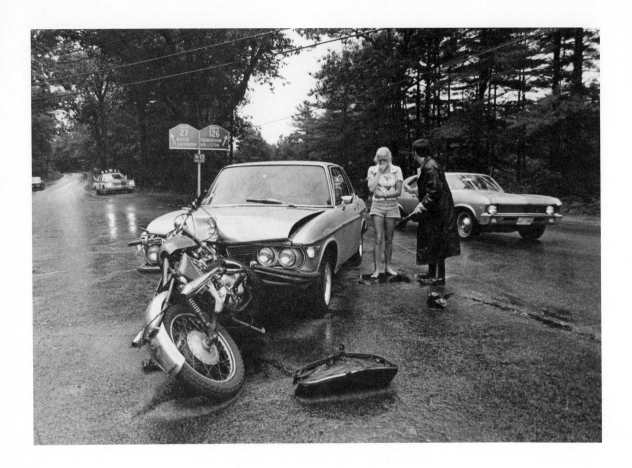

road or highway signs that are unclear or do not provide sufficient advance warning; and lanes that merge in a hazardous fashion. Building roads that avoid these hazards and correcting as many of the existing hazards as possible could significantly reduce the incidence of motor vehicle accidents.

The Car. The lethal potential of the automobile is self-evident. Its speed and force alone are factors that inherently contribute to accidents. It should be noted, however, that the design and construction of the car can significantly affect the rate and severity of motor vehicle accidents.

Before the publication of Ralph Nader's book *Unsafe at Any Speed* in 1966, it was generally assumed that all automobile accidents could ultimately be traced to poor driving. Little or no thought was given to the state of functioning of the vehicle prior to the accident. Brake failure or a faulty steering mechanism, for instance, was rarely suspected. Nader's observations led to the passage of the **National Traffic and Motor Vehicle Safety Act of 1966.** The act resulted in a number of safety improvements being made in automobiles, including collapsible steering columns and energy-absorbing bumpers. In the years that followed, there was a gratifying decline in the death rate from highway accidents.

Drunken Driving

Half of all U.S. traffic fatalities—23,000 deaths a year—are caused by drunk drivers, and over the past few years a lot of people have decided that something needs to be done about it. Until recently, an American's right to drive under any condition has been as sacred as his or her right to breathe, but the carnage on our highways has created strong grassroots pressure to impose stiffer penalties on all drunk drivers and to make it harder for young adults to drive while drunk.

One catalyst in the popular reaction against drunk drivers has been Candy Lightner. Mrs. Lightner's 21-year-old daughter was killed in 1980 by a hit-and-run driver who, though he had numerous drunk-driving charges on his record, had never once had his license revoked. The outraged Mrs. Lightner responded by organizing Mothers Against Drunk Drivers (MADD), which has campaigned for much harsher penalties for driving while under the influence of alcohol.

As a result of MADD's efforts and pressure from several similar groups, a number of state legislatures have toughened their laws against drunken driving. Three basic provisions are found in most of these laws: (1) They make it a criminal offense for a person to drive if his or her blood alcohol content is 0.10 or more; (2) they make a jail sentence of some length mandatory for certain offenses; and (3) they make the drunk-driving offense a permanent part of the driver's record. A number of states have gone even further. Thirty-seven states have begun to enforce "dram shop" laws that hold those who serve alcohol to people who will later be driving responsible for any offenses those people commit. A number of states have established highway "sobriety checkpoints" at which drivers are routinely stopped and given breathalyzer tests to see if they have been drinking. Some large cities have created task forces to crack down on drunk drivers. Some states make the suspension of a driver's license mandatory at the first offense. Some jurisdictions, taking a different approach, give offenders the option of attending therapy sessions as an alternative to some other penalty.

I'M FOR MADD
MOTHERS AGAINST DRUNK DRIVERS

Because drunk-driving incidents are the leading cause of death in the 18-to-20 age group, the drunk-driving campaign has cracked down particularly hard on the young. According to *Time* magazine, "Drivers in this age group are twice as likely as the average motorist to be involved in an alcohol-related crash." For this reason, Congress passed a law in 1984 that required every state to raise its legal drinking age to 21 by 1986 or forfeit part of its federal highway funds; thirty-seven states have complied so far.

The results of the 1984 law and the various state measures have so far been mixed. In some states the accident and fatality rates have dropped sharply, while in others they have showed little change. Proponents of the laws claim that alcohol-related traffic fatalities have declined nationwide by 32 percent since 1980, and the National Highway Traffic Safety Administration estimates that the new higher drinking age is saving 1,250 lives a year. The results have been spectacular in Oregon, where drunk-driving laws have been in effect since 1971. While the number of drivers has increased by 46 percent and the number of vehicles has risen by 62 percent, the traffic fatality rate has dropped by 35 percent.

Critics complain, however, that raising the legal drinking age to 21 is falsely discriminatory because there are almost as many accidents and fatalities in the 22-to-24 age group. In fact, drivers in the larger 20-to-24 group have the highest rates of conviction for drunk driving and alcohol-related accidents of all age groups (the rate generally declines with increasing age).

Students themselves are about evenly divided about the new drinking laws. Many complain that they are being treated simultaneously like children and like adults. They say that it makes no sense to allow a person under 21 to vote, marry, sign contracts, or have an abortion, but not to drink.

Sources: Based in part on "One Less for the Road?" *Time*, May 20, 1985, pp. 76–78; "A New Prohibition," *Newsweek on Campus*, April 1985, p. 7.

The introduction of seat belts, too, has had some effect on the mortality rate from automobile accidents, but not as much as had been hoped because so many people refused to use them. By 1985 states started to pass mandatory seat-belt-use laws, and within a year, because some of the most populous states were the first to act, more than half the U.S. population was covered by such a law. Early results showed a 17 percent drop in auto fatalities in New York, 13 percent in Illinois, and 11 percent in Michigan. Seat-belt use is particularly important to riders in small cars, who suffer three times the injury and fatality rate of riders in larger and more protective automobiles.

In 1986 it was unclear whether some passive restraint, either an **air bag** or an automatic seat belt, would be mandated by the national government. Such a rule had been made by the Department of Transportation, but with the hint that if at least two-thirds of the population were to be covered by mandatory seat-belt-use laws, it might be dropped. The automobile industry, which more than once in the past had succeeded in getting safety regulations modified or dropped, strongly opposed mandatory air bags.

The Driver. In our society driving a car is more than simply a convenient way of getting from one point to another. It is also a psychological symbol, which, at various times and to different individuals, may stand for such things as power, maturity, aggressiveness, competence, and sexuality. It is also a social activity, for the driver must contend with various traffic rules and other cars on the road. Thus the way drivers feel about themselves and others is likely to affect the way they drive. The specific personality traits associated with motor vehicle accidents, such as hostility, alienation, and self-centeredness, have already been described.

Improper driving, particularly speeding and failing to obey road signals or signs, is the cause of more than 72 percent of all motor vehicle accidents. The effect of speeding on the accident toll was dramatically illustrated when the 55-mile-per-hour speed limit went into effect in 1974. Passed as a means of conserving fuel, the measure was not only effective in that respect but also brought about an immediate 17 percent reduction in auto fatalities. There has been a gradual disregard for the 55-mile-per-hour speed limit, however, and as the average rate of speed of the motorist increases, so does the annual number of highway fatalities. The relation of speed to auto accidents is borne out statistically. In a car that is traveling at 70 miles per hour or faster, a motorist has about a fifty-fifty chance to survive an accident. In a vehicle moving at between 50 and 60 miles per hour, the odds of surviving an accident increase to thirty-one to one. The federal Department of Transportation monitors compliance with the speed limit, and in 1986 for the first time withheld some highway funds from states that were not adequately enforcing it.

Although poor training, stress, and the personality traits mentioned above can themselves lead to improper driving, these factors may also give rise to other behaviors that, in turn, make driving much more hazardous. Driving while intoxicated, for example, has been implicated in about half of all motor vehicle accidents. Other unsafe practices that cause accidents are obstructing visibility with decorations, mixing tire types (which results in dangerously reduced traction), failing to use the rearview mirror or directional signals, driving unnecessarily during hazardous road or weather conditions, and failure to give right of way.

Suggestions for reducing driver-caused accidents include: (1) requiring that individuals take a driver education course when they apply for a license; (2) making the process of qualifying for a driver's license more rigorous and including tests of physical ability, such as reaction time and motor coordination; (3) requiring the reexamination of licensed drivers at regular intervals; (4) requiring that driving record receive greater attention during license renewal, so that in certain cases conditional licenses would be issued or a new license would be refused; and (5) suspending or revoking licenses for driving while intoxicated, and also making use of programs of rehabilitation (see box: Drunken Driving).

SUMMARY

1. Accidents are the fourth major cause of death in the United States and the leading cause of death for individuals 1 to 37 years of age. The four major accident categories are *work*, *home*, *public*, and *motor vehicle* accidents. The largest number of injuries occur in home accidents, and the largest number of fatalities are caused by motor vehicle accidents. Most accidents are preventable.

2. *Attitudinal*, *psychological*, *personal*, *equipment*, *cultural*, and *environmental factors* contribute to the incidence of accidents and their severity. Recognizing these factors and dealing with them is necessary before accidents can be reduced. There is a definite relationship between *stress* and vulnerability to accidents. People with chronic personality disorders are particularly accident prone.

3. The largest number of work-related injuries occur in the industries where most people work: services, trade, and manufacturing; the greatest number of work-related deaths, however, occur in the mining industry. A program of prevention must include strengthening of the *Occupational Safety and Health Act*, improvement of the work environment, elimination of hazards, and training of personnel.

4. The major causes of fatal accidents in the home are falls, fires, poisoning, suffocation, and firearms. Their incidence can be sharply reduced by practical measures such as leaving floors uncluttered, storing flammable materials outside the home, properly labeling all substances, and keeping objects that can be swallowed away from children.

5. The single largest cause of public accident deaths is falls. Drowning ranks second; most cases of drowning could be prevented by teaching people how to swim and training them to rescue others. Firearms have become a major public safety problem. Requiring gun registration and sharply upgrading licensing requirements would do much to reduce misuse of firearms.

6. Motor vehicle accidents can be caused by road conditions, the car, or the driver. Improving road surfaces and design would reduce the incidence of road-related accidents. The *National Traffic and Mo-*

tor Vehicle Safety Act of 1966 has resulted in a number of safety improvements in cars, and more than half the population is now covered by seat-belt laws. Improving driver training, upgrading licensing requirements, enforcing the 55-miles-an-hour speed limit, and stiffening the penalties for drunk driving would greatly reduce driver-related accidents.

CONSUMER CONCERNS

1. Though the greatest number of fatal accidents occur on the highways, the greatest number of accidental injuries occur in the home. Many home accidents are caused by faulty or hazardous products such as electrical appliances, tools, chemicals such as cleansers, and children's toys. Are you conscious of the hazard factor in such purchases? How do you exercise caution?
2. As a homeowner or a tenant, are you exercising adequate precaution in respect to your own safety? What equipment do you own, and what precautions have you taken to ensure safety in your home?
3. In the American way of life the automobile is not only a major form of transportation but also a major cause of death. To what degree do you consider safety in the purchase of a car? What precautions do you take to maintain safety in its operation?
4. A modest consumer investment could prevent the improper treatment, or even save the life, of someone with a chronic disability or an allergic condition. What is the wisdom in wearing a Medic-Alert bracelet or carrying some form of card bearing personal information such as blood type and disabilities?

4

Physical Fitness

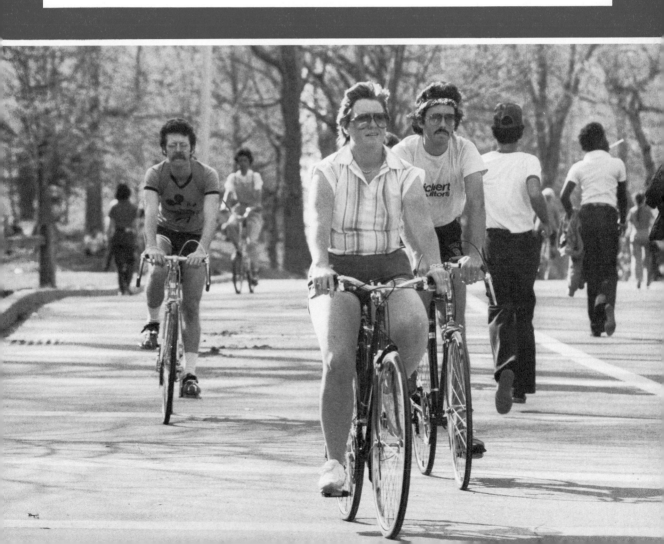

A "fitness boom" has swept over the United States during the past decade and shows no sign of letting up. People all over the country are devoting more and more time and energy to achieving maximum levels of physical well-being. As never before, they are hiking, running, and cycling; playing golf, tennis, racquetball, and handball; lifting weights and jumping rope; skiing, skating, and swimming—to name only some of the more common sports activities. Although Americans have always valued sports, they have only recently begun to change their attitudes toward their own physical fitness. Former spectators are now active participants. Why?

Some thirty years ago studies were conducted to compare American school-age children with those from several continental European countries, Great Britain, and Japan. The results were astounding: When it came to physical fitness, American children were far behind all others. These findings contributed to the creation of the organization now called the President's Council on Physical Fitness and Sports, an advisory group that promotes physical education programs in schools and encourages physical fitness programs in communities and in industry.

Health statistics also prompted an awareness of the need for physical activity. They showed a high death rate in the United States due to cardiovascular impairment; however, those who were physically active were found to have a lower cardiovascular death rate.

Finally, those who were among the first to become more physically active so obviously enjoyed what they were doing that the example they set encouraged others to follow. Tennis, golf, and other traditionally popular sports attracted a growing number of enthusiasts. But suddenly, in the 1960s, more demanding physical activities, identified as **aerobic** (exercises that stimulate heart and lung

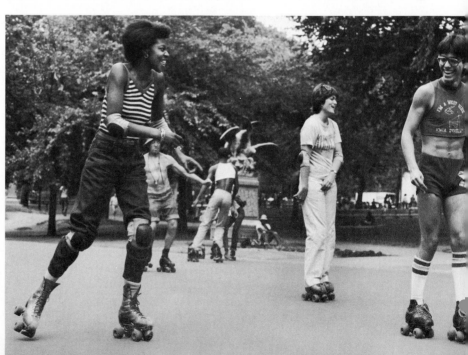

activity), were popularized by Dr. Kenneth H. Cooper. The aerobic concept drew devotees at a rate that suggested a virtual craze. And whereas some activities are short-lived fads and others have cycles of popularity, jogging, the most popular of aerobic exercises, continues to attract enthusiasts to an astounding degree. Today's runners include 30 million Americans, half of them women, and running clubs have multiplied. Cycling lags not far behind, if the sales figures for bicycles are any indication. And ski touring, a relatively unknown winter sport a few years ago, has zoomed in popularity.

The fitness boom is easily documented by sales figures for sports equipment, fitness programs, and related items such as health foods, gadgets, and diet books. Although some of the more than $30 billion a year is spent for fashion instead of fitness (not everyone who wears running shoes is a jogger), the fact that fitness gear is in vogue shows that people value the image highly.

What is the result of this massive effort toward fitness? Those involved are most enthusiastic. They claim their new life style gives them an almost euphoric sense of well-being. And the recent decline in the death rate from cardiovascular impairment gives evidence that this effort has not been in vain.

Not all Americans are enjoying the benefits of the fitness boom, however. Though the number participating in some form of fitness program has doubled during the past twenty years, a nationwide survey by the U.S. Department of Health and Human Services in 1986 showed that 80 to 90 percent of us still do not get enough exercise. In addition, many fitness programs do not meet the standards for achieving physical fitness established by the President's Council on Physical Fitness and Sports. (According to PCPFS, a training program should include, minimally, three sessions per week, each consisting of at least thirty minutes of continuous activity.) Neither have school physical education programs improved, despite the fact that most Americans want strong physical education programs for their children.

Let us look more closely at the interesting and sometimes baffling picture of physical activity. We shall discuss why there is a need for activity, the physical changes it produces, the comparative benefits of a variety of activities, prevailing myths about fitness, changing concepts about aging and activity, and commercial ventures in physical fitness.

WHAT IS PHYSICAL FITNESS?

Physical fitness is usually defined in terms of two main elements: (1) the *readiness* for the complete and efficient release of physical energy and (2) the capacity for sustained activity, or *endurance*. But this definition should also include a person's general state of health, for poor health can interfere with the capacity to perform physically at maximum levels. In order to maintain our well-being, it is important that we eat wisely, sleep adequately, and seek sound medical advice when we need it. There is no universal standard of physical fitness. Each of us must determine what we can do and decide what we hope to accomplish. Most important, our standards must be reasonable enough to lie within our capacities and enjoyable enough for us to maintain interest. Because maintaining a good level of physical fitness requires our constant attention, it is essential that we derive satisfaction and a sense of achievement from our

PROBLEMS AND CONTROVERSIES: Fitness in Childhood and Adolescence

If American schoolchildren and adolescents were less physically fit than their European and Japanese counterparts thirty years ago (see opening section of text), they are in even worse shape today. Half the children in grades 5 through 12 in one recent federal study spent less than an hour a week in any kind of physical activity. Two-thirds of the children in another study could not meet the Amateur Athletic Association's standards for jumps, push-ups, and endurance runs. Many could not even get through ten minutes of moderate aerobic exercise. Skinfold measurements have shown that most children are significantly fatter than they were in the 1960s.

The lack of exercise is taking its toll on children's health. Tests have shown many to have dangerous buildups of fatty plaque in their arteries, high blood pressure, and elevated cholesterol levels—all of which are likely to lead to premature heart attacks and other diseases in adulthood.

School policies and life-style factors are mostly to blame. Most public-school physical education programs steer children into competitive team sports such as football and basketball instead of aerobic activities like jogging, swimming, and cycling—activities that they can pursue alone and carry into adulthood. Furthermore, many school districts have had to cut back on their physical education programs and lay off instructors. Life-style factors also play a large role. Besides eating too much sweet, heavy junk food, the average youngster spends up to seven hours a day in front of a TV set. The availability of transportation also contributes to the problem. If more children walked or cycled to school rather than being driven by their parents or on school buses, they would benefit from this bit of physical activity every school day.

Disturbed by this trend, some school administrators have revamped their exercise programs and obtained dramatic improvements in youngsters' physical and mental health. For example, in several districts children who began a regular aerobic exercise program significantly lowered their blood pressure and blood cholesterol levels. They also scored higher on math and language tests and showed a higher level of self-esteem.

Sources: Adapted from "Failing in Fitness," *Newsweek,* April 1, 1985, pp. 84–87; "The Shape of the Nation," *Time*, October 7, 1985, pp. 60–61.

activities in order to be motivated to continue. Physical exercise also provides psychological benefits, including a tranquilizing effect. Sustained physical activity is known to reduce both anxiety and depression. Older people who exercise have better memories than do those who are sedentary. The mental effects of physical fitness should not be surprising: After all, mind and body function as one and the same.

Physical fitness also includes efficiency of movement as well as a capacity for physical endurance. Therefore the greater the physical fitness of individuals, the longer they are able to continue an activity, the more effectively they can perform, and the faster they will recuperate after the activity has terminated.

All human activity depends on energy produced by the body. The important systems in this respect are the cardiovascular and respiratory systems. Ultimately, a person depends on the efficiency and capacity of the cardiovascular and respiratory systems for the delivery of the two basic ingredients in energy production—oxygen and the fuel provided from the absorption of carbohydrate, fat, and protein—to those areas of the body where energy is being produced and consumed.

The process of energy production begins in the lungs. When we breathe, air enters the lungs; oxygen in the air diffuses into the bloodstream, where it is carried by the red blood cells to the heart. The heart then pumps oxygen-laden blood throughout the vascular systems—the body's network of blood vessels and capillaries—where it is distributed to the tissues. Cells in the tissues consume the oxygen by means of metabolic processes that yield energy, heat, and waste products. One of the metabolic wastes, carbon dioxide, is returned by the bloodstream to the lungs for expiration. The amount of oxygen processed, and therefore the amount of energy produced, depends on: (1) the amount of air the lungs inhale; (2) the number of red blood cells and the total volume of blood; and (3) the efficiency of the heart's pumping action and of the total vascular system.

Physically fit people whose body systems are healthy have greater oxygen reserves and therefore a greater oxygen-intake ability (**aerobic capacity**) than those who are in poor health or a rundown condition. Their lungs deliver more air to the body, and their hearts dispense it with fewer beats and at lower blood pressure. As a result, they are able to indulge in extended and taxing physical activity with less fatigue. As this ability is perhaps the best indication of fitness, the best exercise programs are those that increase aerobic capacity.

Not all vigorous physical activity increases aerobic capacity. Aerobic activities are those in which a sustained and uniform physical effort occurs. In aerobic activities the intake and use of oxygen are gradually increased to meet the demands of the activity and then remain at a fairly stable level, as does the functioning of the entire cardiovascular and respiratory systems. Muscular effort also remains at a constant level. A typical sustained, uniform physical activity would be running or *jogging*; a jogger moves along at a fairly steady pace and, of course, for a reasonable period of time. Other sustained physical activities include rowing, cycling, cross-country skiing, skating, swimming, and rope jumping. The bursts of effort that occur in many popular sports do not fit this pattern. They are not sufficiently constant to produce an increase in aerobic capacity. The sudden efforts involved in pitching a baseball, blocking a football linesman, clearing a high jump, pursuing a tennis ball, dunking a basketball shot, or lifting a barbell occur only for a short time and are discontinued before the body can make its internal adjustments.

HOW PHYSICAL FITNESS AFFECTS THE BODY

As the human organism ages, many body functions begin to degenerate and lose their efficiency. Even cell activity diminishes, as is evidenced by a marked decrease in cell regeneration in certain tissues. Whole organs and systems are affected, giving rise to such conditions as cardiovascular inefficiency, impaired metabolism, and the wasting away of muscle tissue.

The failure to exercise, to keep all body systems operating at peak efficiency, is related to a high incidence of degenerative and organic disease. Abundant evidence exists to support this fact. Inactive people have twice as much heart disease as to active people. Duodenal ulcer and diabetes mellitus are also more common in less physically active people, and at least 80 percent of all complaints of low back pain can be traced to inadequate activity. Emotional problems, inability to cope with stress, neuromuscular tension, and proneness to fatigue often accompany a sedentary life. Physically active people tend to have lower blood pressure and pulse rates and higher breathing capacity than do inactive people.

Exercise for a Longer Life

Moderate exercise . . . can add up to two years to a person's life. In the mid-1960s Dr. Ralph S. Paffenbarger Jr. and his colleagues at the Stanford University School of Medicine recruited [nearly 17,000] Harvard graduates, 35 to 74, and asked them to answer detailed questionnaires about their general health and living habits. Follow-ups carried out until 1978 showed that men who expended at least 2,000 calories per week through exercise had mortality rates one-quarter to one-third lower than those burning up fewer calories. . . . More exercise meant a better chance at a long life—up to a point. A regimen that burned more than 3,500 calories tended to cause injuries that negated most of the benefits derived from exercise. Harvard men who were varsity athletes while in college—and were thus presumed by the researchers to have been starting out life with basically strong bodies—had no advantage over their classmates in terms of survival rates. Indeed, lettermen who subsequently turned soft and sedentary increased their mortality risk. "It's not the kind of activity that you did in college . . . but the amount of contemporary activity that's associated with the longer survival," says Paffenbarger.

Source: Matt Clark with Karen Springen, "Running for Your Life," *Newsweek*, March 17, 1986, p. 70. Reprinted by permission.

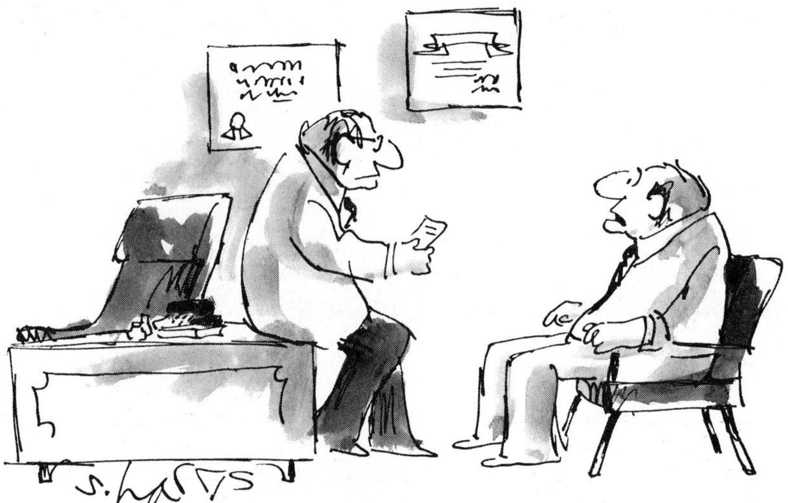

"Jog? What kind of a prescription is 'jog'?"

The Cardiovascular System

The incidence of heart disease, as we have just noted, is lower among those who are physically fit and whose activities increase their aerobic capacity. Furthermore, when physically active individuals suffer a heart attack, they are less apt to die upon the first attack; they generally recover more rapidly; they are less likely to experience a second attack soon after; and they usually have the first attack later in life than nonexercisers.

Among the benefits aerobic exercise affords are the following:

1. An increase in the size and strength of the heart, enabling the organ to pump more blood with each beat and to rest longer between beats—a possible saving of 10,000 to 40,000 beats a day.

2. An increase in the size and pliability of the blood vessels, reducing blood pressure and cutting down on cholesterol levels in the blood.
3. An expansion of the blood supply, including increased amounts of hemoglobin and blood plasma, which streamlines the body's waste removal system and allows more oxygen to saturate the muscles and other tissues; this reduces fatigue and builds endurance.
4. The creation of networks of new blood vessels and capillaries in the cardiac and skeletal muscles, thereby improving the flow of oxygen to all parts of the body.

The Respiratory System

The heart and blood vessels are not the only parts of the body to benefit significantly from the effects of physical fitness. Proper exercise also improves the condition of the lungs and the entire respiratory system. Healthy lungs must be able to process enough air and extract sufficient oxygen to produce the energy required by the body. The amount of air the lungs can take in is controlled by the muscles of the rib cage and diaphragm. During inhalation these muscles contract to expand the rib cage, creating a vacuum in the lung cavity into which air rushes. In exhalation these muscles relax, forcing the air out. Physical conditioning strengthens these muscles: More air can be inhaled, more oxygen can be released to the body tissues, and more carbon dioxide wastes can be removed.

The Muscular System

Though activities such as weight lifting and certain calisthenic movements may increase the size, strength, and tone of specific **voluntary** (or **skeletal**) **muscles** (those over which we have control), they contribute little to the respiratory muscles that control breathing and the vascular muscles that line the blood vessels. Therefore they do little to enhance **endurance**—the capacity to conduct prolonged activity—which is our principal measure of physical fitness. Endurance is promoted only by total fitness exercises that strengthen the **involuntary muscles**—that is, the respiratory and vascular muscles. Such exercises make greater demands especially on the blood vessels; thus they become stronger and more elastic.

Mental Health

Emotional pressures can threaten a person's physical health. They can cause a variety of organic illnesses of the heart, digestive organs, skin, respiratory system, muscles and joints, and other basic systems. Vigorous activity helps the body adapt to strain and keeps it from being overwhelmed by mental stress.

Physical fitness does not necessarily ensure mental well-being, but pleasurable exercise can relieve some tensions that are part of daily life. A healthy body is less quickly overcome by emotional stress. Furthermore, a strong constitution and good health promote a more positive outlook on life and improve one's mental well-being. Most people who exercise regularly report an increased ability to cope, to solve problems, and to think creatively—all of which lends them greater self-confidence.

There is even evidence that many emotional disorders respond to exercise therapy. In one study over 500 students at the University of Virginia were tested for depression. Out of the group 18 percent were judged depressed and

FITNESS SCORECARD

Score

*1. Cardiovascular Health**

0 – Under medical care for heart or circulatory problems.
1 – Such problems exist but medical care not required.
2 – Past cardiovascular ailments have been pronounced "cured."
3 – No history of cardiovascular trouble.

2. Injuries†

0 – Unable to do any strenuous work because of an injury.
1 – Level of activity is limited by the injury.
2 – Some pain during activity but performance isn't affected significantly.
3 – No injuries.

3. Illnesses†

0 – Unable to do any strenuous work because of an illness.
1 – Level of activity is limited by the illness.
2 – Experience uneasiness during activity but performance isn't affected.
3 – No illnesses.

4. First (or Most Recent) Run‡

0 – Able to run less than a half-mile or five minutes without stopping.
1 – Ran between a half-mile and a mile (five to 10 minutes) non-stop.
2 – Completed between a mile and 1½ miles (10 to 15 minutes).

5. Running Background

0 – Have never trained formally for running.
1 – No running training within the last three years or more.
2 – No running training within the last one to two years.
3 – Have trained for running within the last year.

6. Other Related Activities

0 – Not currently active in any regular sports or exercise programs.
1 – Regularly participate in "slow sports" such as golf, baseball, softball.
2 – Regularly practice vigorous "stop-and-go" sports such as tennis, basketball, soccer.
3 – Regularly participate in steady-paced, prolonged activities such as bicycling, hiking, swimming.

the rest normal. A group of subjects, both normal and depressed, jogged regularly for ten weeks. Another group of depressed and normal subjects did not exercise. At the end of the experiment, all subjects were tested again. The depressed patients who jogged had significantly better feelings, whereas depressed subjects who didn't run had no change in outlook. The normal subjects who ran felt even better than they had previously.

Just why exercise improves a person's mental state is not fully understood. Biochemical researchers and brain specialists, however, have noted a correlation between lower levels of epinephrine and norepinephrine (two brain hormones) and a depressive mood. Studies at Massachusetts General Hospital have shown, through blood samples, that norepinephrine levels increase as much as threefold during intensive exercise. Other researchers suggest that exercise may raise mood

7. Age

0 – 50s and older.
1 – 40s
2 – 30s
3 – 20s

8. Weight

0 – More than 25 pounds above your "ideal" weight.
1 – 16 to 25 pounds above your "ideal" weight.
2 – 6 to 15 pounds above your "ideal" weight.
3 – Within five pounds of "ideal" weight (or below ideal weight).

9. Resting Pulse Rate

0 – 80 beats per minute or higher.
1 – in the 70s.
2 – in the 60s.
3 – in the 50s or below.

10. Smoking

0 – A regular smoker.
1 – An occasional smoker.
2 – Have been a regular smoker but quit.
3 – Never have smoked regularly.

Scoring:

Score yourself in each of the 10 areas and add up the total. A score of 20 or higher is excellent. You probably can skip the preliminaries and go directly to a *running* program.

A score of 10 to 19 is average for adults. Start at the *jogging* level.

If you scored less than 10 points, you should forget about running and even jogging for now and concentrate on raising your score by *walking.*

Exceptions:

* = If you have any history of heart or circulatory disease, do not continue with this series; participate in closely supervised activities.

† = If these injuries or illnesses are temporary, wait until they are cured before starting the program applicable to you; if they're chronic, adjust the programs to fit your limitations.

‡ = If you can run continuously for 1½ miles (15 minutes) or more, you may start as high as a running program no matter what your score is; you are fit!

Source: Runner's World, January 1983, p. 27. Copyright © 1983. Reprinted by permission.

simply by increasing the blood flow to the brain, delivering extra oxygen and nutrients.

Body Weight

Physical fitness and weight control are not synonymous. Many people who are physically fit do not conform to the norms for body weight. Nor does physical activity of itself control weight; for example, a person must do fourteen minutes of *fast* running in order to burn off the calories of one candy bar. It is simpler in terms of weight control not to eat the candy bar.

On the other hand, regular exercise is important in any weight-control program. For one thing, the increased metabolic rate that occurs during exercise seems to carry over for several hours after an exercise session, so that the body continues to burn calories at a faster rate even after the exercise has ended.

For another thing, most people report that moderate exercise reduces rather than increases their appetite.

PLANNING A FITNESS PROGRAM

In developing an activity program for yourself, you must consider what type of activity you will enjoy and will therefore be most motivated to continue on a permanent basis. After evaluating the current physical demands of your occupation, daily activities, and recreational pursuits, you can determine what program will add balance and variety to your normal schedule.

Once you have decided on your individual goals, you must undertake the more difficult task of sorting through the multitude of possible activities to find those that most closely meet your requirements. This chore is complicated by the conflicting information offered by commercial promoters, many of whom promise instant fitness and effortless exercise.

The fact is that physical fitness is impossible to achieve without physical exertion. Sitting in saunas or using devices and gadgets that simulate activity will not result in any real improvement in aerobic capacity. Even a regular exercise regimen may accomplish little if the effort it requires is not sufficiently demanding. Yoga exercises, for example, may increase muscular flexibility, a worthy goal in itself, but little more than that. Only a regular, prolonged, and vigorous exercise program will increase *overall* physical fitness.

You should consider several factors in planning a physical fitness program. The most critical of these is your present state of health.

State of Health

Anyone who plans to embark on a physical fitness program—even someone who feels healthy—should first have a medical examination. This is particularly important for those over 35 who have been generally inactive—especially if they have a history of illness or a current health problem. The physician may recommend a modified exercise program or a conditioning program to precede more active participation.

The presence of a degenerative condition does not necessarily preclude physical activity. Certain exercises, especially those that promote aerobic endurance, may actually be prescribed under medical supervision for people with diabetes mellitus, ulcers, emphysema, and certain coronary ailments.

Dr. Kenneth H. Cooper has proposed some general guidelines for physical examinations. For certain age groups, an **electrocardiogram** (EKG)—a record of the electric impulses produced by contractions of the heart—is advised.

- UNDER 30: If within the past year you have received a medical examination and have been found to be in good health, you may start an exercise program.
- BETWEEN 30 AND 39: Within three months of beginning an exercise program you should have a medical checkup that includes an EKG taken while you are at rest.
- BETWEEN 40 AND 59: Within three months of beginning a program you should have a physical, including an EKG taken while you are exercising.
- OVER 59: You should get a medical checkup, including an exercise EKG, just before starting a program.*

*Kenneth H. Cooper, *The New Aerobics* (New York: M. Evans and Company, 1970).

Motivation

Maintaining interest in a physical activity is critical in order to ensure regular participation. An activity performed at irregular intervals does little to promote physical fitness. The following bits of advice may help you maintain your enthusiasm for exercise: If you carry on your normal routine indoors, you might find an outdoor activity such as jogging or tennis appealing. On the other hand, if your working day is spent outdoors, you might find indoor recreation attractive. Group activities may provide companionship, or even good fellowship, and thus stimulate your interest, especially if you spend much of the day alone. Solitary activities are useful, on the other hand, because they do not depend upon the participation of others. Seasonal and local sports in your community or town may provide diversity. Alternating vigorous and moderate, or indoor and outdoor, exercise patterns may also add necessary variety. The person who jogs two or three times a week might enjoy playing tennis or swimming on some days. Many joggers have become ski-touring enthusiasts when conditions permit.

Conditioning

Do not undertake an exercise program without keeping the following principles in mind:

Warm-up. Before starting vigorous exercise, it is essential to spend several minutes limbering up the joints and muscles in order to prevent sprains and to avoid strain on the heart caused by rapidly rising blood pressure. A **warm-up** period will gradually raise the body temperature, which improves the physical work capacity of the large muscles.

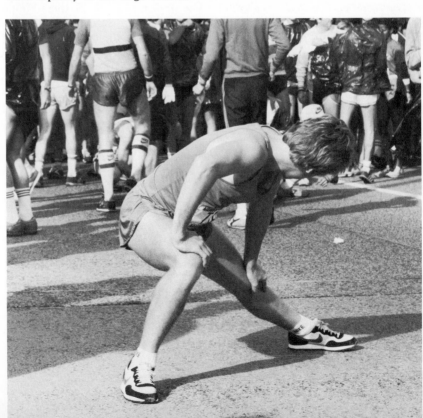

Warming up.

Achieving the Training Level. To be of permanent benefit, an exercise program must be vigorous enough for you to reach what is known as the training level, which is an increase in the amount of oxygen that your body burns during exercise. The **training effect** is achieved when your heart rate, typically measured by your pulse rate, is elevated. Table 4-1 shows the target heart rates needed to achieve the training effect. The lower number of the range is the pulse rate that must be exceeded for the training effect to occur, and the upper number is the rate that should not be exceeded in order to prevent strain. The following formulas provide another way to measure your target heart rate:

MINIMUM RATE = 160 minus your age
MAXIMUM RATE = 200 minus your age

Avoidance of Exhaustion. The general advice for any exercise program is: Start modestly, avoid strain, and guard against exhaustion. Some ambitious beginners defeat the purpose of exercise by tiring their bodies excessively and then becoming discouraged. It is far better to start slowly and progress over several months to more intensive levels. In this way the body gradually increases its ability to provide greater amounts of oxygen for longer periods and more strenuous activities.

There are three methods of determining if you are overdoing an exercise. The first is the *personal stress gauge:* Be alert for any signs of severe breathlessness, chest pain or tightness, lack of muscle control, nausea, dizziness, or lightheadedness. The presence of any of these symptoms should indicate to you that you are exceeding your capacity. A high *heart-rate response* also indicates overstrenuous exercising: If the pulse rate has not returned to normal within five to ten minutes after exercising, you are overexerting yourself. The third guideline is the *breathing-rate response*: If within ten minutes after exercising you are still not breathing regularly (twelve to sixteen breaths a minute), you are overexercising.

TABLE 4-1
Heart-Rate Targets for the Training Effect

Age	Target Heart Rate	Cut-off Heart Rate
20–25	140	167
26–30	134	163
31–35	131	159
36–40	127	155
41–45	124	150
46–50	120	146
51–55	117	142
56–60	113	138
61–65	110	133
66–70	106	129

training range

Source: Bob Glover and Jack Shepherd, *The Runner's Handbook*, p. 43. Copyright © 1978 by Bob Glover and Jack Shepherd. Reprinted by permission of Viking Penguin, Inc.

Do not confuse exhaustion with normal fatigue, however. **Fatigue** occurs when the concentration of lactic acid and carbon dioxide reaches a certain level in the blood, causing a feeling of tiredness. This condition is quite safe and normal, though you should regard it as a warning signal not to exceed your physical limits.

Toning Down. Just as it is necessary first to warm up your body, it is likewise necessary to allow a **toning-down** period in which your body can relax gradually after engaging in exercise. Walking or jogging slowly in place allows the body to recover its normal aerobic condition. Failure to observe this rule may result in dizzy spells and faintness.

Regularity and Consistency. A final principle is to maintain regularity and consistency in your exercise plan. Random exercise, even if strenuous, provides little benefit because it does not build up the body to withstand increasing workloads. As we noted above, a beneficial exercise program requires a minimum of three activity sessons a week. Fewer sessions may burn up some calories,

Pace: The Key to Endurance and Physical Fitness

It is not uncommon for the beginner to launch a training program with too much zeal and too little knowledge. The beginner who attacks early training sessions with uninhibited gusto and schedules training sessions with unreasonable frequency can suffer aches, pains, strains, sprains, stretched ligaments, torn muscles, and inflamed tendons (particularly the Achilles tendon connecting the back of the heel to the calf muscles). Disabilities at this point are often so severe that the beginner becomes disenchanted and discontinues the training effort. A modest, tempered approach, on the other hand, avoids these traumas and allows the beginner to train comfortably within his or her capacities and limitations.

Runners call this modification of effort *pacing*. It is the control of the speed or rhythm with which an activity is conducted. Another word for pacing is *tempo*. Modification of the rhythm or the intensity of effort provides several benefits. It helps prevent extreme exhaustion as well as injuries. A modest pace also enables the performer to conserve energy for the conclusion of the activity or to lengthen the period of activity. The capacity to continue to perform, or to expend energy, is called *endurance*. The aerobic concept is uniquely directed toward the development of endurance.

Many activitiies lend themselves to the development of endurance because they allow a person to determine the intensity at which he or she performs. For example, a woman runner in training may have the capacity to run a mile in seven minutes; theoretically, she could run three miles in twenty-one minutes. However, this effort would leave her totally exhausted and she would not have have exercised for thirty minutes, the recommended minimum standard for a training session. Should she run a mile in ten minutes, on the other hand, she would extend the training session by nine minutes and meet the half-hour standard. This principle of slowing down the pace of an activity in order to continue it longer can be applied to all activities. There is a point, of course, below which the training effect will not occur, and this must be kept in mind. It must also be recognized that different individuals require different intensities of activity to achieve the training level. For some, the equivalent of a modest walk may suffice; others may require a more vigorous activity. In any case, measuring the pulse rate will reveal whether one is within the training range.

By performing at regularly scheduled intervals and by placing modest demands on the body, a person can comfortably and gradually increase the span of a training session. Each increase in the length of a training session represents an increase in aerobic capacity, or endurance; and as endurance increases, so does the level of physical fitness.

but they will not increase overall fitness. During long periods of inactivity the body returns to its former state.

A recent study of twelve nonathletic students at the University of Illinois, however, indicates that a well-conditioned body does not quickly return to its flabby state. All the students ran or biked forty minutes a day, six days a week, for ten weeks. After the aerobic capacity of each had increased at least 20 percent, the students were divided into three groups: Group A exercised four times a week; Group B exercised two times a week; Group C stopped exercising. Fifteen weeks later, Groups A and B were still at least 20 percent above their prior capacity and Group C was 6 percent above. The study showed that the effects of training can be maintained with two to four sessions a week. For capacity to increase and conditioning to improve, though, the demands of the exercise program must increase.

Recovery. Our ability to recover from a period of physical activity depends on the intensity of the activity and our degree of fitness. Age is also a factor in that the older we are, the longer it takes us to recover. Recovery requires a period of rest. Without adequate rest we are not fully prepared to engage in the next session of physical activity.

The most complete form of rest is sleep. The importance of sleep to physical fitness is becoming better understood as research into its physiological aspects continues. Sleep helps us recuperate from daily tensions and muscular fatigue; it provides an environment in which the body cells can regenerate and energy can be restored; and it lowers the blood pressure, pulse rate, and body temperature.

The amount of sleep needed to maintain optimum fitness is a highly individual matter. Although most adults require from six to eight hours of sleep a night, wide variations exist, depending on general health, age, daily activity, emotional state, and sleeping habits. The best measure of whether you are getting enough sleep is the way you feel. You should be rested and ready to face your daily activities within an hour of rising.

DEVELOPING A FITNESS PROGRAM

To help guide you in choosing a personal physical fitness program, we have selected some popular aerobic and sports activities for discussion. In evaluating these activities, ask yourself the following questions:

1. Is the activity sufficiently vigorous to elevate the heart rate to the training level?
2. Will the activity allow the training level, once achieved, to be maintained throughout the exercise?

In this section we shall also consider some of the pros and cons of long-distance marathons, the dangers of muscle strain and other sports injuries, the benefits of regular exercise to people over 50, and some aspects of body building.

Aerobic Activities

If you choose an aerobic activity, you can answer yes to the two questions above: Aerobic activities are sufficiently vigorous and they require an expenditure of energy at a sustained high level. Such activities include hiking, bicycling, ski touring, jogging, and swimming. These activities yield successful results in one of two ways: They can demand a low-intensity effort over a prolonged period of time, as in hiking (or walking); or they can demand a high-intensity effort over a shorter period of time, as in jogging and swimming.

Hiking. Sometimes called trail walking, hiking is a very popular low-intensity activity. Hiking trails can be found almost everywhere: in parks, forests, mountain areas, meadowlands, and along beaches. A trail may be less than a mile long or it may go on for a hundred miles or more. (The Appalachian Trail is 2,000 miles long and extends from Maine to Georgia; the Pacific Crest Trail stretches 2,400 miles from Mexico to Canada.) Most hikes last only a day and range in distance from a few miles to fifteen or twenty. Hiking that extends over several days, weeks, or months is usually known as *backpacking*. Hiking clubs generally schedule outings on weekends throughout the year so that as many people as possible can take part.

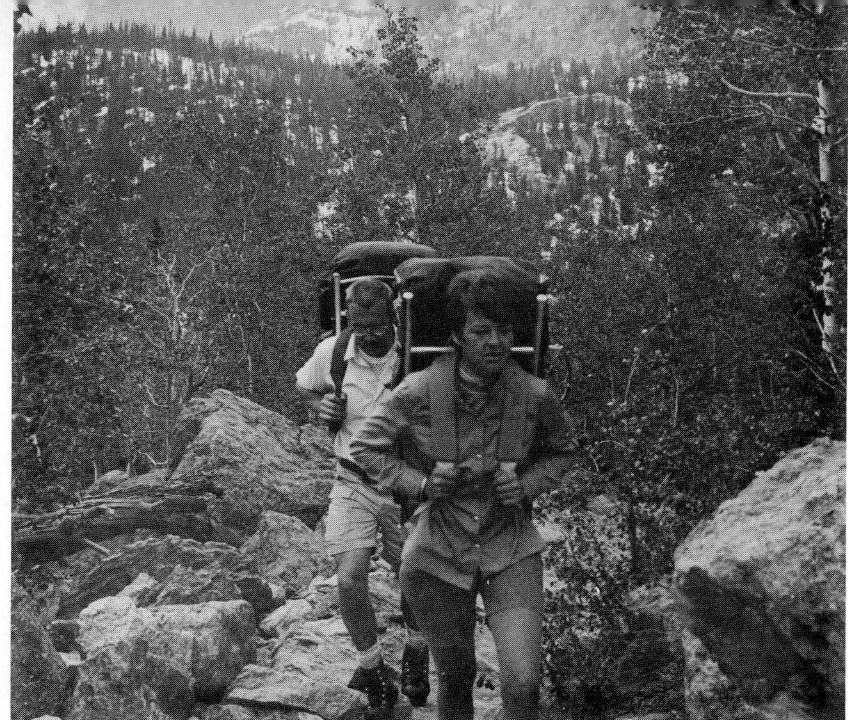

Bicycling. Bicycle sales are booming: More than 10 million bikes are being purchased each year in the United States. On a practical basis, bicycling is becoming an increasingly common means of commuting to school or office, even in urban areas. It helps maintain physical fitness and is also enjoyable as a leisure-time sports activity. More and more cities and towns are setting aside special bikeways or routes to accommodate bicycling's sky-rocketing popularity. New York City's Central Park, for example, is closed to automobile traffic during certain hours and on certain days so that bicycle enthusiasts may safely use its roads. In Iowa an annual event takes place called the *Register's* Annual Great Bike Ride Across Iowa (or Ragbrai). Thousands of bike riders from all over the country join in the amiable week-long 440-mile ride from the Missouri River to the Mississippi, making friends and stretching unused muscles along the way. A word of caution: Nearly a thousand cyclists die in accidents each year, and the number is likely to increase. Bicycle helmets are recommended gear.

Ski Touring. Virtually unknown as a sport in this country until quite recently, cross-country skiing, or ski touring, is experiencing a boom in popularity. With

Aerobic Dancing

Aerobic dancing is a widely popular physical fitness activity, particularly among women, and it is easy to understand why. Put together the companionship that a class provides, the rhythm that the music provides, and the zeal that the instructor provides, and the result is *motion*—and lots of it. If the class is conducted with sufficient intensity and is of sufficient duration, then the benefits that occur are similar to those that result from other aerobic activities. (For guidelines, see Table 4–1.)

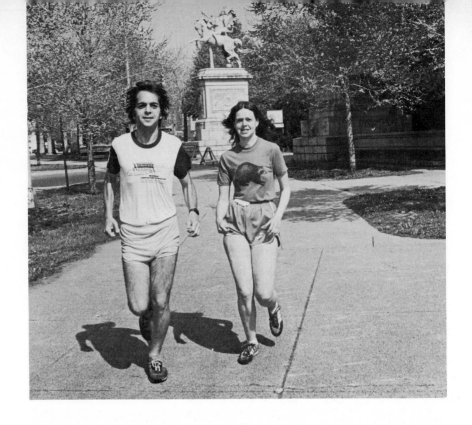

more than 3 million devotees, ski touring is easily the country's fastest-growing winter sport. Summertime joggers, bicyclists, and backpackers are looking at ski touring as an enjoyable way to stay in shape during the winter months, and ski touring can be done anywhere—from cow pastures to city parks, as well as over rougher terrain. Commercialization and competition have helped increase the popularity of ski touring and cross-country racing, but at the same time they have attracted the crowds that many tourers have sought to escape.

Jogging. Considering the number of joggers we see today along our streets, in our parks, and on our beaches, we might conclude that almost everyone jogs. Perhaps the fact that jogging can be done virtually anywhere and requires a minimum of specialized equipment accounts for its popularity. Apart from the jogging shoe itself, clothing need not have any special design. In cold weather several light layers of clothing are recommended, with special thought for covering the head and hands. In hot weather many joggers prefer some light headgear as protection from the sun.

A jog is a moderately paced run. But what is "moderate"? A common measure is the ability to conduct a conversation comfortably while jogging. Because so many people jog in order to improve their physical fitness, let us review some guidelines for starting a jogging program.

The market is flooded with books that outline step-by-step programs for potential joggers. For those who have been inactive for years, a period of increasingly demanding walks should precede any attempts to jog. Jogging should then begin with short runs of 25 to 30 yards, alternating with walks of about the same distance. The running pace should be held in check; in fact, at first it should not exceed the walking pace by much. From then on, one may gradually increase the running portion of the training session, remembering to keep the pace at a modest level.

Swimming. More and more Americans are taking advantage of Masters Swimming, a program of physical fitness and competition for men and women over 25. Since it was started in 1970 in the United States, the program has spread to more than thirty other countries. Local swim meets are held regularly in every part of the country, and two national championship meets are held each year. Competitors are divided into five-year age groups.

For purposes of training and physical fitness, it is recommended that participants swim at least three nonconsecutive days a week and that each workout last a minimum of twenty minutes. The pace at which the swimmer functions should be established by age and a corresponding number of heartbeats per minute. Persons who are overweight or arthritic, and have difficulty bearing their own weight, often find that they can be physically active through a swimming program.

Sports

Sports and games such as tennis, handball, racquetball, basketball, and soccer demand a lot of energy, but since play often occurs in spurts, high-level energy expenditure is not maintained. Though sports requiring this degree of rigor are often a means of maintaining fitness, they usually require a program of

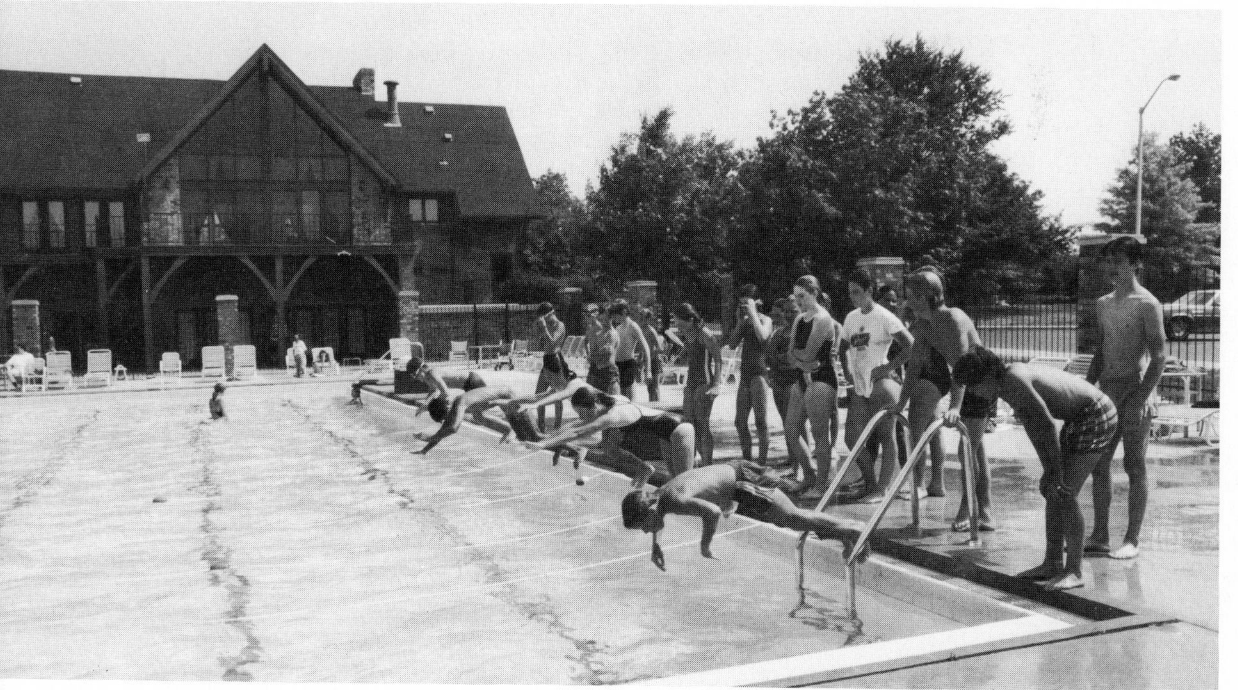

physical fitness before the individual is ready to participate. Other popular activities such as golf, softball, and bowling ordinarily do not place sufficient physical demand upon the individual to produce the training effect.

A physical fitness program based upon a sport has the advantage of motivation, for the individual's interest in the sport encourages continual participation. Being immersed in a sports activity can also stimulate a person to even greater levels of energy expenditure.

Furthermore, the challenge of learning new skills, interaction with other people, the surroundings in which the sports activity takes place, and the element of competition are dimensions of sports activities that are missing from other physical fitness activities. In fact, these elements may be the only ones that can motivate some people to exert themselves. It would be wise for such people to select an appropriate regular sports activity for their fitness program.

The one difficulty with using a group sport as the basis for a physical fitness program is also its advantage—namely, companionship. While it is frequently more enjoyable to engage in a physical activity with other individuals rather than in solitude, it is also more difficult to assemble an adequately motivated and available group of people on a regular basis.

Although sports such as golf and tennis are as popular as ever, activities that are more capable of producing physiological benefits are also enjoying wide popularity today.

Competition

Competition is inspiring. It motivates people to participate in sports, to train, and to exert themselves to maximum capacity during their performance. The question, however, is: Is all of this exertion and training necessary to achieve and maintain physical fitness? The answer from many sources is no.

Physicians at Baylor College of Medicine in Houston stated recently that it does no more good to run six to ten miles a day than it does to run one or two. And we have already seen that three to four activity sessions a week of a half hour's duration are all that is needed to achieve physical fitness.

Nevertheless, the "marathon mania" continues as an indication of the urge

Fitness in a Nutshell

Any physical fitness program should follow three simple principles that apply equally to all forms of physical activity:

1. The intensity of activity must be sufficient to elevate your heart rate into your training zone (see Table 4-1).
2. You must continue the activity at this training level, without interruption, for at least thirty minutes, but there is no need to continue beyond an hour.
3. You must engage in at least three training sessions a week, preferably on nonsuccessive days, in order to maintain or improve your level of fitness.

to compete, and not a week goes by that such an event is not scheduled somewhere. Not only are enthusiasts competing at the official marathon distance of 26 miles 385 yards, but races of 60 and 100 miles are also conducted. So many races of lesser distances are run, such as the Mini-Marathon of New York (6.2 miles), that no one knows the exact number. Many are conducted to raise funds for charities.

The New York Marathon is a barometer of the increasing popularity of marathon running and of competition, as well as a measure of the capabilities of the participants. The New York Marathon, first popularized in 1976 as one activity in the Bicentennial Year celebration, attracted 2,090 entrants. In recent years there have been many times more applicants for a place in the race than could be admitted, and some 16,000 people have completed the run yearly. Nationwide, more than a million Americans have participated in marathons since 1972.

Perils of Exercise

Many of us move too quickly from a life of lethargy to a life of activity and strive to meet the demands of activities far beyond our level of preparedness. The result is a breakdown of the body, usually in the form of a sprain or strain at a vulnerable point: a knee, ankle, elbow, hip, or shoulder. Bruises, blisters, and shin splints are commonplace; but bone fractures and ruptures of the Achilles tendon also occur frequently. These injuries are not limited to beginners but often happen to seasoned competitors who overstrain out of zealousness. The frequency of injury is such that one jogging club reported that half of its members were not able to run at any given time because of some form of athletic injury.

Women in Sports

Boosted by the women's movement, the fitness craze, and various legislative mandates (in particular, Title IX of the Education Amendments Act), women's participation in sports has undergone a near revolution. Not only are more women hitting backhands and swimming laps in the traditionally accepted sports for women, but they are also running, jumping, hitting, and throwing in such sports as jogging, ice hockey, lacrosse, and rugby.

Undoubtedly, sports like tennis and swimming are still the most popular, and participation in them is at an all-time high. The popularity of jogging has made track a highly desirable women's and girls' activity in schools.

Title IX of the Education Amendments Act, passed by Congress in 1972, forbids sex discrimination in any educational institution receiving federal funds. Exactly what constitutes sex discrimination in sports is still open to discussion, but the new law has been responsible for the upgrading of athletic programs for women in schools—either in terms of equivalent women's teams in contact sports or an equal chance to try out for golf and tennis teams.

The evidence is not yet clear as to what degree the anatomical differences between men and women help or hinder their performance in athletic activities. Some say that female swimmers are more buoyant because of the fatty tissue in the lower abdominal area. And although women's speed in marathon running falls short of men's, over very long distances, say fifty miles, women have more endurance. Myths that women should not be strenuously active during menstruation and pregnancy seem to be fading. Women are also taking up weight lifting and body building in increasing numbers. The notion that a well-developed female body is unattractive is quickly losing ground.

Fitness and Aging

From tennis and jogging to ice hockey and even karate, more and more Americans over 50 are taking part in the fitness boom. Some have been active all their lives, while others have been relatively inactive or are becoming active for the first time.

A recent survey showed that over 400 major corporations and many small ones offer employee exercise programs. Many are designed for top-level executives, who are usually in their 50s and 60s. Nearly $5 billion a year is spent on health clubs and corporate fitness programs.

With proper rest and diet and sound medical advice, people in their 60s, 70s, and beyond can engage in daily physical fitness activities and even in competitive sports. As with younger devotees of exercise, older people usually find that their general health improves as a result—and their spirits do too. (See Chapter 10.)

Body Building: Developing Muscular Strength

Weight-training programs are becoming increasingly popular for women as well as men, and are being pursued at home as well as at the local health club or gym. (About $1.15 billion was spent on home gym equipment in 1985.) For people who are concerned with their physique, exercise programs using weights or calisthenic activities can help develop the musculature of the body. The improvement in body appearance that results from these programs can generate a new self-image and impart a significant psychological uplift. Many athletes, too, work out with weights to build up strength and thus improve their performance. The stronger your muscles are, the easier it is for you to perform all sorts of daily tasks as well as sports. Weight training, because it is not sustained, does not usually promote cardiovascular fitness, however.

BUYING PHYSICAL FITNESS

Remember as you spend your dollars to equip yourself for fitness that Madison Avenue has already spotted the tidal wave of American guilt over body flab and sloth. The advertising industry is well aware of your eagerness to reform. It says to you, in effect, "If you want to show that you are serious, then spend money to prove it." Before you purchase a new training suit, another pair of jogging shoes, or other athletic equipment, ask yourself whether you really need it. It's the exercise that counts, not the accessories.

Perhaps you have never been involved in physical fitness, but you have been stimulated by the amount of activity going on around you and encouraged by the enthusiasm of your friends to join the crowd. Maybe you have been attracted by a free pass to a popular health club. Be wary about signing a membership form before understanding fully what is being offered. Leave the premises and in privacy review the program and arrangements being offered.

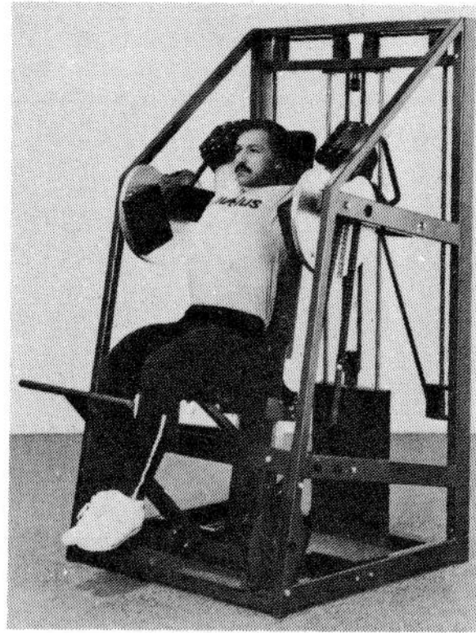

If you are interested in an aerobic activity such as jogging or swimming, a track or a pool of sufficient size should be included among the health club's facilities. Many clubs feature exercise rooms where weight training and calisthenics are virtually the only activities provided. If you are interested in sports, the club should have facilities for activities such as basketball, handball, squash, or tennis. It might be wise for you to find a club designed specifically for the sport you are interested in. In any case, you should always understand the financial arrangements of any club you are considering joining.

Newspapers often carry advertisements for various devices that develop strength or that concentrate on a single activity, such as a stationary cycle or a rowing machine. Keep in mind the limitations of such gadgets, and of your patience. Be sure that your interest in an activity is fairly well established before you make an investment of any kind, whether it be in these devices, membership in a club, or sports equipment. Your initial enthusiasm may wane rapidly.

In fact, fitness need not be a commercial venture at all. Joining a club or enrolling in a commercial program is not your only option. You can design your own training program and arrange a schedule for running, cycling, swimming, skiing, or any other activity to suit your needs.

SUMMARY

1. Today, as never before, people in the United States are devoting time and energy to achieving *physical fitness*. Health statistics, especially those that show a high rate of cardiovascular-related deaths among inactive people, have prompted the current drive toward physical fitness.

2. There is no universal standard of physical fitness. The President's Council on Physical Fitness and Sports has determined that a minimum of three exercise periods a week, each at least thirty minutes long, is sufficient to maintain physical fitness. However, individuals must decide what their capabilities are, what amount of exercise will increase their efficiency, endurance, and general physical and emotional health, and what activities they enjoy enough to sustain their interest.

3. *Aerobic capacity*, or ability to deliver oxygen to the body, affects energy output. Only those activities that place a sustained and uniform demand on the *cardiovascular* and *respiratory systems* can improve aerobic capacity and physical fitness.

4. Physical fitness has been found to improve mental well-being. There is evidence that many emotional disorders respond to exercise therapy.

5. One should have a physical checkup before engaging in an exercise program. During any program it is important to *warm up*, achieve the *training level*, *avoid exhaustion*, *plan a gradual progression* in capacity, *tone down*, *maintain regularity* in participation, and allow for sufficient *recovery* time after each period of physical activity. Good sleeping habits are also an important aspect of a physical fitness program.

6. For an activity session to produce benefits, the level of exertion needed to achieve the *training effect* must be taken into consideration. Although *competition* (with others or with one's own previous performance) is inspiring, it can prompt overexertion and induce injury.

7. The physical fitness boom has encouraged many previously uninvolved groups to participate. Traditionally, *women* have taken a back seat in many sports activities, but the women's movement and new laws have mandated equal facilities in schools; and a virtual revolution is taking place in the training and participation of women in sports. More *men and women over 50* are taking part in physical fitness activities and in competitive sports. Many are enjoying such activity well into their 80s, with a concurrent improvement in general health.

8. Buyers of sports and *body-building* equipment, as well as of *health club* plans, should be wary of high-pressure sales tactics. They should carefully consider what their needs and long-standing interests are before purchasing a fitness plan or expensive athletic equipment.

CONSUMER CONCERNS

1. What athletic clothing and sports equipment do you really need? Can you get along without a jogging suit or gravity boots? Are salespeople reliable sources of information about sports equipment?
2. Do you need to join a health club or participate in a commercial physical program in order to keep fit? What sports activities can you cite that can be conducted on public facilities without paying fees?
3. Would you advise signing a membership contract with a health club on the first visit?
4. Are you sure the person who wrote that book on weight training is really an authority on the subject? What is the author's background? What kind of evidence does the author put forward to support his or her claims or advice?

5

Nutrition

Eating Patterns
The Basic Nutrients
How Much Is Enough?
Calories
The Basic Food Groups
Health Foods and Food Fads
Shopping for Nutrition

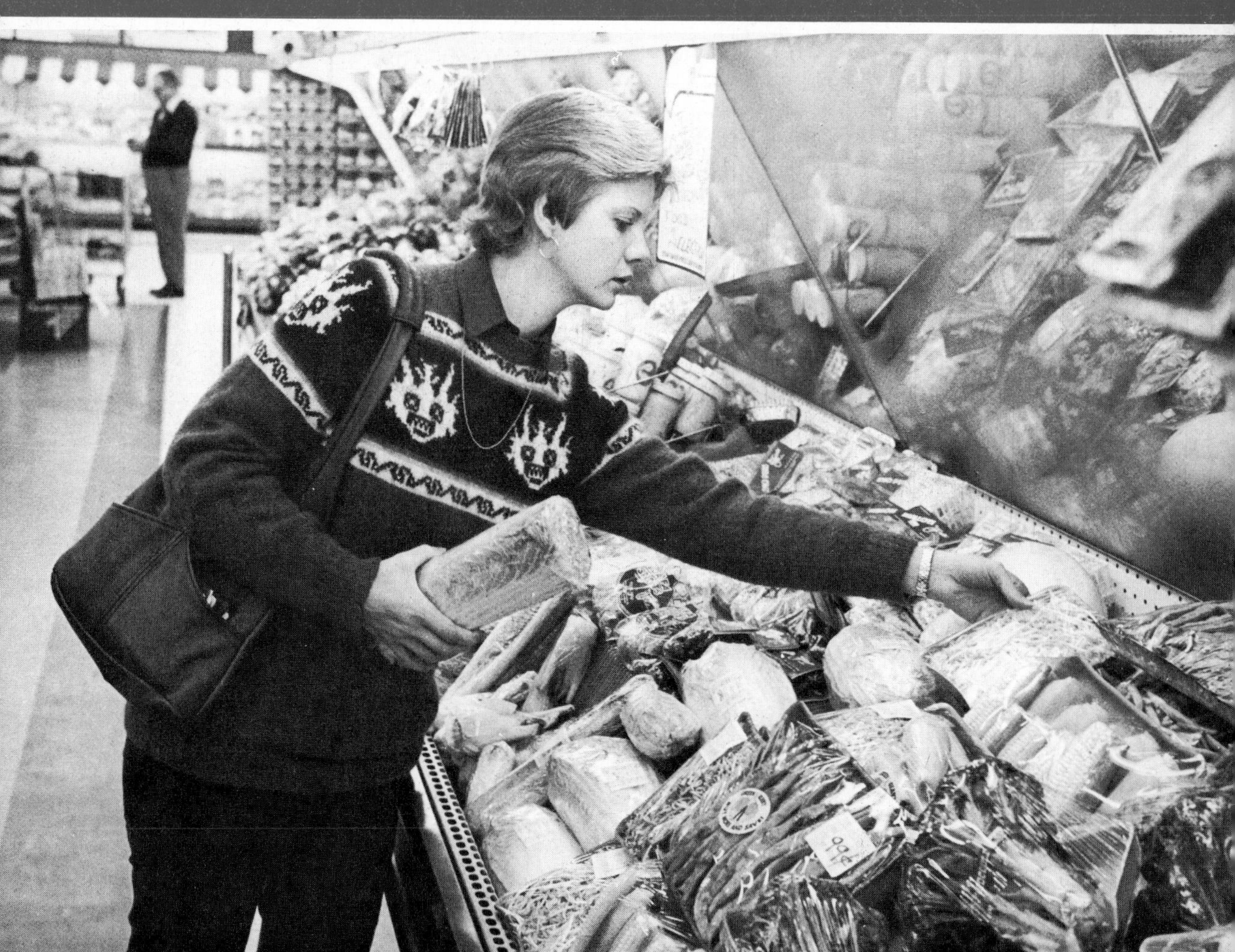

America's eating habits are being guided less and less by nutritionists and more and more by entrepreneurs operating in the vast food industry. Food industry propaganda encourages children to consume sugar-saturated cereals and soft drinks and to ingest salt-laden junk foods. The fast-food industry would have us believe that french fries, onion rings, grilled hamburgers, and hot dogs constitute a balanced diet. And the so-called health-food industry distracts our attention from sensible nutrition by promoting such dubious items as kelp, lecithin, and ginseng.

The search for valid nutritional guidelines is complicated further by the huge number of diet books, newspaper columns, and magazine articles that appear daily. Paid advertisements for commercial products have more influence over our food choices than does the information provided by qualified individuals and agencies. The battle for access to the American stomach—and pocketbook—is quite clearly being won by large business interests.

Countless studies have shown that many Americans do not eat a nutritionally adequate diet for normal growth and development. Americans now eat fewer dairy products, fruits, and vegetables and more baked goods and soft drinks (both full of empty calories) than they did a generation ago. (The consumption of soft drinks has tripled since 1960.) This trend is particularly noticeable among college students, whose eating schedules and food choices are often more influenced by convenience than by nutritional considerations.

The most sensible way to counter these unfortunate trends is to inform ourselves about what nutrients we need and the best way to obtain them. That is the purpose of this chapter.

EATING PATTERNS

Nutritional deficiencies can be found in rural as well as urban populations. As might be expected, people's income levels partly determine whether they receive an adequate diet. Most dietary deficiency occurs among the poor, but this is often a matter of poor eating patterns rather than an inability to purchase enough food.

If we ate only from a desire to provide our bodies with the necessary nutrients, we would have no nutritional problems. But of course we eat for a variety of other reasons. Many of us eat to console ourselves when we are frustrated or unhappy. At other times, we reward ourselves for a job well done by devouring an extra piece of pie. Convenience in food preparation also affects our eating patterns. Many of us do not take the time to prepare adequate and balanced meals. Breakfast may consist of a rushed cup of coffee and a doughnut; dinner, a hamburger and french fries.

People learn their eating habits and patterns early in life. Because parents do not serve varied and balanced meals, children do not develop a taste for green vegetables and other nutritious foods. It takes a determined parent to serve liver and broccoli to a protesting child; most parents take the easy way out and give their children less nourishing food.

Advertising also heavily influences what foods people select. Unfortunately, the most widely advertised foods are often the least nutritious. Commercials aimed at children encourage the consumption of **empty-calorie foods**—that is, foods high in calories but low in proteins, vitamins, and minerals. These foods not only provide little or no nourishment but also spoil children's appetites for more nourishing meals.

As these examples suggest, food choices are influenced by many factors other than nutritional value. Some foods are loaded with emotional overtones and potent memories that make it difficult for us to sort out the propaganda and misinformation we hear about nutritional values. And contrary to the claims of some health faddists, we do not instinctively select an adequate diet because the body creates a yearning for those nutrients that it requires. It is habit, rather than the needs of the body, that creates food cravings. Many of us never appreciate how easy it is to stick to a well-balanced diet that is nutritious, simple to prepare, and satisfying to eat. Ironically, most common nutritional deficiencies may be corrected by merely including more vegetables and fruits in the diet. Putting this simple solution into practice, however, demands a major effort to overcome all the influences that have shaped our present eating patterns.

THE BASIC NUTRIENTS

Nutrition includes the entire process by which our bodies absorb and make use of foods. **Nutrients** are those substances in foods that sustain the body. Food is changed by the digestive process into nutrients, which are then absorbed into the bloodstream and carried to all parts of the body.

Functions of Nutrients

Our bodies use nutrients for three basic functions: (1) to build and repair the body, (2) to regulate body processes, and (3) to furnish energy. Although the principal sources of nutrients can be linked to their main function, as in Table 5-1, each of the three functions is served by more than one category of nutrient. Energy, for example, comes from carbohydrates, fats, and proteins. There is, in fact, a great deal of interrelationship in the ways that the different nutrients nourish the body as a whole.

To Build and Repair the Body. Growth is based on the formation of new cells, for which a continual supply of protein is necessary. Protein in varying chemical combinations makes up the cells and tissues that are as different as blood, muscle, bone, skin, hair, and nerve. Although protein is the essential material of which each cell is composed, the characteristic quality of that cell is affected by the presence of specific minerals and vitamins. Probably the best-known illustration of the absorption of a mineral into the structure of a cell is the degree to which bone tissue is composed of calcium. Vitamins do not become a part of a cell in the same sense as minerals but are necessary to the absorption process. Adequate amounts of vitamin D, for example, are required for the absorption of calcium into the bone structure.

To Regulate Body Processes. Keeping our internal body processes balanced and under control is another function of nutrients. The same nutrients that build and repair the body—vitamins, minerals, and protein—perform this func-

TABLE 5-1
Principal Sources and Functions of Nutrients

Nutrient	Functions	Principal Sources	
Proteins	Build and repair the body Regulate body processes (Furnish energy)*	Beef Veal Pork Lamb Liver Poultry	Fish Milk Cheese Eggs Dried beans Peas
Carbohydrates	Furnish energy	Sugars Syrups Molasses Flour Flour products Bread	Crackers Cereal Potatoes Rice Noodles Other starchy vegetables
Fats	Furnish energy	Butter Lard Vegetable oils Shortening Margarine Salad dressings	Bacon Oils Nuts Cheese Cream Meat fats
Minerals	Build and repair the body Regulate body processes	(See Table 5-2)	
Vitamins	Regulate body processes	(See Table 5-3)	

* Although proteins provide energy, that is not their major function. Carbohydrates and fats are the principal sources of energy.

tion. Vitamins have the major role, and almost all the vitamins in our diet are used for this purpose. Minerals also, often working with vitamins, help regulate many processes; blood clotting is an example. Various forms of proteins are involved in body regulation: as enzymes, in hormones, and in hemoglobin. Enzymes, which are made of protein, do much to regulate the digestive system. Some protein-containing hormones control energy metabolism and other body processes; and hemoglobin, composed largely of protein, carries oxygen in the blood from the lungs to the tissues.

To Furnish Energy. Without energy, our hearts would stop beating, our lungs would cease to function. The energy for these activities and for all our physical actions comes from nutrients, mainly in the form of carbohydrates and fats. Some kinds of proteins are also energy sources. Although their most important role is in building and repairing the body, proteins have about the same capacity for producing heat and energy as do carbohydrates. On a practical scale:

1 gram carbohydrate	= 4 calories
1 gram protein	= 4 calories
1 gram fat	= 9 calories

All three sources—carbohydrates, fats, and proteins—provide energy by combining with oxygen in the cells.

About fifty specific nutrients are known to be required by the cells of the body. These required nutrients are grouped into six categories: proteins, carbohydrates, fats, minerals, vitamins, and water (see Table 5-1).

Protein

About 20 percent of normal body weight consists of protein. Hair, fingernails, eyeballs, skin, red blood cells, antibodies, enzymes, ova, sperm, muscle and nerve fibers—all the cells, tissues, and systems of the body, without exception, consist of protein substances.

What is **protein?** It is an organic compound (a compound containing carbon atoms) that is made up of amino acid molecules. Amino acid molecules, in turn, are composed of carbon, oxygen, hydrogen, and nitrogen atoms, plus very small quantities of other atoms such as sulfur and phosphorous.

We obtain protein primarily from meats, fish, eggs, milk and cheese, and legumes (beans and peas). The digestive system breaks down the proteins in these foods into their constituent amino acid molecules. These molecules then enter the bloodstream and are transported to the cells of the body, where they are recombined to form the body's solid substance.

There are about twenty-four different amino acid molecules in all. From these few building blocks, the cells construct the numerous complex substances that make up the body. The human body, however, can provide only about fifteen of the amino acids using its own chemical equipment. The other nine amino acids must be acquired ready-made in the foods we eat. These nine amino acids are called the **essential amino acids.** Because there is a great similarity between the chemical composition of the human body and that of other animals, eating animal proteins is an efficient method of acquiring all the essential amino acids. Animal proteins include meat, fish, poultry, eggs, milk, and cheese. Such foods contain the essential amino acids in the amounts and proportions required by the human body. They are sometimes called **complete protein foods.**

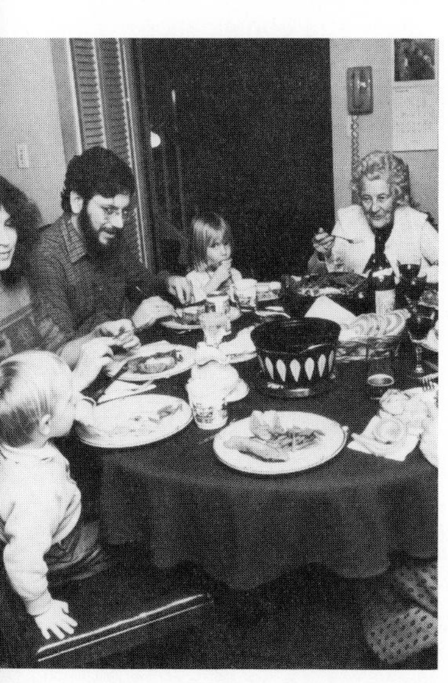

The essential amino acids can also be acquired by eating cereal grains, fruits, and vegetables; but the proportions of the essential amino acids in these proteins differ considerably from the proportions required by the body. It is necessary, therefore, to consume a variety of these foods in relatively large amounts in order to acquire the essential amino acids (see the section Vegetarianism, below).

Any reasonable diet containing meat, fish, legumes, eggs, or milk will provide all the amino acids necessary for good health. Unfortunately, amino acids, unlike carbohydrates and fats, cannot be stored in the body for future use. Proteins that the body cannot use at any given time are excreted. Protein intake, therefore, must be continuous; we need to eat proteins every day.

For most Americans, however, overconsumption, not underconsumption, of proteins is the problem. Nutritionists recommend that we limit our protein intake to about 12 percent of our daily calories, but, in fact, most of us consume twice that amount. Excess protein consumption can put a strain on the kidneys. And because many of the high-protein foods we eat are also high in fat and calories, overconsumption can lead to unwanted weight gain.

Carbohydrates

Carbohydrates are the body's principal source of energy. Chemically, carbohydrates are compounds of carbon, oxygen, and hydrogen atoms. The major sources of carbohydrates in the diet are plant roots, cereal grains, and sweet fruits. Nutritionists recommend that 55 to 60 percent of our daily calorie intake be made up of carbohydrates.

Fruits store their carbohydrates in the form of sugar. Vegetables store excess carbohydrates in their roots as **starch,** which is a complex form of sugar. These roots—potatoes, sweet potatoes, beets, and so on—are excellent sources of carbohydrates. So are the grains of cereal plants like wheat, rice, and corn. Products made from these plants, such as breads and pastries, pasta, and breakfast cereals, also provide carbohydrates.

Dietary fiber, often called roughage, refers to the parts of grains, vegetables, and fruits that cannot be broken down by our digestive system (see box: Dietary Fiber). It is, in effect, nondigestible carbohydrate. Fiber is important to our

PROBLEMS AND CONTROVERSIES: Dietary Fiber

"If eating more fiber prevents cancer, then, believe me, I'm eating more fiber," intones the woman in the prime-time TV ad. For the last decade or so, messages like this have been popping up everywhere in the media, leading millions of Americans to wolf down their morning Raisin Bran with a new earnestness. Health experts have made extravagant claims about the benefits of a high-fiber diet, presenting it as a cure-all for everything from heart disease to colon cancer to schizophrenia.

What lies behind these claims and should you necessarily be eating more fiber? The fact is that the fiber *is* good for you, but it is more often the fiber found in fruits and vegetables such as cabbage, unpeeled apples, and fresh carrots, than that found in grains and cereals. Diets high in fruit and vegetable fibers have been shown to lower blood cholesterol levels, reduce blood pressure, control blood sugar levels in diabetics, and help prevent intestinal ailments such as diverticulosis (an inflammation of pouches in the colon) and constipation. There is some evidence, too, that a high-fiber diet prevents cancer of the colon; it is discussed in Chapter 14.

Too much fiber, on the other hand, can be bad for you. It can give you intestinal and stomach pains, gas, and nausea. It may even prevent your body from absorbing important minerals.

Instead of taking fiber pills or adding special fiber supplements to your diet, you are better off eating plenty of foods that are naturally high in fiber: fruits, vegetables, nuts, breads, cereals, and grains.

Sources: Adapted from Jane E. Brody, *The New York Times Guide to Personal Health* (New York: Avon Books, 1983), pp. 36–39; Barbara Harland and Annabel Hecht, "Grandma Called It Roughage," *The FDA Consumer* (July–August 1977), HHS Publication No. (FDA) 78-2087.

Good Nutrition: What You Can Do

- Make about 55 to 60 percent of your total intake of calories carbohydrates. Be sure that a substantial proportion (40 to 45 percent) comes from complex carbohydrates: whole grains, fruits, and vegetables.
- Keep sugar consumption at about 15 percent of your total intake of calories.
- Reduce overall fat consumption.
- Keep your consumption of saturated fats to about 10 percent of your total intake of calories; unsaturated fats should account for no more than 20 percent. Substitute nonfat milk for whole milk. Eat few foods rich in cholesterol, such as butterfat and eggs.
- Keep salt consumption at about 3 grams a day. (A gram of salt is about one-third of a teaspoon.)
- Eat more fish and poultry than other kinds of meat.

diet because it stimulates the normal action of the digestive system. In addition, bowel movement is aided by the presence of fiber through the retention of water, which softens the feces. The inclusion of fresh fruits, vegetables, and cereals in our daily diet provides an adequate supply of such roughage.

Conversion of Starch and Sugar. The digestive system converts carbohydrates into simple sugar molecules such as **glucose, fructose,** and **galactose.** These molecules are absorbed into the bloodstream and immediately transported to the liver, which controls their distribution through the body.

Glucose that remains stored in the liver is converted into a more compact compound called glycogen. The muscles also store glucose in the form of glycogen; they can quickly convert it into glucose when they need extra fuel.

Glycogen stored in the liver serves as a reserve supply of energy for the entire body. If the intake of carbohydrates is excessive, the reserves build up and excess glycogen is then converted into an even more compact source of energy—fat. The fat passes into the bloodstream, comes to rest within different tissues, and is stored in these tissues as a secondary energy reserve.

Fats

Fats and **oils** belong to the same chemical group. A fat is solid at room temperature; an oil is liquid. Fats and oils are converted into fatty acids and glycerol, which are then absorbed into the bloodstream through the digestive system. Chemically, a fat is solid because all the possible chemical linkages between its molecules are occupied by hydrogen atoms; fats are therefore said to be **saturated.** Oils are liquid because not all the potential chemical linkages are occupied by hydrogen atoms; oils are therefore **unsaturated.**

Like carbohydrates, fats consist of carbon, oxygen, and hydrogen atoms. Also like carbohydrates, fats are a source of energy to the body; but a fat molecule supplies more energy than a carbohydrate molecule. Because of the greater number of calories per unit of weight, people who eat too many fatty foods gain more weight than people who eat the same amount of carbohydrates.

TABLE 5-2
The Principal Minerals

Mineral	Principal sources	Functions	Result of deficiency
Calcium	Leafy vegetables, milk, and milk products	Essential for blood clotting, nerve function, and healthy bones and teeth	Rickets, stunted growth, poorly developed bones and teeth, nerve irritabilities such as cramps, twitching
Iron	Shellfish, liver, meat, legumes, dried fruits, egg yolk	Necessary for hemoglobin in red blood cells, and enzymes of cellular respiration	Iron deficiency anemia
Iodine	Iodized salt, shellfish	Essential to thyroid hormone	Goiter, slow metabolism
Phosphorus	Whole-grain cereals and breads, liver, meat, beans, cottage cheese, milk, broccoli	Essential for cell metabolism, building of bones and teeth, functioning of many enzymes	Rickets, poor tooth and bone formation, stunted growth, loss of weight, weakness
Fluorine	Fluoridated drinking water	Strengthens teeth and bones, protects against tooth decay	

Most of the fats in our diet come from meats and milk or milk products, while most of the oils come from processed corn, olives, cottonseeds, soybeans, and nuts. Vegetable oils are used in shortening, margarine, and cooking and salad oils. Lecithin, which is a part of cell membranes and nerves and which aids in digestion, is produced by the body from fats such as those in egg yolk. (Lecithin supplements purchased at a health food store do not enhance body functions, however, and are a waste of money.) Unsaturated fats are the body's source of a fatty acid, linoleic acid, that is essential to growth. Saturated fats, on the other hand, have been implicated in the high levels of cholesterol associated with heart disease (see Chapter 13). Nutritionists recommend that we get no more than 30 percent of our daily calories from fats, but most of us get much more.

About 10 percent of normal body weight is fat. Fat pads the skin, acting as insulation that helps conserve body heat. The marrow in our bones is largely composed of fat. And fat is packed around the kidneys and other organs, protecting them against shock and injury. The eye sockets are lined with a cushion of fat to help prevent damage to the eyes. The bulging eyes of the very overweight are caused by an excessive buildup of fat within the eye sockets; the hollow eyes of the starving are the result of the disappearance of this fatty cushion. Excess body fat is considered further in Chapter 6, Weight Control.

Minerals

Minerals account for only about 6 percent of total body weight, but they are vital for normal development and for regulation of metabolic processes. So far, fourteen of the minerals found in the body have been proved essential in human nutrition. They are: calcium, phosphorus, iron, sodium, zinc, copper, potassium, sulfur, manganese, magnesium, cobalt, iodine, fluorine, and chlorine. In addition, the body contains traces of such elements as aluminum, silicon, and nickel. From a practical nutritional standpoint, however, we need only be concerned with the three minerals most likely to be deficient in the American diet: calcium, iron, and iodine. If we eat foods rich in these important minerals, we will also be getting adequate amounts of phosphorus, magnesium, sodium, and other essential minerals. The prime sources and functions of the five principal minerals are outlined in Table 5-2.

Vitamins

Strictly speaking, vitamins are not nutrients, since they are not materials the body can convert to energy. Actually, **vitamins** are complex chemical compounds that are necessary for the normal functioning of the body. Many vitamins work with **enzymes,** complex organic compounds that bring about chemical change.

Although the term *vitamin* was not coined until the twentieth century, the fact that specific foods prevent certain illnesses was known in ancient times. Three thousand years ago the Egytpians realized that **night blindness** could be prevented by eating liver (which is rich in vitamin A). In the sixteenth century an Austrian physician discovered that **scurvy,** a disease that affects the gums, teeth, and mucous membranes, could be prevented by eating citrus fruits (which contain vitamin C). In 1795 the English navy first insisted that its sailors drink lime and lemon juices to prevent this disease—hence the popular term *limeys*, used in reference to British seamen. In the 1880s the Japanese navy began to include more meat and vegetables in the diet of its sailors because it was realized that a diet largely dependent on polished rice was the cause of **beriberi,** a painful nerve disease. We now know that it is a shortage of vitamin B_1 that is responsible for this disease.

In the beginning of this century, when deficiency diseases first began to be identified, vitamins were labeled with the letters of the alphabet. As more and more vitamins were discovered, scientists realized that there were probably more than twenty-six vitamins and began referring to them by their chemcial names. There are, for example, at least twelve vitamins included in the vitamin B complex. From a nutritional viewpoint, the most important vitamins are **vitamins A, C, D,** and three of the **B complex** vitamins—**thiamine, riboflavin,** and **niacin.** Table 5-3 lists ten principal vitamins, their chief sources and functions, and the results of their deficiency in human beings.

TABLE 5-3
The Principal Vitamins

Vitamin	A	B_1 or (B), (Thiamine)	B_2 or (G), (Riboflavin)	Niacin
Principal Sources	Milk, eggs, butter, green leafy and yellow vegetables, fish-liver oils, liver	Meat (pork and liver), nuts, egg yolks, potatoes, most vegetables, legumes, yeast, whole grains	Milk, cheese, beef muscle, egg white, liver, organ meats	Liver, organ meats, yeast, peanuts, wheat germ
Functions	Creates healthy skin; necessary for tooth structure, growth, and night vision	Necessary for normal nerve functioning and carbohydrate metabolism; promotes growth	Essential for cell metabolism; promotes general health, good growth	Essential for metabolism, growth, normal skin
Result of Deficiency	Dry skin, poor teeth and gums, slow growth, night blindness, lack of tears in eyes	Loss of appetite, slow growth, improper digestion of carbohydrates, poor nerve function. beriberi	Sensitivity to light, anemia, inflamed lips, weakness	Pellagra, skin irritation, rash, inflammation of tongue, digestive disturbances, diarrhea, nervous disturbances

Water

The human body is about 62 percent water. Although not properly a nutrient itself, **water** allows the chemical machinery and life processes of the body to work. All the chemical reactions of the body take place in a liquid medium. The water content of the body enables the digestive system to break down the foods we eat into their constituent molecules, and then makes it possible for the cells of the body to construct solid tissue from these molecules. Water enables enzymes to transform foods into a form cells can use. Water also makes possible the conduction of nerve impulses and enables the body to maintain a stable temperature. It is the water content of blood that allows nutrients, hormones, and other substances to be transported into the cells and waste products to be removed from the cells.

Though fruits and vegetables supply some water, an adult should drink the equivalent of six to eight glasses of water a day. Soft drinks, artificial fruit drinks, beer, and wine are not satisfactory substitutes. Not only do they add calories, but soft drinks contribute to tooth decay.

HOW MUCH IS ENOUGH?

How much of each nutrient does a person normally need? The latest recommendations of the Food and Nutrition Board form the basis of the RDA (**recommended daily allowance**) labels now required on many food products. They are summarized in Table 5-4.

B_6 (Pyridoxine)	B_{12} (Cyanoco-balamin)	C (Ascorbic acid)	D	E	K
Fish, vegetables, molasses, yeast, liver, whole grains	Liver, beef, pork, organ meats, eggs, milk	Citrus fruits, tomatoes, potatoes, green peppers, cabbage	Sunlight, butter, eggs, milk, fish liver oils	Vegetable oils, lettuce, eggs, cereal products, wheat germ	Eggs, liver, leafy green vegetables, tomatoes
Essential for amino acid metabolism and functioning of cells	Essential for production of red blood cells, growth, and nerve functioning	Necessary for healthy teeth, gums, bones, blood vessels; essential for cellular metabolism	Essential for metabolism of calcium and phos-phorus, normal bone and tooth development	Not known	Essential for blood clotting
Skin lesions, nerve inflammation, anemia	Pernicious anemia, retarded growth, disorders of nervous system	Scurvy, poor teeth, weak bones, bleeding gums, easy bruising	Rickets, badly formed tooth and bone struc-ture, soft bones	Abnormal fat deposits in muscles	Slow blood clotting, anemia

Note that the RDAs are not the *minimum* nutritional requirements for good health, but rather the *average* amounts of nutrients needed in order to maintain good health. The recommendations are broken down by sex and age, and are for a person of "average" weight and height within those groupings. Those whose height and weight differ from the average have to make some adjustments in the nutritional recommendations.

CALORIES

A person needs energy and so burns calories in order to think, eat, sleep, wake, dress, wash, exercise—in other words, to exist. It is possible to measure the energy content of any food by measuring the amount of heat it gives off when it is burned. The unit of measurement used in this calculation is the **calorie.**

Energy requirements vary with the daily physical output of each person. A man of average weight with a physically taxing occupation may require a total of about 4,300 calories or more to meet his energy needs over a full twenty-four-hour day. A smaller man with a sedentary occupation may require only 2,300 calories a day. Table 6-1, on page 135, gives the average daily caloric requirements for people of various ages. Table 6-2, on page 136, gives the average expenditure of calories for various activities.

TABLE 5-4
Recommended Daily Dietary Allowances for Adults

	Males			Females*		
	Age 19–22	*Age 23–50*	*Age 51+*	*Age 19–22*	*Age 23–50*	*Age 51+*
Weight (lb)	154	154	154	120	120	120
Height (in)	70	70	70	64	64	64
Protein (gm)	56	56	56	44	44	44
Fat-soluble vitamins:						
Vitamin A (μg RE)	1,000	1,000	1,000	800	800	800
Vitamin D (μg)	7.5	5	5	7.5	5	5
Vitamin E (mg α TE)	10	10	10	10	10	10
Water-soluble vitamins:						
Vitamin C (mg)	60	60	60	60	60	60
Thiamine (mg)	1.5	1.4	1.2	1.1	1.0	1.0
Riboflavin (mg)	1.7	1.6	1.4	1.3	1.2	1.2
Niacin (mg NE)	19	18	16	14	13	13
Vitamin B_6 (mg)	2.2	2.2	2.2	2.0	2.0	2.0
Folacin (μg)	400	400	400	400	400	400
Vitamin B_{12} (μg)	3.0	3.0	3.0	3.0	3.0	3.0
Minerals:						
Calcium (mg)	800	800	800	800	800	800
Phosphorus (mg)	800	800	800	800	800	800
Magnesium (mg)	350	350	350	300	300	300
Iron (mg)	10	10	10	18	18	10
Zinc (mg)	15	15	15	15	15	15
Iodine (μg)	150	150	150	150	150	150

* Nonpregnant, nonlactating.
Source: Adapted from Food and Nutrition Board, National Academy of Sciences–National Research Council, *Recommended Dietary Allowances*, 9th ed. (Washington, D.C.: National Academy Press, 1980).

THE BASIC FOOD GROUPS

How is it possible to make up balanced and nutritious meals if a person has to take into account so many different nutrients and calories? One widely accepted system is to break down all the foods we eat into four **basic food groups** and then plan our meals to include some from each of these groups. The four major groups are: (1) meats, (2) milk, (3) fruits and vegetables, and (4) grains. The amounts from each group that are recommended for daily intake are listed in Table 5-5.

Meat Group

This group includes all the meats: beef, veal, pork, lamb, poultry, and fish. Included also are eggs, nuts, and legumes, which may be eaten as alternatives to meats.

All foods in the meat group are primary sources of protein. They are also

TABLE 5-5
USDA Daily Food Guide

Milk Group	Vegetable-Fruit Group
No. of servings: 2	*No. of servings*: 4
1 cup milk or yogurt	½ cup vegetable
1⅓ oz cheddar or Swiss cheese	½ cup juice
1 cup cottage cheese	1 typical piece of fruit
Meat Group	**Grain Group**
No. of servings: 2	*No. of servings*: 4
2–3 oz meat, fish, or chicken	1 slice bread
1 cup cooked legumes	1 oz ready-to-eat cereal
2 eggs	1 roll
2 oz nuts	¾ cup pasta
4 tbs peanut butter	

Source: U.S. Department of Agriculture, *Food*, Home and Garden Bulletin 228.

excellent sources of iron, thiamine, riboflavin, and niacin. An outstandingly rich source of minerals and vitamins is liver, followed closely by heart and kidney—three meats that are not very popular in the United States.

Two servings from the meat group should be eaten daily. But note that a serving is not large; two or three ounces of fish, poultry, or lean meat constitute one serving. (An average-sized hamburger contains four ounces of meat; if you had a hamburger for lunch, you have already eaten as much protein as you need for the day.) Two eggs also constitute one serving; so does a cupful of beans or peas. Four tablespoons of peanut butter—as in a thickly spread sandwich—also make up a serving.

Milk Group

The milk group includes cheese and ice cream as well as milk. While the foods in the milk group contain protein, riboflavin, and other vitamins and minerals, they are especially necessary for the calcium requirements of the body.

Children should have three to four cups of milk a day (an ordinary glass tumbler holds one cup.) Teenagers need four or more cups daily, and adults need two cups per day. If you don't care for plain milk, you can blend it into a drink or pour it over cereal or fruit. A piece of cheese roughly the size of two-thirds of a stick of butter is the equivalent of about two cups of milk.

Low-fat and skimmed milk and milk products contain as much calcium as whole milk, and their reduced fat and cholesterol makes them preferable for a healthy diet. Some people cannot digest the lactose contained in milk. This *lactose intolerance*, widespread among blacks, Jews, and Orientals, varies in severity. Some people who cannot tolerate large amounts of milk can eat cheese and yogurt without distress. Lactose-intolerant people can get the calcium they need from other sources (see box: Calcium Supplements, below).

The basic food groups

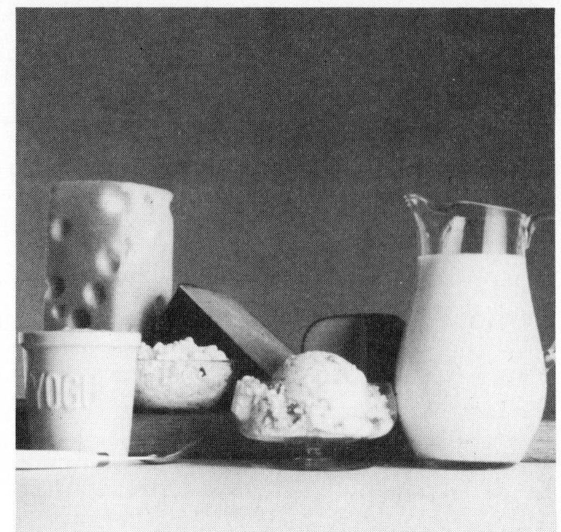

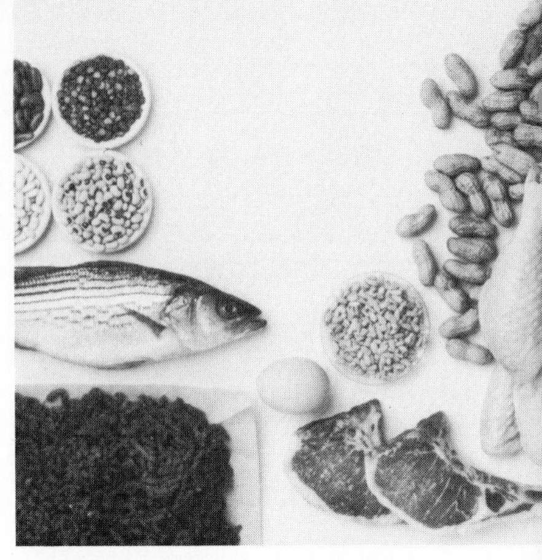

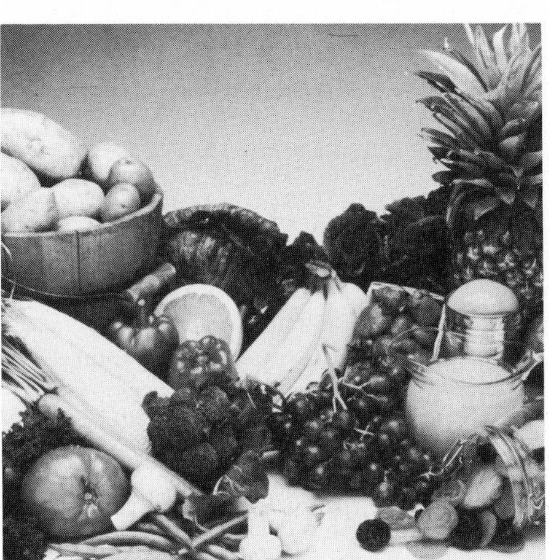

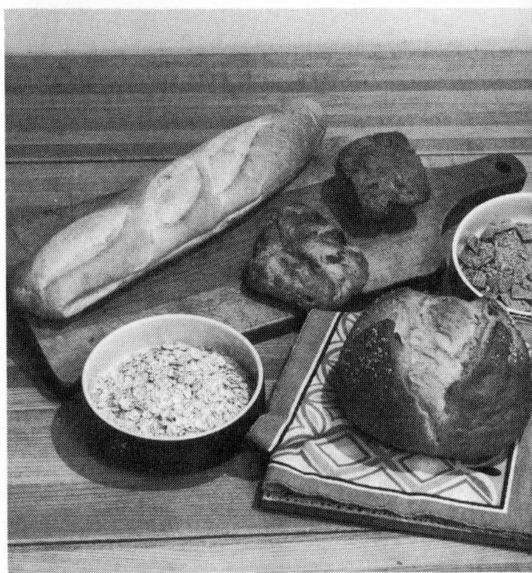

Fruit and Vegetable Group

The fruit and vegetable group supplies us with most of the vitamin A and vitamin C we need. Dark green vegetables generally contain more vitamin A, as well as larger amounts of calcium, iron, and riboflavin, than do lighter vegetables. Spinach, for example, is more nutritious than green beans. Fruits, especially lemons, oranges, and grapefruits, are excellent sources of vitamin C. Both fruits and vegetables are excellent sources of fiber.

Four or more servings from the fruit and vegetable group should be eaten daily. A grapefruit half, the juice of one orange, or about one-half cup of cooked vegetables constitutes a serving. An apple, a banana, a boiled potato, or half a cantaloupe also counts as one serving.

Grain Group

The grain group is an important source of carbohydrates as well as calcium, iron, the B vitamins, and some protein. It is also a source of fiber. Four servings from the grain group should be eaten daily. A slice of bread is one serving, as is one-half to three-quarters of a cup of cooked cereal, macaroni, noodles, rice, or spaghetti.

Meal Planning

Foods from the basic four groups can easily be apportioned into the three daily meals we are accustomed to eating (see Table 5-5). These food groups are also extremely flexible and allow for variety from one day to the next.

Notably absent from the suggestions offered are butter, margarine, oils, and desserts. These foods can be eaten occasionally; but unless you lead a very active life, they contain far too many calories to be eaten in large quantities. They will only turn into body fat.

Another point worth emphasizing is that the three daily meals should contain approximately equal amounts of food value. Too often people skimp on breakfast and save their appetite for a large evening meal. In fact, we need more energy during the day when we are working than in the evening when we are resting.

Varying the diet is in itself a guarantee of good nutrition. The wider the variety of foods we eat, the more assurance we have that we have taken in enough of the essential nutrients. The basic four concept is a guide within which to make our selections.

Eating an Adequate Breakfast

The California State Department of Public Health has identified seven practices that promote good physical health:

1. Sleeping 7 to 8 hours a night
2. Eating breakfast
3. Seldom if ever eating snacks
4. Controlling one's weight
5. Exercising
6. Limiting alcohol consumption
7. Never having smoked cigarettes

It may surprise you to see eating breakfast on the list, but nutritionists tell us that between a quarter and a third of our daily intake of calories and, especially, protein should occur at breakfast. Breakfasts that consist of toast and coffee or a typical cold cereal cannot be considered adequate. The only thing worse is no breakfast at all.

Eating an adequate amount of protein at breakfast provides us with the necessary energy to keep going until midday. Studies conducted on schoolchildren and on workers have come to the same conclusion: Both groups were found to maintain their level of work performance better throughout the morning hours if they had consumed an adequate breakfast.

A nutritious breakfast need not be a mammoth meal. A breakfast of orange juice, a soft-boiled egg, toast, and a glass of milk would be sufficient. (Though eggs need not be avoided completely in an effort to reduce cholesterol intake, nutritionists suggest that they be eaten no more than twice a week.) Cheese is a good protein food, and cottage cheese with fruit is an excellent combination. Chili con carne is as good at breakfast as it is at dinner.

Whatever your choice, keep in mind that breakfast is an important meal of the day.

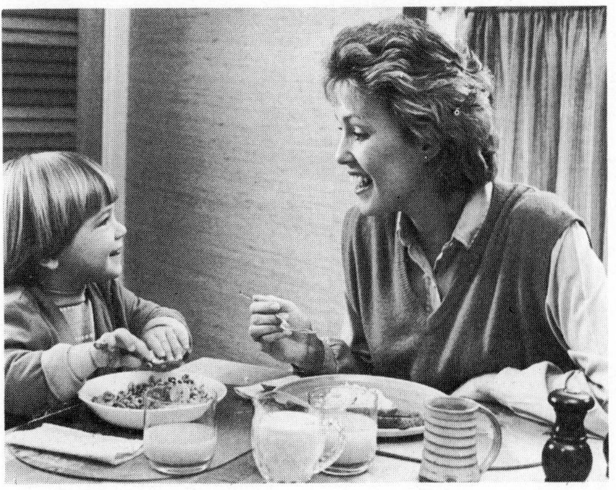

HEALTH FOODS AND FOOD FADS

Once a certain food is eaten, its original form is irrelevant. All proteins are reduced to amino acid molecules; all fats to fatty acid molecules; all carbohydrates to glucose molecules. Yet some people believe that certain foods are transported directly to a special part of the body, where they perform a service that the body cannot otherwise perform for itself. One superstition, for example, is that fish is a brain food. From what we know of digestion, it is obvious that the nutrients in fish could not possibly go directly to the brain. In a sense, all foods are brain foods, or none are.

Some people believe that certain combinations of food are harmful, or that the nutrients in certain foods are blocked if they are eaten in combination

Nutrition and Fast Foods

The nutrient contents of many fast foods have recently been analyzed by diet experts. They report that while most fast-food items *do* provide protein, carbohydrates, fats, and various vitamins and minerals, they also contain:

- Too many calories
- Too much salt
- Too much sugar
- Too much saturated fat and cholesterol from animal sources
- Too little vitamin A and vitamin C

Most fast-food restaurants offer few vegetables, fruits, and whole grains and thus do not provide the requisites for a balanced diet. If you rely on fast foods for most of your meals, you should supplement your diet with foods that give you enough fiber, vitamins, and minerals.

Source: Chris Lecos, "What About Nutrients in Fast Foods?" *The FDA Consumer* (May 1983), HHS Publication No. (FDA) 83-2172.

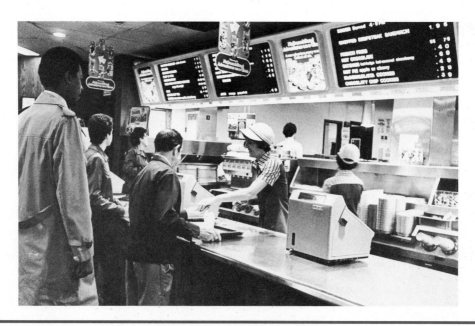

with other foods. Some of these harmful food combinations are said to be fish and milk, milk and shellfish, and buttermilk and cabbage. Although we may balk at eating certain combinations of food, the stomach accepts all good food with impartiality. Fundamentally, people who subscribe to food fads are unusually concerned about their health, and this makes them easy victims of misinformation or fraudulent claims. At various times, blackstrap molasses, wheat germ, honey, vinegar, and yeast have been touted as cure-alls or sources of all the nutrients necessary for health. In fact, the only ailments food may "cure" are those caused by specific deficiencies; and no one food, however nutritious, can supply all the necessary nutrients.

Today Americans are constantly subjected to a barrage of misleading advertising claims. We are told, for example, that we need vitamin and mineral supplements in our diets in order to remain healthy and vigorous. Just how susceptible to such advertising we have become is attested to by the flourishing health-food industry. The mainstay for most health-food stores is the sale of vitamins, which can account for as much as 90 percent of their business. They also carry products of such dubious worth as "natural potato chips" and bee pollen, which will supposedly add vim and stamina to our constitutions. They push claims for such questionable substances as lecithin (a soy product that supposedly unclogs the arteries), kelp, and rose hips. The arguments used by many health-food store supporters are patently absurd, when not downright fraudulent. Some devotees claim that natural foods are better assimilated by the body than processed foods because processors "pulverize the food"—a claim unsupported by any scientific research. Some "no salt" or "saltless" products are actually laced with miso, soy sauce, or some other high-sodium additive.

The very term *health food* is misleading, for it implies that foods bought from common sources are not healthy. When confronted with claims of the superiority of health foods, wise consumers will maintain their skepticism. Any diet that includes proper amounts of foods from the four basic groups will contain more than enough of the nutrients and vitamins necessary for good health. The purchase of such foods is best made in a regular grocery store, where prices are lower than in stores specializing in "health foods" and the variety of foods available is much greater.

We will now examine contemporary nutritional beliefs concerning vegetarianism, organically grown foods, natural foods, macrobiotics, and megavitamins.

Vegetarianism

People become vegetarians for reasons as diverse as a religious conviction about the sacredness of life or the simple belief that animal products are unhealthy. Some studies have shown that people who eat pure vegetarian diets, which are lower in fats than a normal diet, have a lower incidence of heart disease and cancer of the colon. There are degrees of vegetarianism, ranging from the strict **vegans,** who eat only fruits, vegetables, and grains, to the more permissive **lacto-ovo vegetarians,** who accept milk and eggs in their diets. Vegetarians must rely on a balanced combination of legumes, nuts, seeds, and grains for their protein (supplemented by dairy products, if their particular regimen allows them), and on dark green leafy vegetables (particularly if they are vegans) for their calcium. Otherwise their diet does not differ all that much from the mainstream. Frequently, however, people who become vegetarian are extremely health-conscious and impose additional restrictions on themselves, such as eliminating sugar and salt from their diets.

Approximately 5 million Americans practice vegetarianism. If practiced knowledgeably and sensibly, it can provide a perfectly safe and healthful diet, but there is no evidence that a vegetarian diet is in any way superior to a well-balanced diet that includes animal protein. It cannot be emphasized too strongly that vegetarians must carefully balance the amounts of essential amino acids in their meals in order to receive enough protein. In addition, a sufficient number of calories must be included to meet daily needs. If insufficient calories are consumed, protein is used as an energy source, thus depleting the supply that is essential for cell formation.

Even when exercising the utmost care, vegetarians cannot get vitamin B_{12} from a diet lacking any animal protein, and must take vitamin supplements. Pregnant women should be especially cautious because a strict vegetarian diet can impose this and other vitamin deficiencies on their children, not only during pregnancy, but afterward through breast feeding.

Organically Grown Foods and Natural Foods

Organically grown foods have been grown in soil enriched with natural instead of chemical fertilizers, have not been sprayed with pesticides, and have not had any artificial substances added to them. **Natural foods** are foods that contain no synthetic or artificial ingredients, and have undergone no more processing than is generally done in a home kitchen. Certain jams, jellies, baked goods, and so on are called natural foods if they have been made from organically grown products, have received minimal processing, and contain no preservatives or additives other than salt and sugar.

The organic- and natural-food fad started when people began to worry about what effect artificial chemicals might have on their health. However, even organically grown products have been shown to contain traces of artificial chemicals. Some proponents of organic foods claim that these foods are more nutritious than foods grown with chemical fertilizers. In fact, all fertilizers—natural or chemical—are broken down by food plants into the same inorganic elements. If anything, foods grown with chemical fertilizers may be somewhat more nutritious than "natural" foods, because chemical fertilizers are frequently designed to make up for deficiencies in the soil. Organically grown foods are usually more expensive than other commercially grown foods. Some producers of organic foods may have higher costs because, for example, they lose part of their crop to insects—a direct result of not using pesticides. But organically grown foods are often more expensive simply because their distributors want to cash in on this food fad. Fraud is another possibility; investigators have discovered ordinary foods being sold as organic foods—at a higher price.

Macrobiotics

A **macrobiotic diet** is one based mostly on grain, especially brown rice. It is less popular today than it was in the late 1960s and early 1970s. People who follow this diet drink little liquid and eat few dairy products. Meat, milk, and sugar are totally banned.

The macrobiotic diet has some advantages: cheapness, an absence of cholesterol, and a low calorie count. But these advantages are far outweighed by the disadvantages. The diet lacks essential nutrients. People who follow it strictly

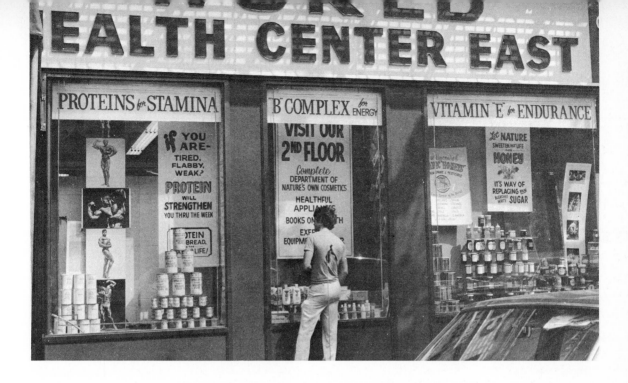

may develop symptoms of severe malnutrition; in fact, there are documented cases of persons on a macrobiotic diet dying from scurvy.

Megavitamins

Can large daily doses of vitamin C prevent the common cold? Will vitamin E supplements increase physical stamina and prevent heart attacks? Does extra vitamin B increase energy and keep hair from turning gray?

Anyone familiar with popular health literature has come across all of these claims (or strong implications of them in advertising.) Unfortunately, they are all unsupported by scientific evidence. As a 1978 Food and Drug Administration (FDA) report cautions, "Consumers should know that elaborate testimonials and miraculous claims result from mere guesswork, confusion, and often outright fraud."

Most vitamin myths are based on the unfounded assumption that if a little does good, a lot will do more good. For example, a vitamin A deficiency is known to cause dry skin; an adequate amount of vitamin A is therefore necessary to maintain healthy skin. This has been proven. But instead of a fantastic complexion, an excessive amount of vitamin A can cause bone damage. Vitamin B deficiency caused the hair of experimental rats to turn gray. When they resumed their normal diet, their hair color was restored. Can we conclude that large doses of vitamin B will prevent human hair from going gray? Alas, the evidence says no. In other studies male rats deprived of vitamin E became sterile, but attempts to treat human sterility with massive doses of vitamin E have proven futile.

But what about vitamin C? It has been widely promoted as a cure or preventative for the common cold. One study, in fact, showed evidence that massive doses may reduce the frequency and severity of colds by about 25 percent. In other studies, however, those who *thought* they were taking vitamin C reported better results than those who actually were taking it.

PROBLEMS AND CONTROVERSIES: Calcium Supplements

On your trips to the drugstore over the last year, you probably noticed that the shelves were awash with every conceivable form of calcium supplement, from dolomite to bone meal to oyster shells. The calcium craze is on: In 1985 alone, Americans spent over $200 million on calcium supplements.

It all started in 1984, when a panel of nutrition and medical experts announced that calcium, along with the hormone estrogen, could help to prevent osteoporosis, a condition in which the bones become porous, brittle, and susceptible to fracture. The disease occurs primarily in older women and it leads to more than a million fractured hips a year.

Authorities disagree over what causes the condition. While people whose diets are deficient in calcium do seem to develop osteoporosis more frequently, the fact that it affects postmenopausal women indicates that estrogen loss is just as important a factor; other experts think that lack of exercise also plays a large role.

Nevertheless, some extra calcium in your diet is no doubt beneficial. Although the RDA is 800 milligrams a day, most Americans take in only about 450 mg to 550 mg a day. Nutritionists are now recommending that this be increased to 1,000 mg to 1,500 mg a day, none of which has to come from a calcium supplement. The full daily complement of calcium can be gotten from a variety of high-calcium foods such as low-fat dairy products (yogurt is one of the best sources); vegetables such as broccoli, kale, and collard greens; and canned sardines with the bones left in. In addition, many packaged breads are now being fortified with calcium.

There are dangers in consuming too much calcium. Many dairy foods, for example, contain too much saturated fat. On the other hand, an overdose of calcium tablets can upset the balance of other vital minerals and cause stones in the urinary tract. Moreover, supplements made from bone meal and dolomite may contain dangerous levels of lead.

The current calcium craze points to a more general, widespread misperception about nutrition. Vitamins and minerals should not be thought of as isolated chemical compounds but as parts of an interdependent nutritional web. By becoming preoccupied with individual nutrients, we stop keeping track of how adequate our total diet is. If we maintain a balance between the four basic food groups and vary the foods within them, we do not need to take any vitamin or mineral supplements.

Sources: Adapted from "The Calcium Craze," *Newsweek*, January 27, 1986, pp. 48–52; Judith Willis, "Please Pass That Woman Some More Calcium and Iron," *The FDA Consumer* (September 1984), HHS Publication No. (FDA) 85-2198.

The vitamin question is far from settled. Research continues, and many more fantastic claims will undoubtedly be made by advocates and marketers of vitamins. So far, however, tests indicate that **megavitamins**—vitamins in abnormally large doses that exceed the nutritional requirements of the body—have little or no value for normal individuals; on the contrary, they may have negative effects. Too much vitamin D, for example, can lead to the deposit of calcium in soft tissue; and large doses of vitamin C have been blamed for causing kidney stones. Vitamin poisoning is a very real danger for individuals who overindulge in the use of vitamins. Children are especially vulnerable. In reality, the ingestion of vast amounts of vitamins is a form of drug abuse. These individuals are literally vitamin "junkies."

In some conditions—pregnancy, for example—people do need vitamin supplements. But most people can get all the vitamins they need simply by eating a balanced diet.

SHOPPING FOR NUTRITION

When faced with the thousands of products on supermarket shelves, nutrition-conscious shoppers may feel bewildered. The first thing to remember is that price is no guide; most foods of the same type have equal amounts of nutritional value. Pound for pound, ground chuck has as much food value as the most expensive filet mignon. It is therefore more sensible to buy cheaper cuts of meat when making hamburger, stews, and pot roasts, and save the filet mignon for special occasions. Organ meats, such as liver, heart, and kidneys, have more food value than the more expensive meats. For example, liver is about four times more nutritious than an equal amount of lamb or ham.

Eggs served scrambled or used in cooking need not be top grade. Grade A eggs are not any more nutritious than those with a lower quality rating. The difference in the size of eggs is frequently due to water content. Therefore smaller eggs are equal in nutritional value to large eggs, and they are at least 25 percent cheaper. Medium-sized eggs are equal in nutritional value to large eggs and are about 12 percent cheaper.

Dry milk has the same food value as whole milk and is much cheaper. Ice cream and cream cheese, on the other hand, are more expensive than whole milk and yet contain only the same food value.

When bought in season, fresh fruits and vegetables offer the best value for the money. Canned or frozen fruits and vegetables necessarily lose some food value. The darker vegetables—deep green or deep yellow—contain larger amounts of vitamin A and offer better food value for the money than lighter ones. For example, there is as much vitamin A in one quarter cup of carrots as in four cups of peas or seven cups of corn. The best fruits for vitamin C are lemons, oranges, and grapefruit. Green peppers, tomatoes, and potatoes are also good sources of vitamin C and may be less expensive. Dehydrated potatoes, however, contain no vitamin C and cost more than fresh ones.

Whole-grain cereals and breads offer greater food value than bread made from white flour, whether bleached or enriched. Many breakfast foods (corn flakes and puffed wheat, for example) have been so overprocessed that they are a very poor value for the money. The vitamins and minerals that manufacturers claim to have added increase the cost of these foods enormously. The best values among breakfast cereals are those made from whole grains. Artificially sweetened cereals and those to which dried fruits have been added cost more per pound and are not worth the added calories or extra money.

Food Additives

An **additive** is a substance blended into food that either restores something lost or represents a supplementary ingredient. According to the FDA, the most common food additives are sugar, salt, and corn syrup. These three, together with citric acid, baking soda, vegetable colorings, mustard, and pepper, constitute more than 98 percent of the food additives used in this country. Though they are harmless in themselves, some of them may be used excessively.

The main reasons for using additives are to improve flavor, give a more appetizing color, extend shelf life by retarding spoilage, and increase nutritional value. Obviously, not all of these objectives are of equal importance. Enhancing the flavor, appearance, and texture of a food may bring added enjoyment to consumers but this is clearly less vital than protection against botulism.

Either intentionally or accidentally, additives are introduced into our food at every stage in its production. Pesticides and chemical fertilizers (intentional additives) as well as radioactive fallout (incidental additives) are introduced

Food Labels

Nutrition labels on many food packages represent the government's and the food industry's current efforts to assist consumers in planning nutritious meals. But nutritional labels are not as easily understood as they might be. One area of consumer confusion is a misunderstanding of the United States Recommended Daily Allowances that form a standard for a part of nutritional labeling policy. The U.S. RDA for a given nutrient as listed on most foods comes from a table meant for children over four years of age and adults; it builds in a margin of safety for the average consumer by being based on the RDA for eighteen-year-old males, the group with the highest nutritional needs.

Federal law requires that when nutritional labeling is used, the following information must be provided in a specific order: serving size, servings per container, and energy, protein, carbohydrate, and fat content per serving. In addition, nutrient values for protein, vitamin A, vitamin C, thiamin, riboflavin, niacin, calcium, and iron expressed as percentages of the U.S. RDA are required. Additional information about some other vitamins and minerals may also be provided but is not mandatory. Manufacturers may also include information about saturated and unsaturated fat content, and cholesterol and sodium content as well.

Ingredient information is required on all manufactured food products, unless these products have a so-called standard of identity (that is, they conform to standard "recipes" that indicate specific levels of mandatory ingredients), such as mayonnaise. Ingredients must be listed on the label in order of decreasing weight in the product—that is, there is a greater amount of the ingredient listed first than the ingredient listed second, and so on down the list.

Source: Patricia A. Kreutler, *Nutrition in Perpective*, © 1980, pp. 420–23. Adapted by permission of Prentice-Hall, Englewood Cliffs, N.J.

NUTRITION INFORMATION PER SERVING

SERVING SIZE — 2 OZ. DRY
SERVINGS PER CONTAINER—8

CALORIES	210
PROTEIN	7 GRAMS
CARBOHYDRATE	41 GRAMS
FAT	1 GRAM

100 GRAMS OR A SERVING (2 OZ. DRY) OF THIS PRODUCT CONTAINS NOT MORE THAN 10 MG. OF SODIUM (MOISTURE FREE BASIS).

PERCENTAGE OF U.S. RECOMMENDED DAILY ALLOWANCES (U.S. RDA)

PROTEIN	10	RIBOFLAVIN	15
VITAMIN A	*	NIACIN	15
VITAMIN C	*	CALCIUM	*
THIAMINE	35	IRON	10

*CONTAINS LESS THAN 2% OF THE U.S. RDA OF THESE NUTRIENTS.

Boxed pasta

NUTRITION INFORMATION PER PORTION

PORTION SIZE	1 TABLESPOON (14 GRAMS)
PORTIONS PER CONTAINER	64
CALORIES	120
PROTEIN	0 GRAMS
CARBOHYDRATE	0 GRAMS
FAT	14 GRAMS
PERCENT OF CALORIES FROM FAT†	100%
POLYUNSATURATED†	8 GRAMS
SATURATED†	2 GRAMS
CHOLESTEROL†	(0 MG/100 G) 0 MILLIGRAMS
SODIUM	(0 MG/100 G) 0 MILLIGRAMS

PERCENTAGE OF U.S. RECOMMENDED DAILY ALLOWANCES (U.S. RDA)

VITAMIN E 15%

CONTAINS LESS THAN 2 PERCENT OF THE U.S. RDA OF PROTEIN, VITAMIN A, VITAMIN C, THIAMINE, RIBOFLAVIN, NIACIN, CALCIUM, IRON.

†INFORMATION ON FAT AND CHOLESTEROL CONTENT IS PROVIDED FOR INDIVIDUALS WHO, ON THE ADVICE OF A PHYSICIAN, ARE MODIFYING THEIR TOTAL DIETARY INTAKE OF FAT AND/OR CHOLESTEROL.

INGREDIENT: CORN OIL.

Corn oil

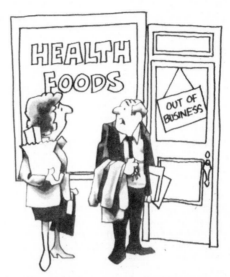

"All of our preservative-free foods rotted."

during the growing stage. At the processing stage nutrient supplements (such as iron, vitamins, or iodine) may be introduced. Also at this stage chemical compounds may be added in the form of nonnutritive sweeteners (or sugar substitutes); preservatives (to prevent spoilage); emulsifiers, stabilizers, and thickeners; flavors and flavoring agents; bleaching and maturing agents; and colors.

Are these chemical elements dangerous to our health? There is evidence that some are. Although the use of any food additive must be cleared with the Food and Drug Administration (except those the agency has already designated *GRAS*, or "generally recognized as safe"), the problem of testing additives is a difficult one. It is only possible to test a substance for known dangers, but unanticipated dangers can show up in later testing—after the substance has been put to use. Nitrites, for example, were widely used, with the FDA's approval, as preservatives in sausages, ham, and other foods until several experiments implicated these substances as possible cancer-causing agents. Sulfites are still widely used to preserve processed fruits and vegetables, breads, and a variety of other foods, but the FDA banned their use on fresh produce in 1985 after they were found to cause allergic reactions in some people.

It is foolhardy, however, to try to avoid using foods with additives or, in the extreme case, to call for a ban on all food additives—although the screening and testing procedures of the FDA must certainly be made more rigorous. Those additives with a purely cosmetic function should be eliminated from foods entirely, but the fact that an occasional substance is revealed to be a suspected carcinogen in experiments does not mean that all additives are hazardous.

On the contrary, the risk of poisoning from contaminated foods would be far greater if it weren't for preservatives. The ability to process, preserve, and

Problems and Controversies: The Irradiation of Fresh Fruits and Vegetables

In 1986 the Food and Drug Administration for the first time allowed the food industry to treat fresh fruits and vegetables with low levels of radioactive material in order to increase their shelf life. Foods are placed on a conveyor belt which travels through a protected area in which they are bombarded with radioactive cesium-137 to kill any insects, molds, or bacteria that might lead to spoilage. The foods themselves do not become radioactive.

There is no question that irradiation works. The FDA had earlier permitted the irradiation of pork to kill trichinae and of dried herbs to prevent insect infestation. But critics charged that not enough is known about the possible cancer-causing effects of the process to be sure that it is safe. They charged that the FDA had acted permaturely and that further tests were needed. Others pointed out that we are already producing tons of radioactive materials each year without adequate storage facilities for them. Is longer shelf life a good enough reason to permit yet another radioactive element to enter our environment?

Source: Adapted from Marion Burros, "Is Radiation the Answer to Spoiled Food?" *The New York Times,* April 16, 1986, p. C4.

transport foods that occurs through the use of these ingredients has enabled us all to enjoy a more varied and nutritious diet than would otherwise be possible.

Instead of worrying about esoteric elements added to our food, it is wiser to recognize the dangers posed by the known and common additives. Because salt and sugar are two of the three ingredients most frequently put in our foods, we can spend our time more productively by concentrating on these.

Sugar and Other Sweeteners

Sugar is the leading additive in American food. The consumption of sugar and other sweeteners in the United States today averages 127 pounds per person per year. According to the sugar industry, that's no more than it was fifty years ago. True, but deceptive. Fifty years ago was a peak time for sugar consumption. Before that it was lower and after that it was lower. Now it's climbing to a new peak.

Americans are not adding all this sugar to their food at home—only 13 percent of it, according to the U.S. Department of Agriculture. The other 87 percent is put into the food for us by the manufacturers. Tomato catsup is 29 percent sugar. Nondairy coffee creamers are over half sugar. Baby foods, hot dogs, salad dressings, frozen vegetables, and peanut butter are all more than likely to contain sugar or other sweeteners.

Of course, manufacturers use so much sugar because we the consumers like their products better that way. Often we don't realize how much sugar we are getting. If a breakfast cereal manufacturer lists the ingredients as rolled oats, sugar, wheat germ, corn syrup, barley, honey, dextrose, and salt, we may not realize that the sweeteners add up to more than 50 percent of the total.

The fact is that we are now getting about 24 percent of our calories from sugar and other sweeteners. Sugar has a definite link to tooth decay, an obvious relationship to obesity, and probably one to diabetes. There is little evidence, however, that sugar contributes to heart disease, except indirectly through obesity.

Sugar-Loaded Breakfast Cereals

The body needs one-third of its daily food requirements in the morning, not an overdose of nutritionally empty sugar. Yet that is what millions of children and adults get when they start the day with a bowl of sugar-coated cereal. Below is a list of ten cereals low in sugar, followed by some of the highest.

Source: U.S Department of Agriculture.

Cereal	*% Sugar by weight*	*Cereal*	*% Sugar by weight*
Lowest:		*Highest*:	
Puffed Rice	0.1	Sugar Smacks	56.0
Puffed Wheat	0.5	Apple Jacks	54.6
Shredded Wheat	0.6	Froot Loops	48.0
Cheerios	3.0	Sugar Corn Pops	46.0
Wheat Chex	3.5	Super Sugar Crisp	46.0
Corn Chex	4.0	Cap'n Crunch's Crunch Berries	43.3
Rice Chex	4.4	Cocoa Krispies	43.0
Kix	4.8	Cocoa Pepples	42.6
Post Toasties	5.0		
Grape-Nuts	7.0		

Nutritionally, there is no significant difference between white sugar and brown sugar (which is simply white sugar sprayed with molasses), corn syrup, honey, and other sweeteners. While none of these has been shown to be toxic in normal amounts, excessive intake of sugar will certainly not do you or your waistline much good.

Salt Salt, or sodium chloride, was probably the first food additive ever used when humans discovered its ability to flavor and preserve meat and fish. Salt is certainly one of the most popular additives, second only to sugar in the total quantity added to food each year.

Americans like salt. Each of us eats an average of ten to twelve grams (two to two and one-half teaspoons) of salt a day, most of it added during food processing. Since salt is about 40 percent sodium, that means that we consume about four or five grams a day of sodium—and it is the *sodium* content of food that is of concern to some people.

Sodium is an essential nutrient; in fact, we could not survive without it. It helps regulate body fluids (including blood) and maintain the balance of fluids and pressure inside and outside the cells. It also plays a major role in nerve impulse transmission, heart action, and the metabolism of carbohydrates and protein.

A daily human requirement for sodium is difficult to establish because the need fluctuates, depending on such conditions as excessive sweating and diarrhea (in which case additional sodium may be called for). Rather than recommend

Do You Use Too Much Salt?

_______ 1. How many times per week do you eat any of the following condiments: pickles, olives, soy sauce, ketchup, steak sauce, mustard?
0. 1 or less 1. 2 to 4 2. 5 to 7 3. 8 or more

_______ 2. On a typical day, how often do you add table salt to your food?
0. Never 1. 1 meal 2. 2 meals 3. 3 meals

_______ 3. Which would you most likely choose for a between-meal snack?
0. Fresh fruits or vegetables 1. Natural cheese 2. Donuts, pastries 3. (Salted) nuts, potato chips, pretzels.

_______ 4. How many times do you eat processed meats (hot dogs, sausage, cold cuts, etc.) in a given week?
0. None 1. 1 to 2 2. 3 to 5 3. Over 5

_______ 5. In an average week, how many times do you use baking soda and/or alkalizers (antacids, seltzers)?
0. None 1. 1 to 2 2. 3 to 5 3. Over 5

_______ 6. Which of the following would you be most likely to have for a quick meal?
0. Green salad without dressing 1. Roast beef or chicken sandwich or salad with dressing 2. Large hamburger or cup of canned soup 3. Ham sandwich or fried chicken

_______ 7. In an average week, how often do you eat any of the following: Canned soups, cubed beef broth, canned tomatoes, tomato sauce, cottage cheese, processed cheese?
0. 1 or less 1. 2 to 4 2. 5 to 7 3. 8 or more

_______ 8. In an average day, how many cans of diet soda do you drink?
0. None 1. 1 or 2 2. 3 or 4 3. 5 or more

_______ **Total**

Scoring: 0–6 points = Safe level of salt for normal healthy adults. 7–12 points = High. Over 5 times the required salt intake. 13–18 points = Very high. Over 15 times the required salt intake. 19–24 points = Dangerously high. Over 20 times the required salt intake.

a specific daily amount, the National Research Council of the National Academy of Sciences has estimated an "adequate and safe" sodium intake to be between 1,100 and 3,300 milligrams a day for adults. (One thousand milligrams equal 1 gram, so the estimate is between 1.1 and 3.3 grams, as opposed to the 4 to 5 grams per day Americans now consume.)

In the past few years the amount of sodium Americans consume has become a source of increasing concern to nutritionists, health professionals, and others who keep watch on the American diet. More and more evidence is linking excessive sodium intake with **hypertension**—high blood pressure—a disease that affects 10 to 20 percent of all Americans. Hypertension has been called a silent killer because it rarely produces warning signals, yet it can lead to stroke, heart disease, and kidney failure. Salt, of course, is not the sole cause of hypertension; rather, experts claim that salt intake should be of special concern to the 10 to 20 percent of Americans who are genetically susceptible to high blood pressure. For such persons, the hidden salt in processed food is a real hazard. For example, a hypertensive patient told by her physician to keep her sodium consumption down to two grams a day would find that a single serving of canned chicken noodle soup (about one and one-half cups) uses up over half her day's allowance of sodium—and to add to her difficulty, she would not find the salt content stated on the can label.

Besides canned and dried soups, some other processed foods that contain large amounts of sodium are canned tuna, canned vegetables, cheese, tomato juice, dill pickles, olives, sauerkraut, frozen dinners, and condiments such as soy sauce, catsup, and salad dressing.

The growing evidence about sodium has prompted public health watchers—such as the U.S. Surgeon General—to advise Americans that a reduction of salt intake would greatly improve their general health.

SUMMARY

1. A great many American eating habits are set by food industry advertising. This makes it all the more imperative that the public become nutritionally informed, particularly since studies have shown that many do not eat a sound diet.

2. *Nutrition* is the entire process by which our bodies absorb and make use of foods. *Nutrients* are those substances in food that sustain our bodies. Nutrients serve three basic functions: (1) building and repairing the body, (2) regulating body processes, and (3) supplying energy. The basic nutrients are proteins, carbohydrates, fats, minerals, vitamins, and water.

3. About 20 percent of body weight consists of *protein*, an organic compound made up of amino acid molecules. We obtain protein primarily from meats, fish, eggs, milk and cheese, and legumes. There are about twenty-four separate amino acid molecules in all, but the human body provides only fifteen of them through its own chemical processes. The other nine must be acquired ready-made in the foods we eat, and these nine are called the *essential amino acids*.

4. *Carbohydrates* are the body's principal source of energy. The digestive system converts carbohydrates into simple sugar molecules such as *glucose*, *fructose*, and *galactose*.

5. *Fats* and *oils* belong to the same chemical group. About 10 percent of normal body weight is fat.

6. *Minerals* account for only about 6 percent of total body weight, but they are vital for normal development and for regulation of metabolic processes. Fourteen of the minerals found in the body have been proved essential in human nutrition.

7. Strictly speaking, *vitamins* are not nutrients, because they cannot be converted to energy. Vitamins are actually complex chemical compounds that are necessary for the normal functioning of the body. In almost all cases, sufficient vitamins for human health can be obtained from a balanced diet.

8. Sixty-two percent of the human body is composed of *water*. Though it is not a nutrient, water allows the chemical machinery and life processes of the body to work.

9. The amount of nutrients people need depends upon each individual's age, weight, and activity. The energy content of food is measured by the amount

of heat it gives off when burned. This unit of measurement is called the *calorie*.

10. The *four basic food groups* are: (1) the meat group, which includes—in addition to red meat and poultry—fish, eggs, nuts, and legumes; (2) the milk group, including cheese and ice cream; (3) the fruit and vegetable group; and (4) the grain group. Foods from all four groups should be eaten daily.

11. Public concern about health issues has given rise to a *health-food industry* that purports to sell foods that promote health more readily than those found in general stores. Such claims must be regarded with great skepticism.

12. *Vegetarianism* is a viable alternative to the standard American diet, but practitioners must balance their nutrients carefully to receive sufficient protein and must supplement their diet with vitamin B_{12}.

13. *Organically grown* and *natural foods* are frequently said to be nutritionally superior, but there is no scientific evidence for it. A *macrobiotic* diet is based mostly on grains, and has proven harmful when adhered to strictly. The practice of taking *megavitamins*—large doses of a range of vitamins—has not been found to promote good health, and sometimes—as in the case of taking overdoses of vitamin A—can actually cause serious harm.

14. *Food additives* are substances that are blended into food in order to restore something lost or to supply an additional ingredient. The most common food additives in America are *sugar* and *salt*, and health experts believe that the overuse of either causes serious health problems.

CONSUMER CONCERNS

1. Do you feel that a person who adheres to the basic four plan of food intake still requires nutritional supplements? If so, why?
2. Have you done any comparison shopping between a health-food store and your supermarket? What differences have you noticed in prices?
3. Have you noticed that the products on the shelves of your grocery store are identified by a unit price and an actual price? How does the unit price information help you to save money?
4. Do you realize that many food items follow seasonal patterns and are priced accordingly?
5. What is impulse buying? How can it be avoided?

6 Weight Control

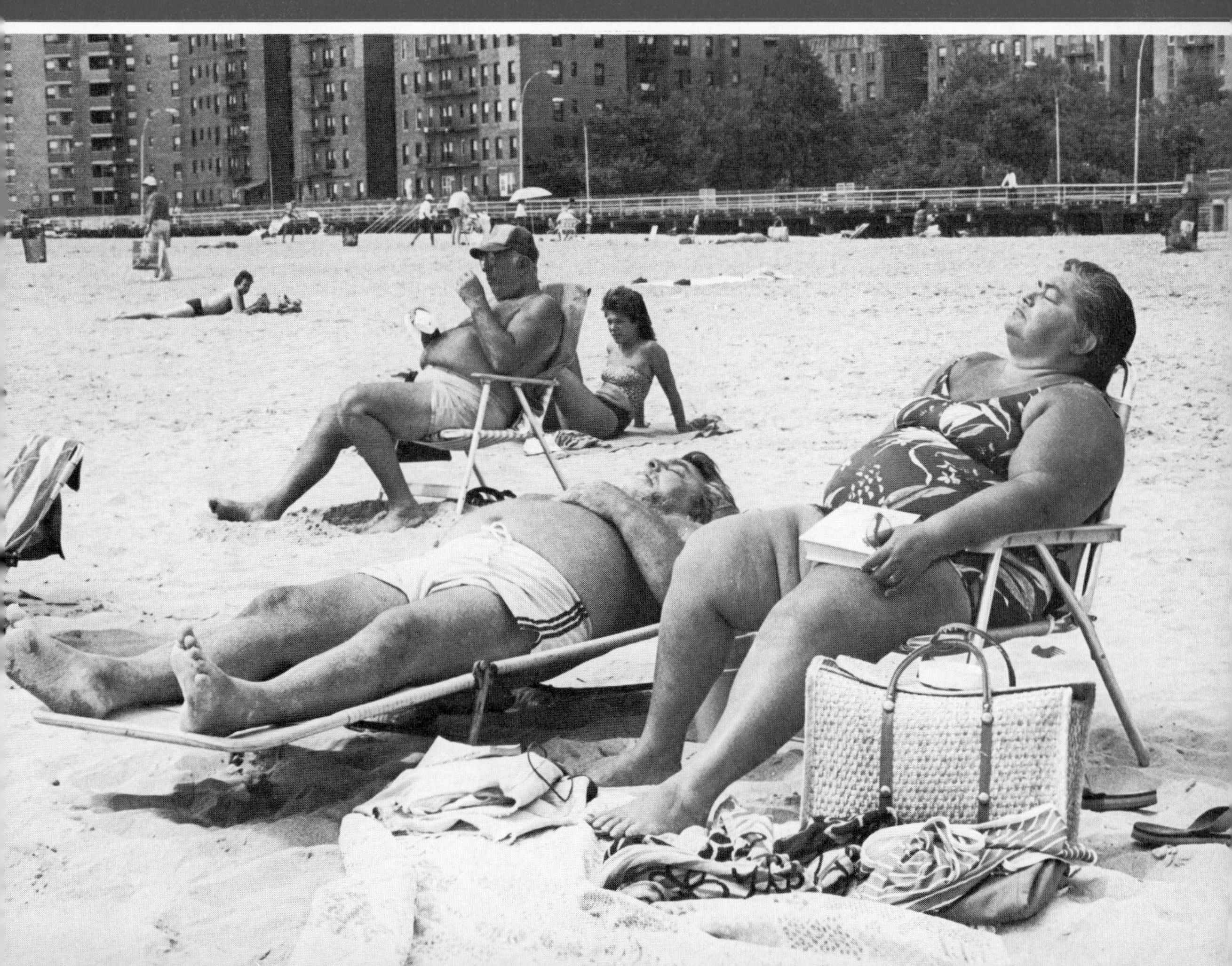

Americans are bombarded by advertisements that promise all kinds of solutions to weight problems. Appetite suppressants, books on fad diets, weight-loss machines, diet clinics, even weight-control vacations—all are extolled in print and on the air. Weight control is big business. Unfortunately, the loss that occurs is usually measured in dollars rather than in pounds. In addition, some approaches and methods are quite capable of impairing health. One of the most serious drawbacks of fad dieting is the disregard for nutritional requirements. It is not necessary to barter one's health for a change in weight.

If we could find a cure for cancer, we could boost overall life expectancy by two years, but a cure for overweight would give us an extra four. Obesity and the diseases that it contributes to account for nearly 20 percent of the mortality rate in our society. In developed, industrialized societies such as the United States, about 35 percent of adults are obese.

Less extensive, and certainly less publicized, is the problem of underweight. For those who suffer from this often debilitating condition, even when it is not carried to the severe limits of anorexia (which we will discuss later), being underweight is every bit as painful as being obese.

In this chapter we shall consider deeply ingrained attitudes toward eating, food, and body image, and offer some practical advice about weight and nutrition. We shall also discuss recommended as well as nonrecommended methods of weight control.

WHAT DETERMINES WEIGHT?

Our body weight is the product of several related factors. It depends in part on the type of body we have inherited from our parents. It depends partly on our rate of metabolism, which may also be inherited. But it depends most of all on the ratio between our intake and expenditure of calories, a ratio we can control by carefully watching how much food we eat and exercising regularly.

Heredity

Scientists are sharply divided over how much of a role heredity plays in obesity. While obesity does run in families (80 percent of the children of fat people are fat), is it because of genetic inheritance or the early learning of bad eating habits? Some recent research seems to support the genetic theory. A 1986 study of 540 Danish adults who were adopted early in childhood showed that those whose biological parents were obese were overwhelmingly likely to be obese themselves. There was no correlation in degree of fatness or thinness between the children and their adoptive parents. Some authorities conclude, therefore, that childhood environment has little or no effect on whether a person will become obese in adulthood; it is all a matter of genetic inheritance. Other authorities cite studies that prove the opposite. They claim that body *proportions* are all that is inherited and that whether an individual is fat or thin depends on life-style factors.

Whichever theory turns out to be true, people can do a lot to prevent and control tendencies toward obesity. The most effective measures are maintaining a vigorous exercise program and keeping a close watch over what and how much food they take in.

Metabolism

Metabolism consists of all of the chemical processes that are involved in converting the food we eat into energy and protoplasm for the repair and growth of cells. Metabolism takes place constantly in the cells of all living organisms. The amount of energy we use to support our basic bodily functions such as breathing, heartbeat, and minimal physical activity such as resting is called the **basal metabolic rate (BMR)**. The BMR varies with sex and with age. Different people of the same age and sex, however, have different BMRs. BMR helps to determine how much body fat a person will store and use: Generally, the higher one's BMR, the more rapidly one's body will burn up food. Quite simply, people with low BMRs have to eat less and exercise more to maintain normal body weight.

The rule of thumb for gaining or losing weight is that 3,500 calories, consumed as food or burned off through cell metabolism and exercise, equal one pound. Some overweight people, however, have been shown to gain a pound for every 2,500 calories, and some underweight people have to eat 4,500 calories worth of food to gain the same pound. Because metabolism changes with age, older people need fewer calories than younger people to maintain the same weight (See Table 6-1).

Physical Activity

Technology has created a sedentary life style for millions of Americans, making them dependent on exercise-robbing conveniences such as the TV set, the escalator, the elevator, and the automobile. Not only does this life style promote obesity and general bad health, it makes it difficult to lose weight. Generally, the best remedy for obesity is a program of regular vigorous physical exercise

TABLE 6-1
Daily Calorie Requirements*

Age in Years	Males	Females
1–3	1,300	1,300
4–6	1,700	1,700
7–10	2,400	2,400
11–14	2,700	2,200
15–18	2,800	2,100
19–22	2,900	2,100
23–50	2,700	2,000
51–75	2,400	1,800
76+	2,050	1,600

* These are average requirements for typical work levels.
Source: Food and Nutrition Board, National Academy of Sciences—National Research Council, *Recommended Dietary Allowances*, 9th ed. (Washington, D.C.: National Academy of Sciences, 1979).

TABLE 6-2
Energy Expenditure by a 150-Pound Person in Various Activities

Activity	Gross Energy Cost in Calories per Hour	Activity	Gross Energy Cost in Calories per Hour
Rest and Light Activity	*50–200*	*Moderate Activity*	*200–350*
Lying down or sleeping	80	Badminton	350
Sitting	100	Horseback riding (trotting)	350
Driving an automobile	120	Square dancing	350
Standing	140	Volleyball	350
Domestic work	180	Roller skating	350
Moderate Activity	*200–350*	*Vigorous Activity*	*Over 350*
Bicycling (5½ mph)	210	Table tennis	360
Walking (2½ mph)	210	Ditch digging (hand shovel)	400
Gardening	220	Ice skating (10 mph)	400
Canoeing (2½ mph)	230	Wood chopping or sawing	400
Golf	250	Tennis	420
Lawn mowing (power mower)	250	Water skiing	480
Bowling	270	Hill climbing (100 ft per hr)	490
Lawn mowing (hand mower)	270	Skiing (10 mph)	600
Fencing	300	Squash and handball	600
Rowboating (2½ mph)	300	Cycling (13 mph)	660
Swimming (¼ mph)	300	Scull rowing (race)	840
Walking (3¼ mph)	300	Running (10 mph)	900

Source: President's Council on Physical Fitness and Sports, *Exercise and Weight Control* (Washington, D.C.: U.S. Government Printing Office, 1979).

and a carefully controlled diet.

Exercise helps us lose weight in a number of ways. First, physical activity itself burns up calories. A walk of a mile a day over the span of a year consumes calories equivalent to ten pounds of bodily weight, and a half hour of vigorous physical activity on a daily basis burns off enough calories to equal sixteen pounds of weight annually. (See Table 6-2 for a list of some common activities and the number of calories they use up in an hour.)

Second—and contrary to what many people think—moderate exercise reduces the appetite. It does this by stepping up the body's metabolism. When the metabolic rate is elevated, fat is released into the bloodstream. The blood-sugar level, however, remains normal, and it is only when the blood-sugar level drops that we feel hungry. Exercise also reduces appetite because it reduces tension; many a needless trip to the refrigerator is made when a person feels false hunger pangs caused by nervous tension.

Third, the weight-reducing benefits of exercise continue long after an exercise session ends. Because the temperature and pulse rate remain elevated for four to six hours after any vigorous physical activity, calories continue to be metabolized at a high rate.

Fourth, exercise causes the body to absorb less food because it increases the rate at which food passes through the intestines.

All the weight-reducing benefits of an exercise program, however, can be undone by injudicious eating. The *intake* of calories, not the expenditure, is the critical factor for most overweight persons. No matter how much exercising you do, it is virtually impossible to burn off the calories acquired by a diet of rich foods and desserts. Consider, for example, that a twelve-ounce milkshake contains 430 calories. It would take an hour's tennis playing or half an hour's running to use them up. For most people, it should be easier not to drink the milkshake in the first place.

Eating Patterns and Obesity

There are people, however, who have a very difficult time resisting that milkshake. Many overweight and obese people have learned poor or inappropriate attitudes about food. Social psychologists have identified two specific eating patterns among the obese.

First, fat people overeat primarily under two conditions: when the food is tasty and when they don't have to work for it. Obese people are less likely than normal eaters to accept food they consider unappetizing. They are also less likely to choose nuts in shells over shelled nuts, to use chopsticks in Chinese restaurants, or to perform other "work" in connection with eating.

Second, the obese are more likely than normal eaters to act on environmental cues rather than on inner signals of true hunger. Fat people tend to be "stimulus bound." Such environmental cues as the sight, smell, or mention of food, the ease of access and amount available, and even the time of day seem to trigger eating in obese people when they are not hungry. These cues are largely ignored by normal eaters, unless they are very hungry.

TABLE 6-3
Weights at Which Men and Women Live Longest, by Height and Body Type*

Men				Women			
Height	*Small Frame*	*Medium Frame*	*Large Frame*	*Height*	*Small Frame*	*Medium Frame*	*Large Frame*
5 ft 2 in	128–134	131–141	138–150	4 ft 10 in	102–111	109–121	118–131
5 ft 3 in	130–136	133–143	140–153	4 ft 11 in	103–113	111–123	120–134
5 ft 4 in	132–138	135–145	142–156	5 ft 0 in	104–115	113–126	122–137
5 ft 5 in	134–140	137–148	144–160	5 ft 1 in	106–118	115–129	125–140
5 ft 6 in	136–142	139–151	146–164	5 ft 2 in	108–121	118–132	128–143
5 ft 7 in	138–145	142–154	149–168	5 ft 3 in	111–124	121–135	131–147
5 ft 8 in	140–148	145–157	152–172	5 ft 4 in	114–127	124–138	134–151
5 ft 9 in	142–151	148–160	155–176	5 ft 5 in	117–130	127–141	137–155
5 ft 10 in	144–154	151–163	158–180	5 ft 6 in	120–133	130–144	140–159
5 ft 11 in	146–157	154–166	161–184	5 ft 7 in	123–136	133–147	143–163
6 ft 0 in	149–160	157–170	164–188	5 ft 8 in	126–139	136–150	146–167
6 ft 1 in	152–164	160–174	168–192	5 ft 9 in	129–142	139–153	149–170
6 ft 2 in	155–168	164–178	172–197	5 ft 10 in	132–145	142–156	152–173
6 ft 3 in	158–172	167–182	176–202	5 ft 11 in	135–148	145–159	155–176
6 ft 4 in	162–176	171–187	181–207	6 ft 0 in	138–151	148–162	158–179

* Figures include 5 lbs of clothing for men, 3 lbs for women, and shoes with 1-inch heels for both.
Source: Courtesy of the Metropolitan Life Insurance Company, 1983.

WHAT IS OBESITY?

Insurance companies have used the factors of height, body type, sex, and age to draw up tables of **desirable weights** for men and women. The tables are based on longevity and blood pressure studies, with ranges of weights differing for different body types. The literature explaining such tables may use the term **overweight** for people whose weight exceeds the range by 10 to 20 percent and the term **obese** for people whose weight exceeds the range by over 20 percent.

Weight tables are at best an approximate measure. In 1959 the Metropolitan Life Insurance Company issued what was to become the standard of desirable or ideal weights—ideal in the sense that they are statistically shown to be the weights at which people of a particular height and body frame live longest. In 1983 the table was revised, and some body types were permitted as much as a ten- to fifteen-pound increase (see Table 6-3). The primary reason for the changes in the chart was that statisticians found that heavier people were living longer than thin ones. And studies made in the past few years do seem to indicate that some weight gain is not harmful past the age of 40. Some researchers have said that the weights listed in the Metropolitan tables are too easy on young people and too hard on the elderly. Many physicians, however, recommend that people aim for weights at the low end of the table, because the likelihood of heart attack, heart failure, and stroke—all major killers—increases with an increase in weight.

Knowing your body type or frame is essential to using the desirable weight tables. To determine your body type, look at your hands and feet: Wide hands and feet usually indicate a large skeleton; narrow hands and feet, a small one.

American Patterns

Using the desirable weight-chart definition (10 to 20 percent above means overweight; over 20 percent means obese), a considerable number of adult Americans are overweight, and many are obese. The Metropolitan Life Insurance Company found that nearly 50 percent of Americans weighed more than the figures in its 1983 table.

For men, most weight gain occurs between the ages of 25 and 40. This is not difficult to explain: Men are usually active during their school years but tend to have sedentary occupations afterward. For women, the pattern is different; most women experience their biggest weight gain after the age of 45. By the time women reach 59 years of age, 67 percent are overweight, and 46 percent (almost one out of two) are obese. This pattern might be explained by the fact that most women have children that keep them active until middle age. As more women become career oriented, however, it is possible that their pattern of weight gain will change.

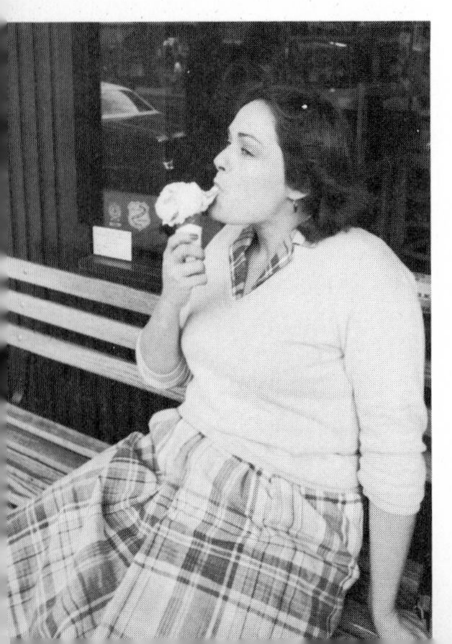

A recently completed study showed that the average weight of men has gone up and that of women has gone down in the past twenty years. Men 20 to 29 are nine pounds heavier than they were twenty years ago, and those 50 to 59 are two and a half pounds heavier. Although women 22 to 24 average five pounds more than they did, those over 30 showed a consistent decline in weight. In the 50 to 59 age category, they are six pounds lighter.

Although the phenomenon of increasing weight with increasing years is common enough to make it seem "natural," it is not inevitable. Though studies seem to show that some weight gain is not harmful in the years past middle

How to Calculate Your Calorie Requirements

To Maintain Your Weight:

1. Take the midpoint of the desirable weight range for your sex, height, and body type from Table 6-3. (If you are a man of medium frame who is 5′ 10″ tall, for example, take the midpoint of the range 151–163, or 157.) Enter that number at the right. ______

2. If you are female, multiply this number by 16; if you are male, multiply it by 18. X ______

   This number represents the approximate number of calories you need per day for rest and light activity. = ______

3. Add from Table 6–2 the average number of calories you spend per day in moderate or vigorous activity. If, for instance, you walk at a moderate rate for an hour a day but do little other exercise, add 300 calories. + ______

   This number represents your approximate daily maintenance-level calorie requirement. If you are gaining weight, you are likely consuming more than this number of calories. ______

To Lose One Pound a Week:

Subtract 500 calories from maintenance calories:

______ maintenance calories
- 500
______ daily diet-level calories

Source: Based on *Food and Your Weight*, U.S.D.A. Home and Garden Bulletin No. 74 (Washington, D.C.: U.S. Government Printing Office, 1977), pp. 3–5.

age, people are usually at their ideal or best weight in their mid-twenties. When they are in their mid-sixties, they should not weigh much more.

Measuring Obesity

Diagnosing obesity means measuring excess fat, not simply body weight. Health hazards and disease are related to excess fat, not to excess muscle.

The **lean body mass (LBM)** measure is taken by subtracting the fraction of body weight taken up by fat-free tissue and its water (about 72 percent). The percentage of excess body fat is then calculated. **Densitometry,** a measure using the principle of water displacement at different fat densities, is based on the lesser density of fat as compared with lean body mass. However, this method requires laboratory facilities to submerge the body in a tank and is therefore not commonly encountered.

The method most often used by physicians is the **pinch test,** or **skinfold**

measurement. A little more than half of all body fat is layered just beneath the skin and is usually measured by calipers at the triceps muscle of the upper left arm. Limits differ for people of different ages and for men and women. The percentage of total body fat carried by adults is about 18 percent for men and 27 percent for women. Adult men have about 11 percent of their body weight in fatty tissue under the skin; adult women, about 18 percent. Skinfold measurement is valued by scientists because it is an independent measure that avoids the tricky connection between the variables of height and body type found in desirable-weight charts.

Lacking calipers, you can give yourself the pinch test on the underside of your left arm. For the college-age group, a fold of more than an inch indicates too much fat. Or take the full-length mirror test. Unless your notions of fatness differ greatly from the standards of your culture or unless you have a false body image, you can probably judge for yourself.

Psychological Typing

Some researchers have classified obesity according to sets of psychological symptoms in the overweight person. Hilda Bruch's classification of obese people as constitutional, reactive, or developmental is widely used. **Constitutional obesity** has its onset in infancy. Children show normal personality development, but their attempts to lose weight usually fail. Genetic or prenatal factors are probably at work, but they have not yet been identified.

Reactive and developmental types both show personality disturbances. The onset of **reactive obesity,** whether in childhood or adulthood, is sudden, and overeating occurs periodically in response to stress and emotional conflict. Bouts of depression, with increasing weight gain and inactivity, are typical. **Developmental obesity** occurs in childhood, and eating patterns are extremely difficult to change over the person's lifetime. Bruch believes that a parent, usually the mother, overfeeds the child to serve her own emotional needs. Since from childhood these persons have confused eating with pleasing a parent, they cannot tell the difference between true hunger and other emotional states once they reach adulthood.

Bruch also recognizes a category called **thin fat people,** people who have lost enough weight to become fashionably thin but who are continually frustrated and preoccupied with food, dieting, and weight. They experience a great deal of stress as a result of worrying about their appearance.

Psychologists also consider a person's **body image**—the physical and emotional picture we have of ourselves and how we appear to others. The body image

Night Eating

Night eating is a widespread disorder that typically leads to obesity. People undergoing stress often have trouble sleeping and think of food as a sedative or tranquilizer. Their raids on the refrigerator—usually between the hour of 11 P.M. and 4 A.M.—result in "snacks" that are apt to total more than 500 calories, or 25 percent of the average daily requirement. Many night eaters say they are desperate to lose weight, but they are notoriously unsuccessful as dieters. The syndrome is dangerous because it is so resistant to treatment.

Anorexia

Anorexia nervosa is a relatively rare, but life-threatening condition in which people, usually young women between the ages of 12 and 18, lose too much weight by refusing to eat, and in severe cases literally starve themselves to death. The death rate from this disorder is between 10 to 20 percent. The condition is diagnosed in a person who has lost more than 25 percent of her body weight when no underlying physical cause can be found. In other words, the individual simply stops eating.

The reasons for this phenomenon are complex and almost wholly psychological. The problem seems to be more common among young upper-class women; the usual explanation is that they are driven by circumstances and by their parents to achieve success. Though it has not been conclusively proven, there does appear to be a relationship between the high-achievement syndrome and the development of anorexia. Many experts say that anorexics believe they are being controlled by a parent (usually the mother) and engage in bizarre eating patterns as a means of exercising authority over their own lives. Also, anorexics tend to have a distorted body image (they believe themselves to be far heavier than they are), enjoy refusing food (they may cook elaborate meals for others while starving themselves), and typically feel a sense of power in "controlling" their bodies. They tend to be perfectionists. Despite their willfulness—and it takes extraordinary willpower to starve oneself—anorexics feel an underlying helplessness and worthlessness. When mild cases are counted, the number of anorexics is estimated to be as high as 1 in every 250 white females in the 12-to-18 age group.

For cases of anorexia, professional help is almost mandatory. Anyone suffering from this disorder should seek both medical and nutritional help, as well as psychotherapy to change her attitude toward food and to help her create a more secure and realistic self-image. The National Association of Anorexia Nervosa and Associated Disorders, Box 271, Highland Park, Illinois 60035, can provide help.

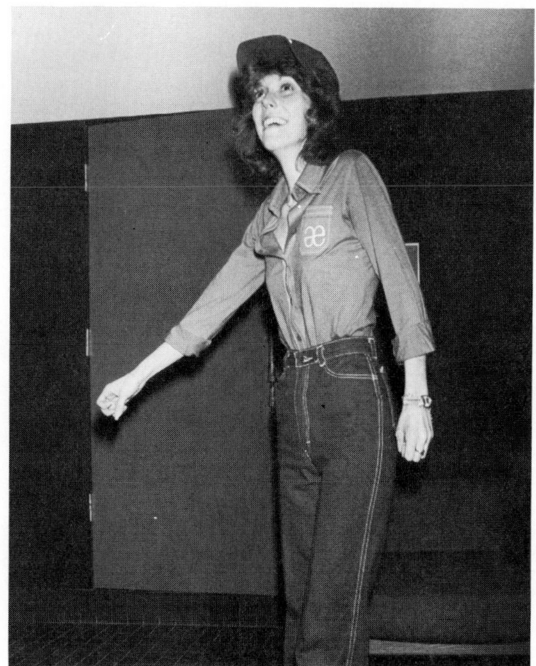

Singer Karen Carpenter in 1980

is usually formed during adolescence and tends to stick throughout our lives. Some people have a false picture of themselves, seeing their bodies as larger or smaller than they really are. However, it is estimated that nearly half of obese people have a true body image. Contrary to popular opinion, many of these people are quite satisfied with themselves. They may be fat, but they are psychologically well adjusted.

Fat Cells and Set Points

The body of a normal adult has between 30 and 40 billion fat cells. The number of fat cells remains constant no matter how much dieting or overeating a person does. What does change is the size of the fat cells. A rich diet and a sedentary life style will add fat to the existing cells; a low-calorie diet and an exercise program will burn fat off.

Unfortunately, however, evolutionary mechanisms in the body have complicated the process of losing weight. Research has shown that the body resists our attempts to slim down. Once we have lost a certain number of pounds by dieting and exercise, the body seems to attempt to return to a certain weight known as the *set point*. It does this by three metabolic processes. First, it lowers the overall metabolic rate by 15 to 25 percent. Thus overweight people are often dismayed to find that in order to keep their weight down, they must eat 25 percent fewer calories than a normal person does to maintain the same weight. Second, the fat cells themselves begin to produce a substance—lipoprotein lipase—that prevents them from shrinking. Finally, the body responds to repeated attempts at dieting by shortening the amount of time it takes to gain weight back after the person goes off a diet.

WEIGHT AND HEALTH

There is a great deal of evidence that being overweight, even to a mild degree, is a hazard to health. It is a real burden for the body to carry excess fat. To get an idea of the strain involved, pick up a five-pound bag of potatoes the next time you are in a supermarket. Then pick up a ten-pound bag, and, if possible, try a twenty-five pound bag. Imagine carrying this extra weight with you constantly, throughout your life, and you will have an idea of the stress being overweight places on your body.

Cardiovascular Disorders

In one study that identified risk factors in coronary disease, increased obesity was found to be associated with increased blood pressure and serum cholesterol. Sixty percent of those who lost weight, however, also regained normal blood pressure. Another study found that high blood pressure occurs more frequently among the obese than the nonobese, that the obese have a greater risk of heart disease, and that obesity combined with hypertension brings a higher risk of death than either obesity or hypertension alone.

Excess fat puts increased strain on the heart and circulatory system in two direct ways. First, the muscles of the body must work harder to carry the extra weight; the circulatory system, in turn, must work harder to meet the increased oxygen and nutritional demands of these muscles. Second, the fat cells themselves require oxygen and nutrients. It has been estimated that each pound of excess fat requires an extra mile of capillaries to nourish it. Thus the heart must work harder to pump blood through an increased number of blood vessels. As it increases its pumping, blood pressure rises.

Other Diseases

Fat people are more likely to develop diabetes, and their death rate from that disease is three to four times that of the normal-weight population. Gallstones and gout also occur more frequently among the obese, largely because of their diet of fatty foods.

The obese are also more prone to chronic diseases and face a greater risk if they require surgery. Pregnant women who are obese are far more likely than women of normal weight to suffer from **toxemia**—a condition in which toxic waste products accumulate in the bloodstream. Its symptoms include high blood pressure, protein loss, excess water retention, and convulsions.

Decreased Life Expectancy

Studies conducted by life insurance companies consistently show that one penalty for being overweight is decreased life expectancy. There is a significant increase in premature deaths as excess body weight increases. For example, a 45-year-old man of medium height and frame weighing 170 pounds can expect to live about one and one-half years less than if he weighed 150 pounds (his best weight). If he weighs 200 pounds, he can expect to live four years less than he would if he weighed 150 pounds.

Fortunately, just as being overweight increases the chances of impaired health and premature death, a reduction in weight results in increased longevity. Studies show that overweight men who have reduced have almost the same mortality rate as those who have consistently kept their weight in the normal range.

Underweight and Health

Though their numbers do not approach the overweight population, quite a few people in the United States are **underweight.** By definition, an underweight individual weighs less than 90 percent of the ideal weight for his or her height and body build.

The medical risks of being underweight are not nearly so severe as those of being overweight. The underweight, however, have a greater susceptibility to infection, including tuberculosis, particularly during adolescence. Overly thin people are also hindered by limited reserves of energy; and during periods of illness or stress, when appetite is diminished, their energy needs must be drawn from lean body mass. Severe underweight may also signal a number of pathological conditions: malnutrition, endocrine disorders, various diseases, hyperactivity, nervousness, drug addiction, or injury to body organs.

Young women who are pregnant and underweight suffer a greater risk, both to their own health and that of their infants. Also, underweight women may have difficulty becoming pregnant, and may experience disturbances of their menstrual cycles.

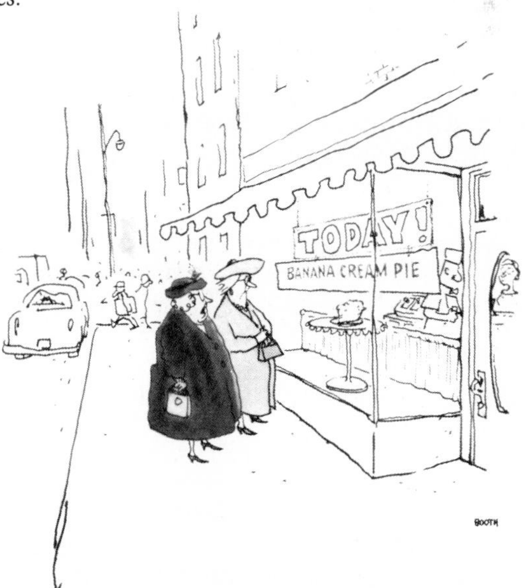

"Let's just go in and see what happens."

PROBLEMS AND CONTROVERSIES: Sugar vs. Artificial Sweeteners

Americans' desire for sweets seems to grow with each passing year. Each of us now consumes 126.8 pounds of sugar a year, as compared to 118.1 pounds in 1976. At the same time, a desire to eat our cake and have a slim body, too, has induced millions of us to avoid sugar and turn to artificial sweeteners. Our intake of foods containing these substances—mostly in the form of soft drinks—has almost tripled in the last ten years. It is easy to see why this has happened. A person who drinks two regular colas a day at 145 calories each will be consuming about 2,000 "empty" calories a week—which adds up to more than half a pound of fat. The same number of diet colas, at 2 calories each, comes to only 28 calories.

What are the advantages and disadvantages of artificial sweeteners?

Saccharin

A coal-tar product discovered in 1879, saccharin contains no calories and is more than 300 times sweeter than sugar. It is widely used by diabetics and others who must restrict their sugar intake. In the 1960s it was combined with cyclamate to eliminate its bitter aftertaste. While studies have shown that very large quantities of saccharin produce bladder cancer in rats, it is still uncertain whether lesser amounts cause cancer in humans. As long as it is accompanied by a warning label, the federal government permits it to be sold to the public.

Cyclamate

Developed in 1937 and widely used in the United States in the 1960s, cyclamate is about thirty times sweeter than sugar. It was banned in 1970 by the FDA after studies showed that the combination of it and saccharin possibly caused bladder cancer in laboratory animals. In addition, cyclamate was thought to be implicated in chromosomal damage and atrophy of the testicles in laboratory animals. While other countries permit it to be sold, cyclamate is banned in Great Britain and the United States.

Aspartame (NutraSweet)

Aspartame is composed of natural amino acids and thus is not really "artificial." While it contains the same number of calories as sugar, only 1/200th the amount needs to be used to obtain the same degree of sweetness. The substance began to be widely used in soft drinks in 1983. Although it is generally regarded as safe, consumer groups have complained that it has caused headache, nausea, rashes, and even brain damage in a few users. Some experts maintain that further testing of aspartame's effect on the brain will be necessary before it can be declared absolutely safe.

But, assuming that artificial sweeteners are safe, will they help you to lose weight? In one study a group of overweight people was first put on a diet high in sugar and then switched to one using aspartame. This step should have reduced their intake of calories by 25 percent. But the subjects partly compensated for the lost sugar-derived calories by eating 10 percent more calories from unsugared food. Artificial sweeteners may thus be of only limited use in a low-calorie diet.

Source: "America's Sweet Tooth," *Newsweek*, August 26, 1985, pp. 50–56. Condense from Newsweek. Copyright 1985.

PLANNING A WEIGHT-CHANGE PROGRAM

A weight-change program of any significance should be undertaken only after consultation with a physician or other similarly competent individual. Cases of extreme underweight or overweight may be reflections of other physical or emotional problems. Changes in diet to influence weight should be undertaken with proper advisement. It is important to remember that, ordinarily, a weight-control program need not and should not be conducted at the expense of proper nutrition.

Some Practical Advice

The most difficult part of any diet is the need for the constant exercise of willpower. For a weight-change program to succeed, the person must be well motivated. People must realize that their eating habits will have to change permanently. **Crash diets,** for example, followed by a return to old eating habits will produce a pattern of weight loss and gain called the *yo-yo effect*, which may be unhealthy and is certainly self-defeating, as we have seen. Crash diets are all too common among Americans. Instead, realistic goals must be set. If the goal is weight reduction, a loss of one or two pounds a week is realistic. At this rate a loss of fifty pounds in six months to a year can be achieved. If the goal is to put on weight, the gain should be steady and gradual.

Some people find it helpful to chart their weight changes. Since weight fluctuates from day to day, it is generally more encouraging to check your weight only once a week—on the same scale, at the same time, and with the same amount of clothing (or nude). A significant weight loss may not show on the scales for one or two weeks. But this is only because water has replaced the fat that has been burned up. When the water leaves the tissues, the scale registers a most satisfactory sudden drop in weight.

If you are a moderately active adult, a simple rule of thumb can help you determine about how many calories you normally need during the day: Multiply your ideal weight in pounds by 16 if you are a woman, by 18 if you are a man. (See box: How to Calculate Your Calorie Requirements.) Average daily calorie requirements for various groups are shown in Table 6-1. If you engage in vigorous daily activity, you will probably use more calories. If you are relatively inactive, you will use fewer.

Low-Calorie Diets. As we have seen, it takes 3,500 calories to put on one pound of weight and a total deficit of 3,500 calories to lose one pound of weight. People who wish to lose at least one pound a week must reduce their daily caloric intake by 500 calories below normal or burn off 500 calories through exercise (see Table 6-2).

For example, if you usually consume 2,400 calories a day, you will probably lose one pound a week by restricting yourself to 1,900 calories a day, and two pounds a week by restricting yourself to 1,400 calories a day. A low-calorie diet for women is generally 1,000 to 1,500 calories per day. For men, it is 1,200 to 1,800 calories per day. In dieting, each meal is important. Nutritionists advise taking in one-fourth to one-third of your calories at breakfast and the same amount at lunch. Avoid between-meal snacks, and particularly avoid empty calories.

Planning a Weight-Gain Program

To gain weight, simply reverse the procedure for losing it, but continue a fitness program. For example, if you follow a **high-calorie diet** and increase your caloric intake by 1,000 calories a day, you will gain an average of two pounds per week. Most people gain weight satisfactorily on a 3,000- to 3,500-calorie diet.

If you are underweight, you are probably consuming fewer calories than you need. You may not be able to consume the amount of food listed in high-

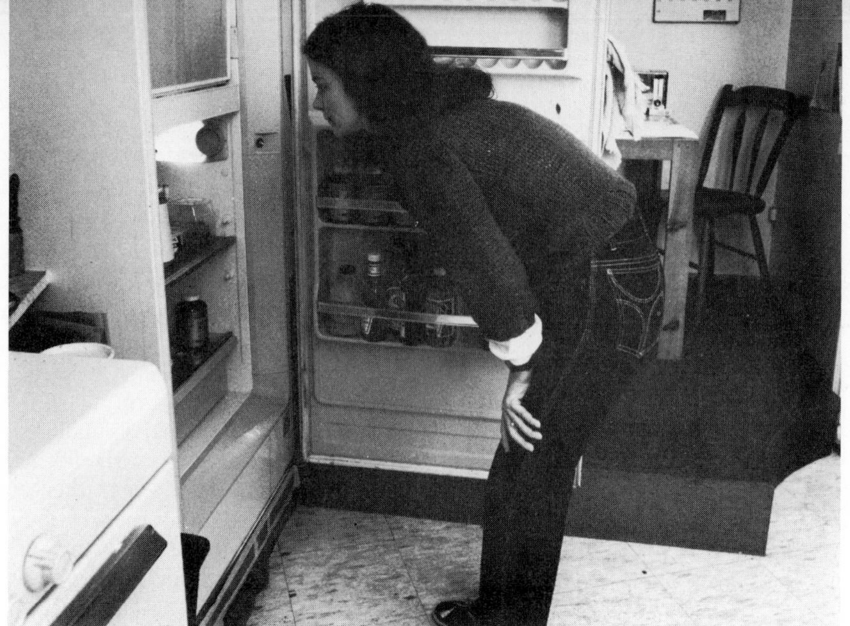

One way to maintain a weight loss is to avoid between-meal snacks.

calorie diets, so start by eating foods that are low in bulk but high in calories. Raw fruit and salad, for example, will add bulk, but not substantial calories; and they may satisfy the appetite before an adequate amount of energy-yielding food has been eaten. Therefore it is recommended that the underweight eat fat-rich, low-bulk foods such as cheese, cream, butter, and mayonnaise. Here one has to be cautious, because excessively fatty or sweet foods at meals can depress the appetite even further.

It is especially important for the underweight person to eat regular meals and to eat every meal. If it seems impossible to eat the required number of calories on a three-meal schedule, you might try frequent small meals or between-meal snacks. And since the underweight person is frequently overactive, it is advisable to conserve calorie consumption by getting plenty of sleep.

Weight Maintenance

The sequel to a weight-loss or weight-gain program is weight maintenance. Therefore weight control is on ongoing, year-round program, not a spasmodic two-week effort. A lifelong program must take into consideration more than the mere concern for the consumption and expenditure of calories. It must also satisfy the nutritional requirements of the body. Some foods you can easily avoid because they have little or no nutritional value; other foods you cannot afford to avoid because of the nutrients they contain.

Eating Slowly

A surefire way to gain weight fast is to gulp your food down and then immediately have a second helping. To lose weight and keep it off, you must acquire some new eating habits, one of the most helpful of which is eating slowly. The reason for this is that the stomach needs time to inform the brain that it is full. By taking small bites, chewing your food much longer than usual, and laying your fork or spoon down between bites, you are giving your stomach time to send the "satiety signal" to your brain. For the same reason, it is a good idea to wait twenty minutes before deciding whether or not to have a second helping; by that time your hunger will probably have disappeared.

Source: Jane Brody, *Jane Brody's Nutrition Book* (New York: W. W. Norton & Company, Inc., 1981), p. 312.

TABLE 6-4
Caloric Values of Some Beverages and Snack Foods

Food	Approximate Serving	Calories
Beverages		
Coffee	6 oz	5
Cranberry juice cocktail	8 oz	147
Iced tea, made from mix presweetened with sugar	8 oz	80
Milk, skim	8 oz	90
Milk, whole	8 oz	160
Orange juice, made from concentrate	8 oz	120
Soft drinks, cola type, regular	12 oz	145
Soft drinks, diet	12 oz	2
Beverages, Alcoholic		
Beer, regular	12 oz	150
Beer, light	12 oz	100
Gin, Vodka, Whiskey (80 proof)	1½ oz	100
Wine, table	3½ oz	85
Wine, dessert	3½ oz	140
Cake and Doughnuts		
Angel food cake	1 slice	135
Cheesecake, plain	1 slice	250
Chocolate cupcake, iced	1 cake, 2½″ diam.	130
Doughnut, cake type, plain	1 average	125
Doughnut, jelly	1 average	225
Pound cake	1 slice	130
Candy and Popcorn		
Chocolate bar, plain	1½ oz	240
Chocolate coated peanuts	1 oz	160
Fruit chews	1 oz	110
Fudge	1 piece	115
Peanut butter cup	1 piece	100
Popcorn, made w/oil	1 cup	40
Popcorn, caramel coated	1 cup	130
Yogurt coated raisins	1 oz	120
Chips and Pretzels		
Corn chips	1 oz	150
Nacho cheese chips	1 oz	145
Potato chips	1 oz	155
Pretzels	1 oz	110
Cookies		
Brownie, made from mix	1 oz	130
Chocolate chip	1 cookie	50
Fig bars	1 cookie	50
Dairy Products		
American cheese	1 oz	90
Cheddar cheese	1 oz	115
Cottage cheese, 4% fat	4 oz	120
Cottage cheese, 1% fat	4 oz	90
Cream cheese	1 oz	105
Ice cream, vanilla	1 cup	255
Sherbet with milk	1 cup	260
Swiss cheese (domestic)	1 oz	100
Yogurt, plain, 1½% fat	8 oz	150
Yogurt, fruit	8 oz	260
Fruits and Vegetables		
Apple	1 medium	70
Banana	1 medium	100
Carrot	5½″ by 1″	20
Corn on the cob	1 ear, 5″ by 1½″	70
Lettuce	2 large leaves	10
Orange	2½″ diameter	65
Strawberries	1 cup	55
Tomato	3″ diameter	40
Watermelon	1 wedge, 4″ by 8″	115
Miscellaneous		
Bagel, plain	1 whole	150
Chicken nuggets	6 pieces	250
French fries, cooked in oil	10 fries	155
Granola bar, w/nuts & raisins	1 bar	130
Hot dog on roll	2-ounce	290
Hamburger patty on roll	3-ounce	365
Pizza, frozen cheese	4-oz slice	240
Wheat germ	1 ounce	110
Nuts		
Almonds, shelled	1 cup	850
Mixed, shelled	8 to 12	94
Peanut butter	1 tablespoon	95
Peanuts, shelled, roasted	1 cup	840
Walnuts, chopped	1 cup	790
Pies		
Apple	4″ sector	350
Cherry	4″ sector	350
Lemon meringue	4″ sector	305
Pumpkin	4″ sector	275
Salad Dressings		
Bleu cheese	1 tablespoon	75
French, commercial	1 tablespoon	65
Oil and vinegar	1 tablespoon	110
Thousand Island	1 tablespoon	80
Soups (Commercial, Canned)		
Chicken noodle	4 oz	70
Green pea	4 oz	160
Minestrone	4 oz	80
Vegetable	4 oz	60

Sources: U.S. Department of Agriculture, *Nutritive Value of Foods* (Home and Garden Bulletin No. 72); consumer research by Julie Turko.

Restrictions you should follow for weight maintenance are as follows:

1. Avoid the **empty-calorie** foods. These are foods with high caloric value and little or no nutritive value. The extreme examples of these are soft drinks, candy, and drinks containing alcohol. A secondary category consists of such foods as pies, cakes, and cookies. Included in this category are many of the breakfast cereals and snack foods such as potato chips. (See Table 6-4.)
2. Those who are overweight should avoid certain high-calorie foods despite their nutritive value; other sources of such nutrients are available. Foods in this category include mayonnaise, most salad dressings, butter and its equivalents, pork products, and nuts and nut products. (Underweight people, of course, can eat as much as they want from this category.)
3. Remember that the manner in which food is prepared is also important. Frying food, for example, adds calories and destroys vital nutrients. Foods served in rich sauces are similarly high in calories. It is much better to eat broiled meats and fish and pressure-cooked or steamed vegetables.
4. Finally, the overweight must be very cautious about food portions. Though the body requires a variety of nutrients, relatively small amounts of each are all that is necessary.

It is essential to remember that in the ongoing effort to maintain your weight at the desirable level you must adhere to the principles of good nutrition. The recommended guide for this is the "basic four" food groups (see Chapter 5: Nutrition). You may increase or decrease the amounts of food you consume from each of the four categories to fit your needs, but selections from these categories should be represented in each meal. In addition, varying the particular selections from each category will ensure a balanced diet.

Reducing Clubs

Many people have found that **reducing clubs,** such as Weight Watchers and TOPS, provide needed group support. Reputable clubs teach you to prepare tasty, well-balanced, low-calorie meals. In addition, they provide a sense of belonging that helps dieters overcome feelings of guilt and shame.

There is usually a fee involved in joining such groups (they are profit-making organizations), and they are not designed for the person who is only a few pounds overweight. But for obese people who have trouble in staying on a diet, the reducing club may be an answer. These persons should be certain to check any weight-loss program with their physician beforehand, because most reducing group leaders are not qualified to judge a person's medical condition or nutritional requirements.

FAULTY WEIGHT-LOSS METHODS

Since there is so much anxiety attached to being overweight, it is inevitable that a whole industry of mostly ineffective systems and plans has sprung up to help the fat grow thin. (There has been no corresponding surge to reverse the process—that is, to help the underweight put on pounds.) The following is a discussion of some of the more dubious methods that are regularly touted.

Bulimia

Bulimia is an out-of-control cycle of binge eating followed by purges. The victim may gulp down food containing thousands of calories in less than half an hour, then immediately throw it up. Ostensibly the reason is to maintain normal body weight.

The extent of the problem is unknown; some estimate that 15 to 30 percent of young women occasionally binge and purge, while 1 to 4 percent do it all the time. About 5 percent of bulimics are male. Most sufferers are white and come from middle- and upper-class families. The vast majority are in their teens and 20s. Some have been bulimic for more than ten years and are suffering serious health problems, yet cannot stop themselves.

Bulimics may consume 10,000 to 20,000 calories at one time, then take laxatives and diuretics, vomit, or do an abusive amount of exercise to unload the excess before it turns to body fat. Usually the food ingested is junk food such as cookies, candies, pastries, and fried foods.

Experts are not certain whether the problem is a habit, an addiction or compulsion, or an emotional disorder. They do know that bulimia usually starts when a person goes on a rigorous diet, and then breaks it with an eating binge. A severe guilt reaction follows, and this leads to a purge.

Most bulimics share the same psychological and social characteristics: They are usually perfectionists, with high expectations of themselves; they feel ineffective and lack self-esteem; and they have a strong need for approval from other people.

The health consequences of bulimia can be severe. The teeth and gums can be damaged from repeated exposure to acidic vomit. Also binging and purging may damage the esophagus, throat, and stomach. Victims usually pursue their bulimic behavior in private, and they become increasingly isolated.

The problem almost always requires professional help.

Fad Diets

Many popular **fad diets** are unsound when judged by the basic principles of nutrition. The Complete Scarsdale Diet, popular in the late 1970s, was a fourteen-day diet consisting of a strict regimen from which virtually no deviations were allowed. The diet called, for example, for the same daily breakfast of half a grapefruit, one slice of protein bread, and black coffee or plain tea—a breakfast that did not provide the recommended daily intake of protein. The Scarsdale Two-Weeks-On, Two-Weeks-Off Program not only prevented the development of a stable weight-maintenance program but also established a yo-yo pattern of weight control. And the pound a day that the developers of the program said was the average amount of weight lost is severe when compared to the pound or two a week that nutritionists and physicians generally recommend.

One-Emphasis Diets. **One-emphasis diets** claim that individuals will lose weight if they eat only certain foods daily; they are even more nutritionally deficient than the Scarsdale Diet. Advocates of such diets assert that a single food has special metabolic effects that produce a rapid loss of weight. However, almost all nutritionists deny that any one food has this special property.

A dramatic example of a one-emphasis diet was the Beverly Hills Diet, published in 1981. Adherents to this diet were required to eat nothing but fruits—and certain fruits in a certain order—for the first ten days. They were allowed as much of the fruit as they liked, but nothing else. The diet was exceedingly high in fiber and caused diarrhea, which in turn caused dehydration and the loss of essential vitamins and minerals. It was also seriously deficient in protein.

Other examples of one-emphais diets include the banana-and-skim-milk diet; the grapefruit, or Mayo, diet (which is not endorsed by the Mayo Clinic) and its successor based on "grapefruit super pills"; the egg diet; the buttermilk diet; the shrimp-and-lettuce diet; and the fish-and-tomato diet. In all these diets the important factor is not the emphasized food but the lack of other essential nutrients.

Fasting. **Fasting,** or starvation, is the oldest and quickest way to lose weight, but it is also the most dangerous. When the body is deprived of food, it uses its own excess fat to keep going—the result the dieter hopes for. But fasting also reduces vital protein meant for tissue and cell maintenance and repair. Prolonged fasting can result in cardiac irregularities and damage to the heart, muscles, and brain. Prolonged fasting can also cause death. Because of these dangers, it should never be attempted without strict medical supervision.

Low-Carbohydrate Diets. **Low-carbohydrate diets** instruct dieters to drastically reduce the number of carbohydrates they consume each day and to take in an unlimited amount of high-protein foods. These diets, which include the Dr. Atkins' Diet Revolution, the Doctor's Quick-Weight-Loss Diet, the Drinking Man's Diet, and the Air Force Diet (which is not recommended by the U.S. Air Force), are designed to produce quick weight loss by causing the body to burn fats at an accelerated rate and excrete substances called ketone bodies, along with minerals and vitamins. Despite these claims, experts contend that unless dieters reduce the number of calories they take in each day, no real weight loss will occur. Moreover, a host of debilitating symptoms, including nausea, fatigue, low blood pressure, and kidney problems, may plague dieters as they futilely try to lose weight.

Each year newly marketed diet books are prominently displayed in booksellers' stalls (see box: The "Immune Power" Diet). They promise quick cures for overweight, but their primary success is in making money for publishers. The one "diet book" that would truly help people lose weight and stay healthy is not likely to appear on bookstore shelves. It would consist of perhaps a single sheet of paper that explained proper nutrition and the principles of metabolism outlined in this chapter. It would state that the loss of a pound a week is sensible and is achieved by eliminating 3,500 calories per week through lower calorie intake and exercise.

Drugs and Reducing Pills

In general, there are two types of **reducing drugs: appetite depressants,** such as tranquilizers and amphetamines ("pep pills"), and **diuretics** (drugs that cause water loss by increasing the body's excretion of urine). **Tranquilizers** act to relax an individual and thus are supposed to reduce appetite caused by nervousness. However, it has not been proved that appetite is really affected by these pills. **Amphetamines** do reduce appetite, but for a short time only. Diuretics do cause excess water to be eliminated from the body. However, fluid retention is usually caused by an overabundance of carbohydrate reserves in the body,

PROBLEMS AND CONTROVERSIES: The "Immune Power Diet"

Any fad diet promoter who wants to make a financial killing has to keep up with the times. Since the AIDS epidemic has put millions of Americans in a panic about the state of their immune system, what better time than now for a diet that promises not only to help you lose weight but also to strengthen and "revitalize" your immune system?

The first of these to appear—more are bound to follow—is Dr. Stuart Berger's "Immune Power Diet." In his book by the same title, Dr. Berger—educated at Tufts and Harvard—claims that the immune system is damaged by allergic reactions to many common foods. These reactions are said to include everything from asthma, insomnia, hives, headache, anxiety, heart palpitations, and cramps to more serious disorders like ulcers and arthritis. Such an all-encompassing list ensures that millions of worried, gullible people will diagnose themselves as food-allergic and therefore immune-damaged.

Dr. Berger claims that his plan repairs the immune system in three ways. First, it identifies the foods that are causing the reactions—usually by means of a very expensive set of allergy tests—and then eliminates them from the diet. Second, since fat is said to impede the immune response, it puts the food-allergy sufferer on a low-fat diet. Third, it bolsters the allergy-ravaged immune system with an expensive array of vitamins, minerals, and food supplements. Some bonuses of this last intervention are relief from jet lag and premenstrual tension and the prevention of prematurely graying hair.

Because the First Amendment guarantees freedom of speech, anyone in the United States can publish all sorts of false, even outrageous, claims. What distinguishes the Immune Power Diet from other dubious and fraudulent diets is the author's credentials from Tufts University, which has a renowned nutrition department, and the Harvard Medical School, one of the best in the world. The prestige of these institutions is invoked repeatedly in advertising for the book. But neither Tufts nor the Harvard Medical School has endorsed Dr. Berger's claims in their well-known health newsletters. In fact, the Harvard newsletter has termed the plan quackery and has cited numerous errors and misrepresentations in the book.

Medical and nutritional authorities at these two schools agree that as yet no known single food or combination of foods and vitamins strengthens (or damages) the immune system, nor can high dosages of vitamins and special food supplements help the body ward off disease. They also deny that millions of people are allergic to certain foods. Food allergies, they say, are relatively uncommon, and when they do appear, they usually cause skin rashes and digestive problems, not arthritis, insomnia, ulcers, and heart palpitations. Furthermore, any physician who makes such claims is not just a quack, but a dangerous quack, because he or she may delay a patient from seeking proper diagnosis and treatment.

Diets and diet books have long been big business, and by the time you read this Dr. Berger's may be out of fashion. But there is sure to be another on the best-seller list. There alway is. Diet is a lucrative business.

Sources: "Power Failure for the 'Immune Power' Diet," *Consumer Reports*, February 1986, pp. 112–13; Judith Willis, "Diet Books Sell Well But . . ." *The FDA Consumer* (March 1982), HHS Publication No. (FDA) 82-1093.

which diuretics leave unaffected. Aside from being ineffective, these drugs can also be hazardous. Amphetamines may cause insomnia, dizziness, irritability, and headaches. After prolonged use, they also produce symptoms that imitate those of paranoia. Physicians no longer prescribe them widely. Diuretics may remove certain vital substances from the body, such as potassium. The risks involved in using these drugs must be weighed by each individual and his or her physician.

In 1981 pills called "starch blockers," made from kidney-bean extract, became another diet rage. Starch blockers were marketed as a "natural" product that would slow down the digestion of starchy foods and thus allow people to eat

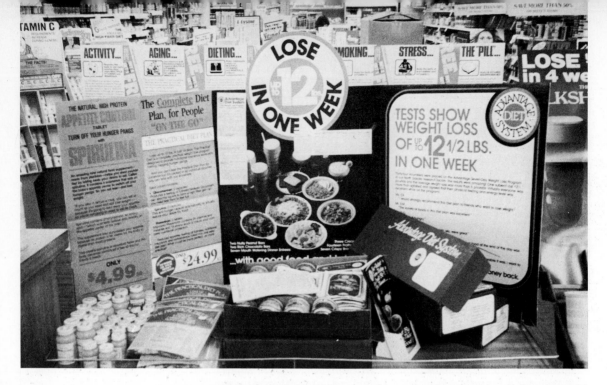

more starch and eliminate it from their systems by excretion before it could be metabolized and added to body weight. The trouble was that the pills caused nausea, vomiting, abdominal cramps, and diarrhea, as well as flatulence. Millions of dollars' worth of the pills were sold before the FDA took them off the market in 1982.

Other Ineffective Weight-Loss Methods

Saunas or Steam Baths. The weight loss occurring through exposure to extreme heat, as in a sauna or a steam bath, can be very impressive. Unfortunately, it is also temporary. Weight loss by this means simply amounts to the weight of the water being perspired. It will be restored as soon as more liquids are drunk—a process that should not be avoided. Exposure to extreme heat over a prolonged time may also cause the body to lose essential salts. These also must be replaced.

Massage and Spot Reduction. Having your fat massaged away is a concept that is advertised frequently. Unfortunately, the only person who might lose weight in this process is the masseur. The only way to burn up the calories required for weight loss is through physical activity, and being massaged does not require activity. "Cellulite parlors" make false claims about spot reduction (see box: Cellulite: The Hard-to-Budge Pudge).

Gadgets and Programs. Extravagant claims are made for exercise programs that will take the weight off specific parts of the body through spot reduction—abdomen, thighs, or other areas, according to our preference. Many gadgets are marketed for the purpose of selected, specific weight loss. Such programs and gadgets are based on false notions, since fat cannot be absorbed selectively.

Cellulite: The Hard-to-Budge Pudge

Cellulite, the waffly looking fat found in dimpled patches on women's hips and thighs, has caused a good deal of body-image anxiety over the last several years. It has also fattened the purses of many purveyors of dubious products and treatments.

Cellulite (pronounced "sell-you-leete") is a pseudo-scientific term for fat that has "gone wrong." Said to be composed of fat, water, and toxic wastes the body cannot get rid of, cellulite accumulates in unsightly deposits on thighs and buttocks that, according to advertisers, "stubbornly resist dieting and exercise." The advertisers also claim that cellulite is found on four out of five women—and only women, because of their unique physical characteristics and hormone balances.

Because it is claimed to be an unusual kind of fat that collects only in specific areas of the body, unique "spot-reducing" treatments and compounds are said to be required to get rid of it. Accordingly, the back pages of women's magazines continue to be crowded with advertisements for " 'loofah' sponges, cactus fiber washcloths, horsehair mitts, creams that 'dissolve' cellulite, vitamin-mineral supplements with herbs, exercise books, liquids to be used in the bath, massagers, rubberized pants, brushes, rollers, and toning lotions." Most of these products cost $20 or more; treatments can run into many hundreds of dollars, with no guarantee of effectiveness.

Before you spend any money on cellulite products or treatments, you should be aware of a few important points. First, there is no such thing as cellulite. Fat is fat, no matter what its texture or where it is located on the body. "Cellulite" fat, therefore, has to be lost the way all fat does: through diet and exercise. As for spot reducing, no nonsurgical treatment, exercise, or equipment can remove fat from any specific area of the body. As one weight-control expert stated, "The only way to get rid of fat on your thighs is to get rid of it all over your body."

Source: Based on *The FDA Consumer* (May 1980), HHS Publication No. (FDA) 80-1078.

Conclusion In planning either a weight-loss or a weight-gain program, the same principles apply: Eat a well-balanced diet from the basic four food groups and develop exercise and sleep patterns that enable your body to operate at peak performance and that give you the relaxation and sense of well-being that you need.

SUMMARY

1. Body weight can usually be controlled by regulating the intake of food and through physical activity. Severe weight problems may reflect other physical or psychological conditions.

2. Usually people who surpass their ideal weight by 10 to 20 percent are considered overweight, and those who surpass it by more than 20 percent are obese. Ideal weights compiled from mortality statistics have been revised upward in the last few years, but there is controversy over the statistical methods used; most physicians recommend that people keep their weight toward the lower end of any given range of ideal weight.

3. In the United States most men gain weight between the ages of 25 and 40; most women after the age of 45. Over the last few years the average weight of men has gone up, that of women down. Most people are at their ideal weight in their mid-20s, and this is the weight they should keep all their lives.

4. Excess fat can be calculated by various means,

such as the *lean body mass* (*LBM*) measure, *densitometry*, and *skinfold measurements*; the last is the most commonly used because it is the most convenient.

5. Obesity has both psychological and physical aspects. Bruch's categories of *constitutional obesity* (arising in infancy and probably caused by prenatal factors), *reactive obesity* (a response to stress and emotional conflict), and *developmental obesity* (caused by childhood eating patterns) are widely used. In addition, there are *thin fat people*, who slim themselves down but are continually preoccupied with food and dieting. Our *body image*, the physical and emotional picture we have of ourselves, is formed during adolescence and exerts a lifelong influence.

6. Obesity produces a change in the size, not the number, of the body's *fat cells*. The body tends to defend its weight at certain *set points* beyond which it is difficult to lose weight despite constant effort.

7. Because excess fat strains the heart and circulatory system, overweight and obese people are very susceptible to cardiovascular diseases, especially hypertension. In addition, they are more likely to develop diabetes, gallstones, and other chronic diseases. Their life expectancy is also significantly reduced.

8. An individual who weighs less than 90 percent of the ideal weight for his or her height and body type is defined as being *underweight*. There are fewer diseases linked to this condition than to overweight; primarily there is a greater than normal susceptibility to infection.

9. A proper diet is the key to losing or gaining weight. A deficit of 3,500 calories is necessary to lose one pound, and the same number of calories is required to gain one pound. Whatever one's goal—to gain or lose—the "basic four" food groups should serve as a nutritional guide.

10. Also to be avoided are the many systems and plans that capitalize on people's anxieties about being overweight. Fad diets and reducing pills, gadgets, and salons for special spot reduction of fat are all ineffective methods to lose weight. The best way to achieve and maintain proper weight is to eat a well-balanced diet and develop exercise and sleep patterns that enable your body to function properly.

CONSUMER CONCERNS

1. From whom might you seek reliable advice about your weight and your health in general?
2. What would be your reaction to an advertisement for weight reduction that guaranteed you would lose five to ten pounds a week and "keep it off"?
3. If you were to plan a food regimen for yourself that would enable you to control your weight, what would be your basic concern?
4. Are the two-week weight-control programs conducted at a desert retreat or on an ocean cruise of any value for permanent weight control?
5. What is the medical evidence in respect to the effectiveness of appetite suppressants as a means of weight control?

7

Reproduction and Birth Control

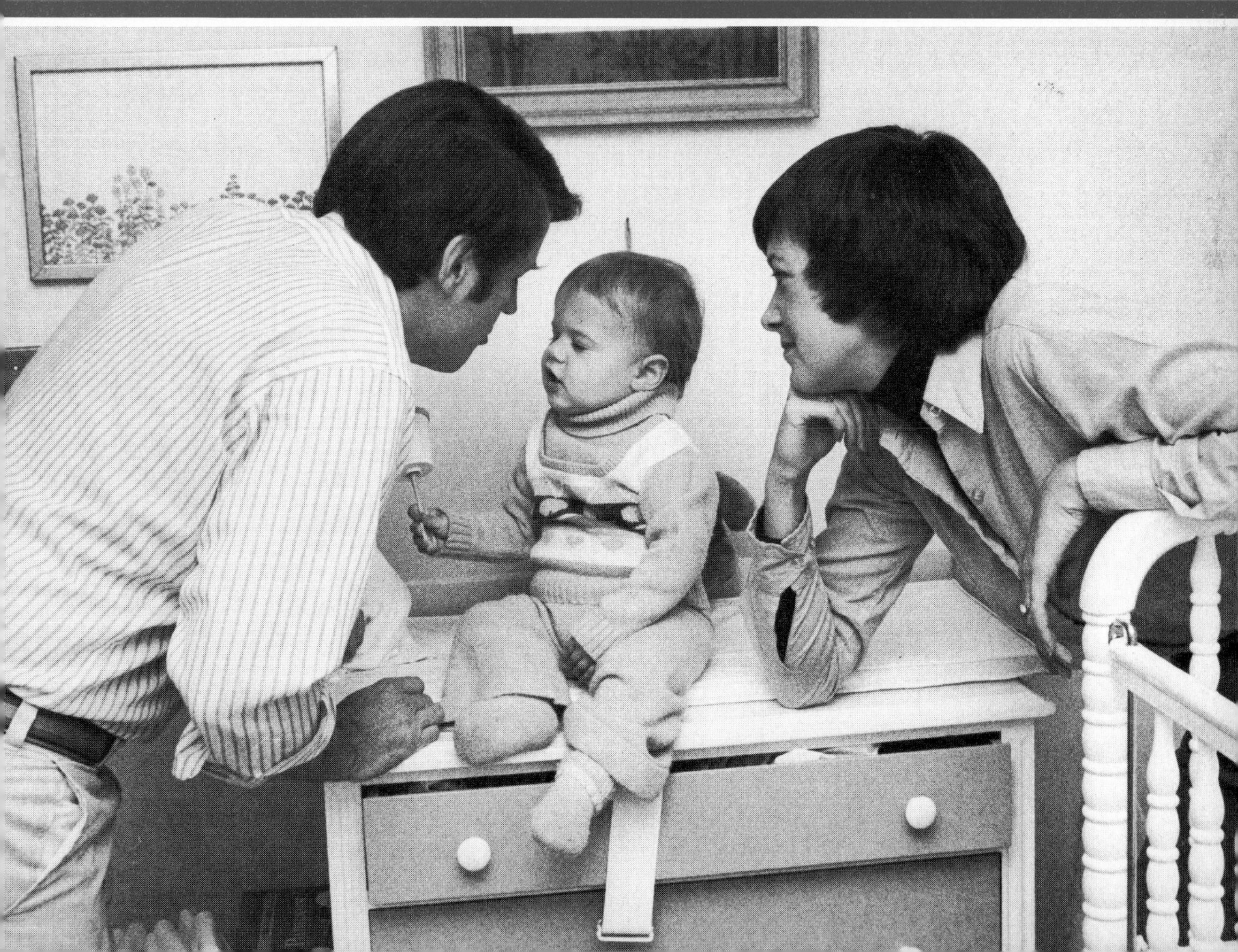

Think for a moment about the technological advances made during the past twenty years. We have placed men on the moon, conquered diseases, developed sophisticated diagnostic tools to save lives, and computerized our nation. Ironically, these "miracles" of science do not compare with a process many of us take for granted: the process of human reproduction.

Recently, after several years of stability, both the *birth rate* (the number of live births per 1,000 population) and the *fertility rate* (the number of live births per 1,000 women of child-bearing age) have begun to increase in the United States. Percentage increases have been concentrated in the later years of childbearing (the thirties and early forties), but the numbers of children actually born have increased most to mothers of younger years, because these are the years at which most women bear children. Increases overall, however, have been very modest, primarily for two reasons. First, many women are marrying much later in life than before, and they are having fewer children. Second, there is a widespread acceptance of birth-control programs and a general concern about the effects of overpopulation on the quality of life.

In this chapter we shall discuss the birth process, beginning with an explanation of the male and female reproductive systems. We will see how a fertilized egg develops in the uterus and how the mother's body adapts to pregnancy. We shall examine the process of birth, what occurs during a miscarriage or abortion, the causes of infertility, and how heredity affects the developing fetus. We shall look at some of the major inherited disorders and discuss some genetic screening methods that can be performed before and during pregnancy. Finally, we shall examine how different birth control methods are employed to prevent reproduction.

THE MALE REPRODUCTIVE SYSTEM

The male reproductive system includes: the spermatozoa, or sperm, which are the male reproductive cells; the male sex hormones; the testes, or testicles, in which sperm and hormones are produced; and the penis, the male organ of copulation. (The act of sexual union, during which the male penis is inserted into the female vagina, is called **intercourse, copulation,** or **coitus.**) The ducts through which sperm travel on their journey from the testes to the penis and the accessory glands that empty their secretions into the ducts are also a part of this system (see Figure 7-1).

The Testes

The **testes** (or **testicles**) are two egg-shaped glands, each about one inch in diameter and one and one-half inches long. They are contained within the **scrotum,** a thin-walled sac of skin and muscle that hangs between the legs behind the penis. Each testis is supported by a **spermatic cord,** a thick tube containing blood vessels, nerves, and ducts leading to and from it.

Since sperm cannot survive in the relatively high temperatures of the inner abdominal area, the testes must rest in the scrotum, where the temperature is usually about two degrees lower. To maintain the optimum temperature during hot weather, the muscles within the scrotum relax, and the scrotum hangs more loosely between the legs. In this position it can release more heat

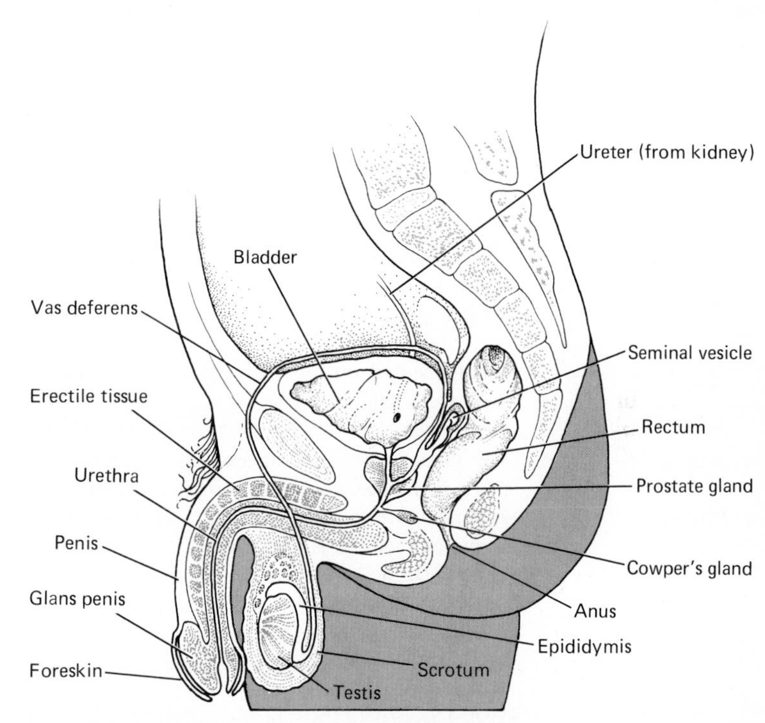

FIGURE 7-1

The male reproductive system.

than if it were located more closely against the body. In cold weather the muscles within the scrotum tense, drawing the scrotum closer to the body and thus increasing the temperature of the testes.

Each testis is divided into about 250 compartments that resemble segments of an orange. Each compartment contains from one to three extremely fine tubes called **seminiferous tubules,** which lie elaborately twisted and coiled within the compartment. Spermatozoa are constantly being produced by special cells that make up part of the walls of the tubules.

All the tubules within each testis deposit mature sperm into common ducts located on the upper side of the testis. Each collecting duct, in turn, leads into an **epididymis.** Sperm are stored within the epididymis until they move toward the penis.

Each epididymis merges into a duct known as the **vas deferens.** Sperm are conducted through these ducts to the point where they connect with two glands called the seminal vesicles; the sperm then flow to the prostate gland via the **ejaculatory ducts.** In the prostate gland the urinary tract from the bladder joins with the two ejaculatory ducts to form a single duct, the **urethra,** which passes to the tip of the penis. Urine or semen flows out of the penis through the urethra. Without an ejaculation, sperm may take up to sixty days to make the journey from the tubules through the penis. During ejaculation, however, muscular contractions move sperm from the tubules through the ducts and out of the penis in a matter of seconds.

The Accessory Glands

The **seminal vesicles** are a pair of glands, each about two inches long, located below the bladder. They secrete a clear fluid that forms part of the **semen.** The secretion from the seminal vesicles appears to increase the sperm's *motility* (capacity to move). At the point where the ejaculatory ducts merge with the urethra, there is a spongy gland about the size of a walnut. This is the **prostate gland,** which secretes a thin, milky fluid that makes up the bulk of the semen. This fluid has an important function: It neutralizes the normally acidic environment of the urethra and vagina, thereby increasing the motility and viability of the sperm.

During their journey through the male ducts the sperm are inert and are passively carried along. When they come in contact with the prostatic fluid, however, they become highly active. Their tails begin lashing back and forth vigorously, and this motion will enable them to propel themselves through the passageways of the female's reproductive system.

A third pair of glands, the **Cowper's glands,** also empty their secretions into the urethra whenever the male is sexually excited. The secretion of the Cowper's glands is a lubricant that facilitates the passage of the sperm through the urethra; it also helps neutralize the acidity of the urethra.

The Penis

The **penis** consists of three cylindrical masses of tissue, two of which lie alongside each other, with the third lying below and between the upper two. The urethra passes through the center of the lower column and emerges at its tip. The bell-shaped head of the penis, which is larger in circumference than the shaft, is called the **glans penis.**

The penis is covered by a loose layer of skin that is a continuation of the skin covering the scrotum; the skin is attached to the penis just behind the

Circumcision

Normally the head of the penis (the glans penis) is covered by a fold of skin called the foreskin. The foreskin conceals the sensitive tip of the penis; it can be drawn back, however, to expose the glans penis.

The foreskin can be removed in a surgical procedure known as *circumcision*. Although there are rare occasions when circumcision is performed for medical reasons, it is most often done because of religious or social customs. All male Jews and Muslims, for example, are circumcised as a religious requirement; in American hospitals about 80 percent of baby boys are routinely circumcised.

The value of routine circumcision is debatable. The operation is sometimes botched, leaving a deformed penis. There is some risk of infection and hemorrhage; and the operation, done without anesthetic, is painful. The presence or absence of a foreskin has no effect on sexual sensitivity. It is true that when the foreskin is intact, a white secretion called *smegma* can accumulate underneath it. Unless this is washed away regularly, the area under the foreskin can become irritated, inflamed, and even infected. There is also a link between smegma and cancer of the penis in men, and a possible (though disputed) link between smegma and cervical cancer in women. Circumcision, however, seems a radical substitute for bathing.

glans penis. A fold of the skin extends forward to cover the glans penis. This fold is the **prepuce,** or **foreskin.** The inner side contains glands that secrete a lubricant called **smegma. Circumcision**—the surgical removal of the foreskin—is performed on many males soon after birth (see box: Circumcision).

The three columns of tissue making up the penis consist of what is called **cavernous,** or **erectile, tissue.** This tissue contains a large number of hollow spaces. Because these spaces are normally empty, the penis usually hangs limply from the body. When the male becomes sexually aroused, however, the arteries that supply blood to the penis expand in size, which increases the rate at which blood enters the penis. This extra quantity of blood begins to flow into the spaces of the cavernous tissue. The tissue swells, and the exit valves of the veins in the penis close, thus restricting the flow of blood out of the penis. As a result, the cavernous tissue becomes engorged with blood and the penis grows rigid, a condition known as **erection.**

Sperm are discharged from the penis during **ejaculation,** a process in which a series of muscular contractions expel semen (containing sperm and glandular fluids) from the penis. The subjective sensation of pleasure and release experienced at the height of the sexual act is called **orgasm.** While in the vast majority of instances ejaculation and orgasm occur almost simultaneously, each can take place independently.

THE FEMALE REPRODUCTIVE SYSTEM

The female reproductive system includes: the ovum, or egg, which is the female reproductive cell; the female sex hormones; the ovaries, in which the ova and hormones are produced; the oviducts, or fallopian tubes, through which the egg must pass to reach the uterus; the uterus, in which a fertilized ovum evolves into an embryo; and the vagina, into which the sperm of the male are deposited during intercourse (see Figures 7-2 and 7-3).

The Ovaries

The **ovaries** are small almond-shaped glands about one and one-quarter inches long. Each ovary is located close to the inner side of the pelvis and is held in place by a thin sheet of connective tissue attached to the pelvis by ligaments.

Each ovary consists of two sections: an inner tissue layer called the **medulla,** and a thinner outer layer known as the **cortex.** Each cortex contains about 200,000 microscopic cells called **primordial ova,** each of which is enveloped by a layer of cells. A primordial ovum, together with its covering layer of cells, is called a **primary follicle.**

After a female reaches puberty—which usually occurs between 10 and 15 years of age—one of the 200,000 primary follicles (occasionally two or more) migrates toward the surface of an ovary on an average of every twenty-eight days. The primary follicle develops into a large fluid-filled structure called a **Graafian follicle,** which contains the maturing ovum. The mature ovum is subsequently released from the Graafian follicle.

During the course of a woman's reproductive life, which lasts from puberty until she is about 45 to 51 years old, between 300 and 500 ova will mature and be discharged from her ovaries; the primary follicles that do not mature are gradually absorbed by the body.

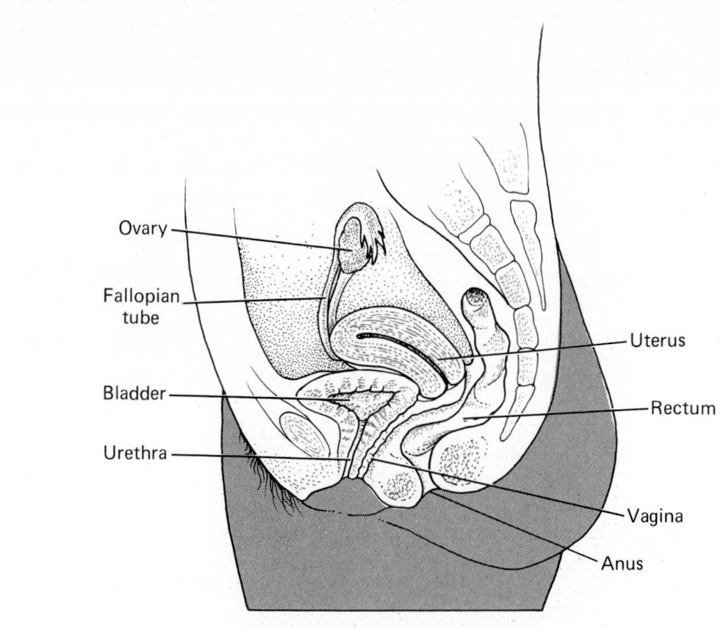

FIGURE 7-2

Placement of major female reproductive structures.

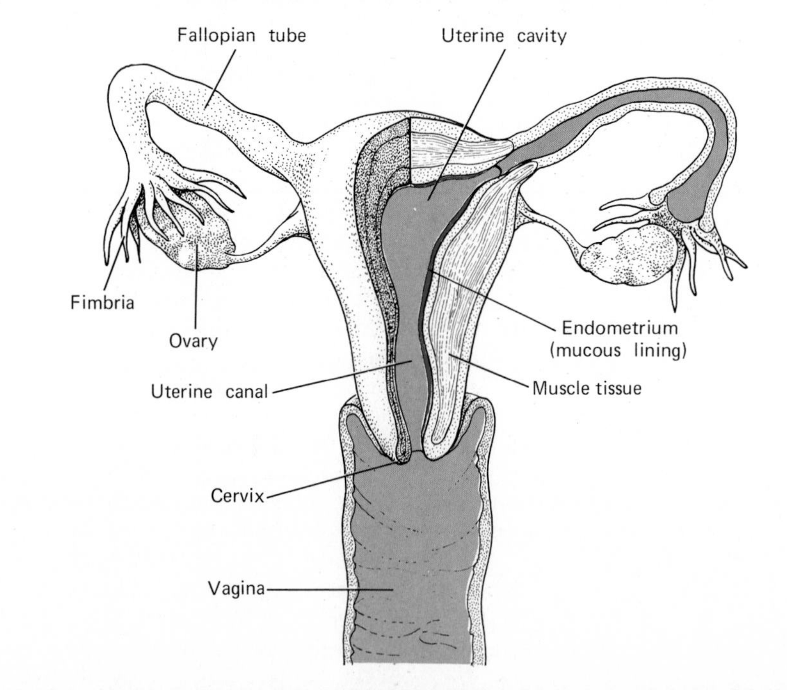

FIGURE 7-3

The female reproductive system.

The Fallopian Tubes

The **fallopian tubes** are the connecting link between the ovaries and the uterus. Each tube is about four and three-fourths inches long. Layers of muscle tissue wrapped around each fallopian tube contract to move an ovum along the tube to the uterus. The fallopian tubes are not attached directly to the ovaries. As an ovum is released from an ovary, the open end of the fallopian tube moves until it covers the ovary like a funnel. Then **cilia,** hairlike projections on the inner lining of the fallopian tubes, produce wavelike motions that draw the ovum into the fallopian tube. The ovum's monthly journey through the fallopian tube to the uterus usually takes about seventy-two hours.

The Uterus

The **uterus** is located a little above and to the rear of the bladder. It resembles a flattened, inverted pear about two and one-half inches long and about one and three-fourths inches across its widest part. The large portion of the uterus, into which the fallopian tubes open, is known as the **fundus.** The smaller, necklike portion at the bottom of the uterus is the **cervix,** which opens into the vagina.

The uterus is the organ that harbors the fetus before birth. Its walls consist of thick layers of muscle tissue. These muscles have the extraordinary ability to stretch to about one hundred times their normal size during pregnancy. Special qualities of the uterine muscles enable the uterus to bear the strain of carrying a fetus during pregnancy and of expelling the baby during birth.

Midway through the menstrual cycle, as an ovum moves along a fallopian

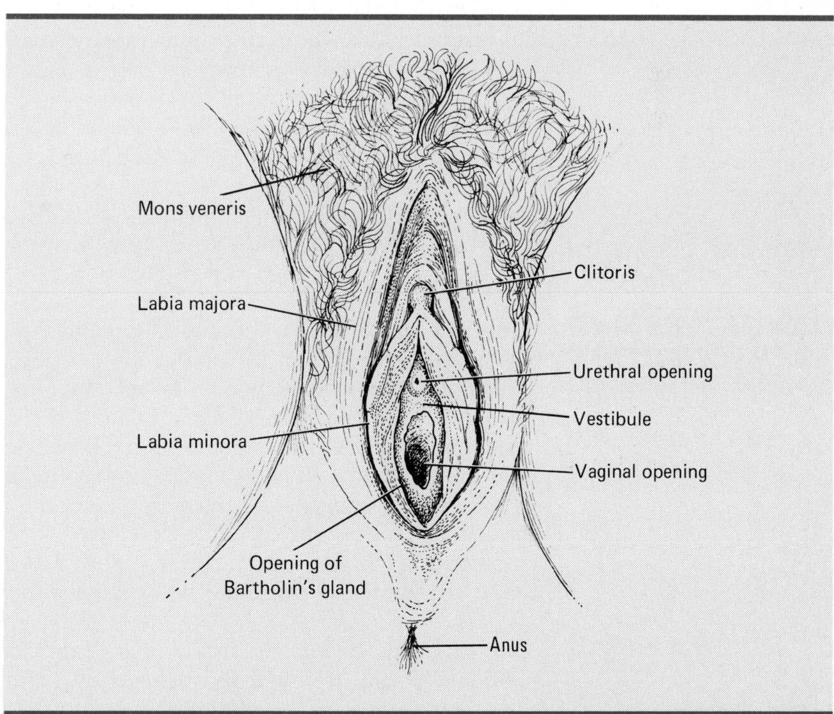

FIGURE 7-4
Female external genitalia

tube, the inner lining of the uterus, the **endometrium,** prepares to receive it by gradually thickening and becoming filled with small pools of blood. If the ovum has been fertilized, it will adhere to the thickened endometrium and be nourished by it. If the ovum has not been fertilized, this layer of cells dies and is shed from the body in the menstrual flow. When this happens, the endometrium is replaced by a new layer of cells.

The Vagina and External Genitalia

The **vagina** is a thick-walled tube about three inches long. The wall of the vagina consists of muscle tissue that can be stretched greatly. The entrance to the vagina is protected by a ring of muscle that can be contracted voluntarily. A thin membrane called the **hymen** partially closes the vaginal opening.

Just outside the vagina are several structures that are collectively called the external genitalia, or the **vulva.** These include the labia majora (outer lips), the labia minora (inner lips), the vestibule, the clitoris, and the mons veneris (mons pubis) (see Figure 7-4). All these tissues are sensitive and excitable.

The **labia majora** are two fatty folds of flesh about two and one-half inches long that lie on either side of the vaginal opening. Extending from within these folds are two thin, sensitive lips of flesh called the **labia minora.** The labia minora form the borders of the vestibule and meet at its top to enclose the clitoris. When they are not sexually stimulated, the labia minora remain pressed together, covering the vaginal opening. The **vestibule** surrounds the vaginal opening and the opening of the urethra. Two glands within the vestibule, called **Bartholin's glands,** secrete a fluid during sexual excitement.

The **clitoris** is a small cylindrical mass of erectile tissue. It is almost completely buried within the folds of the labia minora where they meet at the top of the vestibule. Like the penis, the clitoris becomes engorged with blood when the woman is sexually aroused. It stiffens and swells up to twice its resting size when sexually stimulated, but relaxes and withdraws during the plateau phase and is not even visible during climax. A large number of sensitive nerve endings are located on or around the clitoris; it is the most sexually excitable area of a woman's body.

Above the vulva is a thick mound of fatty tissue covered by skin and pubic hair. This is called the **mons veneris** and serves to protect the genital area.

HORMONES AND REPRODUCTION

The Pituitary and Adrenal Glands

About the size of a pea, the **pituitary gland** is suspended below the brain by a short stalk. It regulates the production of the male and female sex hormones and stimulates the production of the sperm and egg cells. (In fact, the pituitary controls all the hormone-producing glands of the body.) The rear portion of a women's pituitary gland secretes several hormones that causes uterine contractions during childbirth and the secretion of breast milk during nursing.

The **adrenal glands** are located atop each kidney. Hormone secretions from the adrenal cortex influence the development of primary and secondary sex characteristics. If the adrenal cortex is not functioning properly, the hormones that it produces may overstimulate or understimulate sexual development.

The Gonads

The sex glands, or **gonads** (ovaries and testes), produce not only the primary reproductive cells (ova and spermatozoa) but also the hormones that regulate the reproductive systems and keep them functioning. In the male these hormones, called **androgens,** not only aid in the maturation of the reproductive system but also play a vital role in the development of secondary sex characteristics (facial hair, for example). The hormones secreted by the female gonads are the **estrogens** and **progesterone.** Through their reciprocal effect on pituitary hormones, these female sex hormones regulate the monthly cycles of menstruation and ovulation and play a role in the development of secondary sex characteristics.

Hormones and Puberty

Puberty is the period in life when secondary sex characteristics develop and the capacity to play a role in reproduction becomes possible. In females this stage begins on the average at the age of 11, while males usually enter puberty about two years later. In both males and females puberty is initiated when the pituitary gland begins to secrete hormones in a quantity sufficient to stimulate the gonads.

In the Male. With the onset of puberty in the male, hormones produced by the pituitary gland stimulate the cells in the testes to produce **testosterone,** the primary male sex hormone. Testosterone influences the maturation of the male reproductive system and also stimulates the development of the secondary sex characteristics: broadening of the shoulders; deepening of the voice; the growth of hair over the face and chest, under the armpits, and around the genitals; and the enlarging of the penis to its mature size.

The secretions of the male sex hormones are also responsible for the male sex drive. Stimulated by hormones from the pituitary, the testes begin producing sperm. At the same time, the accessory sex glands enlarge and begin to secrete their fluids, which mix with the sperm cells to produce semen.

In the Female. In the female the release of certain pituitary hormones and the corresponding stimulation of estrogen production initiate puberty. The estrogens in turn initiate and control the menstrual cycle; and the female then experiences her first menstrual flow, called **menarche** (pronounced "MEN-ar-key"). Ovulation itself, which involves progesterone, may not start until as much as a year later.

The female sex hormones are also responsible for the secondary sexual characteristics that appear at puberty. The female's pelvis enlarges, and fatty tissue builds up under the skin around the hips and within the breasts. In addition to increasing in size, the breasts also become more sensitive. The female's voice loses the piping tones of girlhood, and hair begins to grow under the armpits and around the external genitalia.

The Menstrual Cycle

When a period of menstruation terminates, a new phase of the menstrual cycle begins. An ovarian follicle begins to increase in size, stimulated by a pituitary hormone. This Graafian follicle, containing the ripening egg, begins to release estrogen. The estrogen causes a thickening in the endometrium (uterine lining) so that the uterus will be prepared to receive the egg if it is fertilized. At approximately the fourteenth day from the start of menstruation, the Graafian follicle ruptures and the ovum and estrogen-rich liquid within the follicle are released. The moment when the egg is released is called **ovulation.**

The Dark Ages

A recent poll reveals that:

- Twenty-two percent of the public believes that menstrual pain is psychosomatic.
- Sixty-six percent of the public finds menstruation an unfit topic for the office and for social conversation.
- Twenty-five percent deem menstruation unacceptable for discussion by the family.

After ovulation the remainder of the Graafian follicle seals itself off to form the **corpus luteum** ("yellow body"), which is a yellowish mass of endocrine tissue. Stimulated by another pituitary hormone, the corpus luteum begins to secrete progesterone. This hormone prepares the uterus for egg implantation by causing it to store **glycogen** (a type of sugar) and to grow thicker. The glycogen will provide nourishment and the thickened uterus a bed for the egg should the egg be fertilized.

If the ovum is not fertilized, the high level of progesterone signals the pituitary to reduce its secretion, causing the corpus luteum to regress slowly and its secretions of estrogen and progesterone to decline. Decreasing amounts of these hormones cause the endometrium to begin breaking down. The degenerated endometrium is expelled from the body in the menstrual fluid.

During the breakdown of the endometrium the corpus luteum continues its own degeneration. Soon it ceases to produce any progesterone at all. The lack of progesterone secretion, together with the low levels of estrogen, causes the pituitary to start secreting certain hormones and a new menstrual cycle begins.

Ovulation generally occurs in the middle of the twenty-eight-day menstrual cycle. Therefore menstruation begins approximately fourteen days after ovulation. **Menstruation,** or the **menses,** is the flow of blood, mucus, and cells of the newly developed uterine lining. This flow usually lasts from four to seven days.

The twenty-eight-day menstrual cycle is only a convenient average. Some women menstruate about every thirty-one days, while for others the period may be roughly every twenty-six days. Still others menstruate with greater irregularity and may even skip a cycle. Strong emotional events such as anxiety or fear of an unwanted pregnancy, or a minor illness such as a cold, may bring menstruation on unexpectedly or cause it to be delayed.

For many women, menstruation is accompanied by mild physical complaints—headaches, abdominal cramps, a feeling of emotional tension or depression. In addition, the breasts may become fuller, the body tissues slightly bloated, and the labia minora irritated. The appearance of these symptoms often signals the beginning of menstruation. For some women these symptoms are fairly acute and may be accompanied by lethargy, irritability, and depression. These women are said to be suffering from **premenstrual syndrome.** Other women, however, never experience any of these discomforts. Still others feel ill one month but not the next.

CONCEPTION

The development of a fetus begins the moment a single **spermatozoon** (or **sperm**) deposited into the female's reproductive system penetrates a mature **ovum** (or **egg**). In a normal ejaculation between 200 million and 400 million sperm are discharged into the vagina. All but a few thousand remain within the vagina and die, usually within three days. Those sperm that manage to make their way into the body of the uterus move toward the fallopian tubes by a vigorous thrashing motion of their tails and may reach the fallopian tubes within a half hour from the time they are deposited in the vaginal tract.

The spermatozoa that reach the ovum in the fallopian tubes encounter a solid layer of cells surrounding the outer surface membrane of the egg. The substance that binds these cells together is broken down by an enzyme found within the heads of the spermatozoa. A single spermatozoon does not contain enough of the enzyme to loosen the cementing substance, but several thousand spermatozoa pressing together against the ovum do. Their combined enzyme

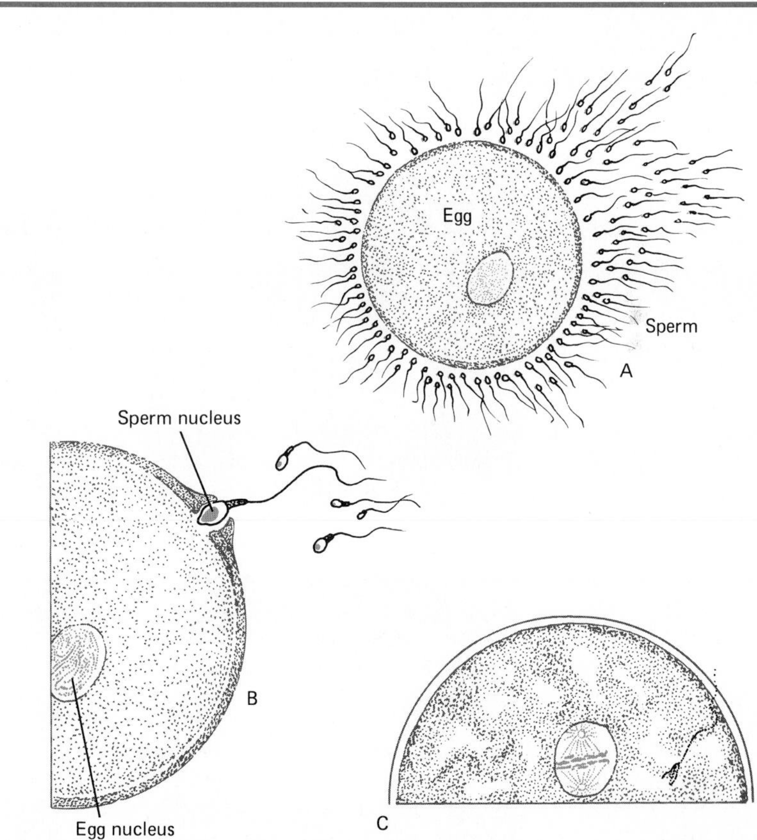

FIGURE 7-5

Events of fertilization. A. An egg cell is surrounded by numerous sperm. B. A single sperm penetrates the membrane and enters the ovum. C. The sperm tail gradually disintegrates, but the head reaches the egg nucleus and initiates the process of cell division.

FIGURE 7-6

Fertilization and implantation. The mature egg leaves the ovary and is fertilized in the fallopian tube. The fertilized egg continues through the tube to the uterus, where it implants itself in the endometrium.

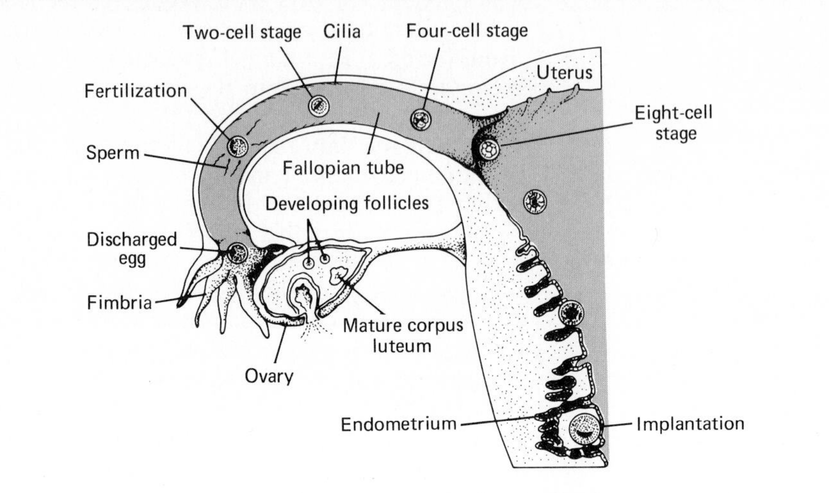

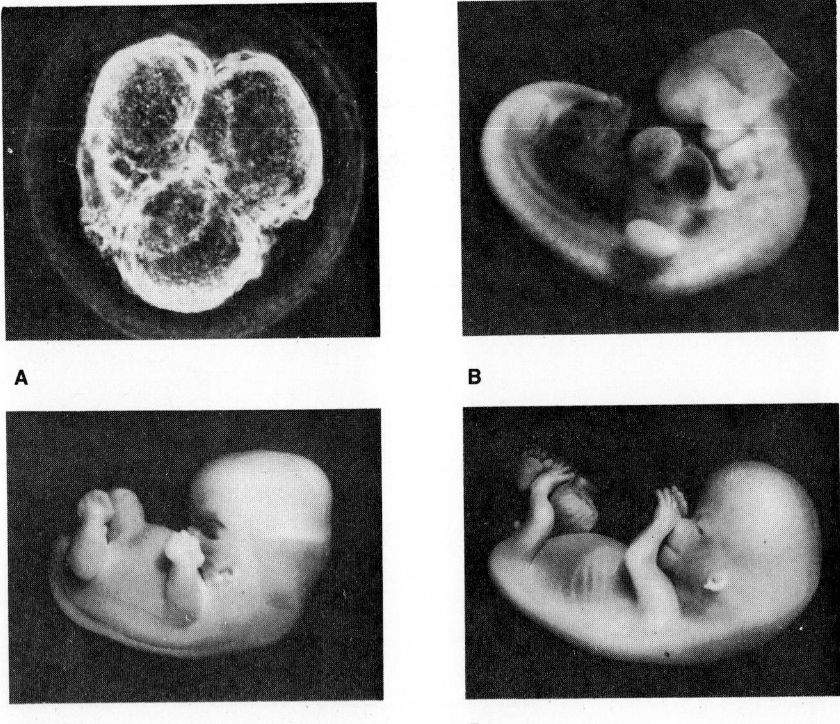

The development of a human embryo. A. The zygote about 3 days after conception. B. The embryo at 5 weeks. C. The embryo at 6 weeks. D. The embryo at 8½ weeks.

loosens the cells. One—and only one—spermatozoon then penetrates the membrane and enters the ovum. The ovum membrane hardens in some unknown way when a sperm penetrates, preventing others from entering (see Figure 7-5).

PREGNANCY

First Stages of Development

An ovum is generally fertilized within a fallopian tube during its journey from the ovary to the uterus. As the fertilized ovum, now called a **zygote,** continues toward the uterus, it undergoes a series of cell divisions. In four days it becomes a cluster of cells and reaches the uterus.

The zygote comes to rest in the lining of the uterus and buries itself in the endometrium. This process of **implantation** is completed by the eleventh day after fertilization (see Figure 7-6).

Prenatal Development

The plan of prenatal development is contained within the chromosomes that are part of the nucleus of each cell. As the cells divide and redivide during the embryonic stage, differentiation and specialization occur, programmed by the hereditary message contained within the chromosomes.

The Embryonic Period. The first two weeks after conception are called the **zygote stage.** The next six weeks—the third to eighth weeks after conception—are called the **embryonic period.** During this time three membranes—the amnion, the chorion, and the placenta—develop around the embryo (see Figure 7-7).

The **amnion** is a thin membranous sac filled with a light, straw-colored liquid called **amniotic fluid.** This fluid insulates the embryo, acts as a protective cushion by absorbing any physical shocks or blows against the woman's abdomen, and permits the embryo to change position.

Within the endometrium, and surrounding the amnion, is a thick membrane known as the **chorion.** This membrane develops fingerlike projections called **chorionic villi,** which connect the separate circulatory systems of the pregnant woman and embryo. Through the walls of the villi, nutrients, vitamins, antibodies, and other substances are diffused from the woman's blood into the embryonic circulatory system, and waste material from the embryo, chiefly nitrogen compounds and carbon dioxide, is diffused into the woman's circulatory system. These waste products are then excreted in the woman's urine and through her lungs.

The embryo, at this time, is attached to the endometrium by a thick stalk. About the third week after conception the first blood vessels appear in the embryo's body. The blood vessels extend themselves along the stalk and continue their growth into the villi. The **vascular tissue** of the endometrium in which the villi are embedded eventually surrounds the chorion. This tissue, with its network of tiny blood vessels, is known as the **placenta.** It eventually links the chorionic membrane with the endometrium. The stalk that connected the embryo with the endometrium is now known as the **umbilical cord.** It contains three large blood vessels that transfer blood between the embryo and placenta.

By the end of the fourth week after conception, the primitive heart has already begun pulsating spontaneously at the rate of sixty beats per minute. Shortly thereafter limb buds appear, as do the rudimentary eyes, ears, nose,

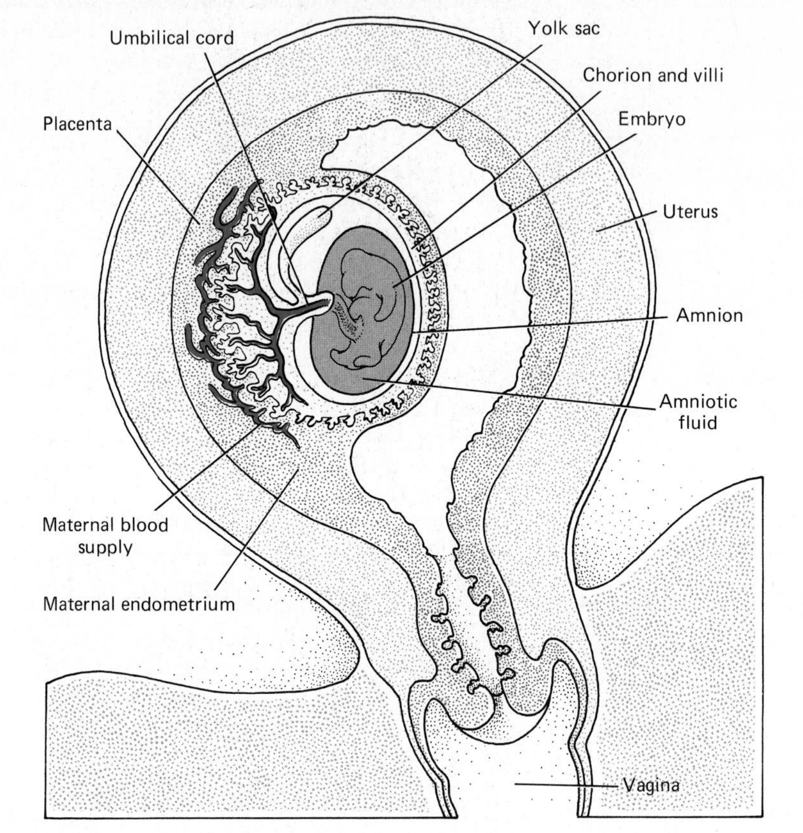

FIGURE 7-7

An early human embryo and its supportive membranes—the amnion, the chorion, and the placenta.

and mouth. Next, rudimentary hands and feet form on the ends of the limb buds during the sixth week. And by the end of the seventh week, fingers and toes appear, tooth buds form in the mouth, and the first bone cells appear and begin to manufacture red blood cells.

At the end of the embryonic period the embryo is about an inch long. Its nervous and muscular systems are so well developed that it can move its arms and legs very slightly, though the movements are unperceived by the mother.

Fetal Stage. The embryo is now called a **fetus.** During the **fetal stage,** from the ninth week to birth, the embryonic structures mature and assume their final forms and functions.

During the third month the fetus becomes capable of moving its limbs, opening and closing its mouth, and swallowing. Genitalia can also be distinguished at this time.

By the end of the fourth month, the fetus is about five and one-half inches long, and it fills the entire uterus. Fetal movements ("quickening") may be felt at this time, and a heartbeat can be detected. During the last month of pregnancy the fetus descends farther down into the pelvis. In late pregnancy the uterus begins to prepare for the expulsion contractions of labor. These contractions may sometimes simulate real labor, but are distinguished from actual labor by their irregularity.

The fetus gains most of its weight, about five pounds, during the final three months of pregnancy. A fetus that is born before the sixth month rarely survives. If birth occurs during the seventh month of pregnancy, the fetus has a 50 percent chance of surviving. At eight months the chance of survival is 90 percent. And at the full nine months the chance of survival is 99 percent.

First Indications of Pregnancy

Usually a woman first suspects that she may be pregnant when she misses a menstrual period. However, this by itself is far from conclusive evidence, since a menstrual period may be skipped for a number of reasons.

Other indications of possible pregnancy are seen a short time after the missed menstrual period. The woman's breasts may become swollen and tender. She may begin to feel slightly ill or nauseated in the mornings—so-called **morning sickness,** which may, in fact, occur at any time of the day.

A physician can usually tell if a woman is pregnant by examining her reproductive organs. The color of the vagina will have become darker as a result of the increased flow of blood through the reproductive system. In addition, the juncture between the cervix and the body of the uterus will have softened. Additional confirmation is provided by testing samples of the woman's urine in the laboratory. These tests check for the presence of a special hormone that becomes detectable about two weeks after the missed menstrual period.

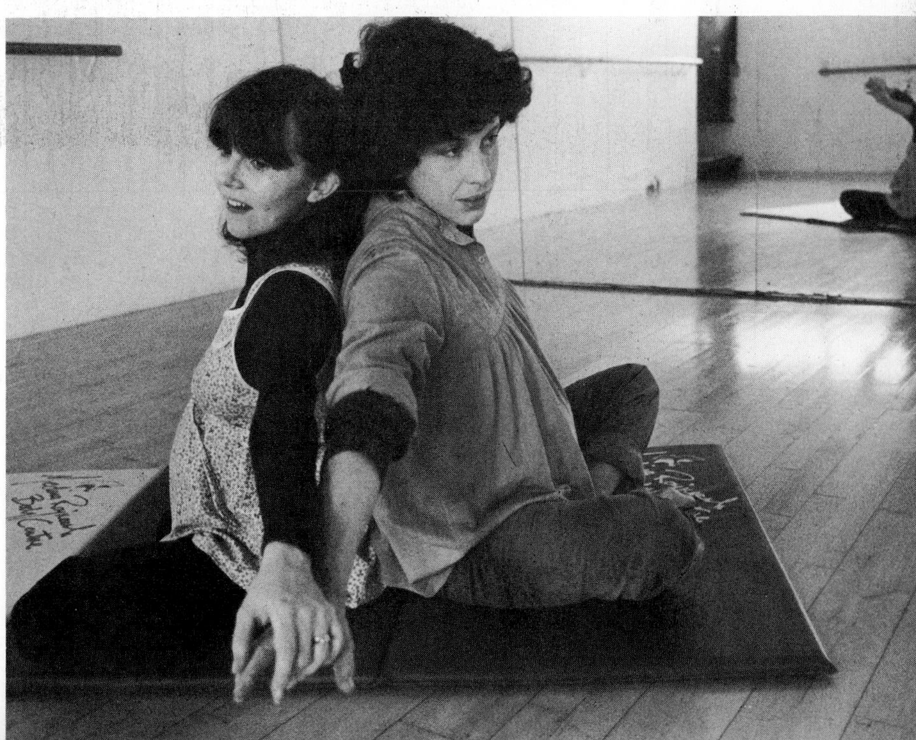

Some women join exercise classes to keep fit during pregnancy.

Self-administered pregnancy-testing kits that have FDA approval are also available, as over-the-counter products.

From the moment of conception, widespread physical changes occur in the woman's body. The most obvious change is the gradual increase in the size of the abdomen, with a concurrent increase in weight. The total weight gain by the time the fetus is fully matured is approximately seventeen to twenty-four pounds, of which about seven pounds is the fetus itself. Much of the remaining weight is due to the collection of fluids in the woman's body.

Care During Pregnancy

Medical Care. It is extremely important for a woman to have frequent medical checkups during pregnancy, not only for her own health, but also for the health of the fetus. Over 90 percent of all cases of mental deficiency in children, for example, are caused by events that occur during the prenatal period, rather than by hereditary factors. The following schedule of examinations is recommended for the pregnant woman: once a month for the first twenty-eight weeks; once every two weeks from the twenty-eighth to the thirty-sixth week; and weekly from the thirty-sixth week on.

During the visit in which the pregnancy is confirmed, the physician makes a thorough examination and also learns the woman's medical history. If it is her first pregnancy, the physician will estimate the size of the space enclosed by the bones of the pelvis. A small pelvis may mean a difficult birth, for a full-term baby may not be able to pass easily through the birth canal.

The urine is tested for sugar level and for any indications of abnormal metabolic or kidney function. A blood sample is taken to determine the woman's blood group (in case a transfusion is necessary during labor); to check for syphilis; to test the hemoglobin level of the blood; to find out whether the woman is anemic; and to determine if her blood contains the **Rh factor.**

A dangerous reaction may occur when a mother who has no Rh factor in her blood (indicated as **Rh negative**) conceives a child who has the factor (**Rh positive**), transmitted through inheritance from the father. Normally, the first child to be born escapes damage. But following delivery, **sensitization** occurs; that is, antibodies are developed in the mother's blood that may attack the red blood cells of subsequent fetuses possessing the Rh positive factor. Unless one or more massive blood transfusions are administered to the infant, anemia, jaundice, or even death could result. The drug Rho-GAM, or other immune globulin, may be administered to the mother soon after delivery to prevent the formation of antibodies that would attack a future fetus.

Diet. The old saying "You are eating for two now" has more sentimentality behind it than reason. As long as a woman is healthy and within the weight limits desirable for her height and body build, she does not need to increase her intake of food during the first four and one-half months of pregnancy. It is indeed more important for her future health that she avoid overeating and gaining unnecessary weight.

The woman should carefully follow the diet recommendations of her physician. In general, the best diet to follow during pregnancy is one that is low in carbohydrates and salt and high in proteins and minerals; it should also contain a sufficient, but not excessive, amount of vitamins. (Birth defects, for example, may result from too much vitamin D.) Liberal amounts of fruits, vegetables, and lean meats should be included in the diet.

As for general physical fitness, exercise is not only permissible but beneficial during pregnancy. Women are becoming increasingly more active during pregnancy.

A pregnant woman needs a greater amount of sleep than she does normally. In addition to eight hours of sleep at night, she may need a rest period during the day. Such a rest, preferably with the feet elevated, will also prevent or limit the severity of varicose veins.

Because of the fetus's need for calcium, small cavities in the woman's teeth may worsen quickly and should therefore be filled in early pregnancy. Inflammation and bleeding of the gums are also frequent.

Heartburn or indigestion in the later months of pregnancy is caused by the baby's increased size. Only preparations recommended by a physician should be taken for these complaints. Constipation may also result from changes within the pregnant woman's body. Drinking large amounts of water, eating additional fruits and vegetables, and exercising may help to alleviate constipation.

In addition to the physical alterations that take place in pregnancy, there may be psychological changes. Some pregnant women experience enormous mood swings—they may feel depressed one moment and elated the next. Others report feelings of peace and harmony throughout pregnancy. Whatever anxieties expectant parents have should be aired instead of suppressed.

LABOR AND CHILDBIRTH

First Stage of labor

For a woman having her first child, the first stage of **labor** may last up to sixteen hours. This time period decreases with each subsequent pregnancy. The first stage of labor usually begins with a mild backache. Gradually, the aching sensation shifts toward the front of the body, where the uterus has begun to contract.

A physician, nurse, or midwife judges the stage of labor by directly feeling to what degree the cervix has dilated: A fully dilated cervix signals the end of the first stage of labor. Labor often begins with the passage of a small amount of blood-stained mucus from the vagina. In about 10 percent of births the amnion ruptures and the amniotic fluid escapes. These signs indicate that labor is imminent. As the first stage of labor progresses, the contractions occur more frequently and the pain becomes more intense. Most women enter the hospital or alternative birth setting when contractions are occurring about every twenty minutes.

As the end of the first stage approaches, the contractions occur about once every eight to ten minutes. If the amnion did not rupture earlier, it will usually do so at this time. As the uterine contractions become increasingly strong, the woman may be given an analgesic or painkilling drug if she wishes. Throughout the following stages of labor, carefully monitored amounts of anesthesia may be administered to her, although the current trend is to avoid the use of general anesthetic gases.

Second Stage of Labor

The second stage of labor begins when the baby's head enters the fully dilated cervix; it ends when the baby is finally born. This stage lasts about one and

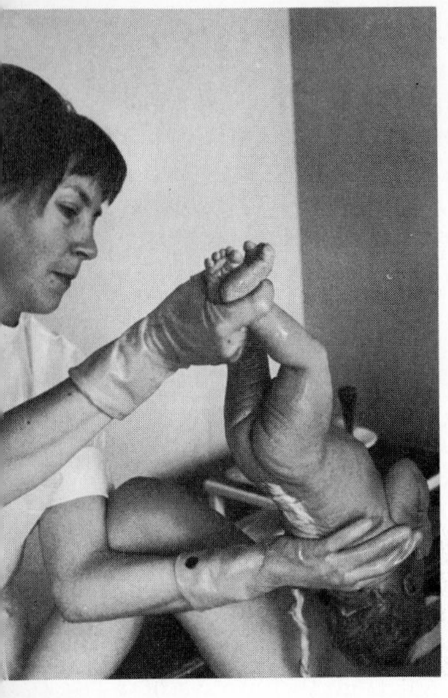

three-fourths hours in the case of a firstborn and a somewhat shorter time if the woman has previously given birth.

It is during the second stage of labor that the mother adds her voluntary abdominal contractions to the automatic contractions of the uterus. Every time she feels a contraction coming on, she takes a deep breath and contracts her abdominal muscles so they exert a constant, steady pressure as long as the uterine contractions last. Her voluntary efforts almost double the force of the uterine contractions and substantially reduce the length of the second stage. With each labor contraction, the baby descends lower, until its scalp is visible at the entrance of the birth canal.

During this stage of labor the **perineum** (the tissue between the vagina and the anus) must stretch to accommodate the infant's head. To avoid possible vaginal tears from the pressure and stretching, most obstetricians perform an **episiotomy,** which is an incision in the perineum. Episiotomies, if necessary, are more often required for first births.

As the baby's head passes through the **birth canal,** it is carefully guided by the physician (or by the birth attendant for women who choose to deliver in their homes or other birth settings). After the head has emerged, the professional feels for the umbilical cord to make sure it is not wrapped about the baby's neck. He or she supports the weight of the child, which, once the head has emerged, rapidly continues its egress from the mother's body.

Once the baby is delivered, the physician or birth attendant uses a rubber tube to suck fluid out of the baby's throat and nose, permitting it to take in its first breath of air. Its first cries help the lungs to expand fully.

The physician or birth attendant then clamps the umbilical cord shut and ties it. Afterward the cord is severed and a stalk about two inches long is left. The stalk withers off in about two days; what remains is an involuted piece of skin called the **navel.** Medical practitioners will wash the baby's eyes with an antibiotic solution immediately after birth to prevent infection, should the mother have gonorrhea. The process of birth is illustrated in Figure 7-8.

Kinds of Delivery. In about 97 percent of all births the head of the baby precedes the rest of the body. This is called a **cephalic presentation.** If the feet or buttocks appear first, it is called a **breech presentation.** If a shoulder or the chest appears first, it is known as a **transverse presentation.** Physicians can usually manipulate the position of a baby between contractions so the head appears first. If they cannot, and if it appears that the baby might become jammed in an unmovable position that endangers both it and the mother, they will deliver the baby through an incision made in the mother's abdomen and uterus. This is known as a **cesarean delivery.** Cesarean delivery is also used when the mother's pelvis is too small and for other medical reasons (see box: Cesarean Births).

Third Stage of Labor

The third stage of labor begins shortly after the baby's delivery. During this stage, which lasts just a few minutes, the **afterbirth**—consisting of umbilical cord, placenta, and the remnants of the chorion and amnion—is expelled from the uterus. The physician, nurse, or midwife may hasten the expulsion of the

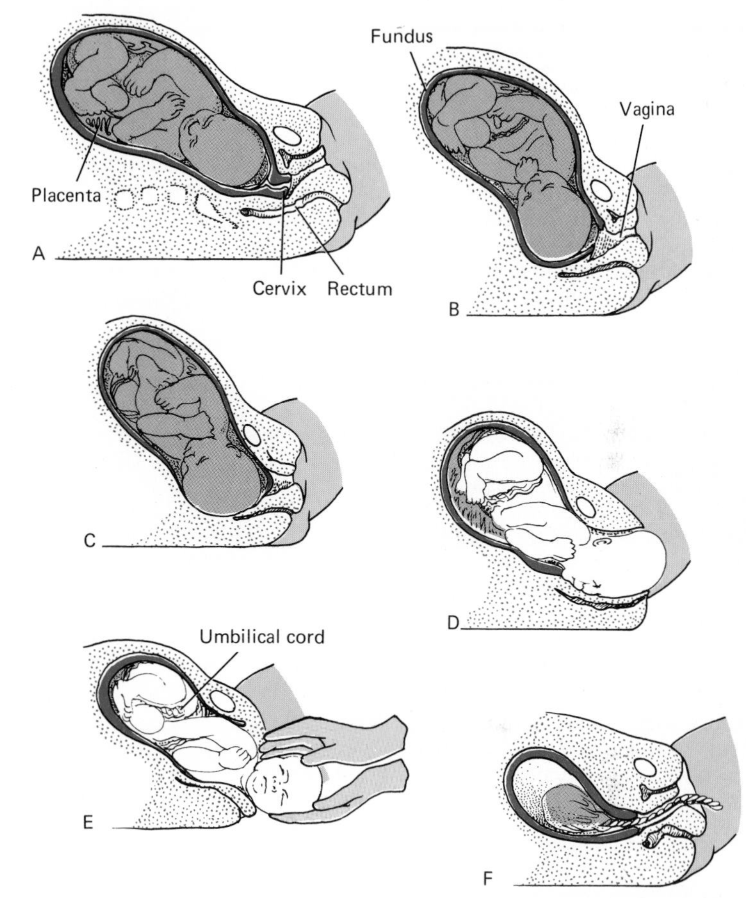

FIGURE 7-8

The process of birth. A. The uterus before the dilation of the cervix. The baby is still enclosed in the placenta. B. The cervix dilates as the uterus contracts. C. The cervix is fully dilated as the baby begins to leave the uterus. D. The baby has left the placenta; its head emerges from the birth canal. Note how the head has become elongated. E. The physician (or birth attendant) guides the baby through the remainder of the delivery. F. The afterbirth—the placenta and cord—are expelled.

afterbirth by pressing down on the mother's distended abdomen to force it from the uterus.

The placenta is then examined to make sure no fragments have remained attached to the wall of the uterus. If they have, there is a possibility of hemorrhage. After the removal of any fragments, the episiotomy is repaired and the process of birth is complete.

Postnatal Period

An enormous quantity of fluid is discharged from the mother's body in the first twenty-four hours after delivery. As much as three quarts of urine will be eliminated the first day. The abdomen remains soft and flabby for several months until the abdominal muscles can return to their original size and regain their tone. The process can be aided by doing special exercises that utilize the abdominal muscles. The cervix slowly shrinks to its former state, and the vagina and uterus contract almost to their original size.

Problems and Controversies
Cesarean Births

One out of every five American babies is now being delivered by cesarean section. (The procedure was named for Julius Caesar, who is said to have been born by this method.) Fifteen years ago it was one out of twenty. The mothers of those babies often feel sad, guilty, and angry over having been deprived of the profound emotional experience of a natural birth; they also criticize doctors for resorting to the procedure too quickly.

Nevertheless, doctors continue to perform the operation for various reasons. Many believe that once a woman has had a cesarean, she should have one for every following birth; they fear that a normal delivery will cause the original incision to break. Others point to the fact that more and more women are waiting until their thirties to have their first child and are thus more likely to have difficult deliveries. They also say that small-framed women often have an increasingly difficult time in childbirth because later babies tend to be bigger.

Many mothers, on the other hand, complain that the procedure is often unnecessary. They point to the fact that, thanks to improved surgical techniques that involve a smaller incision, over half the women who have undergone one cesarean can go on to have later children by vaginal delivery. They say that doctors perform most cesareans just to save themselves time.

Others claim that physicians perform most cesareans in order to avoid malpractice suits. Because juries are now holding physicians responsible for any injury an infant or mother suffers in the course of a natural delivery, many physicians quickly resort to a cesarean the moment any sign of birthing trouble begins. The act of performing a cesarean seems to convince juries that a doctor has done everything possible to avoid a bad outcome.

Pressures to reduce the number of cesareans have grown stronger in recent years. In spite of claims that the procedure is as safe as a tonsillectomy or an appendectomy, twice as many women die as a result of a cesarean as from a natural birth, owing mostly to complications from anesthesia, not surgery. Federal authorities, worried over soaring Medicaid costs, are pressing for fewer cesareans because the operation requires the mother to be hospitalized twice as long as for a normal delivery.

Sources: Adapted from Sandra Blakeslee, "Doctors Debate Surgery's Place in the Maternity Ward," *New York Times*, March 24, 1985, Sect. 4, p. 24; "Still Too Many Caesareans?" *Newsweek*, December 31, 1984, p. 70.

The first menstrual period after childbirth usually occurs approximately six weeks after delivery. The physician schedules the patient for a checkup at about that time. Sexual intercourse and douching are prohibited until this checkup; but after the examination all normal activities, including intercourse, may be resumed. Precautions should be taken against a subsequent pregnancy, however, until the mother has had adequate opportunity to recover.

Some women may have a psychological sensation of anticlimax following delivery. The anticipation is over, the child is here. **Postpartum depression** is the common name for this feeling. Generally, the depression disappears after a few weeks when a routine of child care is established.

Natural Childbirth

On a worldwide basis, most children are born out of hospitals by the simplest of all methods: by allowing normal uterine contractions to carry out the process. During the birth process the mother supplements the force of labor contraction by exerting pressure at appropriate moments. If she receives any professional assistance during delivery, it is usually from a **midwife,** a layperson or nurse trained especially to perform these duties.

The traditional childbirth practices in the United States have been quite different. Here babies are usually delivered in hospitals under operating-room conditions in which the mother is anesthetized, at least to some degree. Criticism of this method of child delivery centers around the effects of anesthesia upon both the fetus and the mother. A general anesthesia can quickly traverse the placenta, enter the bloodstream of the fetus, and cause some impairment. Any form of anesthesia renders the mother less capable of consciously assisting the childbirth process, thereby necessitating the greater use of forceps upon the fetus. Brain damage and other injuries have been attributed to the use of forceps. These factors contribute to our **infant mortality rate.**

The concern of many parents over the welfare of their children, as well as their desire to participate fully in the experience of childbirth, has led to an increasing interest in the natural childbirth method. The most popular of these approaches is the Lamaze method, developed by a French obstetrician, Ferdinand Lamaze. The Lamaze method requires the prospective mother, accompa-

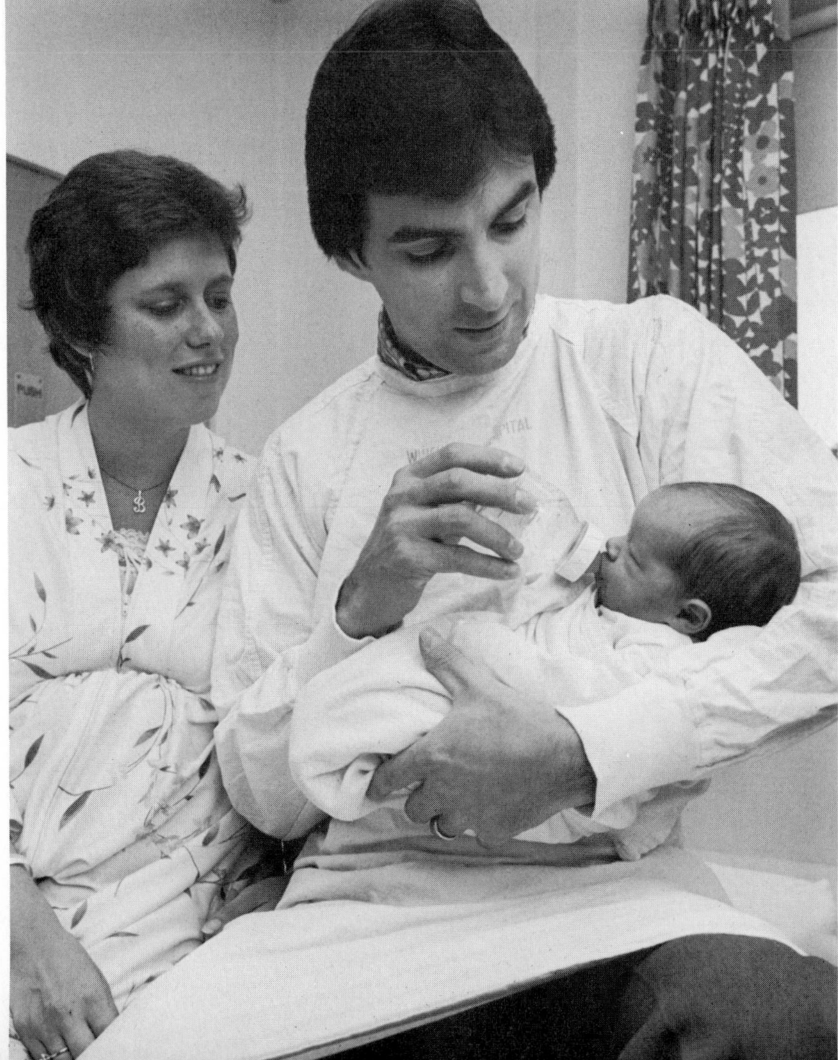

nied by the father or another person, to enter a specialized program during her last months of pregnancy. The program is physical and psychological.

The physical aspects of the program are designed to develop the muscle tone of the pelvic and abdominal areas of the pregnant woman's body so that she will be able to contract these muscles at will. She is also taught to regulate her breathing in order to minimize the pain of labor contractions.

As for the psychological aspects, the mother learns positive attitudes toward the process of childbirth. Being well informed about the birth process, having a very specific role to perform, and gradually acquiring confidence in her ability to perform this role—all help the mother develop a favorable attitude toward childbirth. This positive outlook, combined with the distraction of being occupied with the birth process, serves to reduce nervous tension and subsequent muscular tension—an ultimate cause of pain. The role of the father or other person is supportive: to coach the mother and provide encouragement and reassurance during the birth process.

A mild painkiller may be administered to the woman in labor, but the use of general anesthetics is avoided unless at some point she determines that she does not wish to continue with the Lamaze method.

Natural childbirth may be conducted in specially designated hospital facilities called *birthing rooms*, or in newer institutions created for this purpose, called *childbirth centers* (see box: Alternatives to Hospital Birth). Midwives generally assist in these facilities. In addition to the personal satisfaction that parents derive from participating in the natural childbirth method, there is a financial benefit as well. Natural childbirth in a childbirth center often costs much less than a traditional hospital delivery.

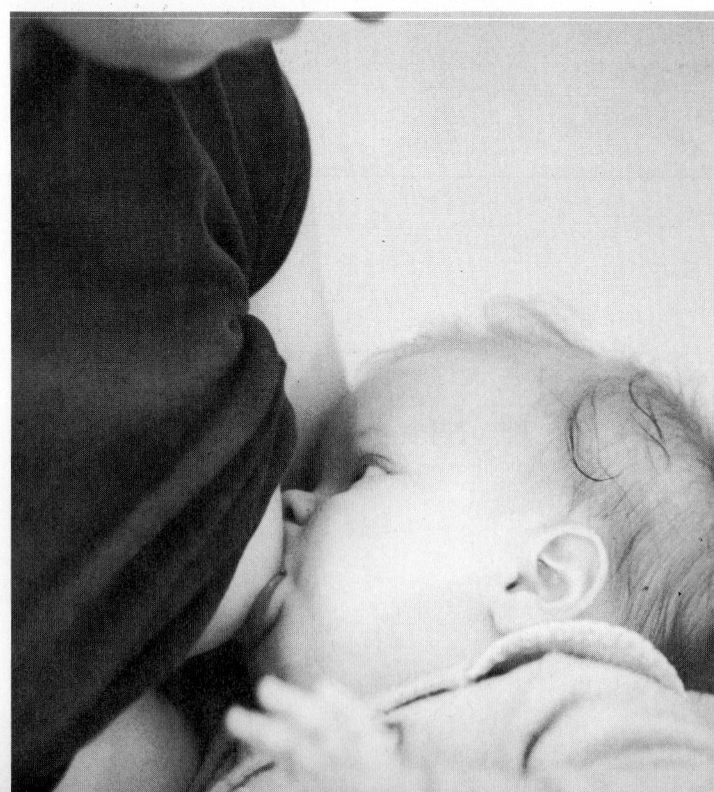

Nursing The first fluid secreted by the **mammary glands** in the breasts is not milk but **colostrum.** It is a thin yellow liquid that often has a gentle cathartic effect on the baby's intestines. The flow of colostrum lasts two or three days before it is replaced by milk.

If the accumulating milk is not drawn from the breasts, the swelling of the blood vessels and mammary glands can be quite painful. Thus mothers who do not breast-feed are given an injection of testosterone and estrogen to suppress **lactation** (milk production) and enlargement of the breasts. For mothers who nurse, the breast swelling subsides within two or three days, partly as a result of the baby's sucking at the nipples. The sucking sensation stimulates the nervous system, which in turn triggers the secretion of a hormone produced by the pituitary gland. The hormone causes the smooth muscles in the mammary glands to contract and expel the milk.

A mother who intends to nurse her child must increase her intake of essential nutrients so that her body can produce enough milk. Between two and a half and three and a half cups of milk are secreted per day, more than enough for a newborn child. As the child grows, the amount of milk produced by the mammary glands increases proportionately, to a maximum of about a quart and a half a day. Gradually, the amount of milk produced becomes inadequate for the nutritional needs of the growing child, whose diet must be supplemented.

With the current interest in doing things the natural way, nursing is once again becoming a widespread practice. (It has been estimated that half of American mothers with twelve or more years of education nursed their babies during the 1970s). One of the pioneer organizations promoting the back-to-breast-

Alternatives to Hospital Birth

While only 1.5 percent of American women have their babies outside a hospital, a growing number of them are becoming dissatisfied with the impersonal nature of traditional hospital facilities and personnel. They are choosing instead to give birth under the supervision of a midwife at a birthing center or at home. (A midwife is a childbirth assistant who remains with a mother throughout labor. Most midwives have spent a year or more studying obstetrics and related subjects in hospital training programs in addition to their years in nursing school.)

Childbirth centers are relatively new institutions in which women can give birth with a midwife attending in comfortable, homelike surroundings. Fathers, mothers, and newborns often stay together in the same room. The women usually receive little, if any, medication and are often able to leave the next day. The cost is about half that of a hospital stay.

Women who give birth at home have the advantage of being surrounded by supportive friends and family members; they are also able to keep their babies with them constantly.

Whether she chooses a birthing center or a home birth, a prospective mother must be in good health and must expect an uncomplicated delivery. It is essential that she watch her nutrition carefully and obtain good prenatal care. In some states women who give birth at home with a midwife must either be under the care of a physician or visit a clinic at least three times during their pregnancy. Pregnant women over 35 are advised to have their children in a hospital.

Source: Adapted from Robin Warshaw, "The American Way of Birth: High-Tech Hospitals, Birthing Centers, or No Options at All," *Ms. Magazine,* September 1984, pp. 45–50, 130.

feeding trend is the La Leche League. More than any other group, it has been responsible for reeducating American women about the benefits of nursing.

Nursing has numerous physiological and psychological advantages. It is an important means of bonding between mother and child, ensuring regular, close contact between the two and giving the child an initial feeling of security. Mother's milk, and colostrum in particular, is full of antibodies that protect the baby against allergy and disease. Breast milk is easy on the baby's sometimes delicate digestive system, and it does not cause constipation or diarrhea, as some mixed formulas do. Advantages to the mother include helping her to relax and to take time to enjoy her baby. Nursing also helps the womb return to its normal size more quickly.

Although some people are still squeamish about mothers nursing in public, such activities are becoming more readily accepted as people accept their own sexuality more completely.

MISCARRIAGE AND ABORTION

The word **miscarriage** is commonly used to mean a spontaneous or involuntary termination of pregnancy before the fetus can survive outside the uterus. The term **abortion** is frequently used to mean a termination of pregnancy that is artificially induced. Medically, however, the term *abortion* refers to *any* termination of pregnancy—whether it occurs spontaneously or is induced—before the fetus can live outside the uterus.

Spontaneous Abortion

About one out of every ten pregnancies terminates in a spontaneous abortion at a point before the fetus can survive outside the uterus. Most of these occur before the twelfth week of pregnancy, with only 25 percent occurring between the twelfth and twenty-eighth weeks.

Some of the causes of spontaneous abortion are: (1) poor physical condition

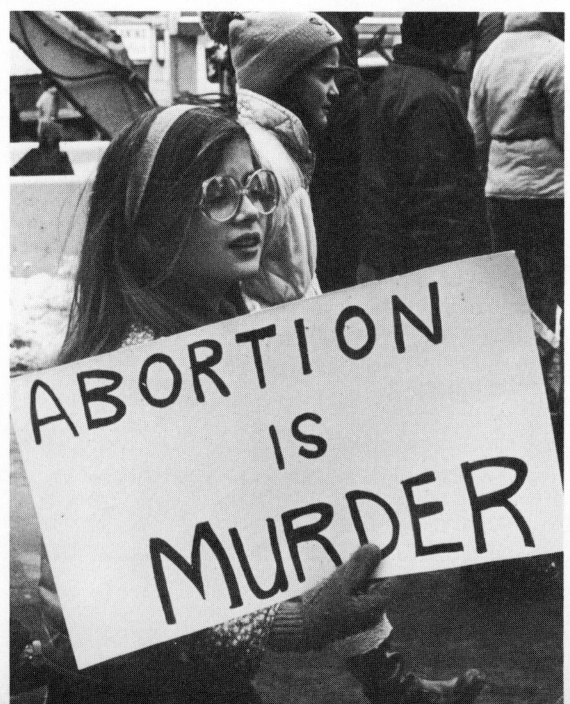

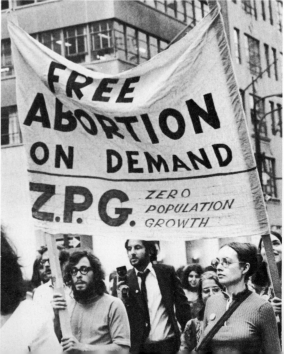

of the mother's uterus; (2) congenital malformations of the reproductive organs; (3) certain illnesses, such as diabetes mellitus or syphilis; (4) a defect or abnormality in the fetus; and (5) an unfavorable uterine environment. Contrary to popular belief, abortions are not caused by overstrenuous activity such as vigorous exercise, travel, sexual intercourse, or a fall.

Induced Abortion

Moral and religious objections to induced abortion have existed since earliest times, and laws against it were passed down from generation to generation. Ancient Christians and Jews considered abortion a sin against God's commandments and his wish for human beings to "be fruitful and multiply." Since old civilizations were periodically faced with a severe problem of underpopulation, abortion was considered not only a sin in a religious sense but a threat to the survival of a people as well.

Today some religious philosophies still condemn abortion, and many individuals consider it an act of murder against a human being, even though it is yet unborn. The fear of underpopulation, however, no longer applies—the world is rapidly becoming overpopulated. For this reason, many people have come to regard birth control and abortion as the only viable alternatives to a disastrously overcrowded environment. Others have supported abortion as part of the inalienable right of women to control their own lives. These new attitudes and changing environmental conditions are slowly being reflected in our abortion laws.

Until rather recently, most state laws stipulated that the only reason a woman could legally have an abortion was in order to save her life. Some states also permitted abortions if the pregnancy resulted from rape or if the child would be born with a severe birth defect. In 1973 a Supreme Court decision liberalized the laws concerning abortion. This decision declared that every woman is eligible for a legal abortion anywhere in the United States.

The sole legal requirement during the first trimester (through the twelfth week of pregnancy) is that a licensed physician perform the abortion. During the second trimester (the thirteenth through twenty-sixth weeks), a state may determine the abortion procedure used. During the third trimester, state laws would remain in effect under most conditions. Essentially, however, a woman may now obtain a legal abortion at any time and for any reason during the first six months of pregnancy.

The liberalized abortion laws have led to a sharp decrease in the number of abortion-related deaths. Prior to the Supreme Court ruling, it is conservatively estimated that from 300 to 800 deaths occurred each year as a result of illegally performed abortions. In fact, legal abortions are much safer than childbirth. The safest time to have an abortion is between the eighth and tenth weeks of pregnancy. Under no circumstances should a woman who desires an abortion go to anyone except a qualified physician.

Before the Supreme Court's 1973 ruling, some 200,000 abortions were being performed in the United States each year. The number is now about 4,000 a day; more than one pregnancy in four is ended by abortion. The large number of abortions now being performed has made the issue more controversial. Many "right-to-life" groups have been formed, with the aim of convincing the Supreme Court to reverse its decision. Congress has voted restrictions on government-paid abortions. And the fact that fetuses can be kept alive at increasingly earlier ages because of advances in medical research has further complicated the abortion issue.

Many states circumvented the intent of the Supreme Court's decision by legislative requirements that made abortions more difficult to obtain. The Supreme Court has struck down many of these statutes, reaffirming the basic principle "that a woman has the fundamental right to make the highly personal choice whether or not to terminate her pregnancy." It is not until the third trimester that the state can intervene to protect the life of the fetus. In respect to state laws requiring parental consent, the Court ruled that such laws must be sufficiently flexible to allow a minor to show that she is mature enough to make the decision on her own or that the abortion is in her best interest.

Abortion Methods. The following methods are generally used in abortions up to the sixteenth week of pregnancy, although after the twelfth week they are likely to be done on an inpatient basis.

Dilation and curettage can be performed under local anesthesia. The cervix is dilated, and the physician then scrapes the embryo from the inner lining of the uterus with an instrument called a curette.

Uterine aspiration is largely replacing dilation and curettage for early abortions. In this procedure the cervix is dilated and a suction tube removes the contents of the uterus. The method takes about five minutes.

Menstrual extraction is similar to uterine aspiration but does not necessitate dilation. It is sometimes performed as early as two weeks after a missed period, even before pregnancy has definitely been diagnosed.

The following three methods are hospital procedures, used in late-term abortions.

Saline instillation or **injection** is a procedure in which a tube is inserted through the abdominal wall and into the amnion. A pint of amniotic fluid is then replaced by a saltwater solution. Spontaneous abortion occurs within 6 to 96 hours, with most occurring about 36 hours after the operation.

An **open hysterotomy** is a major surgical procedure in which an incision is made through the abdominal wall and the fetus removed. This operation is performed only for advanced cases of pregnancy, in which the fetus is too far developed for the other methods to be used safely.

All of these processes must take place under strict medical supervision in case of shock or hemorrhage and to prevent infection.

INFERTILITY

The vast majority of couples will conceive a child within two years if birth control methods are not used. It has been estimated, however, that there are perhaps 3.5 million couples in the United States who want children but who are infertile. Infertility was once believed to be the exclusive fault of the woman, probably because she is the one who bears the children. Actually, in about 40 percent of all childless marriages the infertility is due to the male's inability to produce or deposit viable sperm.

Infertility in Women

Fertility in women depends on a number of general factors: normal good health, a normal reproductive system, a normal ovarian cycle, the absence of any infections or inflammations of the reproductive tract, and the absence of any psycho-

Female Fertility after 30

It has long been observed that a woman's fertility is highest during her 20s and then falls off in her 30s. Many have disputed, however, whether the decline reflects a true biological change in reproductive capacity. It has been argued that the drop in pregnancy rates after 30 is the result of such factors as reduced sexual activity or a decline in male fertility.

A recent study appears to rule out such possibilities. The study covered pregnancy success among more than 2,000 women who underwent artificial insemination because their husbands were sterile. The conception rate was 73 percent for women under 25, and 74 percent for those between 26 and 30. But pregnancies among women 31 to 35 showed a sharp drop to 61 percent, and for those over 35 it fell to 53 percent. The reason for the decline in fertility remains unknown.

logical barriers to bearing children. Psychological factors that suppress menstruation, poor health, a hormone imbalance or hormone deficiency, the presence of an infectious disease, or the development of scar tissue in the fallopian tubes because of a past infection blocking the passage of the ovum (see the section Pelvic Inflammatory Disease in Chapter 15)—any of these conditions might impair the normal fertility of a woman.

A physician can learn from the normal secretions of the cervix whether the ovaries are functioning correctly. If these secretions are examined under a microscope at various stages in the monthly cycle, they demonstrate very distinctive patterns that change with the progression of the cycle.

Any possible blockage of the fallopian tubes is checked by injecting into the uterus an opaque dye that can be detected by X-ray. If the tubes are not blocked, the dye will travel through them, and the X-ray will reveal the outlined uterus and fallopian tubes. Surgeons may be able to repair blocked tubes through delicate microsurgery. But often this cannot be done, and the ovum cannot travel down the fallopian tube.

A hormone imbalance is usually obvious and can be confirmed by analysis of the woman's blood and urine. Fertility pills have been developed to correct hormone imbalances. One such pill supplies a hormone that mimics the action of a pituitary hormone by artificially stimulating the production of ova by the ovaries. In fact, it may cause several ova to mature simultaneously. This increases the chances that sperm will fertilize an ovum and sometimes results in multiple conceptions.

Infertility in Men

Fertility in men, as in women, depends on several general factors: normal good health, a normal reproductive system, the production of viable sperm by the testes, the absence of any infections or inflammations of the reproductive tract, and the absence of nervous strain or fatigue.

In general, fertility requires a minimum of 20 million sperm per milliliter of semen. At least 70 percent of the sperm must be active and must travel at a minimum rate of speed; and at least 70 percent of the sperm must be normally shaped. The sperm can be counted and checked for abnormalities by examining a fresh sample of semen under a microscope.

Overheating of the testes is perhaps the most common reason for failure to produce viable sperm. Normally, the temperature of the testes is about two to three degrees below body temperature. In some men, however, the scrotum may habitually be too close to the body, which causes the testes to become overheated and decreases the number of viable sperm produced. It is also possible that an otherwise normal male who is addicted to prolonged soaking in hot baths, to steam rooms, or to saunas may unwittingly sterilize himself for days or weeks because of overheating the testes.

In some infertile men a swollen vein, or **varicocele,** has developed within the scrotum. Warm blood accumulates in the vein and increases the overall temperature within the scrotum. As a result, the production of viable sperm is diminished. This condition can be corrected by surgery, but fertility is not guaranteed.

The absence of sperm in the seminal fluid indicates a blockage in one of the sperm ducts. A blocked duct can often be opened by a surgical operation. In a very small percentage of men an organic defect of the testes may result in an inability to produce mature spermatozoa.

Infertility in the Couple

Even though a man and woman may have nothing individually wrong with them, as a couple they may be unable to conceive children. For example, a woman who exhibits low fertility may be able to conceive with a man who has a high sperm count but unable to conceive with a man who has an average or low sperm count. (This particular condition may be corrected if intercourse is avoided until the sperm count is raised.)

The position of the woman during and after intercourse may also prevent conception. It takes some twenty to thirty minutes for the semen to liquefy completely, which increases the probability that sperm will enter the cervix in sufficient numbers. Therefore if the woman does not lie recumbent for about thirty minutes after intercourse has been completed, the sperm may not be given maximum opportunity to enter the uterus.

The possibility that some women develop an allergic reaction to their husband's sperm is being studied. It may be that an antibody reaction in the vaginal secretions of some women will destroy the sperm in much the same way that any other foreign object in the body is destroyed by antibodies. Hormonal treatments offer a possible solution to this problem.

Overcoming Infertility

If the man's sperm is normal but is produced in insufficient quantities, his semen may be collected and stored so that a concentrated sample can be injected into the woman. If the man is infertile, a childless couple may choose to have the woman impregnated with the semen of a donor. Both of these methods of fertilization are called **artificial insemination.**

If a donor is sought, he is often chosen on the basis of demonstrated fertility and known hereditary traits. Very often a doctor will try to match the donor's physical appearance with the husband's. The anonymity of the donor is assured by the physician.

Sometimes infertility occurs when a blocked fallopian tube prevents the egg from descending to the uterus, or the sperm from reaching it. When the condition cannot be corrected by surgery, the woman's egg cells may be removed from the ovary by means of a small incision in the abdomen and put in a glass dish, where they are fertilized by the man's sperm. After the embryos have undergone a few cell divisions, two or three are injected into the woman's uterus, where they may become implanted in the endometrium and continue to develop normally.

The process is properly called **in vitro** ("in glass") **fertilization.** *Test-tube baby* is an inaccurate and misleading term because the embryo spends only a few hours in a glass dish and the next nine months in the normal environment of the uterus.

When all else fails, but the man's sperm is still normal, the couple may seek the services of a **surrogate mother.** A surrogate (substitute) mother is a woman who agrees to be artificially inseminated with the husband's sperm, carry the child full term, give birth to it, and then turn it over to the contracting couple. (Surrogate mothers and couples rarely, if ever, meet.) For these services, she is paid a sum of money and has her medical, legal, and insurance costs covered by the couple. She signs a contract in which she agrees to surrender custody of the child to the man and his wife.

The practice of surrogate motherhood has raised complex legal and moral questions. Some critics condemn it as a form of adultery, others as a form of baby selling. As for the surrogate mothers themselves, most feel that they are performing an invaluable service and, being contented mothers with children of their own, take joy in making other couples happy.

HEREDITY

Heredity is that aspect of the reproductive process that involves the transmission of the characteristics of parents to their offspring. We usually think of these characteristics as physical traits, such as hair color, eye color, facial features, and so on. It may well be, however, that some personality traits are also transmitted through heredity.

To see how heredity operates in determining a person's characteristics, let us start with conception, the point when the female's ovum is fertilized by the male's sperm cell.

Chromosomes

The nucleus of each cell of our bodies, except our reproductive cells, contains forty-six particles in twenty-three matching pairs called **chromosomes.** Because of a process of reduction during their formation, reproductive cells (sperm and egg) contain half the usual number, or twenty-three single chromosomes. After the sperm has penetrated the ovum, the new cell carries twenty-three matching pairs of chromosomes, or a total of forty-six chromosomes.

Genes

Chromosomes are composed of complex chemical packets called **genes.** Genes are the basic units of heredity and direct the formation of every part of the body. The basic chemical of the gene, **deoxyribonucleic acid (DNA)**, carries all the information of heredity (**genetic code**). DNA is considered to be the memory of the cell. The genetic code is transmitted from DNA in the nucleus to the cytoplasm of the cell by a chemical messenger, **ribonucleic acid,** commonly called *RNA*.

Dominant and Recessive Genes

The physical characteristics of the child are the result of its receiving combinations of genes for each of the traits manifested. The genes may be *dominant* or *recessive*. For a given trait, the child may receive a dominant and a recessive gene, two recessive genes, or two dominant genes. If the child receives either two dominant genes or one dominant gene and one recessive gene for a particular characteristic, the dominant gene will determine the trait that appears. If, however, the child receives two recessive genes, it will manifest the recessive characteristic. Those traits that are manifested are known as the *phenotype*—the observable characteristics of the individual. The *genotype* is the total genetic constitution of the individual; it includes the dominant as well as the recessive traits. Thus an individual manifesting a dominant trait, but carrying both dominant and recessive genes, may pass the recessive gene on to his or her offspring.

There is yet another possibility regarding the inheritance of dominant and recessive genes. Certain physical traits are due to combinations of several types of genes. For example, the child might inherit several pairs of genes for different shades of light or dark hair color. In this case, the manifested characteristic will often be some modification of completely blond hair (a recessive characteristic) or completely black hair (a dominant characteristic); possibly the child will have sandy-colored or reddish-blond hair.

Determination of Sex

Chromosomes determine an individual's sex. When sperm and egg join, the twenty-third pair of chromosomes is responsible for sex determination. The sex-determining chromosomes are the only pair whose members are dissimilar in appearance. The larger member is called an X chromosome; the smaller one is the Y chromosome. Each male cell (sperm) contains either an X or a Y chromosome. Each female cell (ovum) contains an X chromosome.

When sperm cells are formed, one-half of them receive an X chromosome and the other half a Y chromosome. When egg cells are formed, they receive an X chromosome in every case. If a sperm cell containing an X chromosome fertilizes an egg cell, the fertilized ovum will carry two X chromosomes (XX), and the baby will be a girl. If the sperm cell carries a Y chromosome, the cell produced by fertilization will carry an X and a Y chromosome (XY), and the baby will be a boy.

Theoretically, a fertilized ovum has a 50 percent chance of becoming a female. However, there are approximately 105 male births for every 100 female births. This may occur because the sperm that carry the Y chromosome move slightly faster than those that carry the X chromosome (perhaps because the Y chromosome is smaller). It is therefore more likely that a sperm carrying the Y chromosome will fertilize the egg. An equal sex ratio in the population is achieved because infant mortality is higher for boys than for girls.

Sex-Linked Characteristics

The X chromosome carries a number of genes for which there are *no* corresponding genes on the Y chromosome. These genes produce what are known as **sex-linked characteristics**—that is, the chances of exhibiting these particular characteristics strongly depend upon one's sex. Hemophilia, color blindness, and childhood muscular dystrophy are examples of sex-linked characteristics.

If a gene for a sex-linked characteristic is recessive, a woman would have to inherit the gene on *both* her X chromosomes in order to manifest the trait. The odds against this happening are high, since each parent would have to be a **carrier** of the gene. A man, however, would have to receive only *one* recessive gene in order to manifest the trait, since he has only one X chromosome in a pair (as noted, the Y chromosome bears no corresponding trait that might offset the recessive gene). For this reason, males have a greater chance of inheriting an X-linked recessive characteristic.

The woman who inherits a gene for a recessive sex-linked trait will not manifest that trait; she will, however, function as a carrier and may pass on the recessive gene to her offspring. If they are males, there is a 50 percent chance that they will manifest the recessive trait.

GENETIC COUNSELING

Genetic counseling is a new medical procedure that can tell a couple whether their offspring is likely to inherit a disease or disorder, or even whether a high-risk pregnancy may develop. The methods used for determining this information are varied and can be applied both before and during pregnancy. In fact, genetic counseling can actually start before a couple marries, because it is possible to administer tests to find out whether one or both prospective parents carry genes of an inherited disorder.

Inherited Disorders

As we have seen, some X-linked recessive disorders are carried by the mother and passed on almost exclusively to male children. Other inherited disorders are passed on to a child only if both parents carry the gene for it. Four of the more common disorders transmitted in this manner are sickle-cell anemia, Tay-Sachs disease, thalassemia, and cystic fibrosis.

Sickle-cell anemia, in which an abnormality in the production of the red-cell protein hemoglobin distorts the red blood cells into a "sickle" shape, is most commonly found in blacks. The child whose parents are both carriers and who inherits both recessive genes (about 1 child in 400 or 500) usually dies before the age of 20.

Tay-Sachs disease is an inborn error of metabolism affecting the brain and terminating in death, usually by age 4. It is most prevalent in people whose ancestors were Eastern European Jews. In order to be afflicted, a child must inherit two recessive Tay-Sachs genes (one from each parent), and the chances are one in four that this will happen if both parents have a recessive gene for the disease. Current estimates are that one in every thirty Jews is a carrier. Carriers can be detected by a simple blood test.

Thalassemia is a type of anemia in which the red blood cells do not have sufficient hemoglobin; there are two types of thalassemia: alpha and beta. The disease was originally discovered among people whose forebears came from areas near the Mediterranean. More recently, this condition has been found to be even more prevalent in Asia.

Cystic fibrosis affects 1 of every 1,000 babies born in the United States. It damages the lungs and digestive system, and generally kills its victims before they reach the age of 20. The group at highest risk of bearing infants with the disease are whites. Carriers of this disease can be detected by a simple test measuring the amount of salt in perspiration.

Testing During Pregnancy

Once a high-risk pregnancy occurs, there are several methods for determining whether the offspring will be normal. A diagnosis can ease parents' fears, or it can alert them to the probability of a serious birth defect and allow them to choose either to end the pregnancy or to take prenatal and postnatal measures to minimize the effects of the abnormality.

Amniocentesis is a procedure usually performed in the obstetrician's office during the fourteenth to eighteenth week of pregnancy. Using local anesthesia, the physician inserts a hollow needle through the abdominal wall into the uterus and withdraws a small amount of amniotic fluid. The physician can then detect any abnormalities by examining the fetal cells in the fluid. Nearly all chromosomal abnormalities can be diagnosed by this method. It is also possible to determine the sex of the baby with an accuracy close to 99 percent.

One common reason for performing amniocentesis is to rule out **Down's syndrome** (mongolism). This nonhereditary defect may result in a severely mentally retarded child. The victims of the disease also have heart disorders and respiratory problems that often result in death before adulthood. Down's syndrome occurs at the rate of 1 in 3,000 births when the mother is under 30; 1 in 600 when she is aged 30 to 34; 1 in 280 when she is between 35 and 39; 1 in 80 when she is aged 40 to 44; and 1 in 40 when the mother is older than 44. Because of this increased risk with age, many physicians recommend that all pregnant women over age 35 undergo amniocentesis to determine the presence of Down's syndrome.

Ultrasound, or pulse-echo sonography, is frequently an adjunct of amniocentesis. High-frequency sound waves are directed into the abdomen of the pregnant woman to produce a picture of the uterus, placenta, and fetus. This method

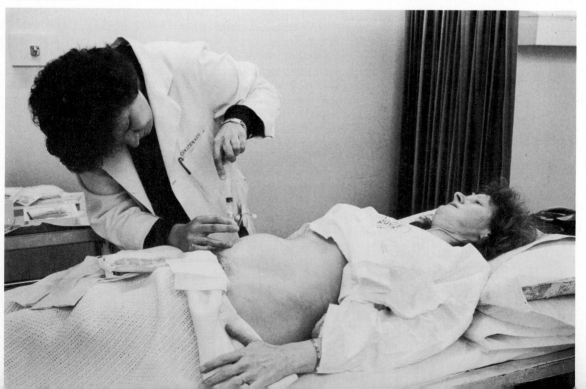

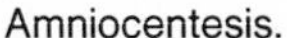
Amniocentesis.

causes no discomfort and reduces the necessity for X-rays or radioisotope (radioactive tracer) scanning.

Ultrasound can be used to locate fetal structures, the umbilical cord, and the placenta, and to determine if the fetus is alive. Sometimes it may be used to corroborate a diagnosis obtained by amniocentesis.

Alpha-fetoprotein (AFP) testing helps diagnose neural-tube defects by measuring the level of AFP (a normal fetal liver product) in the mother's blood and amniotic fluid. High levels of AFP may indicate the fetus has *anencephaly* (a defective formation of the brain that invariably results in the death of the baby shortly after birth) or *spina bifida* (abnormalities in the spinal column requiring surgical correction after birth and possibly also resulting in paralysis and mental retardation). The incidence in the United States of anencephaly and spina bifida is 1 to 2 per 1,000 births. However, elevated AFP levels may also indicate a multiple pregnancy or a fetal death.

Fetoscopy and **placental aspiration** are even newer techniques of gaining information about the fetus. At present both are still considered experimental. In fetoscopy a small device is inserted through the woman's abdomen, enabling the physician to directly view the fetus and placenta. Placental aspiration is a method of sampling fetal blood. The physician inserts a needle into the inner surface of the placenta and aspirates, or draws up by suction, a sample of fetal blood. Both methods are useful mostly for diagnosing hemophilia, beta-thalassemia, and cases of sickle-cell anemia that cannot be diagnosed by amniocentesis.

Congenital Birth Defects

Birth defects may be caused by occurrences during the prenatal period. These may be such varied factors as drugs, disease and infection, radiation, alcohol, and smoking. Drugs taken during pregnancy pass from the mother's bloodstream into the placenta. An infant can be born addicted to heroin if its mother was a heroin abuser during her pregnancy; it can be brain damaged from the effects of painkilling drugs and anesthetics administered at the time of delivery; or it can be the potential victim of cancer from the effects of DES (diethylstilbestrol). (During the late 1940s and early 1950s DES was given to pregnant women to prevent miscarriage. The daughters of women who took DES have a high risk of vaginal cancer.) During the late 1950s and early 1960s thousands of children born to mothers who used thalidomide in the early months of pregnancy were born impaired, most often with flipperlike arms. If a woman has rubella (German measles) during the first trimester of pregnancy, her child may suffer from deafness, heart defects, cataracts, glaucoma, and other serious medical problems. If the mother is infected with syphilis, the child may be born with bone malformations and infections in many of the body organs; if she has gonorrhea, the child may become blind.

Alcohol may cause severe growth deficiencies, mental retardation, and heart defects (see Chapter 11). Smoking is linked to low birth weight, a factor that greatly affects a baby's chances for survival. Ingestion of cocaine by pregnant women has resulted in severe defects in their babies (see Chapter 13). It is estimated that one baby in thirty born in the United States suffers from birth defects due either to genetic causes or to bad health practices during pregnancy.

If, for whatever reason, there is any suspicion of fetal malady, it is now possible to do more than wait despairingly for what may be a tragic birth. Genetic counseling can give parents information that was undreamed of only a few years ago.

BIRTH CONTROL

Many people, for religious or personal reasons, have expressed opposition to the use of birth control devices or drugs to prevent pregnancy. Some people, on the other hand, have viewed the availability of these birth control methods as part of their right to sexual freedom. Many are concerned about overpopulation, which they feel threatens human welfare, and they regard birth control as a commonsense solution to the problem of a burgeoning population.

People who use birth control devices or drugs do so because they provide an effective and convenient means of preventing or spacing pregnancies. If individuals do choose to practice birth control, it is wise for them to consult a physician or birth control clinic to be sure they are choosing the method most suitable for them.

Oral Contraceptives

Oral contraceptives function by maintaining a high level of progesterone ("progestin-only pills") or both estrogen and progesterone ("combined pills") in the body. The high level of sex hormones maintained throughout the menstrual cycle by oral contraceptives prevents the development of a mature ovum. And without an ovum, of course, no fertilization—and thus no pregnancy—can take place.

It has been estimated that 30 percent of all American women between the ages of 18 and 44 use oral contraceptives as a means of birth control. If used properly, they are virtually 100 percent effective in preventing conception.

The decision to opt for the Pill as a birth control method should not be made without a clear understanding of its advantages and disadvantages. For example, women who use the Pill seem to be protected against certain forms of cancer. The Pill also regulates the menstrual cycle and may eliminate the discomfort associated with menstruation. However, women who use the Pill are also at a higher than normal risk for heart attacks, strokes, and the formation of blood clots. According to the latest findings, 450 American women die every year from the effects of the Pill on the circulatory system and heart. However, both the Centers for Disease Control in Atlanta and the Royal College of General Practitioners in Britain have conducted studies showing that half of these deaths would not have occurred if the women had not been smokers. Still, Pill users are three times more likely to have fatal heart attacks than nonusers. Among 100,000 Pill users age 20 to 29, 3 are likely to have a heart attack each year, with 2 out of 3 attacks attributable to the Pill. Among 100,000 Pill users age 40 to 44, 75 are likely to have a fatal heart attack, with 2 out of 3 attacks again attributable to the Pill. Additional drawbacks include: blood clots, which may result in death if they break away and travel to the lungs; a slight risk of increased blood pressure; and a very slight risk of gallstones.

Women choosing to use the Pill should have a complete and thorough medical checkup beforehand. Since birth control pills can be acquired only through a physician's prescription, a medical examination can easily be performed at that time.

Mechanical Device: The IUD

Intrauterine devices (IUDs) are coils or loops that are inserted into the uterus. The IUD does not prevent sperm from fertilizing an egg; it is believed to prevent pregnancy by slightly irritating the endometrium so that a developing embryo cannot implant. IUDs must be inserted by a physician, and the woman must return to the physician at intervals to make sure that it is still fitted correctly and that no harmful reactions have occurred. IUDs used alone are second only to the Pill in their contraceptive effectiveness, and they are simple to use. Once inserted, they require little further attention on the part of the woman.

But, like oral contraceptives, the IUD has some serious drawbacks. Some women are unable to tolerate an IUD, and their bodies expel it. Other women may normally tolerate an IUD, but may, on occasion, expel it. It is important, therefore, that women check themselves regularly to make sure the IUD is in place, in order to prevent an unintended pregnancy. An IUD can also perforate the uterus and enter the abdominal cavity, requiring surgery to remove it. IUD users have also been found to be at greater risk of pelvic inflammatory disease than nonusers (see the section Pelvic Inflammatory Disease in Chapter 15). And studies in 1985 reported a possible link between IUD use and female infertility, so that women who have not already borne as many children as they desire might consider some other method preferable.

One early IUD, the Dalkon Shield, caused other problems and was removed from the market in the 1970s. After a flood of lawsuits forced its manufacturer to declare bankruptcy, manufacturers of other IUDs found it difficult to obtain liability insurance and chose to take their devices off the U.S. market in 1986, even though they had not caused the problems of the Dalkon Shield. The IUD thereupon became difficult to obtain in the United States, though it is still widely available elsewhere (see the box Birth Control: Decisions, Decisions, on page 194).

Chemical Methods

Vaginal Insert. Recently, an effective new method of contraception has been introduced to the American market after four-year trials in Western Europe. A small white oval tablet, the **vaginal insert** is placed in the vagina and pushed up toward the cervix with the finger. Within ten minutes, the tablet melts from the heat of the body and effervesces into a protective foam. The ingredients include a spermicide, but no hormones—so there is no danger of harmful side effects. The vaginal insert is convenient and easy to use, and the spontaneity of sex is minimally interrupted. Protection begins after ten minutes and lasts for up to two hours for each act of intercourse. As with the spermicidal foams, jellies, and creams, douching should not take place for at least six hours after intercourse.

Reliability of the vaginal insert has been demonstrated in a West German survey in which only 43 pregnancies were reported among 10,017 women who used this method for an average period of six months each. As with most methods of contraception, much of the effectiveness in preventing pregnancy depends on correct and consistent use.

By Choice, Not by Chance

T or F

______ 1. The purpose of birth control methods is to allow people the right to determine when they wish to enter parenthood.

______ 2. Preventing an unwanted pregnancy is an equal responsibility of both partners.

______ 3. A pregnancy will not result from any single act of intercourse.

______ 4. Natural methods of birth control present no problems of side effects but are less reliable than other methods.

______ 5. Douching is not a good method of birth control because sperm enter the uterus within seconds after intercourse.

______ 6. Withdrawal as a birth control method is about 75 percent effective.

______ 7. A female can have intercourse during her period without fear of pregnancy.

______ 8. Foam and a condom, used together, are about as effective as the pill.

______ 9. A very important factor in favor of the sponge, condom, and foam is their ready availability.

______ 10. A unique characteristic of the condom is that in addition to being an effective birth control method, it also provides a barrier to the spread of venereal disease.

______ 11. People are sterilized so that they cannot engage in sexual intercourse.

______ 12. A woman can verify the presence of her IUD by feeling the string at her cervix.

______ 13. The IUD may cause side effects because it is a foreign body.

______ 14. The contraceptive pill provides protection against venereal disease.

______ 15. The success of any birth control method is affected by the motivation of the people using it.

Scoring: Statements 1, 2, 4–6, 8–10, 12, 13, and 15 are true; 3, 7, 11, and 14 are false. The goal should be a perfect score.

Source: Adapted in part from *Growing Awareness*, 2nd ed. (Rochester, N.Y.: Planned Parenthood, 1979).

Foams, Jellies, Creams, and the Sponge. Spermicides in the form of foams, jellies, and creams can be inserted into the vagina by means of a plastic applicator. Foam has the advantage of being less messy than creams and jellies, and it forms a physical barrier to the cervix more rapidly, but no evidence demonstrates that foam is more effective than creams or jellies. The foam must be inserted high into the vagina near the cervix; it must be inserted no more than twenty minutes before intercourse; it must be newly applied before each act of intercourse; and douching should not take place within six hours after intercourse. The reliability of contraceptive foam is increased when it is used together with a diaphragm or condom.

Since 1983 a nonprescription contraceptive, the spermicidal sponge, has been available. It is 80 to 87 percent effective in preventing pregnancy for twenty-four hours after insertion into the vagina. It has few serious side effects, the most common being irritation and allergic reactions in fewer than 4 percent of the users. Toxic shock syndrome (a bacterial infection that causes reddening of the skin, fever, diarrhea, and vomiting) has occurred with the use of the sponge, but only at the rate of 1 case out of every 3 million—about the same as that which occurs with the use of standard tampons. According to the FDA, the risk can be virtually eliminated by following the directions that come with the product.

The sponge's effectiveness can be increased considerably (possibly to the level of the Pill) if the male wears a condom. This step also provides protection against sexually transmitted diseases. The particular virtue of this method is that it does not require a prescription and thus may be used by people who do not want to go to a physician and therefore use no contraceptive method at all.

New Drugs. Scientists are at present attempting to develop new types of contraceptive drugs. Among them is a birth control pill that contains no estrogen, thus minimizing the possibility of side effects. A "morning-after" pill has also been developed, but it is used only in emergency cases, such as rape, because its large estrogen dose can make a woman very ill. Time-release capsules that can be implanted in the vagina are among the other contraceptive devices now being tested. For men, most drugs that have been tested have caused side effects; but researchers are working on new, harmless, effective drugs that will stop the production or ejaculation of viable sperm.

Barrier Devices

The Diaphragm. The **diaphragm** is a cuplike device made of rubber that fits inside the upper vagina in order to prevent sperm from entering the uterus. It must initially be fitted by a physician and from then on periodic checkups are necessary so that the physician can confirm proper fit. The woman herself should examine the diaphragm regularly for perforations.

The diaphragm is inserted into the vagina by the woman before intercourse takes place. She fills the diaphragm with a jelly or cream **spermicide** (sperm killer). Since sperm may have a life span of several hours, the diaphragm should not be removed until six to eight hours after intercourse.

Until the advent of the Pill in the 1960s, one-third of all American couples practicing birth control used the diaphragm. Now it is again gaining popularity because people have become alarmed by some of the dangers of birth control pills. From the point of view of a person's health, the diaphragm is one of

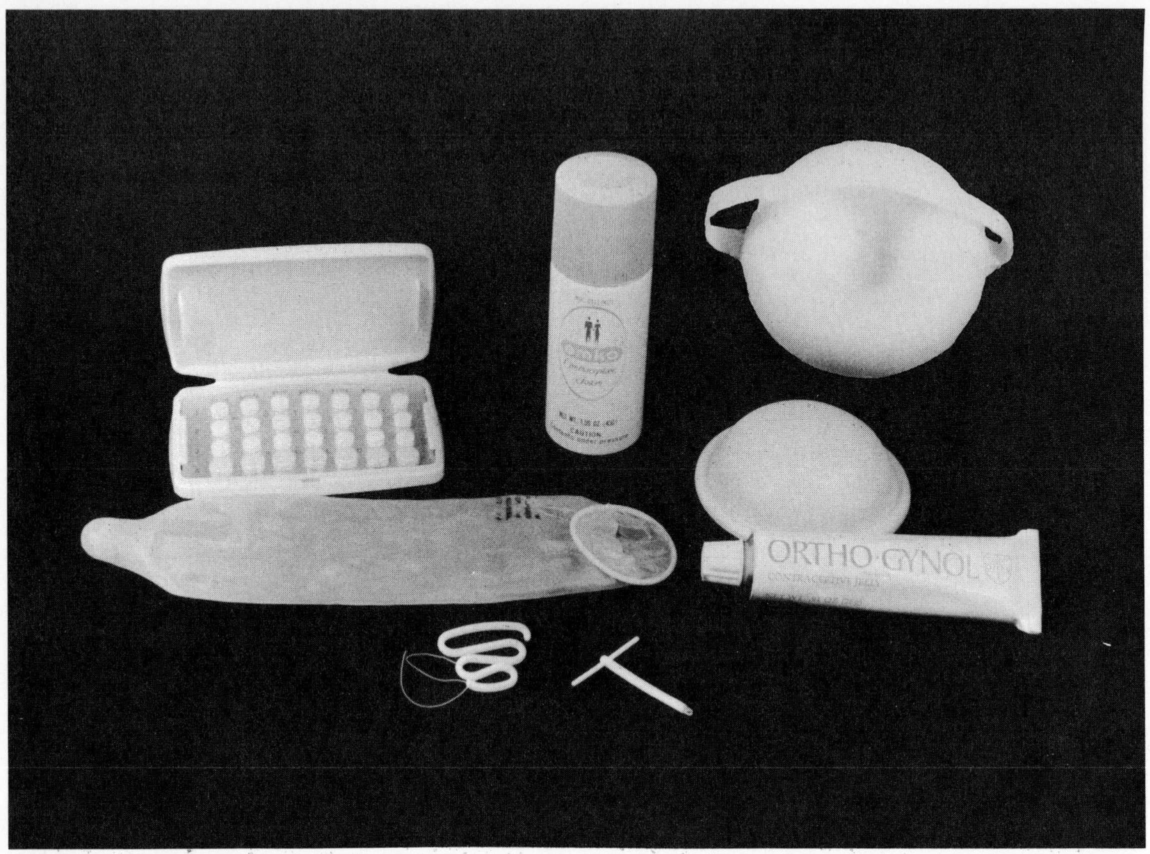

Contraceptive methods. Clockwise from top left: birth control pills; contraceptive foam; spermicidal sponge; diaphragm; contraceptive jelly; intrauterine devices (IUDs); condom.

the safest means of contraception; and if used properly and routinely before sexual intercourse, it is 96 percent effective, or higher. Most women find the diaphragm comfortable to wear, and it can be inserted in advance so that foreplay before intercourse need not be interrupted. It is also generally comfortable for the male partner, who usually cannot feel its presence.

The Cervical Cap. The **cervical cap** is similar to the diaphragm, in that it blocks the passage of sperm through the cervix. The cap fits over the cervix and is held in place by suction. Invented in 1838, it has been used widely by European women with satisfactory results; it has only recently been introduced in the United States and is being used by about half a million women. Most women find the cervical cap more comfortable than the diaphragm and just as reliable when used with spermicide.

The Condom. The **condom** is one of the most frequently used contraceptives in the world, and like the diaphragm, it has no harmful side effects. It is a long sheath made of very thin rubber or animal tissue, which is rolled onto the penis after erection and before intercourse. For maximum effectiveness, it is important that the erect penis not come near the vagina before the condom has been applied. Application can be done by the man—or by the woman as part of foreplay. During ejaculation the semen collects in the condom and is thus prevented from entering the vagina.

The effectiveness of the condom depends on how carefully it is used. The risk of pregnancy from a defective condom is slight because of the rigorous testing required by the Food and Drug Administration. When used in combination with vaginal foams, condoms are as effective in preventing conception as are oral contraceptives. An additional advantage of the condom is that when used properly it also may act as a barrier to sexually transmitted diseases.

There are no recognized side effects with the use of a condom. Some men complain that the condom reduces the sensitivity of the penis, although this can be an advantage to an easily excited man who wants to sustain an erection until after his partner achieves orgasm. The newer lubricated condoms may actually enhance a man's penile sensitivity.

TABLE 7-1

First-Year Failure Rates of Birth Control Methods

Method	Lowest Observed Failure Rate (%)[a]	Failure Rate in Typical Users (%)[b]
Tubal sterilization	0.4	0.4
Vasectomy	0.4	0.4
Combined birth control pills	0.5	2
Progestin-only pill	1	2.5
IUD	1.5	5
Condom	2	10
Diaghragm (with spermicide)	2	19
Sponge (with spermicide)	9–11	10–20
Cervical cap	2	13
Foams, creams, jellies, and vaginal suppositories	3–5	18
Coitus interruptus	16	23
Fertility awareness techniques (basal body temperature, mucous method, calendar, and "rhythm")	2–20	24
Douche	—	40
Chance (no method of birth control)	90	90

[a] Designed to complete the sentence: "In 100 users who start out the year using a given method and who use it correctly and consistently, the lowest observed failure rate has been ________."

[b] Designed to complete the sentence: "In 100 typical users who start out the year using a given method, the number of pregnancies by the end of the year will be ________."

Source: Robert A. Hatcher et al., *Contraceptive Technology, 1986–1987*, 13th rev. ed., p. 102 © 1986 by Irvington Publishers, Inc. Adapted by permission.

Birth Control: Decisions, Decisions

Preferred methods of contraception vary widely from culture to culture because of differing laws, traditions, and levels of development, but an estimated 319 million people worldwide use modern methods of birth control.

Country/Region	Tubal Ligation	Vasectomy	Pill	IUDs	Condoms	Other Modern Methods*
U.S.	23.2%	11.4%	30.0%	7.9%	12.9%	14.6%
China	37.5	12.9	4.8	41.1	2.0	1.6
India	40.0	40.0	2.9	8.6	5.7	2.9
Latin America and the Caribbean	36.8	2.6	36.8	5.3	7.9	10.5
Middle East and Africa	14.3	0	57.1	14.3	7.1	7.1
All developed countries†	13.0	7.4	26.9	11.1	24.1	17.6

* Includes injectable contraceptives, other steroidal methods, the diaphragm, and spermicides.
† Includes Western Europe and the United States.
Source: *Newsweek*, March 11, 1985, p. 70.

Douche. **Douching** is a technique in which a woman washes the vaginal tract with water or a spermidical solution immediately after intercourse. It is not a recommended method of contraception, since it is very likely that at least a few sperm will have entered the cervix seconds after ejaculation and before douching takes place.

Other Methods

Rhythm Method. The **rhythm method** is a relatively unreliable method of contraception. It is based on the fact that a woman can conceive for only a few days during her menstrual cycle, and that abstaining from intercourse during this time may prevent impregnation. A woman's fertile period usually falls somewhere between three days before and five days after ovulation. By counting the days from her last menstrual period, the woman can calculate her *approximate* time of ovulation and thus her approximate "safe" period.

As an aid to determining the time of ovulation, the woman may keep a chart of her body temperature taken every morning with a special basal temperature thermometer. From this chart she then calculates her probable infertile period. During ovulation body temperature drops slightly. A day or two after ovulation body temperature increases slightly, perhaps half a degree or less. If a woman has a regular pattern of temperature changes, she may be able to calculate her safe days more precisely.

One disadvantage of the rhythm method is that unless the woman has a regular menstrual cycle, she will not be able to calculate her infertile periods with any degree of certainty. Often the body temperature changes are irregular or impossible to detect. In addition, since the efficiency of the method also depends on abstinence, it is unsuitable for couples who cannot or do not wish to control their desire for intercourse.

Withdrawal (Coitus Interruptus). In the **withdrawal** or **coitus interruptus** technique, the male removes his penis from the female immediately before

Reproduction and Birth Control: Where to Go for Help

Family Planning/Sex Information

The Alan Guttmacher Institute
360 Park Avenue South
New York, NY 10010
(212) 685-5858

Association for Voluntary Sterilization
Suite 2300
703 Third Avenue
New York, NY 10017
(212) 986-3880

National Clearinghouse for Family Planning Information
P.O. Box 2225
Rockville, MD 20852
(301) 881-9400

Planned Parenthood Federation of America, Inc.
810 Seventh Avenue
New York, NY 10017
(212) 541-7800

Fertility

American Fertility Society
Suite 101
1608 13th Avenue South
Birmingham, AL 35256
(205) 933-7222

Genetic Diseases

March of Dimes/Birth Defects Foundation
1275 Mamaroneck Avenue
White Plains, NY 10605
(914) 428-7100

National Clearinghouse for Human Genetic Diseases
Suite 500
805 15th Street
Washington, DC 20005
(202) 842-7617

National Sickle Cell Disease Program Division of Blood Diseases and Resources
National Heart, Lung and Blood Institute
National Institutes of Health
Room 504, Federal Building
7550 Wisconsin Avenue
Bethesda, MD 20205
(301) 496-6931

National Tay-Sachs and Allied Diseases Association, Inc.
122 East 42nd Street
New York, NY 10168
(212) 661-2780

Source: The Columbia University College of Physicians and Surgeons Complete Home Medical Guide (*New York: Crown Publishers, Inc., 1986*). Reprinted by permission.

ejaculating. This practice can be frustrating to both partners, and it requires a great deal of self-control on the part of the man. A drop of semen in the vagina can result in pregnancy; in fact, the first few drops ejaculated contain the highest concentration of sperm. Even the lubricating fluid that precedes ejaculation contains some sperm.

Sterilization

Sterilization is the process of surgically rendering a person incapable of reproduction. For a man, sterilization requires an operation (called a **vasectomy**) in which the vasa deferentia are either tied off or severed. The actual operation is minor, requiring only a small incision into the scrotum, and it can be performed in fifteen minutes in a doctor's office. There are no aftereffects, and the operation alters neither the male's ability to have intercourse nor his sex drive. However, once the procedure is done, it takes extreme surgical skill to rejoin the two ends of the vas deferens, and even then fertility is not guaranteed. Therefore a man should regard sterilization as permanent when deciding whether or not to undergo this operation. Men anticipating a vasectomy can have some of their sperm frozen and stored in a sperm bank. In this way, a sterlized man can become a father by means of artificial insemination if he should decide later that he wants children.

In a woman sterilization is a more complex operation. It requires an incision through the abdomen or vagina and involves tying off the fallopian tubes (**tubal ligation**) or severing them entirely from the uterus by cauterization (burning). The sterilization has absolutely no effect upon a woman's ability to have intercourse or upon her sex drive; nor does the operation interfere in any way with the normal hormonal balance of her body. But once the operation has been performed, the odds are small that fertility can be restored. However, a newer method of sterilization now being tested may permit fertility to be restored. It involves blocking the fallopian tubes by means of clips or rings that can be removed if a child is desired.

Sterilization has become the most widely used form of contraception in the United States over the last twenty years. Almost 28 percent of the nation's couples in which the wife is of childbearing age have chosen sterilization as the means of limiting their families, according to a 1985 study by the National Center for Health Statistics. (The study also noted that twice as many wives as husbands had been sterilized.) The greatest number of sterilizations occurred among older couples aged 40 to 44, who felt they had had enough children. Other reasons for sterilization include fears over the potential side effects of the Pill and the fact that many couples in all age groups have decided not to include having children as part of their life plan.

SUMMARY

1. The male reproductive system includes the *testes*, *penis*, and accessory glands and ducts. Sperm are produced in the seminiferous tubules of the testes and move to the epididymis and then through the vas

deferentia to the seminal vesicles and the prostate gland. They then pass into the urethra and out of the penis.

2. The female reproductive system is composed of the *ovaries*, *fallopian tubes*, *uterus*, *vagina*, and external genitalia. Each month an ovum is expelled from a *Graafian follicle*, which develops from a primary follicle and eventually becomes the *corpus luteum*. The ovum moves down the fallopian tube toward the uterus, where the *endometrium* (uterine lining) prepares to receive it. If fertilization does not take place, the ovum and uterine lining are expelled during menstruation.

3. Hormones play a crucial role in sexual maturation (puberty) and and in the functioning of the *reproductive system*. In the male *testosterone* influences the development of the reproductive organs and maintains sex drive; pituitary hormones initiate the production of sperm and stimulate testosterone production and sperm cell maturation. In the female *estrogens*, *progesterone*, and the pituitary hormones are important in regulating the monthly menstrual cycle. In addition, the estrogens influence the development of secondary sex characteristics.

4. Fertilization occurs when a *spermatozoon* breaks through the membrane of a ripe ovum in a fallopian tube. The fertilized egg is called a *zygote*; the two weeks following fertilization are called the *zygote stage*. The zygote undergoes cell divisions and implants itself in the endometrium.

5. The second to eighth week of pregnancy is the *embryonic period*. Three membranes form around the embryo: the *amnion*, the *chorion*, and the *placenta*. The final developmental stage is the *fetal stage* (ninth week to birth); in this stage body structures assume their final form.

6. Pregnancy is accompanied by physical and psychological alterations. Proper prenatal care is important. The pregnant woman should see a physician regularly and be checked for complications such as *Rh factor* incompatibility. Her diet should be high in protein and low in carbohydrates and salt. Drugs, tobacco, and alcohol should be avoided.

7. Labor has three basic stages. The first stage begins with regular uterine contractions, dilation of the cervix, and discharge of the *amniotic fluid* from the vagina. The second stage begins when the baby's head enter the cervix and ends when it is born, after passage through the birth canal. Delivery of the *afterbirth* is the third stage of labor.

8. *Natural childbirth* involves delivery with little or no medication. Couples enter a program that prepares them to participate consciously and actively in the birth process. Many women are choosing to have their babies in *childbirth centers* where *midwives* usually take charge of the delivery.

9. An involuntary termination of pregnancy is called a *miscarriage*, or *spontaneous abortion*. The voluntary termination of pregnancy, by one of several methods, is called an *artificially induced abortion*.

10. *Infertility* in women and men may result from hormonal, congenital, structural, psychological, or disease-related causes. It may also be due to poor health habits.

11. *Artificial insemination*—the injection of the husband's or a donor's sperm into the woman—may be used to counteract infertility. In *in vitro fertilization*, another technique for overcoming infertility, the woman's egg cells are removed from the ovary and fertilized in a glass dish by the man's sperm; the resulting embryos are injected into the uterus, where they may develop normally. Finally, *surrogate motherhood* involves a contract between a woman and a couple whereby the woman agrees to be artificially inseminated with the husband's sperm, carry the child full term, give birth to it, and turn it over to the couple.

12. *Heredity* involves the transmission of characteristics through *genes* contained within *chromosomes*. The *genetic code* in the *DNA* is carried to the cell cytoplasm by *RNA*. The gender of the offspring is established by the chromosomes that pair at the time of fertilization. Genetic counseling enables couples to tell whether their offspring will be likely to inherit a disease. Some abnormalities that may be inherited are Tay-Sachs disease and sickle-cell anemia. *Birth defects* may also be caused by such factors as drugs, disease and infection, smoking, and alcohol. Maternal age influences the risk of giving birth to an infant with Down's syndrome.

13. The availability of numerous birth control methods allows everyone to select a suitable and effective way of preventing or spacing pregnancies. Common methods are: *oral contraceptives*, *intrauterine device*, *diaphragm*, *condom*, various *spermicides*, *rhythm method*, *coitus interruptus*, and *sterilization*.

CONSUMER CONCERNS

1. Government funding helps to finance voluntary agencies such as Planned Parenthood. Of what significance would it be should this funding be discontinued?
2. Family planning is an important issue medically, socially, and economically. Therefore shouldn't family planning counseling be a routine aspect of medical services?
3. There is a constantly growing body of knowledge pertaining to maternal health practices during pregnancy, but is this information disseminated adequately?
4. Birth control items are pharmaceutical products that fall within the jurisdiction of the Food and Drug Administration (FDA). Does the judgment exercised by the FDA meet with your satisfaction? Do you think FDA standards for these products might be even more stringent? Or perhaps less stringent?
5. Do you know whether the nurse-midwife is a licensed professional in your state? Do you favor the licensing of midwifery?
6. The issue of voluntary abortion is probably the most explosive political question that we face. In addition to political and moral points of view, there is also an economic issue involved. How do the legal decisions related to legal abortions become consumer issues?

8

Sexual Behavior

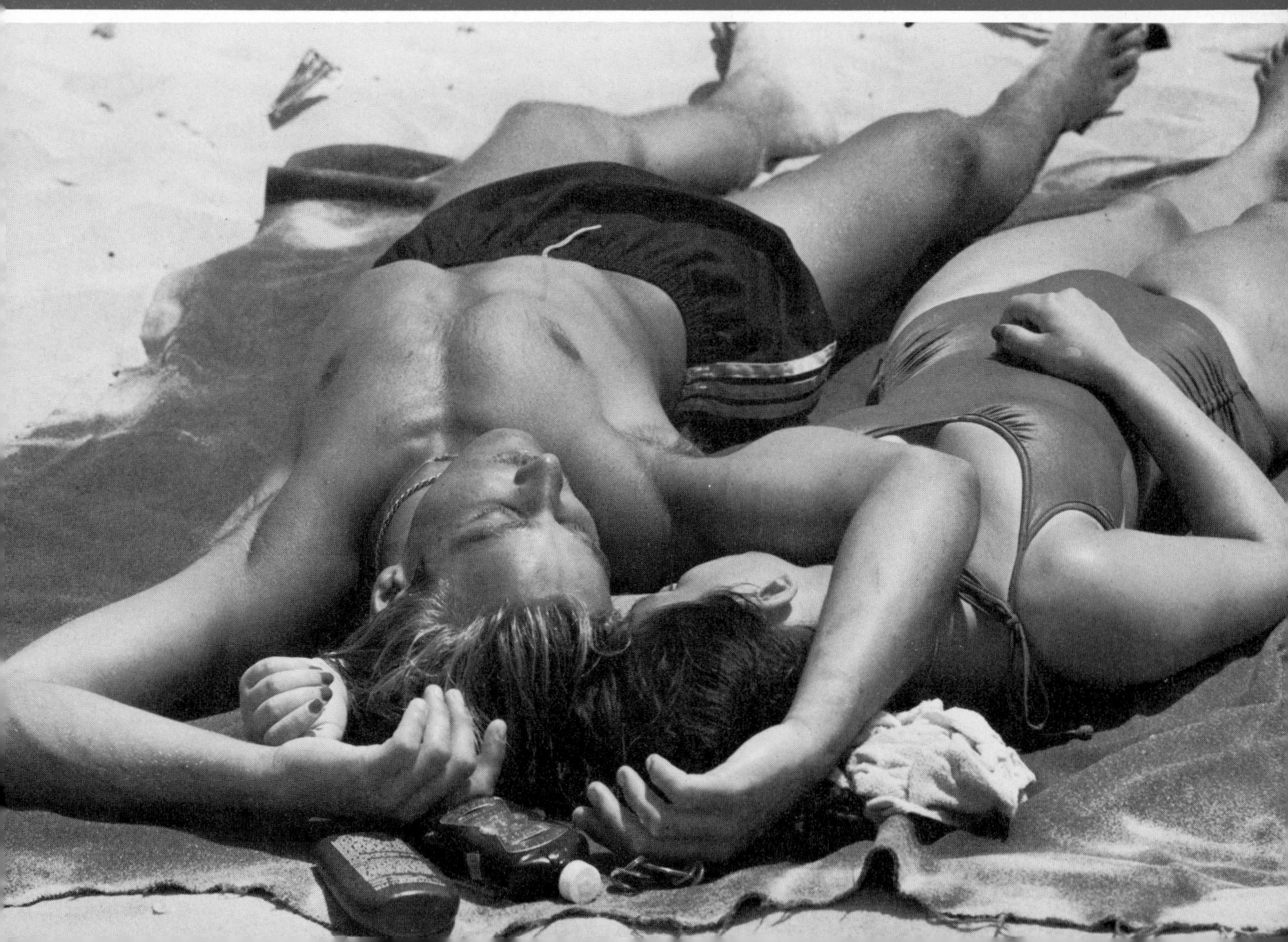

Things are not always what they seem. The vaunted "sexual revolution" of the late 1960s and early 1970s was at least partly an invention of the media. Statistical reports are inconsistent regarding changes in American sexual behavior patterns. For instance, it is generally assumed that the percentage of sexually active young women has greatly increased in the recent past. But is this really the case?

According to one study of young female college students, their responses indicated that they believed 75 percent of their classmates to be sexually active. But when each student was personally polled regarding her individual behavior, only about 20 percent turned out to be sexually active.

On the other hand, the results of two nationwide surveys of teenage female sexuality conducted by staff members of Johns Hopkins University revealed that by age 16, one in five of these young women had engaged in sexual relations and by age 19, two-thirds had had such experience.

Many people in the United States endorse the traditional moral code and at the same time violate it knowingly. Sexual themes are commonplace in our books and literature, but paradoxically only 10 to 20 percent of American parents discuss sexual matters with their children. (Yet, in the face of this glaring neglect, young people are continually condemned for mishaps due so often to sexual ignorance and misinformation.)

In films and books, as in "real life," profane language is regularly used; but in stark contrast to this permissive trend, many people are reluctant to use words such as "urinate," "masturbate," "menstruate," "penis," or "vagina" when they are appropriate. Individuals who appear to be comfortable in the scantiest of bathing suits at a public beach are deeply embarrassed when caught unexpectedly in their underwear by a member of their own family. These are, indeed, conflicting values.

In view of such inconsistencies and distorted perspectives, our society obviously needs to provide all people with the opportunity to acquire an education in human sexuality that will enable them to function more constructively and comfortably in their personal lives.

An effort directed toward enlightenment, rather than suppression, would be a more effective approach toward the resolution of our personal and social problems.

SEXUAL ATTITUDES

Where do our attitudes toward sex and sexual behavior originate? There is no simple answer. We are all influenced not only by our own particular needs and personalities but also by our culture, our parents, and our friends.

Sexuality in America is often tinged with guilt and embarrassment. Our Puritan heritage (which spread westward with the country's expansion) and repressive Victorian standards are still influencing our sexual attitudes and behavior.

Among many groups in the United States young people are expected to abstain from sexual intercourse until marriage, despite the fact that they are becoming physically mature at an earlier age than previous generations. The sexual needs of people, both young and old, are often ignored because American sexual codes are slow to change.

SAT (Sexual Attitudes Test)

There are no right or wrong answers in this test. Its purpose is to provoke you to think about some areas of sexuality in which people are often either uncertain or disturbed.

1. Are you comfortable with the manner in which you are conducting your sexual life?
2. Do you feel you are the best judge of your own sexual behavior?
3. Is the question of conformity a problem for you? Are the expectations of society, or the standards of your peers, a concern for you?
4. Do you experience feelings of guilt about any aspect of your sexual life? Have you been able to explain these feelings to yourself satisfactorily?
5. Do you have anyone with whom you can discuss sexuality freely? Do these discussions enable you to cope with your concerns?
6. Do you feel that there should be strong feelings of affection between people who engage in sexual intercourse with each other?
7. Does your sexual code make allowances for the sexual code of others?
8. Does your sexual behavior reflect a sense of responsibility?
9. Sexuality can be exploitive. Does it disturb you if people exploit the sexuality of others, or exploit sexuality for personal gain?
10. Do you agree with the reform of the law, which has occurred in many states, which exempts persons engaging in sexual acts from penalties of the criminal code so long as the individuals involved are adults who are acting of their own free will and the acts are conducted in private?

Restrictions such as age limits, legal status, and standards of propriety and respectability combine to inhibit sexual expression in the young. Sex information is inadequately transmitted, and the undue guilt and complexes of many individuals are often the unfortunate consequences of ignorance and misinformation. In addition, attitudes in our society may militate against sexual expression among other groups such as elderly singles, the widowed, and institutionalized persons (married or single).

Sexual attitudes begin to form at an early age. Children are extremely sensitive to gestures and tone of voice, and it is in this manner that they obtain a quick grasp of the emotional dynamics of a household. When punished for genital exploration, children interpret this an an expression of sexual taboo, a feeling that is further reinforced when parents and adults refer to genitalia and bodily functions not by their actual names, but by code words and euphemisms. Children acquire the idea from their parents that the body is a shameful thing. Sexual segregation and the veiled references of adults contribute to a view that sexuality is something forbidden, but also endlessly fascinating.

Children begin to ask questions when they are still quite young. They are extremely curious about birth, sexuality, and bodily functions, but their curiosity is rarely satisfied because most parents and teachers shy away from the duty

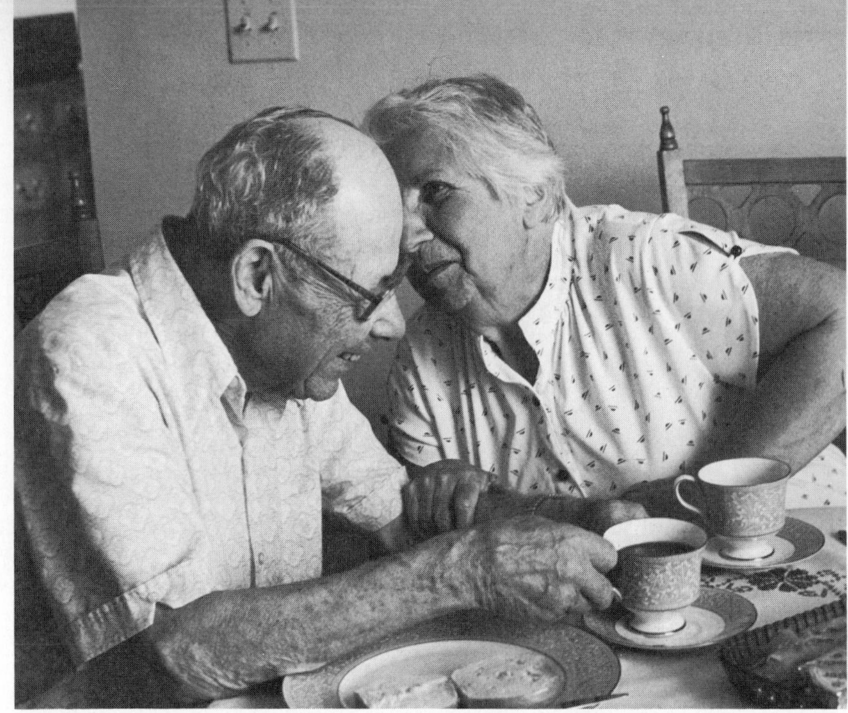

The need to share our lives with others is not limited by age.

of informing children about such matters. Children's questions are too often met with falsehoods, admonitions to mind their own business, or merely an embarrassed silence. Most parents in the United States do not discuss sex frankly with their offspring, and too few of the nation's schools have an adequate sex education system.

Most American parents still have extreme difficulty in communicating sexual information to their children. A recent study revealed that out of 1,461 parents interviewed, a mere 12 percent had spoken to their offspring about intercourse, premarital sex, or sexually transmitted disease. However, almost all of the parents supported the concept of sex education, and 80 percent of these thought that the subject should be taught in schools.

Whereas attitudes toward male sexual expression are relatively permissive in the United States, young females are under far greater social pressure to remain celibate. Fear of an unmarried daughter's possible pregnancy turns many parents into excessively strict disciplinarians. Such parental attitudes and prohibitions may be partly responsible for the early difficulties in sexual fulfillment experienced by many American women. Early acquired negative attitudes often come into conflict with later beliefs and produce guilt, thereby inhibiting sexual performance.

Many American males have grown up feeling that "real men" should be capable of sexual performance at all times. Such a belief can make occasional failure to achieve an erection seem a sign of a lack of masculinity, which can lead to sexual problems.

Understanding a partner's needs and desires is essential to sexual fulfillment. Partners can receive pleasure, for instance, by hugging, caressing, and kissing. Touching also serves to indicate feeling, caring, affection, and love—all of which enhance sexual gratification.

THE SEXUAL LIFE CYCLE

Human sexual response begins virtually from the moment of birth. An evident manifestation of sexuality occurs during breast feeding, when the newborn child takes pleasure and comfort from the sheer physical proximity of the mother. It has also been recorded that newborn babies have displayed all the visible and somatic signs of orgasm: tumescence (erection), increased rates of blood circulation and heartbeat, changes in breathing, and flushing of the skin.

The physical self-exploration that children carry on throughout early childhood indicates that a considerable degree of pleasure is obtained by means of the sense of touch. Sexual exploration of other children also begins at this stage. Young children manifest a high level of curiosity about, and a developing awareness of, the anatomy of other persons—adults as well as children. This alertness also extends to words, gestures, and other cues that have sexual connotations. Instead of using this innate curiosity and taking advantage of the opportunity the home environment provides for imparting information, many parents, following tradition, chastise the child.

Increased sexual awareness and exploration, together with a number of other experiences during the middle years of childhood, combine to form the child's sense of gender identity. Most children are gradually programmed for sex-role identification through selected clothing and toys, teachings, confrontations, and parental models.

The developmental stage of puberty is significant in all respects, and the appearance of the secondary sex characteristics is perhaps most significant of all. (Hormonal changes during puberty are discussed in Chapter 7.) The capacity to produce reproductive cells first occurs during this stage. On the average, girls experience the onset of menstruation at about age 12, but ovulation does not begin until approximately one year later. At about age 13 or 14, boys normally begin to be capable of ejaculation, although a number of them have already been experiencing satisfying sexual play.

Any distinctive departure from the norm regarding the size of the adolescent breasts or penis may cause an individual acute embarrassment and suffering. Adolescent boys and girls prefer to remain inconspicuous at this stage of development and to appear as much like their companions as possible. Although today's youth are often considered to be more worldly and precocious than their counterparts in the decades before the 1960s, adolescence nevertheless continues to be a period of confusion, embarrassment, and sometimes fear. Some young females are kept in such total ignorance about their sexual development that their first menstrual period is a surprising, if not terrifying, event.

Their capacity to ejaculate having begun a year or two earlier, 95 percent of all boys will have experienced orgasm by the age of 15. Usually by age 16, and rarely later than 17, a frequency of orgasm is established that will remain unsurpassed throughout the entire life span. For some males, the frequency at this time may be several times a week; for others, it is several times a day. For most males this frequency of orgasm establishes a pattern that will continue for the next thirty years. Then, at about age 45, a significant number of males begin to experience a decline. At present there is no explanation for this phenomenon.

The sexual development of girls begins earlier than that of boys, but their involvement in expressive, orgasmic sexuality occurs much more slowly. By the age of 15, only 23 percent of females have achieved orgasm. The capacity to achieve orgasm does not occur for many women until they have reached their 30s or 40s, and sometimes beyond. It is also during this age span that women experience the peak of their sexual drive, and it remains at a rather uniform level of intensity until their late 50s and 60s. The range of individual female response is broader than that of men, extending from the number of women who report never achieving orgasm to those whose orgasmic capacity is many times that of the most responsive male. Women also have an ability to endure periods of abstinence from sexual activity that may extend for years.

There is no physiological explanation why women should achieve full sexual maturity, in the sense of orgasmic response, so late in life. It is possible that the repressive attitudes toward sexual expression imposed upon young women create psychological barriers toward sexual fulfillment that women find difficult to overcome until later in life.

Menopause, or the **climacteric,** usually begins among women when they are between the ages of 46 and 51. Menopause is the gradual cessation of the menstrual cycle. The process lasts about two years. Depression often accompanies menopause because a number of women unfortunately misinterpret the termination of their ability to reproduce as the virtual end of their womanhood. Such women experience a marked decline in sexual interest. Other women feel liberated from the threat of pregnancy and develop new and greater levels of sexual responsiveness.

There is nothing comparable to menopause in men's sexual experiences; no vital physiological process suddenly stops functioning. Instead, the male climacteric takes the form of an almost imperceptible decline in many of the physical aspects of sexual function. Although some men begin to lose sexual interest earlier, actual physical changes are not generally noticeable until around the age of 55. At that point, the amount of semen ejaculated may begin to decrease, erections take longer to achieve, orgasm becomes less intense, and the period of time between orgasms become greater. Changes in mood may accompany these physiological transformations, but it is not usual for the male climacteric to have any sudden and direct effect upon the sexual drive.

Sexual activity should continue well into the later years of life, diminishing only somewhat, as do other bodily capacities. There are no physical reasons why both men and women should not continue to enjoy expressing their sexuality well into their later years. Statistics reveal that, on the average, one out of five women is sexually active in her 60s and that some men 75 and older report experiencing orgasm about once a week. There have been many instances of sexual activity continuing into the 90s (see Chapter 10).

Some men and women report an increase in sexual interest as they grow older. Perhaps this is because they have learned to fulfill themselves, rather than society's expectations of them. It has also been shown that those who lead active, satisfying sex lives in their earlier and middle years are more likely to remain vigorous and interested further into old age.

Human sexuality, however, is far more than a series of orgasms. From infancy to old age, we all have the need to love and be loved and to enjoy acceptance

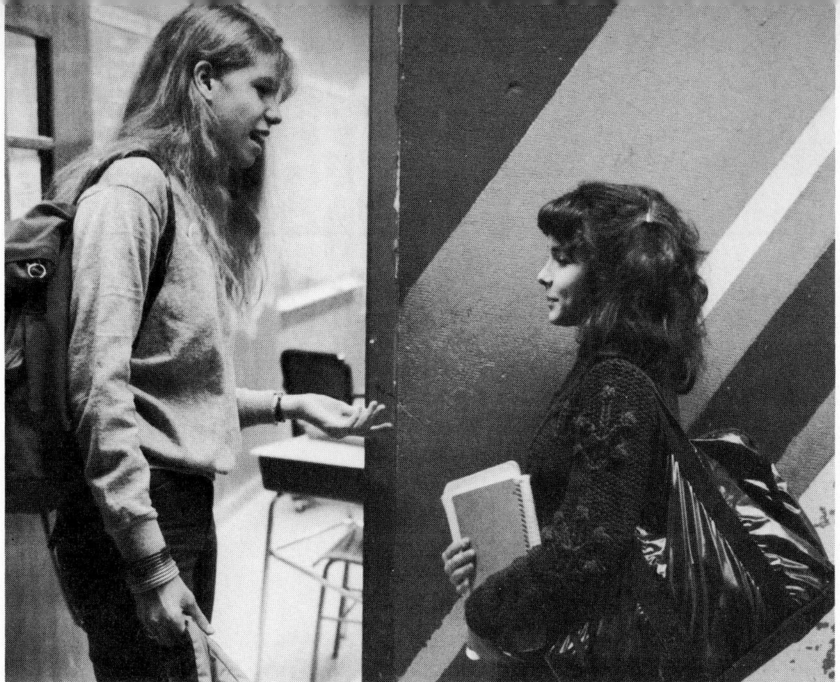

and affection. The need and desire to express our emotions and sexuality, and to share our lives with others, is essential to persons of all ages.

HUMAN SEXUAL RESPONSE

The reproductive structures and roles of the two sexes are quite different. Because of this, it has been presumed that vast differences must exist in sexual expression as well. Recent studies indicate, however, that there are far more similarities than differences. This should be no surprise; the two sexes are not, after all, separate species.

Both men and women react favorably to kindness, sensitivity, verbal endearments, and caresses. Conversely, both can be inhibited by depression, anger, anxiety, or guilt. Men and women have **erogenous zones**—areas that, when stimulated, cause sexual arousal. These areas are analogous in both structure and sensitivity. To have lips, face, neck, breasts, back, or abdomen touched by someone's lips or hands is exciting to members of both sexes. The genitalia of both sexes are the most responsive to touch and provide the most intense erotic pleasure. Both the penis and the clitoris become erect during periods of sexual excitement. Furthermore, the rhythmic pelvic movements that typically occur during intercourse result from a natural reaction that is shared equally by both sexes.

The four physiological phases of sexual expression identified by William Masters and Virginia Johnson—excitement, plateau, orgasm, and resolution—are also remarkably similar for men and women. The only differences, in fact, involve the capacity of women to experience multiple orgasms and the greater length of time women require to achieve orgasm during intercourse.

Female Sexual Response

In women sexual arousal—the **excitement phase**—causes an increase in heart rate, blood pressure, and muscular tension. An increased volume of blood flows

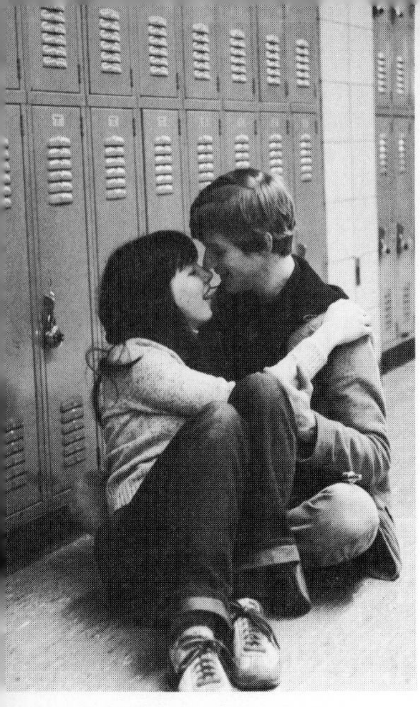

to the breasts, external genitalia, and vagina. The breasts increase in size by about 20 percent, and the nipples may become erect. Most women in the excitement phase also exhibit a **sex flush** over the abdomen, breasts, and throat. At the same time, the entire vaginal passage becomes lubricated by a sweatlike secretion given off by the cells that make up the inner wall of the vagina. A few droplets may also be discharged by the Bartholin's glands.

As sexual excitement becomes more intense, the clitoris, labia minora, and uterus increase in size, and the vaginal walls expand. When the plateau phase nears, the enlarged uterus is pulled upward, widening the innermost part of the vagina. The expanded vaginal passage accommodates the erect penis, and the new position of the uterus probably facilitates the entry of sperm into the cervix.

In a favorable mood and setting, the excitement phase can be made more intense by prolonged stimulation of the erogenous zones. Because they contain a high concentration of nerve endings, the nipples and external genitalia are extremely sensitive to touch. Many women respond most to rhythmic stroking of these areas.

Once the penis has entered the vagina, its to-and-fro motion against the erogenous zones of the vulva increases a woman's excitement. (Because the inner two-thirds of the vagina contain few nerve endings, the size of a man's penis has little effect on a woman's sexual response or pleasure, though many in our society place an erotic premium on large penises.) During the **plateau phase** the sex flush spreads to most of the body surface and the breasts reach their maximum enlargement. The heart rate continues to rise, and muscular movement and tension become more pronounced. The outer third of the vagina becomes congested with blood, and the vaginal muscles begin to tighten around the penis. The clitoris withdraws almost completely into its hood, so that it is no longer visible. Finally, the labia minora change color from pink to bright red as the level of excitement increases and they become filled with blood.

Despite the **orgasmic phase** heart rate, blood pressure, and muscular tension reach a peak. According to Masters and Johnson, the vagina contracts strongly around the penis every four-fifths of a second. If stimulation is continued, more than one orgasm can be achieved. Some women report that the additional orgasms are increasingly pleasurable.

According to a current survey of American female sexual attitudes and behavior, most women require more than coitus to achieve orgasm. The number of women who achieve orgasm regularly during sexual intercourse has been estimated to be as low as 26 percent. Because of this, manual excitation of the clitoris during sexual intercourse is quite common among women who seek orgasm.

According to Masters and Johnson, Sherfey, and others, there are no separate vaginal and clitoral orgasms. Every orgasm is the result of direct or indirect stimulation of the external genitalia and the muscles surrounding the vaginal opening. However, the sensation of orgasm itself is not restricted to the genital area; the entire body may become involved in the release of sexual tension and the sensation of pleasure.

Following orgasm, the woman enters the **resolution phase,** when the physiological changes that occurred during intercourse gradually reverse themselves.

(She may, however, remain in the excitement phase for a relatively prolonged period of time.) Unlike a man, the woman does not enter a long refractory period. If stimulated during the resolution phase, the woman can quickly return to the excitement phase or even to the plateau phase and again achieve one or more orgasms.

Male Sexual Response

During the excitement phase a man's heart and respiratory rates and blood pressure increase. Erection occurs, although over a prolonged excitement phase the erection may be partially lost and regained repeatedly. A muscle contraction tightens the scrotal sac and brings the testicles up near the base of the penis. The nipples of most men also become erect during this phase.

During the plateau phase a sex flush may develop, and the glans penis may become purple. Muscular tension, heart and respiratory rate, and blood pressure increase. The testes fill with blood and become 50 percent larger. The testes and scrotal sac remain in an elevated position, and if sexual stimulation is maintained, orgasm will occur.

The penis contains a large number of highly sensitive nerve endings, especially in the skin just below the glans penis. The rhythmic friction of the penis against the walls of the vagina greatly increases the excitability of these nerve endings. When the pitch of excitement reaches a certain level—the orgasmic phase—the muscles surrounding the epididymis contract, forcing sperm into the vas deferens. At the same time, the muscles surrounding Cowper's glands, the prostate gland, and the seminal vesicles contract peristaltically, forcing the glandular secretions into the ejaculatory ducts and urethra.

Then, triggered by nerve impulses transmitted from the central nervous system, all the muscles surrounding the accessory sex glands and the ducts undergo several convulsive contractions. These contractions cause semen to spurt through and out of the penis. The total volume of semen discharged during **ejaculation** amounts to about a teaspoonful of liquid. This fluid ordinarily contains between 200 and 400 million spermatozoa, only one of which is needed for fertilization.

During ejaculation the man experiences the subjective sensations of orgasm. The heart rate reaches a peak and muscle tension becomes extreme. Once orgasm occurs, the man enters a **refractory period** during which he is temporarily incapable of achieving another orgasm. The length of this period varies with age, frequency of intercourse, and intensity of renewed sexual stimulation. During this time the glans penis is usually very sensitive to the touch.

In the resolution phase almost all the physiological changes that occurred during sexual activity are rapidly reversed. The man feels pleasantly exhausted. Gradually, the heartbeat resumes its normal rate and the penis returns to its prearoused condition.

Individual Differences

These events in the sexual response cycle do not always occur as described for all men and women. Individuals may have different responses, and responses within the same individual may vary at different times or according to different states of mind. Preferences as to how the coital act is performed may also vary. In general, worrying about "performance" or "technique" inhibits enjoyment; communicating one's desires frankly and being sensitive to the desires of one's partner lead to mutual satisfaction. It should be added that sexuality is often only one aspect of a relationship between two people. There are many ways of sharing experiences and expressing affection. Focusing attention on intercourse may cause a couple to ignore possible fulfillment—or real problems—in other areas.

FORMS OF SEXUAL EXPRESSION

Nocturnal Orgasms

Erections are not usually under a man's conscious control, though he can often cause an erection by deliberately engaging in sexual fantasies. Most men in their teens and early twenties have frequent spontaneous erections because of the sexual excitability that exists during those years. Erections that occur during sleep, however, are not always the result of erotic dreams; they may simply be caused by certain phases of the sleep cycle.

Some men may also experience *nocturnal emissions*, or **wet dreams,** while they are asleep. A "wet dream" is a spontaneous discharge of semen accompanied by the sensation of an orgasm. The orgasm usually results from a dream with sexual content. Most women also have erotic dreams, and about half of these women have accompanying orgasms, though, of course, there is no discharge or emission.

Masturbation

Masturbation—self-manipulation of the genitals to induce orgasm—has been censured by Judeo-Christian moral codes since biblical times. The "spilling of seed" was considered a sin because it supposedly diverted sexual expression from its original purpose—procreation. The condemnation of masturbation became extremely prudish and hysterical during Victorian times, when masturbation was presumed to cause physical disorders, insanity, and eternal damnation.

Victorian attitudes toward masturbation are still widespread. Today many parents induce fear or guilt about masturbation in their children. They may communicate their own discomfort about sexual matters in general, or they may react harshly to their children's genital play. Whatever the form prohibitions against masturbation take, mental anguish, guilt feelings, and fears of abnormality invariably result.

The fact is that masturbation is a perfectly normal, healthy act, practiced by over 95 percent of males and 65 percent of females. It is the principal introductory sexual act in our society and continues to be the most frequently used method of attaining orgasm by unmarried men and women. Far from being an adolescent act, as some believe, masturbation is first practiced by most women when they are already adults. In fact, women initiate the practice in increasing numbers up to the age of 40, and both men and women continue masturbating through middle and old age. Nor is masturbation practiced exclusively by the unmarried. Many married men and women continue to masturbate throughout their lives. Recent surveys have shown that masturbation is a common sexual practice among all groups. About one-third of men and women in almost every age group, married and single, masturbate more than once a week.

Many psychologists today feel that masturbation is a positive form of sexual expression and gratification. It provides a healthy release for sexual tensions and fantasies, particularly for those who have no other outlet available; it permits greater variety in sexual activity; and it helps some people lose their sexual inhibitions. Individuals in sex therapy take an important first step toward achieving satisfactory intercourse when they learn to respond fully to their own self-stimulation.

Petting

Petting is any form of sexual contact between individuals that does not involve intercourse. (Petting that precedes intercourse is known as **foreplay.**) Thus petting may include any of a wide range of activities: kissing, manual or oral stimulation of any part of the body, caressing, and hugging.

In general, petting is a reflection of a person's sexual attitudes. A reluctance to caress one's partner or an inability to enjoy being caressed might indicate sexual guilt or confusion. Of course, many persons who are sexually well adjusted engage in no petting. There is, however, considerable evidence that some petting experience plays an important role in developing sexual maturity and the ability to function effectively in a sexual relationship.

The degree to which petting is used as a source of sexual satisfaction varies among individuals and the stage of the relationship. Couples sensitive to each other's needs and sexual attitudes respond accordingly in determining what is considered acceptable. Generally, petting becomes increasingly intimate as the couple becomes more involved in the relationship and the expression of their affection for each other.

Mutual Masturbation. Couples who, for whatever reason, are reluctant to engage in full intercourse may satisfy each other by means of various forms of mutual masturbation. Heterosexual or homosexual couples may bring each other to orgasm by simply massaging each others' genitals. Many women, in fact, reach orgasm only when the clitoris is stimulated by hand. In situations where the male cannot maintain an erection and copulation is not possible, mutual masturbation can provide a satisfying form of sexual expression. And many people engage in mutual masturbation simply as a variant form of sex.

Oral and Anal Sex. Sexual expression can include various kinds of oral-genital contact. Using the mouth and tongue to stimulate a woman's genitals is formally referred to as **cunnilingus:** to stimulate a man's, **fellatio.** When both partners wish to stimulate each other orally at the same time, they must assume what is popularly known as the "69" position. Partners should make sure their genital areas are clean before an act of oral sex.

Like the genitals, the anus in both sexes is highly erogenous. In spite of persisting Victorian mores, at least half of all men and women enjoy some form of anal stimulation. Both the active and passive partner may derive pleasure from anal stimulation, but it should be recognized that it is not without risk of transmission of infection.

Mutual pleasure is the only reason for engaging in any of these forms of sex play. Neither partner should ever be compelled to perform or made to feel guilty or inadequate if unwilling to do so.

Sexual Intercourse

Before Marriage. Nowhere has the so-called double standard in our society operated with greater force than in the area of premarital intercourse. While our moral code forbids premarital intercourse to men and women equally, our

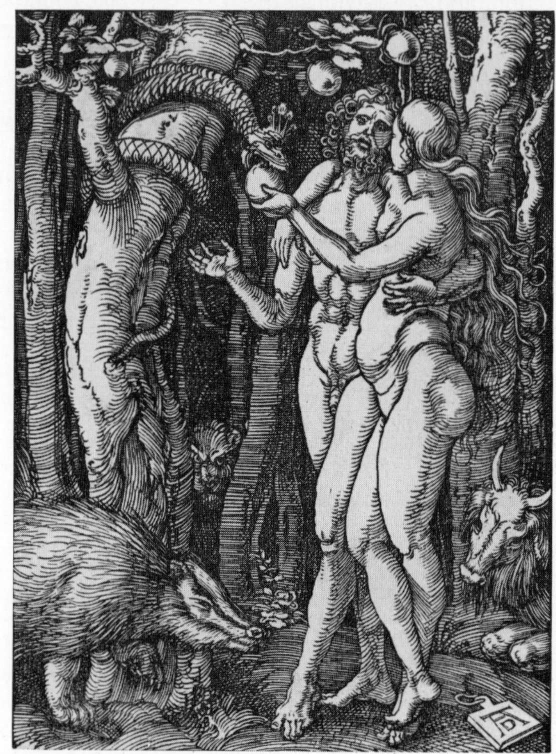
Adam and Eve: a woodcut by Albrecht Dürer.

culture in fact has been quite permissive, if not encouraging, toward male sexual behavior. Women, on the other hand, have been expected to conform to Victorian standards of chastity.

In recent years, however, the traditional roles of women have undergone a radical change. This transformation is reflected in the increased participation of women in sexual activities, including premarital intercourse. While studies between 1945 and 1965 indicated that somewhat fewer than 30 percent of college women had premarital intercourse, recent studies show that between two-thirds and three-fourths of college women have intercourse before marriage. (The rates vary enormously, as might be expected, however, between liberal Eastern universities and certain church-affiliated colleges.) The rate for college men has remained more nearly constant: From six to eight out of ten college men have intercourse before marriage.

Although sexual standards have become somewhat more permissive, they do not signal that a "sexual revolution" has taken place—at least not in the sense that a great number of people have become more promiscuous. Most young people have intercourse in a relationship of mutual commitment—often with the person they intend to marry.

Many experts feel that premarital intercourse with a loved and loving person can be a meaningful and healthy experience. However, the growing acceptance of premarital sexual behavior has undoubtedly created difficulties for many.

The weakening of parental and societal guidelines for behavior has meant that young people must make choices they are not always prepared to make. Some people, for example, who feel it is morally wrong to have premarital intercourse may come to believe that disregarding their own feelings is the price they must pay for peer acceptance. Others may engage in intercourse before they are mature enough to accept the responsibility for contraception, venereal disease prevention, and pregnancy. The new sexual freedom brings with it not only increased possibilities for individual self-fulfillment but also new responsibilities. As we noted at the opening of this chapter, sexual freedom has also resulted in fears and worries about sexual competence and performance.

Laws and Customs. It is no mere coincidence that marital sexual intercourse is the only form of sexual expression that has had universal acceptance. In view of high mortality rates until very recently, the human race has required high birth rates in order to survive. Therefore sexual acts not directed toward reproduction were considered threatening and were condemned. But notwithstanding its significance as the means of propagation, marital intercourse, too, has traditionally been subject to restriction. Taboos formerly existed with regard to intercourse during menstruation, and even the position of the partners during the act has been regulated by dogma. Today the laws governing sexual intercourse are less punitive than they once were, and are usually not enforced. In many states recent legislation exempts from criminal prosecution sexual acts conducted in privacy between consenting adults. In most states, however, criminal prosecution, as well as civil suits, may result from acts of nonmarital intercourse, and about two states in five still outlaw heterosexual sodomy.

To perform the act of intercourse, the male may enter the female from a variety of positions: lying, kneeling, sitting, or standing; from a position above, beneath, or alongside the female; and from a frontal or rear approach. The position that a couple assumes is generally dictated by comfort and personal satisfaction. Practical considerations such as obesity, the size of the penis, or an infirmity of one of the partners may influence this selection as well.

Bisexuality

A growing number of psychologists embrace the concept that people are capable of very fluid sexual responses. By this they mean that a person's sexual response and behavior may not necessarily be uniform throughout life; instead, they may vary, depending on time and circumstances, far more than has been traditionally assumed. Masters and Johnson's study *Homosexuality in Perspective* supports the thesis that bisexual desire is a possibility for everyone: Among the group studied, sexual fantasies almost invariably included persons of both sexes.

How such desires are expressed, of course, depends largely on the permissiveness of the society in which they arise. There is a developing consensus, however, that everyone is potentially bisexual, both behaviorally and emotionally, and that large numbers of people have at least experimented with that potential.

In view of the realization that the human being is capable of sexual expression with either gender, it would seem appropriate to employ the terms *homosexual* and *heterosexual* to refer to the sexual act conducted between individuals rather than to the individuals themselves.

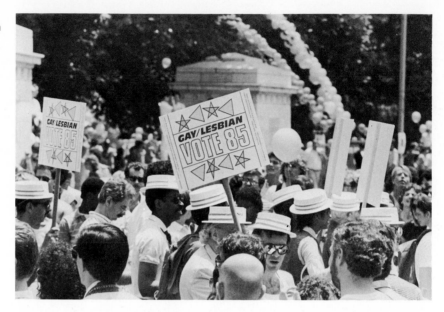

In some cities where homosexual groups have been politically active, discriminatory practices have been outlawed.

The decision may also reflect the customs of a country or an ethnic group. For example, in the United States the partners generally assume a face-to-face position, with the male resting upon the female. In the Soviet Union it is customary for the male to enter the female from behind, while she crouches upon her knees, head downward, in the "crayfish" position.

It should be mentioned again that sexual intercourse is not necessarily as satisfying to the female as it is to the male. This is because stimulation of the clitoris may be minimal during intercourse and insufficient to excite the female to the degree reached by the male. For this reason, many females stimulate the clitoris manually during intercourse so that they may achieve satisfaction along with their partners.

Homosexuality

The terms *gay*, *straight*, and *bisexual* have come into everyday usage, and homosexuality is no longer a forbidden subject. Despite this apparent knowledgeability about homosexuality, however, we may question whether the perceptions of the public are accurate, and whether openness on the topic has had any effect upon attitudes.

Until recent years an individual was thought of as either exclusively **homosexual**—interested only in sexual relations with members of his or her own sex—or exclusively heterosexual. Today the concept of **bisexuality** is fairly well recognized, as we have come to realize that there are people whose behavior pattern includes both homosexual and heterosexual expression. There are also persons who have homosexual fantasies but live exclusively as heterosexuals. The Kinsey studies, carried out some forty years ago, revealed a much greater incidence of homosexual behavior than had been generally recognized. They also revealed that a significant percentage of the population had had homosexual as well as heterosexual experiences at some point in their lives. Though many had engaged in homosexual acts, relatively few had done so exclusively.

Kinsey developed a seven-point scale for dividing his study population into groupings according to the percentage of their sexual experiences that were heterosexual and homosexual. He found that while the overwhelming majority of his study population considered itself heterosexual, 37 percent of the men he studied and 13 percent of the women had had at least one orgasm with a partner of the same sex.

Subsequent research has confirmed Kinsey's findings on the incidence of homosexuality. According to John Money and Claus Weideking, over 3 million American males are predominantly homosexual. The number of female homosexuals (called **lesbians**) is estimated to be a third to half that number.

Although homosexual acts have traditionally been categorized as deviant or unnatural, there is no evidence that they are any more or less so than heterosexual acts. It appears that a person's sexual preference results from his or her personal experiences and not from biological predetermination. Hormone levels in most homosexual and heterosexual individuals are the same. Nor has a hereditary predisposition to homosexuality or heterosexuality been found. It has also been impossible to identify any experiences that will definitely lead to homosexuality. For example, many individuals who have had a seductive parent of the opposite sex—traditionally considered a cause of homosexuality—still consider themselves to be heterosexual.

One of the most persistent myths about homosexuals is that they can be easily identified on the basis of appearance, speech, personality, or occupation. Homosexual men are supposed to lisp or otherwise act in an effeminate manner, and homosexual women are expected to look masculine. Numerous studies have indicated that the vast majority of homosexuals do not conform to these popular stereotypes. Homosexuals may be found in any occupation (even in those forbidden to them by law) and in any ethnic, religious, or cultural group. And while the popular notion is that homosexuals are emotionally disturbed, several carefully controlled studies have shown that they are no more so than heterosexuals. Most homosexuals prefer their orientation; they may, however, experience greater stress because of society's attitude toward them.

In 1973 the American Psychiatric Association voted to stop classifying homosexuality as an abnormality. In the lexicon of experts in sexuality, homosexuality is no longer considered a deviant but a variant form of sexual expression. (See the section Homosexual Relationships in Chapter 9).

Homosexuality and Society. Throughout the ages societies have expressed a full range of reactions toward homosexuality, from total acceptance to absolute rejection. In some societies where homosexuality has been accepted, homosexual rites have existed as a part of the culture and homosexuals have been among the most highly esteemed individuals. In most societies, however, perhaps because it is considered threatening to the birth rate, homosexuality has been disparaged. Our Judeo-Christian heritage condemns and even prosecutes acts of homosexuality. Laws in almost half the states, whose legality was upheld

Variant Sexual Behavior

The variations that can be played upon the sexual act are seemingly endless. Through the ages different forms of sexual expression have been either encouraged, tolerated, or proscribed, depending upon complex social factors. The following list is a brief, and by no means complete, sampling of some of these variations.

Incest: Every known present-day society has an incest taboo that prohibits sexual relations between close relatives. On the other hand, incest within royal families—most often between brother and sister—was expected in ancient Mayan, Inca, Hawaiian, and Egyptian societies.

Pedophilia: Pedophilia ("love for children"), sexual gratification with children, is prohibited in our society; it is, in fact, one of our strongest taboos. Girls are far more likely than boys to be victims of sexual abuse, contrary to popular opinion. While many cases of child molestation in day-care centers have been reported in recent years, it has been difficult to establish guilt. That some children have been coached to accuse innocent adults has complicated the situation.

Voyeurism and *exhibitionism*: A voyeur is a person whose principal source of sexual pleasure is in looking at the bodies of others and watching sexual acts. An exhibitionist is someone who finds it erotically pleasurable to display the nude body or its parts, or to be observed obtaining sexual gratification.

Sadomasochism: Sadists derive sexual gratification from inflicting pain upon their partners; masochists find sexual pleasure in receiving pain. Sadomasochistic ("S & M") sex is usually performed by willing partners who understand each other's role and particular form of pleasure. Such acts, however, have sometimes led to the death of a participant.

Promiscuity: In our culture promiscuity—sex with many different partners—is generally frowned upon, though more so for women than for men.

Nymphomania and *satyriasis*: A nymphomaniac is a woman who presumably has an insatiable, uncontrolled sex drive. Satyriasis is the male equivalent of nymphomania.

Fetishism: Fetishism is the transfer of sexual interest to objects (such as shoes or lingerie) or parts of the body (such as the foot) that would not ordinarily be considered erotic.

by the Supreme Court in 1986, outlaw homosexual acts even between consenting adults within their own homes. Under more liberal laws in other states, however, individuals who engage in homosexual acts enjoy the same protection from criminal prosecution as those who engage in heterosexual acts, provided that the sexual act is conducted in privacy and between consenting adults.

Other laws and customs attempt to deny persons identified as homosexual the rights enjoyed by heterosexuals. It has been the practice to exclude homosexuals from teaching, from the military, and from various government positions. Discrimination has been practiced in housing regulations. Gay bars and baths have been raided or closed. In addition, homosexuals suffer from hoodlums who prey upon them, are sometimes the victims of extortion schemes, and are subject to entrapment by the police.

Homophile organizations in many communities have been successful in ending discriminatory practices in housing and employment, and in general, the social and legal harassment of homosexuals has seemed in recent years to be subsiding. Whether the widespread fear of AIDS (see Chapter 15) will cause a reversal of this trend is uncertain, but there is much evidence that it has affected many people's attitudes.

RAPE AND VIOLENCE

Sex educators and psychologists consider rape to be an act of assault and violence, not an act of sexual lust. The distinction is important. Seen in this light, rapists are not people searching for sexual gratification: They are persons committing a vengeful act of assault. The motives may range from inhibitions and guilt about sexuality to paranoid fear of, or hatred for, women.

The rapist's past experiences with women may have been characterized by ineptitude, impotence, rejection, embarrassment, or anger. Violent assault, then,

Problems and Controversies: Acquaintance Rape

Violent crimes against women are on the increase all over the country. Authorities estimate that each year between 1.5 million and 2 million women in the United States are victims of rape or attempted rape. Most of the victims are young, between the ages of 15 and 24, and the average age is 18. The finding that surprises most people is that more than half of the rape victims either knew their attacker well or were at least acquainted with him.

The problem is reaching crisis proportions on the nation's campuses, where one out of four women have experienced some form of violent sexual assault. The crime is most likely to occur not in a darkened alley or vacant lot, but in a dormitory room, a bachelor pad, or the front seat of an automobile. The attacker is most often not a "loser" but an attractive young man who, up until the critical moment, has been attentive and well behaved—even charming. The scene then takes an ugly turn, the woman is forced into sex against her violent protests, and she then is often quietly escorted home, sometimes after being made to promise another date. Women who have undergone such experiences often have difficulty admitting or realizing that they have been raped, and their attackers find it almost impossible to see themselves as rapists or to characterize what they have done as rape.

Nevertheless, women who have been "date-raped" may suffer even greater emotional and psychological damage than those who have been assaulted by a stranger. Most blame themselves for their partner's uncontrollable behavior and do not report him to the authorities. Instead, they develop a "fear of the familiar" and wonder whether they can trust any male acquaintance or friend. If a woman does report the incident, she is often in for an especially difficult time. Frequently she is persuaded by prosecutors not to bring charges against her attacker because the attacker is not likely to be convicted. The attacker is seen as a "nice decent guy" who simply let his urges momentarily get out of hand. If it does come to a trial or hearing, the woman is often perceived to be a willing participant in a romantic situation in which the boundaries of petting and more intense lovemaking are unclear.

The situation of these women is not helped by a cluster of prevailing social attitudes toward rape victims and toward women in general. Many men, for example, continue to believe that a woman's "no" actually means "yes" and that all women expect men to be aggressive. Surveys show that an alarming number of high-school boys and girls think that it is all right to force other persons to have sex against their will. As for rape itself, many men still think that most women lie about rape, that they actually like it and are not harmed by it, and that they deserve it.

Perhaps the most important need is for young adults to reexamine their beliefs and expectations about sex. Many need to be reeducated in the rudiments of intimacy, starting with holding hands. Men need to realize that when a woman says "no" she means it, and many women have to learn how to become more convincing about it.

Sources: Adapted from Ellen Sweet, "Date Rape: The Story of an Epidemic and Those Who Deny It," *Ms. Magazine*, October 1985, pp. 56–59, 84–85; "The Date Who Rapes," *Newsweek*, April 9, 1984, pp. 91–92.

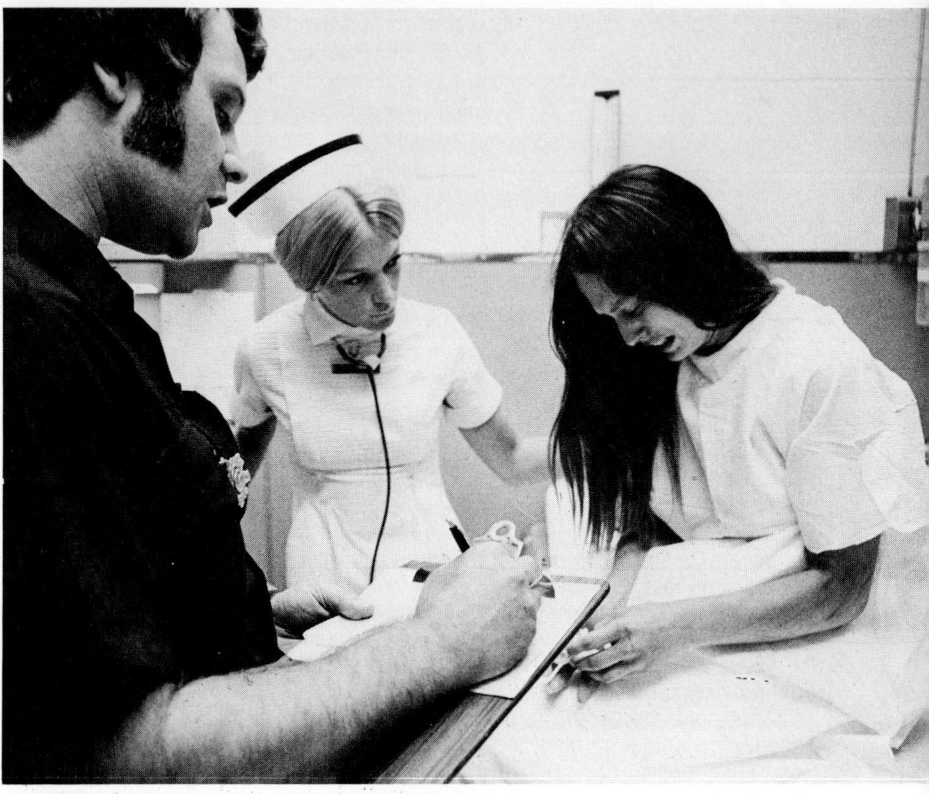
Many women do not report being raped, fearing that they will be thought to have invited the assault. Both laws and attitudes have changed for the better in recent years.

is the way a rapist chooses to assert his superiority in some way and take revenge; it is not an expression of sexual desire.

Until quite recently, courts have been slow to follow the psychologists' lead. Courts have traditionally held that the victim "must have asked for it" by her provocative actions or manner of dress; this attitude is less prevalent today among judges and juries than in the past.

Lately the public has become more aware of the phenomenon of homosexual rape, often through exposés of prison conditions. Less sensational forms of both homosexual and heterosexual rape often go unreported, some because they occur between family members. The rape of a woman by a man with whom she is out on a date has become a matter of recent concern; it is discussed in the box titled Acquaintance Rape. Gang rape, a group sexual assault by males perpetrated upon a female or another male, further illustrates the violence and aggression inherent in these acts. The gang situation also permits individuals to mask or overcome their own inhibitions, ineptitudes, or other problems of adjustment.

Opinions differ on what a woman should do to protect herself against rape and on how she should best respond if she is attacked. Some widely respected advice, though, is contained in the box titled Rape: How to Protect Yourself.

Rape: How to Protect Yourself

Knowing that a crime *could* happen is the first step toward protecting yourself. Self-defense courses are available at many women's centers, YWCAs, and rape-crisis centers, but short of taking a course, there are ways to work on your own assertiveness, vigilance, and preparedness.

On the Street

- Walk near the curb or in the street, facing traffic, not next to walls, parked cars, or hedges.
- Walk with a purpose. If you look as if you know where you're going, people are less likely to bother you.
- Wear flat shoes or sneakers in case you need to run.
- Don't be afraid of insulting a friendly stranger; if he is really friendly, he'll understand your caution.
- If something feels wrong about a situation, trust your gut feelings and get out of it.

If You Are Attacked

- If possible, run away as fast as you can.
- If you can't flee, then scream, yell, punch, and kick. Pleading and crying are very ineffective defense strategies.
- The earlier in an attack you start to defend yourself, the more likely you are to escape rape. Women who resist their attackers are more likely to suffer *minor* injuries such as scrapes and bruises, but no more likely to suffer *serious* injury than women who do not resist.

Source: Susan Grossman, "How to Protect Yourself," *Glamour*, February 1986, p. 213. Courtesy *Glamour.*

SEXUAL DYSFUNCTION

Most men and women at one time or another find that their efforts to achieve sexual satisfaction are unsuccessful. An occasional disinterest in sex, a failure to maintain an erection, or an inability to achieve orgasm are perfectly normal phenomena. When such problems occur repeatedly, however, the affected individual is said to be suffering from **sexual dysfunction.**

According to Masters and Johnson, some form of sexual dysfunction or inadequacy occurs among at least 50 percent of the married couples in the United States. About three-quarters of those who seek help from psychotherapists or marriage counselors manifest sexual difficulties. These problems are almost always psychological, rather than physiological, in origin. They can be the result of an inadequate or nonexistent sex education, an overly rigid religious upbringing, or fears about sexual performance or intercourse.

The lack of proper sex education can cause sexual difficulties in several ways. Some couples may never have been taught the fundamentals of human anatomy. More often, individuals or couples have a set of false ideas about the sexual act and find themselves unable to cope with its reality. A woman may grow up to believe that "it's all up to the man" and may be totally unprepared to deal with a man who is as inexperienced as she is. Or because of false notions about masculinity, a man may feel required to perform sexually even when he is not in the mood to do so; if he fails to achieve erection, he may suffer a psychological blow that will inhibit him in future encounters. Perhaps most important, persons who have received little or no sex education may find it hard to communicate or even comprehend their own needs and desires. Achieving a satisfactory sexual relationship is difficult when sexuality itself is clouded by ignorance, confusion, and misunderstanding.

A healthy—or unhealthy—sexual orientation begins in childhood. For this reason, parental influence is extremely important. Some parents who are overly moralistic or inhibited inculcate unhealthy sexual attitudes in their children. They may, for example, fail to make a clear distinction between sexuality itself and sex outside religious or social tradition. A person who is taught that "sex is dirty," instead of "sex is good, under the right conditions," may experience sexual difficulties later on. Also, some parents are uncomfortable with their own sexuality and find it difficult to provide their children with a sound sex education.

Fears about sexual performance or intercourse are almost always related to feelings of inadequacy. A typical pattern of sexual dysfunction begins when an individual approaches intercourse lacking self-confidence. His or her anxiety may inhibit a normal sexual response—that is, the person may fail to achieve erection or orgasm because he or she expects to fail. This initial lack of success may cause increased anxiety during the next sexual encounter, making another failure almost inevitable.

Male Sexual Dysfunction

Impotence. **Impotence** is the inability of a man to achieve or maintain an erection sufficient for the act of coitus. Any man may have an episode of impotence when he is tired or ill, when something is worrying him or distracting his attention, when he is "turned off" by his partner, or when he is under the influence of alcohol or drugs. An occasional episode of impotence caused by realistic factors such as these is called **functional impotence.** Most men experience functional impotence at one time or another.

Aphrodisiacs: The Love Potions

Throughout history, and from all parts of the world, come tales of magic elixirs that stimulate the sex drive to the point of frenzy, or prolong the waning libido of the aged or infirm. These love potions have included all imaginable substances. The demand in some Asian countries today for pulverized rhinoceros horn is such that it has all but caused the extinction of the animal. The ginseng root has its advocates in many parts of the world. In the United States it is commonly believed that eating raw eggs or oysters stimulates the sex drive. Others insist that alcohol and other drugs can produce the magic effect. And, in recent years, purveyors of health foods have used the lure of an "increased sexual drive" to promote some products.

Unfortunately, there is not a shred of scientific evidence for believing that any food or chemical substance has the capacity, in and of itself, to stimulate the sex drive. Intoxicants, for instance, are more apt to induce sleep than sexual desire. As James Leslie McCary put it, "All in all, good health, plenty of rest and sleep, an adequate amount of exercise, and freedom from emotional tension remain the most effective aphrodisiacs."*

* *Human Sexuality* (New York: Van Nostrand Reinhold, 1967), p. 311.

Masters and Johnson have defined **primary impotence** as a condition in which a man has *never* been able to achieve or maintain an erection sufficient to accomplish coitus. **Secondary impotence** is defined arbitrarily as the condition that exists when a man is unable to achieve or maintain erection in 25 percent of his sexual encounters. Often he has had successful experiences a number of times but is unable to respond to certain situations or at a certain period in his life. New sexual liaisons, for example, may cause anxiety about performance and lead to secondary impotence. As suggested earlier, a single occurrence of impotence may be enough to initiate a cycle of failure in sexual performance.

Secondary impotence can be caused by any one of a number of disturbances, in addition to those already mentioned. A man may harbor fear or resentment toward women in general or toward his specific partner; he may have a deep-rooted sense of inferiority; he may fear being compared to other men; or he may have a history of premature ejaculation. Sometimes, too, a partner's overly dramatic or intense reaction can turn a temporary inability to maintain an erection into a case of impotence. (It should be noted that erection is an *involuntary* response; an impotent man cannot will an erection to occur.)

Premature Ejaculation. There is a great deal of disagreement as to what constitutes **premature ejaculation.** Some researchers believe that only ejaculation that occurs prior to penetration can be considered premature. Others believe that a premature ejaculation is one that occurs uncontrollably within a minute of penetration. When one considers that about 75 percent of American men ejaculate within two minutes of vaginal penetration (according to Kinsey), it is clear that "premature" is a difficult concept to define. According to Masters and Johnson, a man is a premature ejaculator if he cannot delay ejaculation long enough to satisfy a normally responsive partner in at least half of his sexual counters.

Occasional premature ejaculation is normal and should not become a cause for alarm. A man who is tired or highly aroused, for example, or who has been without sexual release for several days, may be unable to delay his ejaculation. If overexcitement is the cause of the problem, the man can usually engage in a second, more prolonged act of intercourse.

When premature ejaculation occurs often enough to be considered a sexual dysfunction, the cause is almost always psychological. However, premature ejaculation may also be the result of conditioning. For example, repeated experiences with prostitutes, who usually try to rush the coital act, may accustom a man to early ejaculation. A pattern of premature ejaculation may also be set if intercourse, for one reason or another, must frequently be hurried.

Female Sexual Dysfunction

Orgasmic Dysfunction. **Female orgasmic dysfunction** is defined by Masters and Johnson as the inability to go beyond the plateau phase in sexual response. (The word *frigidity* is no longer used by these and other experts because it is an imprecise and negative term.) An occasional inability to achieve orgasm is normal; fatigue, mental distraction, or an unappealing partner may inhibit full sexual response. When the problem occurs repeatedly, however, a dysfunction may be said to exist. Masters and Johnson distinguish between a woman who has never had an orgasm (primary orgasmic dysfunction) and a woman who has achieved orgasm in the past but is no longer able to do so (situational orgasmic dysfunction).

Like impotence, the inability to achieve orgasm may be caused by certain diseases or hereditary disorders. In the vast majority of cases, however, the cause is rooted in an emotional conflict. The woman may consider her mate to be unacceptable; she may harbor resentment toward men in general; she may feel guilty about sex or fear getting hurt during the sexual act; or she may approach intercourse with the idea that she *has* to have an orgasm. If one does not occur (as is likely, since she is self-conscious about it), the woman may become too anxious to have orgasms in future sexual encounters.

American social attitudes have much to do with female sexual dysfunction. Women are usually made to feel more guilty or ambivalent about having sex than are men (particularly about having premarital intercourse). They are therefore more likely to suppress their sexual feelings and come to see sex as something unpleasant or threatening. Men, for their part, are often taught that sensitivity, kindness, and consideration are not "masculine." A man who is indifferent to a woman's physical or emotional needs should not be surprised if he finds her sexually unresponsive to him.

Dyspareunia. **Dyspareunia,** or painful coitus, occurs far more frequently among women than among men. Typically, the affected woman feels pain either in the external genitalia or in the vagina upon penetration by the penis. Physical factors are usually responsible for this disorder. The woman may still have an intact hymen or be suffering from a vaginal infection, or she may secrete an insufficient amount of vaginal lubricant. Sometimes an anatomical abnormality in the reproductive organs may cause coital pain. The vagina may also be irritated or obstructed by a contraceptive. Psychological factors that may cause dyspareunia are similar to those responsible for other female sexual dysfunctions.

Vaginismus. **Vaginismus** is a powerful and often painful contraction of the vaginal muscles, making penile penetration difficult or impossible. Fear of sexual intercourse caused by a rigid upbringing, a brutal partner, or terrifying sexual experiences may bring on vaginismus. Often the woman has a partner who has failed repeatedly at intercourse, either because of impotence or premature ejaculation. She will subconsciously prevent further frustration by shutting the vaginal opening.

Treating Sexual Dysfunction

Much sexual dysfunction might not occur if partners were more sensitive to each other's needs and desires and more attentive to satisfying these needs. A greater emphasis on foreplay and the enjoyment of acts not necessarily directly designed to produce orgasm would reduce tensions and preclude at least some sexual problems. The preoccupation with orgasm creates a tension-producing situation that interferes with what should be a time of relaxation.

The most immediate "treatment" for a sexual dysfunction is understanding and reassurance. If the affected person is not made to feel a failure and is instead caressed or otherwise made to feel desirable, intercourse may become possible. At the very least, severe emotional trauma will be prevented.

Sexual and Sex-Related Problems: *Where to Go for Help*

Community Sex Information, Inc.
P.O. Box 2858
Grand Central Station
New York, N.Y. 10017

National Rape Task Force Coordinator
National Organization of Women Legislative Office
1107 National Press Building
Washington, D.C. 20004
(202) 347-2279

Association of Women in Psychiatry
Women's Studies Dept.
University of Delaware
34 W. Delaware
Newark, Delaware 19711

Association of Gay Psychiatrists
P.O. Box 29527
Atlanta, Georgia 30359
(404) 231-0751

Homosexual Community Counseling Center, Inc.
30 E. 60th St.
New York, N.Y. 10022
(212) 688-0628

National Coalition Against Sexual Assault
c/o Fern Ferguson
8787 State St., Ste. 202
East St. Louis, Ill. 62203
(618) 398-7764

Source: Adapted from Charles G. Morris, *Psychology*: *An Introduction*, 5th ed., © 1985, p. 470. Adapted by permission of Prentice-Hall, Inc., Englewood Cliffs, N.J.

If the dysfunction persists, a physician's examination is required, since the problem may have a physiological basis. If the underlying cause is psychological in nature, highly effective treatments are available. Masters and Johnson have developed therapeutic programs aimed specifically at each type of sexual dysfunction. Several principles form the foundation of their approach: (1) It is preferable to treat both the affected individual and his or her partner, since a sexual dysfunction involves both. (2) A therapy team consisting of a man and a woman is best suited to understand and treat the problems of both sexes and guarantee that each patient will have a sympathetic listener. (3) The patient should be given an opportunity to reawaken natural, positive attitudes toward pleasure without having to "perform" sexually. Typically, the affected individual and his or her partner are given a brief, sound sex education to eliminate false ideas about sexuality. They are then told to practice tender touching, stroking, and embracing over a period of several days without having intercourse. In this way, the couple can be actively involved in rediscovering sensuality without being inhibited by the fear of failure. When the therapists feel the couple is ready, intercourse is allowed to take place.

In addition to following these general guidelines, the couple is trained in techniques appropriate to the particular dysfunction. If a man is impotent, for example, he is stimulated to erection repeatedly until he becomes more confident of his ability to respond. Similarly, a woman with an orgasmic dysfunction is repeatedly stimulated to the point of orgasm before intercourse is attempted.

Individuals interested in therapy should keep in mind that a multitude of disreputable "sex clinics" claiming to use the "Masters and Johnson method" have sprung up all over the United States. These clinics often do great emotional harm.

SUMMARY

1. Our sexual attitudes and identities are formed by influences from our culture, our parents, our friends, and our own individual needs.

2. The *sexual life cycle* extends throughout the human life span. Expressions of sexuality have been observed both in newborn infants and people in their 90s. Sexual expression is necessary to old and young alike.

3. In adolescence males establish a pattern of orgasmic frequency that continues usually into their 40s, at which time many men experience a decline. Orgasmic sexuality occurs more slowly in females, peaks in their 30s or 40s, and remains at a uniform level into their 50s and sometimes 60s. The range of individual response is greater in women than in men.

4. The physical changes brought about by *menopause* or the *climacteric* need not cause a diminution in sexual response; a satisfactory sex life can be maintained throughout old age. *Masturbation* (self-stimulation to induce orgasm) is a perfectly healthy act, engaged in by almost all men and women of all ages.

5. Four phases of male and female sexual response have been identified: *excitement*, *plateau*, *orgasm*, and *resolution*. In general, these are similar for men and women, except that men experience a temporary *refractory* period during which they cannot achieve *orgasm*, while women usually require longer to achieve orgasm in intercourse and also have the capacity for multiple orgasms.

6. *Nocturnal orgasms* during sleep occur in some men and women, usually because of erotic dreams.

7. *Petting* is any form of sexual contact between individuals that does not involve intercourse. Petting that precedes intercourse is called *foreplay*.

8. Marital sexual intercourse is the only form of sexual expression that has had universal acceptance. But sexual standards have become more permissive in recent decades and there is growing acceptance of premarital intercourse.

9. *Homosexuality* is sexual activity with a member of one's own sex. A significant part of the population experiences orgasm in a homosexual circumstance at some time in their lives. *Bisexuality* is the experience of sexual gratification with people of both genders.

10. Sexual dysfunctions such as *impotence*, *premature ejaculation*, *orgasmic dysfunction*, *dyspareunia*, and *vaginismus* are most often psychological in origin. They may result from inadequate sex education, an overly rigid upbringing, feelings of inadequacy, or fears related to the sexual act. Treatment may involve psychotherapy or techniques aimed at correcting the dysfunction itself.

CONSUMER CONCERNS

1. Do the public schools in your community provide a family living program? Is it effective?
2. Is your physician at ease with topics pertaining to human sexuality? Does your physician make you feel comfortable in discussing sexually related concerns?
3. Would you be able to verify the professional credentials of a sex counselor or sex therapist should you need to?
4. How can the public be protected against the false claims of products advertised to enhance virility?
5. It seems that many articles on the subject of human sexuality that appear in popular magazines are written to entertain rather than to inform. But do they also misinform?

9

Life Styles

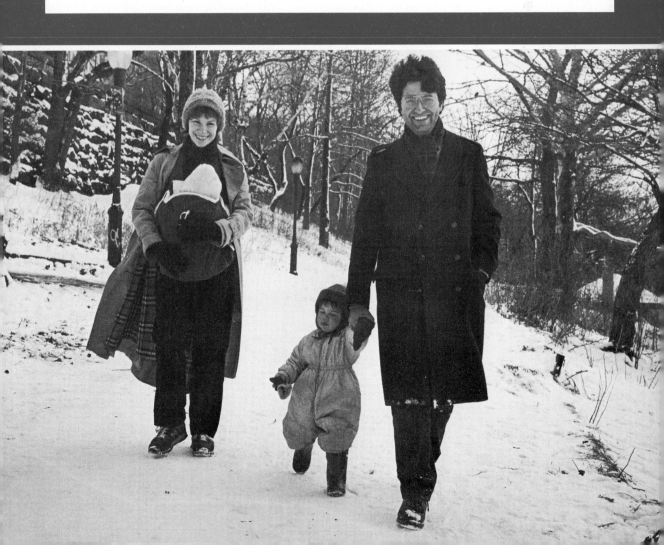

For more than a century, the traditional concept of marriage in the Western world has been that of the love match. The popular view has been that love should be sanctified by marriage and that children should be a natural outcome of marriage. However appealing this simple and romantic concept may have been, many Americans are now choosing to remain single; many love without marrying; many marry for other reasons; and many divorce and wed more than once. In addition, a number of Americans have established compatible relationships with members of their own sex.

The traditional family as we once perceived it may be on the way to becoming an anomaly in America. Families are noticeably smaller than they once were, averaging less than two children each. This has resulted from American women having fewer children than ever before and from their postponing having children until later in life. The additional fact that many couples have decided not to have children has brought about a leveling off of the birth rate.

There are more one-parent families than ever before. More singles, as well as couples, are adopting children. And more and more families include children from more than one marriage.

TODAY'S FAMILY

Most Americans today live in **nuclear** rather than extended families. While extended families include three or more successive generations living in one household, nuclear families contain only two successive generations: parents and their children. In addition to producing children and socializing them—the two primary functions of all families—extended families served several other critical functions in agrarian societies. According to sociologist William Ogburn, they gave economic support, conferred social status, supplied educational and religious training, cared for the sick, provided leisure-time entertainment, and lent emotional support. In industrial societies most of these functions have been assumed by educational, religious, and medical institutions. Moreover, young people today usually spend their leisure time with same-age friends outside the home. Their social status, especially in high school and college, depends more often on community, academic, or athletic achievements than on family prestige. Emotional and economic support, however, are still central functions of the family, especially for children living at home. **Modified nuclear families**—single parents and their children or childless couples—are becoming increasingly common. The single parent has the burden of giving both economic and emotional support to her children (in nine out of ten cases, the single parent is a woman). Single parents themselves need emotional support and often financial support from their own parents, whose grandparenting role in this kind of family structure is very important.

Now even the patterns of the relatively recent nuclear family appear to be undergoing extensive change. The modern family is not bound by the traditional spirit of self-sacrifice, but rather by the ideal of self-fulfillment. A marked preference shown for freedom rather than authority, self-fulfillment rather than commitment, and duty to self rather than duty to others is a hallmark of what has become known as the "me generation." Members of the "me generation" tend to regard children (at least during the early stages of a marriage) as an encumbrance and an interference with their personal pursuits.

Although a recent study showed that 57 percent of American families with one or more children under 13 generally held to the traditional family values and ideals of strict child rearing, 43 percent did not. This "new breed" appears to be as loving as the traditionalists but much more self-oriented. Concerned with personal freedom, they advocate freedom for their children, saying in effect that since they do not sacrifice for their children, they will not expect major sacrifices of those children. But, uncertain of their own new values, new-breed parents tend to teach their children traditional values.

Two-Earner Families. Values and outlooks are changing, nevertheless. The traditional American family, consisting of working husband, housewife, and children, now accounts for a mere 18 percent of households in the United States. Fifty percent of married-couple families are *two-earner* families. Both husband and wife in such families have jobs. Pressures on the partners are usually greater, but so are the rewards, among them fewer financial worries.

The massive entry of women into the labor market has had a tremendous economic impact upon American society. For the first time in the country's history, half its women are in the labor force. At present, they hold 42 percent of all jobs in the United States. While most women work primarily for financial reasons, few working wives—as opposed to single women—are in the higher income brackets. Regardless of their income bracket, however, wives who have completed college are more likely to be employed than those who have not.

Two-Career Couples. Sociologists distinguish the two-earner family, in which the wife typically works only part time or from time to time for various reasons such as helping to pay bills, from **two-career couples,** where both partners are pursuing careers and working full time over a period of years. This new

The American Family in the Year 2000

Because of the recent sharp changes in marriage and family life, the life course of children and young adults today is likely to be far different from what a person growing up earlier in this century experienced. It will not be uncommon, for instance, for children born in the 1980s to follow this sequence of living arrangements: live with both parents for several years, live with their mothers after their parents divorce, live with their mothers and stepfathers, live alone for a time when in their early twenties, live with someone of the opposite sex without marrying, get married, get divorced, live alone again, get remarried, and end up living alone once more following the death of their spouses.

Source: Andrew Cherlin and Frank F. Furstenberg, Jr., "The American Family in the Year 2000," *The Futurist*, June 1983, pp. 7–8. Reprinted by permission.

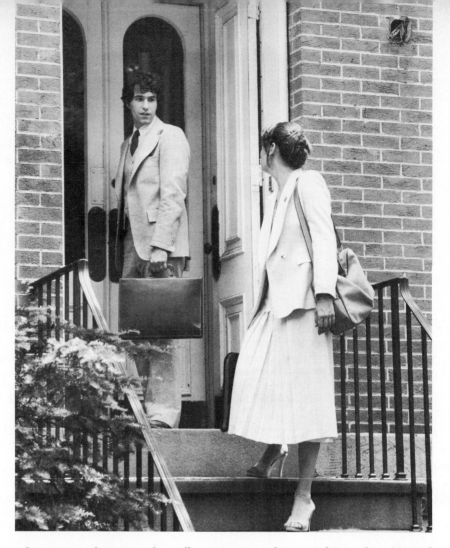

subgroup, numbering in the millions, consists of "marrieds" in their 30s and 40s whose combined incomes place them close to, or in, the upper middle class. Both husband and wife work not only for money but also for professional satisfaction. Problems may develop, however, when a wife whose career may be just as prestigious and demanding as a husband's cannot get her husband to share household and child-care duties. Problems also develop when the competitive values of the workplace infiltrate the marriage, making each spouse protective about money, prestige, and power. Marriage counselors often tell such couples that they should not expect to be perfect parents, spouses, and professionals all at once.

The Day-Care Problem. A major problem for working women is finding affordable, reliable day-care facilities for their preschool children. The problem is a major one because there are now 8 million working wives and single mothers in the United States who have children under 6, and there will be a great many more in the future. (It is estimated that there will be 38 million children under 10 by 1990.)

TABLE 9–1
Median Age at First Marriage, 1940–1983

Year	Male	Female
1983	25.4	22.8
1975	23.5	21.1
1965	22.8	20.6
1955	22.6	20.2
1940	24.3	21.5

Source: U.S. Bureau of the Census.

The United States is one of the very few developed countries that have no national day-care system, nor is there likely to be one soon in view of recent cuts in federal funding for day-care programs. Instead, women must rely on relatives, neighbors, baby-sitters, or privately owned facilities in homes and day-care centers. The costs of child care range from under $50 to over $100 a week and, depending on the number of children, can absorb up to 25 percent or more of a family's income.

The quality of private day-care facilities varies widely. Ideally, a facility should provide a child with a high level of social and intellectual stimulation and a consistent source of emotional support—requirements that can be met only by facilities that have a low child-caretaker ratio and low staff turnover. Many parents are wary, however, of putting their children in any type of day care for a variety of reasons, including the high rates of infectious diseases reported in some and the sexual abuse reported in others.

A growing number of corporations have found it cost-effective to provide on-site or nearby day-care facilities for their employees' children. Employees who feel secure in the knowledge that their children are nearby and are being well cared for perform better on the job, take far fewer days off, and change jobs far less often than those who must seek outside care.

Later Marriages, Fewer Children. Although male and female roles in modern society are changing, most Americans continue to seek their greatest opportunities for intimacy and sharing through the institution of marriage. Nearly all Americans marry at least once, and about 80 percent of all divorced persons marry again.

Despite these figures, the marriage rate has declined slightly since reaching a high in 1972. People are marrying later (see Table 9-1) and having fewer or no children. Of women between 20 and 24, the number remaining single has risen from 36 percent in 1970 to 56 percent in 1983 and the percentage of unmarried men in that age group has increased from 54 percent to 73 percent.

The Changing Role of Women

As the role of the family has changed, so also has the role of marriage. Today there is a great deal of questioning about the roles that men and women should play in our technological society; and with this questioning have come changes in how men and women view themselves and their roles in the context of marriage.

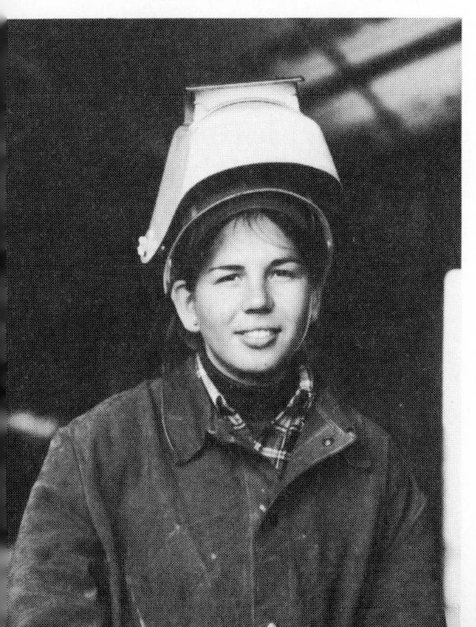

No longer bound by the imperative of the family, many women in America have ventured outside their traditional place within the home to demand and fill positions in business and industry heretofore held by men as the exclusive providers for the family. Because they have become increasingly important as wage earners, women now find themselves with greater financial freedom. However, as a group, they still earn only 69 cents for every dollar men earn. With the shift of interest from family life to professional life, women now focus more and more on their individual needs for personal fulfillment and for partnerships founded first and foremost on love and mutual respect. As economic freedom is reinforced by sexual freedom and as their emphasis in life shifts toward self-realization, many women find their goals in conflict with traditional role expectations that persist in regarding wives primarily as homemakers and mothers. A significant number of women enter marriage today with goals quite different from those of their mothers or grandmothers.

The Changing Role of Men

Two decades ago the average middle-aged American male saw himself ideally cast in the role of husband and father, holding authority over his wife and children as family head, and shouldering full responsibility for the material welfare of his family. Today, however, authority and responsibility are increasingly shared between men and women. Although statistics show that the vast majority of American men pursue marriage as a desirable goal, a significant number of them are attempting to redefine their marriage roles in terms of changing social expectations. This process is proving difficult, mainly because our culture still stresses the traditional male roles. But many men are finding that while a marriage based on equal partnership means a diminution of traditional male authority, it also means that the traditional male burden of providing for the family can now be shared.

APPROACHING MARRIAGE REALISTICALLY

Society demands no training for marriage. In fact, most people avoid premarital counseling and sex education, two kinds of "training" that greatly increase the chances of marital success. Instead, many people enter marriage in a rush of intense feeling but with little careful thought.

Evaluating Personal Readiness

Readiness for marriage requires *emotional maturity*—that is, a healthy self-image and a strong sense of personal identity. One sign of emotional immaturity is dependence on a parent. Young people may expect a husband or wife to be a substitute father or mother. But it is unrealistic—and harmful to one's own development—to expect a spouse to fill a parental role. It is wise, therefore, to test your independence by living away from home for a time.

Readiness for marriage also requires a capacity for compassion and sexual expression. You should ask yourself: Can I put my partner's feelings on the same level as my own? Am I ready to share my body sexually with another? If you are preoccupied with what you can get from marriage and not with what you can give, you are not ready to express love. Moreover, to give fully, you must feel that you have something to give in the first place—and this implies a sense of your own worth.

Financial independence is also important to marital readiness. A couple should be able to meet its financial obligations and have a plan for doing so. Will both partners work? How much can they expect to earn? Will they be able to afford to have children? If not, are they willing to postpone parenthood until their economic condition improves? Many marriages succeed despite financial hardships, but the couple must be willing to work together and to make sacrifices.

The box on page 232 provides questions that can help individuals judge their readiness for marriage. You might like to answer them before you read the following sections.

Evaluating Motives

Motives for marrying should be assessed. Today there is less reason to yield to social pressure than before. The mere fact that one's friends are marrying is no reason to follow suit. It is unwise, too, to use marriage to boost one's prestige or as a concession to parental needs. The desire to get away from home is another common but faulty reason for marriage. Marrying for wealth may produce a life poor in all other respects. "Marriage on the rebound" may be nothing more than a gesture of bravado or an attempt to recover self-esteem. Marriage because of unexpected pregnancy often results in unhappiness for all concerned—the husband and the wife, as well as the child. The decision to marry should be grounded in the conviction that one's personal fulfillment will be achieved in a life of shared experience and mutual commitment.

Choosing a Marriage Partner

Marriage partners are often chosen on the basis of strong feelings and unconscious drives. For example, people generally tend to choose a marriage partner whose life experiences and values are similar to their own, although they may be unaware of this tendency in themselves. We are spontaneously attracted to certain physical types and personalities and often fail to consider how different factors affect the chances of marital success.

Physical Attraction and Sexual Compatibility. Physical attraction is an important part of love and marriage. *Physical attraction* usually refers to the sensual and sexual feelings one person arouses in another; but it also refers to the pleasurable emotional and aesthetic feelings that are aroused. For most people,

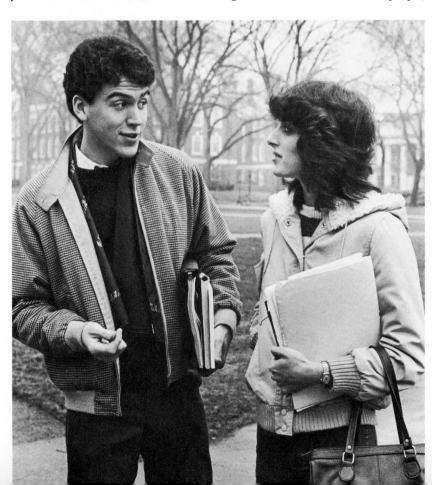

a good sexual relationship is essential to the success of a marriage. Not only is sexual activity satisfying in and of itself, it also opens up avenues of intimate communication.

People vary, however, in the intensity of their sexual needs, and assessing and accepting your own needs and those of your partner is an essential first step in establishing a marital relationship. A fully satisfying sexual relationship takes time to develop. But candor and openness play an important role in achieving compatibility.

Personality Traits. People with similar personality traits feel more attracted to one another and achieve more stable marriages than do those whose personalities differ. In a life of constant proximity, personality differences often create confusion and hostility. Any attempt to change a partner's personality traits is misguided and unrealistic. Bad habits such as excessive drinking at parties or not calling home when late can be changed, but basic traits such as procrastination or fears of social interaction are not likely to change and must be accepted.

Intellectual Compatibility. For some couples, shared interests may be more important than intellectual compatibility. Serious intellectual inequality, however, will hinder communication at every level, including domestic problems. Further schooling may make up for lack of knowledge, but differences in innate capacity often create insurmountable obstacles in marriage.

Social Background, Family Values, and Religious Differences. Marriages succeed more often when partners come from similar backgrounds and when parents are not opposed to the union. Childhood and cultural experiences affect attitudes, values, and behavior patterns, and marked differences in these areas can cause serious conflicts.

While religious differences—particularly in attitudes toward sexual behavior, family planning, and children's education—may seem trivial during courtship, they can cause serious rifts in daily married life. A couple should therefore assess their religious commitments before marriage to see whether their beliefs will engender conflict.

Race. Interracial marriage in the United States is still frontier territory and requires maturity and pioneer fortitude of both partners to succeed. They must pit the strength of their personal bond against the strength of social attitudes and squarely face any opposition they and their children meet. However, if the social barriers in one community are insurmountable, the couple would do well to move to a less hostile one.

Age. It is hazardous to choose a marriage partner until you have established your social and occupational goals in life. Studies indicate that the younger the couple, the poorer the chances of marital success. People who choose partners much older than themselves are often looking for a parent figure. Marriage may not be the solution for this problem.

Financial Resources. Financial resources are a major problem in many marriages and a frequent cause of divorce. A realistic assessment of earnings and living standards is an essential ingredient in marriage. Money problems often arise when a couple has children, for parenthood may have the double effect of increasing expenditures and at the same time decreasing income if one partner must discontinue work.

Health. Couples who plan to marry should be examined by a physician, not only for sexually transmitted disease (as required by law) but for health factors that may affect their marriage. Problems with the ability to have children and with genetic factors do arise, and these should be frankly discussed by the couple and their physician.

Overcoming Unrealistic Expectations

The expectations of marriage are often influenced by idealized childhood memories, TV dramas, and romantic novels and films. Love is idealized by many Americans, who see it as the simple answer to the complex and often adverse aspects of real life. A few common misconceptions about married life are described here.

Marriage Is a Perpetual Romance. Marriage is not an endless, dreamlike romance. The constant physical proximity and intimacy of marriage exposes all the unromantic traits of both partners that were not apparent during courtship. In any lasting partnership, one must be free to reveal one's complete self—not merely one's best self—and partners should encourage such openness

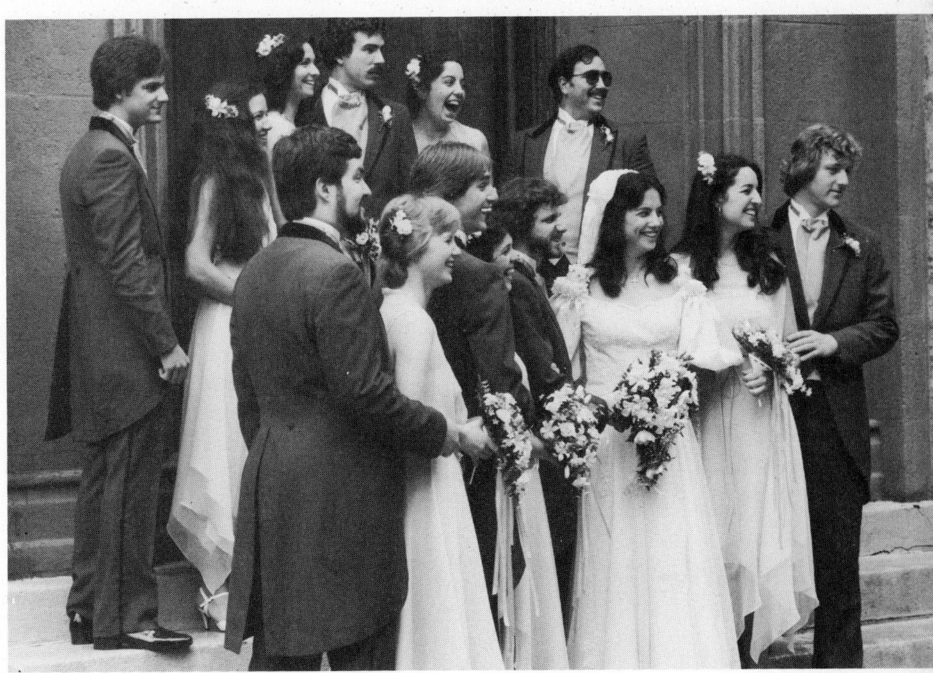

Are You Ready for Marriage?

The following questions should stimulate thought about readiness for marriage. Answer by drawing a circle around the "?", the "Yes," or the "No." Use the question mark only when you are uncertain. After you are through think about the meaning of your answers, and if possible discuss them with someone. The questionnaire assumes you are now considering some specific person as a possible marriage partner.

Yes No ? 1. Even though you may accept advice from your parents, do you make important decisions for yourself?

Yes No ? 2. Are you often homesick when you are away from home?

Yes No ? 3. Do you ever feel embarrassed or uneasy in giving or receiving affection?

Yes No ? 4. Are your feelings easily hurt by criticism?

Yes No ? 5. Do you enjoy playing or working with small children?

Yes No ? 6. Do you feel embarrassed or uneasy in conversations about sex with older persons or members of the other sex?

Yes No ? 7. Do you have a clear understanding of the physiology of sexual intercourse and reproduction?

Yes No ? 8. Do you understand the psychological factors determining good sexual adjustment?

Yes No ? 9. Have you had the experience of using some of your earnings to help meet the expenses of others?

Yes No ? 10. In an argument, do you lose your temper easily?

Yes No ? 11. Have you and your fiancé(e) ever worked through disagreements to a definite conclusion agreeable to both of you?

Yes No ? 12. Can you postpone something you want for the sake of later enjoyment?

Yes No ? 13. Are you normally free from jealousy?

Yes No ? 14. Have you thought carefully about the goals you will strive for in your marriage?

in each other. Ideally, as partners become more aware of each other's needs and limitations, their mutual understanding will grow and deepen.

Marriage Will End All Loneliness. Two people can live in the same house and sleep in the same bed for years and yet still feel very lonely. The root source of much loneliness is difficult to unearth. A person may feel so inadequate that he or she goes into a self-imposed exile. A person may feel lonely as a result of a partner's rejection or indifference. Furthermore, people vary in their needs for closeness, and a desire for solitude should not be interpreted as loneliness or as a sign of rejection.

Problems or Arguments Will Not Occur. During courtship, couples often avoid arguing. However, pressures build up in the daily routine of married life. Evenings may bring out the tensions and troubles of the day. Furthermore, when two people contract to live together, they do not discard their individuality. Conflict is therefore bound to arise between individuals who have their own opinions, attitudes, likes, and dislikes.

Togetherness Is Always Necessary. Love is supposed to be deepened by total sharing. In the ideal state of togetherness, individual preferences are suppressed,

Yes No ? 15. Do you sometimes feel rebellious toward facing the responsibilities of marriage, occupational or family life?

Yes No ? 16. Have you been able to give up gracefully something you wanted very much?

Yes No ? 17. Do you think of sexual intercourse chiefly as a pleasure experience?

Yes No ? 18. Do you find it difficult to differ from others on matters of conduct or dress, even though you disagree with what they think?

Yes No ? 19. Do you often have to fight to get your way?

Yes No ? 20. Do you often find yourself making biting remarks, or using sarcasm toward others?

Yes No ? 21. Do you find yourself strongly emphasizing the glamor aspects of marriage, e.g., the announcement, congratulations, showers, the wedding?

Yes No ? 22. Have you and your fiancé(e) associated with each other in a variety of non amusement situations, e.g., caring for children, in a work project, in time of stress?

Yes No ? 23. Have you and your fiancé(e) discussed matters which might cause marital conflict? For example: (Underline those you have discussed) religious differences; plans for having children; attitudes toward sex; differences in family background; financial arrangement in marriage; basic values in life.

Scoring: An answer of no to questions 2, 3, 4, 6, 10, 15, 18, 19, 20, and 21 and of yes to the others is an indication of readiness for marriage

Source: Lester A. Kirkendall and Wesley J. Adams, *The Students' Guide to Marriage and Family Life Literature: An Aid to Individualized Study and Instruction*, 8th ed. (Dubuque, Iowa: Wm. C. Brown Company, Publishers, 1980).

and experiences that cannot be shared are avoided. One partner, for example, may give up old friends because the other dislikes them. Truly loving people, however, encourage self-expression in their partners and, in turn, expect their partners to support their independence. If marriage is shared experience, then the freedom of two intimate individuals is a vital part of that experience.

There is no formula for a successful marriage. How couples define their individual roles and purposes is very much a matter of choice. But given the essential elements of respect, compassion, sensitivity, and concern, and combining these elements with candor and flexibility, a married couple should be able to work out a relationship tailored to their individual needs and expectations.

HANDLING CONFLICTS IN MARRIAGE

All couples, no matter how well-adjusted, are bound to have conflicts. There are three general patterns for handling such conflicts.

The first pattern is characterized by *aggression* on the part of one partner and *retreat* on the part of the other. The aggressive partner out-shouts, out-threatens, and out-insults the other, who grudgingly gives way to the aggressor. When his or her fury is spent, the aggressor harbors feelings of guilt, while the victim is consumed with resentment. This pattern sets the stage for a bitter and lasting cold war.

In the second pattern frequent *mutual combat* prevails. Both partners fight forcefully, no decision is ever reached, and open bouts of hostility are the rule. Ironically, some marriages are maintained by the force of such continuous conflict. However, constant and disproportionate hostility is nearly always a sign of deeply thwarted needs and desires. The enormous energies spent in marital combat might be used more productively in self-examination and mutual adjustment.

Family violence in the form of wife or husband abuse may be part of these two patterns of handling marital conflict. It is estimated that over 3 million women and nearly 1 million men are victims of abuse by their spouses. Victims are found in all socioeconomic classes and ethnic backgrounds. In the past several years recognition of this problem has become so widespread that many states have passed laws against **spouse abuse.**

In the third pattern conflicts are resolved through *reasoning*. The couple restrains hostility, each partner listens to what the other has to say, and both try to express honest thoughts and feelings, while at the same time wounding as little as possible. If, despite reasonable efforts, a genuine disagreement persists, the couple tries to find an acceptable compromise. Maturity and restraint are required to resolve conflicts through reasonable confrontation, but such an approach usually turns the conflict into a source of deepened understanding.

Certain techniques may be used to keep conflicts reasonable. One is to make criticism as objective as possible. Statements like "You are a stupid fool" or "You've spoiled everything, as usual" are guaranteed to produce resentment instead of an examination of the mistake made. It is helpful simply to suggest alternate ways of handling a situation rather than pronounce a negative judgment: "I think you should pull over and wait for the rain to stop" is better than "Only an idiot would keep driving in this rain." Another wise approach is to be sure that what is said expresses what is meant: "This marriage doesn't make sense anymore" may simply be a poor way of saying that the couple should start to approach things sensibly. Marital conflict can be successfully resolved if the good of the marriage as a separate entity is put ahead of victory for either partner.

MARRIAGE COUNSELING

In cases where there is an impasse or where an adjustment seems unlikely, a professional marriage counselor may be of help. It is preferable, though not essential, that both partners visit the counselor—either together or separately. Some couples hesitate to seek outside help because of embarrassment or a belief that doing so represents weakness and failure in solving one's own problems. On the contrary, seeking counsel is almost always a sign of good judgment and maturity.

As a disinterested third party, the counselor can objectively view the destructive games being played by the couple. Situations are rarely as hopeless as the couple imagines, and it is probable that the marriage counselor has dealt with similar problems before. Marriage counselors also recognize that not all marriages should be saved. They will encourage the couple to express their true feelings, to assess the problem, and to decide on their own whether to attempt an adjustment or to apply for divorce.

DIVORCE

The ending of any intimate relationship is painful. *Divorce*, the legal termination of a marriage, is especially so, because marriage merges two lives on many levels of experience. For some individuals, divorce is an unbearable personal defeat; for others, the termination of an unsatisfactory marriage represents an opportunity for personal growth. Whatever its emotional impact, divorce inevitably presents a series of practical and social problems: the division of property, the establishment of new living quarters for at least one of the partners, the setting forth of financial obligations, the working through of emotional responsibilities toward any children, and the simultaneous adjustment to single status.

The divorce rate in the United States showed a steady increase starting in 1955, reaching an all-time high of 5.3 per 1,000 population in 1979 and 1981. Since then, it has declined slightly, to 4.9 per 1,000 population in 1984.

Variations in the divorce rate occur by geographic region and by variables such as social class and age at marriage. Divorce rates are higher in the southwestern and western states than in the Northeast. They are also higher among the poor, whose marriages are constantly stressed by economic troubles. High divorce rates occur among partners who marry in their teens, a statistic that also relates to social class. Middle-class people are likely to marry in their twenties, whereas most low-income people marry in their teens. The length of marriage is an important predictor of success or failure. One out of four couples separate or divorce in the first three years, and half of all divorces occur within seven years of marriage.

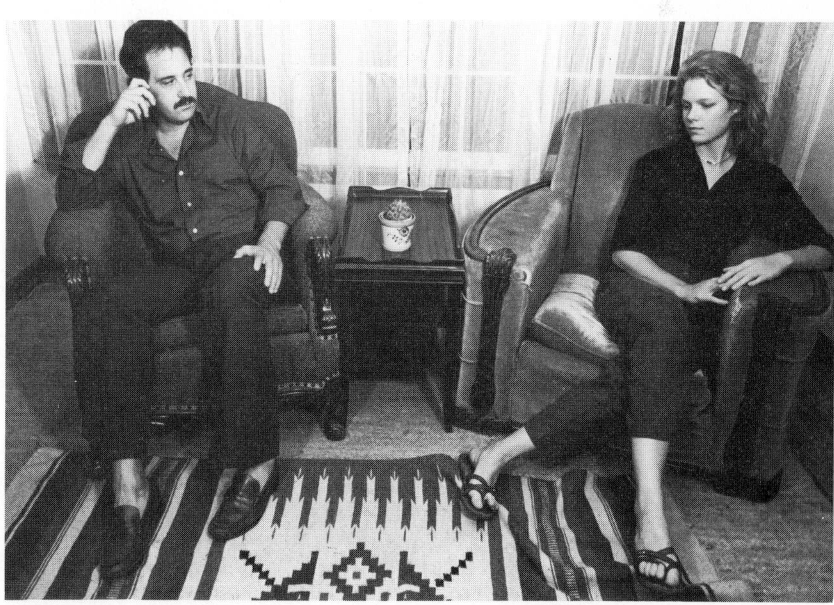

Marriage Problems: Where to Go for Help

Two national agencies that can provide a list of professional marriage counselors in your region are:

- American Association for Marriage & Family Therapy
  1717 K Street NW
  Washington, D.C. 20006
  Telephone: (202) 429-1825
- Family Service America
  44 East 23rd Street
  New York City, N.Y. 10010
  Telephone: (212) 674-6100

There are many reasons for the increase in the rate of divorce. More and more people emphasize the "here and now" and are therefore less likely to remain in a situation that makes them unhappy. Divorce is becoming a more acceptable procedure in our society, even among the very religious. Legal barriers to divorce have been lowered in recent years, and divorced individuals have become more socially accepted. Perhaps most important, modern couples expect much more from their marriages than their parents or grandparents did. Greater expectations—realistic or not—make feelings of failure less tolerable and divorce more likely.

In most states a person can obtain a divorce only by proving that he or she is an innocent party and that the partner is guilty of one of the "faults" the state has listed as "grounds for divorce." According to the U.S. Department of Health and Human Services, about three-quarters of all divorces are granted for either desertion, nonsupport, or cruelty (physical or mental). A more liberal and realistic approach is found in the "no-fault" divorce laws of states such as California, Colorado, and Oregon. These laws make it possible to obtain a divorce without a lawyer and for a nominal fee. All that is required is that the husband and wife live apart in accordance with a decree or judgment of separation for a given period of time and that both live up to the terms and conditions of the agreement. Great variations exist among states regarding not only grounds for divorce but also residency requirements, which range from two years in Rhode Island to six weeks in Nevada to no requirement at all in Washington State. To cope with the increasing divorce rate and the legal problems involved, many states now have separate divorce courts attended by special judges, counselors, and investigators (the last to ensure that the facts of the cases are heard).

Child custody is perhaps the most agonizing issue for all concerned. The child is often involved in the tension and conflict between the adult partners. This conflict frequently continues in renewed fights over custody of the child or visiting rights, or in efforts to win the child in one-sided emotional commitments. During the transitional period of divorce, both parents would do well to consider the special needs of the child. In particular, they should assure the child that the divorce is in no way the child's fault, for many children are prone to feel guilty for the marital failure of their parents. Parents should also keep in mind that it is far better for a child to be raised in a home by one loving parent than in a home filled with conflict.

Mothers obtain custody of their offspring in nine out of ten cases. Today, however, as sex roles are changing in society, so are ideas about custody. Since about 60 percent of divorced women work, and more men are sharing domestic responsibilities, the concept of *joint custody* is gaining in popularity. The courts are slower to agree, but several states already have laws regarding joint custody and others are considering related legislation.

When the mother is granted custody of the children, the divorce settlement typically provides that the father must pay money for their support. But more than half of divorced fathers fail to provide the full amount of such payments, leaving the family impoverished and obliging the mother to seek welfare assistance. A federal law passed in 1985 provides for the mandatory garnisheeing of wages of delinquent parents, and may help to relieve what is a major problem for divorced mothers.

In the past divorced persons were socially stigmatized and often thought to be less virtuous and less mentally healthy than their married counterparts. Inasmuch as the goal of the family is to provide psychological well-being and happiness for all its members, divorce now seems a reasonable solution when this goal is not achieved. Divorced persons are no longer at a social disadvantage. National statistics indicate that more than 90 percent of those divorced between the ages of 20 and 30 succeed in finding new mates. In fact, of all couples issued marriage licenses, almost a third include at least one partner who has been divorced.

FAMILIES OF REMARRIAGE

The high rate of remarriage has created millions of *blended families*. A typical blended family (or stepfamily) might be composed of two previously married adults, their children from previous marriages, and the children they have together. While these new family configurations present a complex array of possible tense relationships, they may also provide many social and emotional benefits to both adults and children.

For a number of reasons, relationships between stepparents and children are often strained. For example, children often experience painful loyalty conflicts when a stepmother tries to establish a bond as intense as the one they had with their original mother. The problem is especially acute between a stepmother and stepdaughter because of the traditional close ties between daughters and their biological mothers. A stepdaughter may also fear that her stepmother will jeopardize her relationship with her father.

Because 90 percent of all children live with their mother after a divorce, problems between stepfathers and stepchildren are far more common. Many stepfathers tend not to regard their stepchildren as true family members and thus resist establishing close ties with them. Many stepmothers likewise resist close ties to their husband's children when the children remain with the biological mother.

A particularly delicate situation often exists between new and former wives. The new wife often resents the alimony and child-support payments her husband must make to his former wife. At the same time, she does not want to create difficulties for another woman, particularly one who is most likely to be living on a much reduced income.

In spite of all the strains and tensions, second marriages and families are often much happier than first ones. The experience of an unhappy first marriage often leads to a new maturity of outlook. Instead of seeking out physical attractiveness or occupational prestige in a spouse, people now look for qualities such as thoughtfulness, shared interests, and emotional stability. An unhappy first marriage has often taught them to communicate more openly and tolerate differences more willingly. Such psychological and emotional changes can produce a happier family life. Large, tolerant blended families can provide both adults and children with a broader base of emotional support and an expanded social network. Children are especially apt to benefit from the new arrangement. Many of them had been "latchkey" children living with a single parent; now they never find themselves in the house alone.

COLLEGE MARRIAGE

A successful college marriage is an achievement against difficult odds. Nonetheless, marriage among college students has become commonplace. The greatest problem college couples face is financial: having sufficient money for an independent home, school expenses, and the birth and support of children. Most students

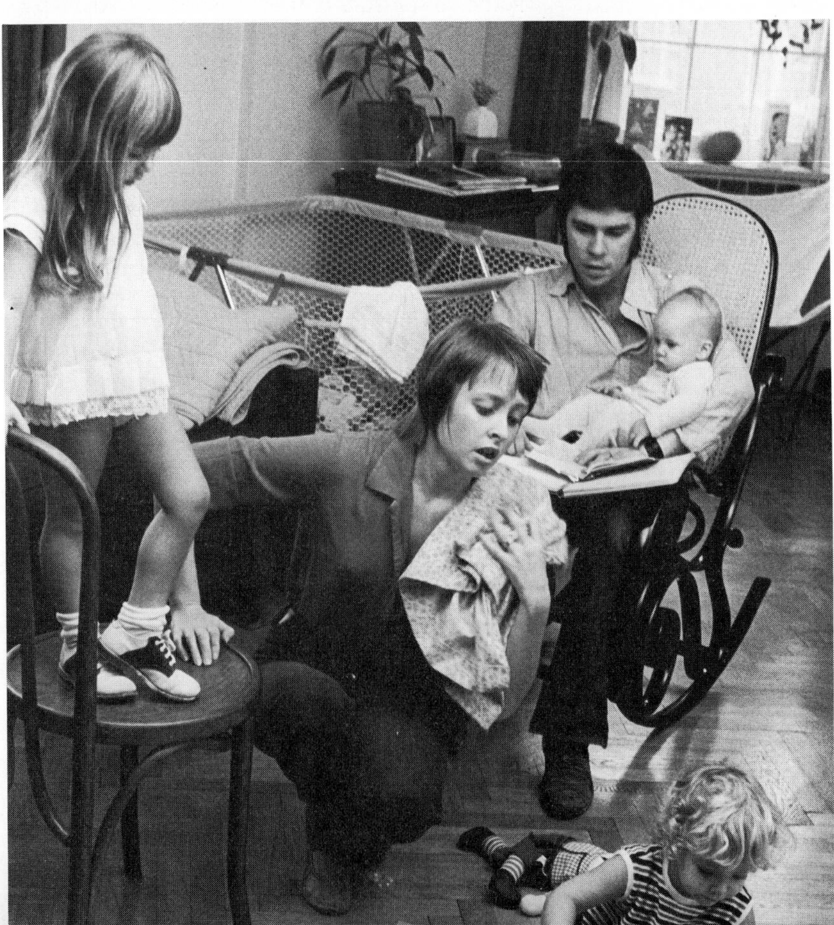

The birth of children to a college couple adds to the burden of an often difficult situation, but many such marriages survive.

depend on their parents for at least part of their support. Parents, however, are often reluctant to help their children once they are married; and young couples are often reluctant to accept help. Some parents feel their children have assumed adult privileges prematurely and should be forced to accept the responsibilities that go with them. Some withdraw support in disapproval of the partner. In any case, most students manage to get by—with parental help or by part-time work. Students who have to earn a living and also spend long hours studying must give up something—usually companionship, sexual activity, and leisure-time pursuits. A wife may have to give up her college education if she is the one who has to work while her husband finishes school. If children are born while one or both partners are still in college, the complications multiply. If a wife does not return to school while the children are young, her world consists mainly of home duties and child rearing. The husband must divide himself between work, school, and his family—a triple burden that leaves little time or energy for any one of the three. Many couples find their marriages cannot survive these strains. Those that do, however, seem to look back on these days with special pride in their efforts and accomplishments.

OTHER LIFE STYLES

Contrary to what many people believe, most Americans do not live in the traditional single-breadwinner nuclear family. Only 18 percent of American households fall into this category. Many more people are choosing alternate life styles, and some of the most common will be discussed here.

Staying Single

Today Americans feel free to shape highly individual marriage patterns that suit their specific needs. It is now possible, with less social discomfort than before, to experiment with alternative married life styles or simply not to marry at all. Whereas single persons were once considered social failures or psychologically inadequate, it is now realized that the single life can itself be socially productive.

According to recent census figures, an unexpectedly large number of people have found this alternative attractive. The number of Americans living alone or with roommates has climbed spectacularly during the last fifteen years. However, they are not living the freewheeling, sexually active life usually associated with singles. Many of those who lived through the years of the sexual revolution. are now in their forties, perhaps still single, but looking for something more fundamental than instant gratification. While they still resist the idea of a permanent commitment, they are no longer indulging in casual sex. Indeed, many single people in all age groups feel a need for a mature relationship of some kind and are no longer making sex the primary goal of their socializing. Furthermore, time and energy that used to be spent experimenting with sex and drugs are now being channeled into a career.

Success in the single state depends on emotional maturity and a clear understanding of one's personality and needs. A prime indicator of such success is happiness; and while social science researchers find it extremely difficult to measure levels of "happiness," their studies have shown marked differences between single men and women, differences that challenge many of our stereotypes.

Although cultural values are changing, the single male is still at a disadvantage in the world of work, particularly if he is a career man or professional. The corporate world, for example, has unwritten codes by which young, upwardly mobile employees are evaluated. Many employers consider unmarried men less responsible than married ones, especially for high-level positions. Both married and unmarried men rank work satisfaction very high for personal happiness, yet single professional men often report less happiness than married ones. Single males also have more emotional illness and die younger than married men.

In contrast, single women live longer and score higher on emotional well-being than married women and both single and married men. A survey of female managers found that all were single during their twenties, as they were building their careers. Commitment to career is not the only reason such women do not marry. Traditional values of male superiority probably limit their field considerably. In the past men have often rejected women whose achievements were equal to or higher than their own, and such women tend to reject men of a lower achievement level than their own. The small number of superior males still in bachelor status helps account for the fact that so many women who are high achievers remain single.

As cultural values and standards change, it is likely that single men will show an improved health profile. Positive attitudes toward staying single will reduce the stress and stigma that many singles still face today. As sex-role attitudes change, many more people will probably choose spouses of equal education and income level, and more satisfying, equal-partner marriages may result.

Living Together

One trend that seems firmly estalished, particularly among young people of college age, is **nonmarital cohabitation,** or living with a person of the opposite sex outside of marriage. In the 1970s the number of households classified as "living-together arrangements" had doubled. A survey of 1,100 undergraduates at Pennsylvania State University found that one-third of the sample had cohabited for a period of time. Efforts to differentiate students who have cohabited from those who have not have failed to disclose distinguishing characteristics in family, background, or emotional and intellectual maturity. Cohabitors do, however, seem to be more liberal in general outlook and more interactive socially. Most of these arrangements occur casually as one partner gradually moves in with another. Some do not involve sexual relations for some months, if at all. Usually the couple does not regard the partnership as a trial marriage, but more as a test of what it is like to live with another person on a daily basis. Changes in sexual codes and the availability of contraceptives have contributed to the rise of cohabitation.

For most young people, cohabitation does not represent a rejection of marriage, but rather a restructuring of the traditional dating, engagement, marriage sequence. Less binding and more intimate than the traditional engagement, cohabitation allows couples the chance to know each other in a way that is similar to marriage in many respects. Many couples sign a "cohabitation contract" that sets the rules they must follow while they are living together and if they separate. The contract may specify how the couple will handle their income and expenses, property, and household duties, and what will happen to their money and belongings if their relationship ends. The chief disadvantages of this arrangement include the disapproval of family and friends and, in the long run, the possible lack of future stability for the relationship.

In addition to the young, many middle-aged people also live under this arrangement; and senior citizens have also found cohabiting to be a convenient way of life, in part because of the tax advantages in remaining unmarried.

Extramarital Affairs

One of the most important problems in married life is the loss of sexual interest between partners. Ideally, sexual interest should increase with sexual fulfillment during marriage. Often the opposite is true. In some men, for example, sexual boredom may result from "a kind of psychological fatigue born of gradual accommodation to the lesser apparent sexual interests of their wives and the lack of novelty in their marital relationships." In some women frustration may occur in the middle years of marriage when they have reached a high level of responsiveness and want more attention than their husbands are prepared to offer. Often the extramarital affair becomes the solution. In addition, men and women who want homosexual experiences may have extramarital affairs, since they cannot fulfill such desires in marriage.

Sexual infidelity in America generally takes the pattern of a small number of relatively short affairs at wide intervals, rather than a string of episodes. A 1969 study by Johnson of one hundred American families found that in 28

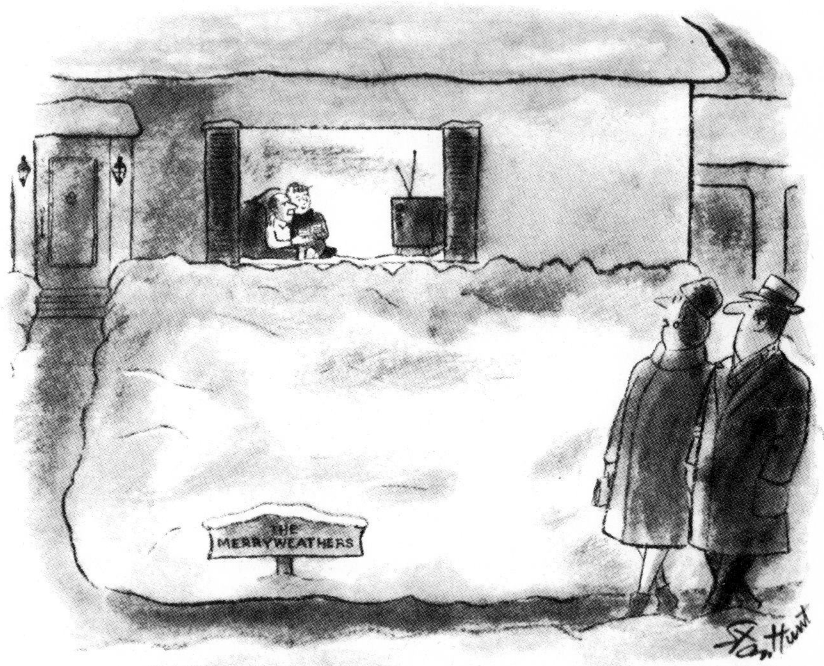

"Apparently, The Merryweathers have a very good relationship—although, come to think of it, I don't believe that's Mrs. Merryweather."

percent of the marriages, one partner had been involved in at least one affair. While most of the husbands and wives were reasonably satisfied with their marriages, 40 percent—most of them men—had taken advantage of opportunities that had arisen. Polls conducted by popular magazines in the early 1980s showed that 34 to 54 percent of married women were willing to do the same. In its own poll the Institute for the Advanced Study of Human Sexuality found that 43 percent of married women were unfaithful. These polls have been criticized, however, for being biased toward liberal, sexually sophisticated Americans and therefore not being representative of the norm. Whatever the true percentage, the marriage partner usually never learns of the infidelity and the marriage is not affected. The discovery of the affair, however, may precipitate painful marital and personal crises.

Homosexual Relationships Over the last fifteen years the gay pride movement has had a profound effect on homosexual men's and women's image of themselves; in addition, the attitudes of parents, friends, and society in general have become more favorable.

Sexual Freedom: Laws and Customs

"Men and women have always invented elaborate refinements upon the simple 90-second act of penetration and ejaculation that fertilizes the egg, as required by nature," says Lawrence Stone, a Princeton historian. The history of sexuality in the Western world has shown great shifts over time in attitudes toward what sexual practices are permitted, and to whom. In the past, sexual permissiveness has been approved mostly for a narrow elite. Only in our day, says Stone, has sexual freedom become so widespread.

Will this trend continue? Sexuality, Stone believes, "is a cultural artifact that has undergone constant and sometimes dramatic changes over time, and there is every reason to suppose that there are still more surprising transformations in store for us in the not too distant future."

We are living in a period of quite unprecedented sexual toleration, and of sexualization of all aspects of everyday life from sea-bathing to the selling of automobiles. . . . It may well not last much longer, in view of the deepening moral tangle about abortion, as medical technology makes the problem of what is and what is not a viable fetus a more and more unanswerable question; the rising tide of anti-pornographic feminism; and the steady expansion of "moral majoritarian" prudery and demands for sexual control. There is also growing public anxiety about the social consequences of the apparent disintegration of the traditional family, now that the divorce rate has reached 50 percent and the illegitimacy rate is creeping up close to 20 percent. The appearance of so far incurable new venereal diseases such as AIDS and herpes makes it impossible any longer to regard promiscuous sex as a cost-free and victimless form of entertainment. Larger and larger numbers of households are today composed of single persons, or pairs of diverse genders living together outside formal marriage. This is not a new phenomenon, but the scale on which it is now occurring and its spread to all social levels are certainly unprecedented. Whether these trends are temporary or permanent has yet to be seen, and the degree to which they are the cause of social instability and of maladjusted children is still unproven. What is certain is that these trends do not seem to be increasing the sum of human happiness, as was anticipated when the sexual revolution began in the 1960s. Sexual liberation is forging its own new chains.

Source: Lawrence Stone, "Sex in the West," *The New Republic*, July 8, 1985, pp. 25–37. Reprinted by permission.

The result is that thousands of people at all levels of society now openly proclaim their homosexuality.

Studies done in the 1970s identified five major kinds of homosexual relationships: (1) *close-coupled* homosexuals, who had a monogamous relationship that was very similar to heterosexual marriage; (2) *open-coupled* homosexuals, who were committed to each other but participated in a wide variety of sexual relationships; (3) *functionals*, who led carefree lives as singles and enjoyed casual sex with many partners; (4) *dysfunctionals*, who were also sexually active but had sexual problems and often regretted being homosexual; and (5) *asexuals*, who were not sexually active and often tried to hide their homosexuality.

These studies made it clear that homosexuals were just as capable as heterosexuals of having fulfilling personal relationships and that very few of them were problem-ridden misfits. In fact, almost all of the subjects in the studies had had long-lasting relationships that involved a deep emotional commitment of the kind that many heterosexual couples have (see the section Homosexuality in Chapter 8).

The fact remains, however, that a great many homosexual men in the 1970s and early 1980s chose to keep their options open and enjoy a wide variety of sexual partners. Then came the AIDS epidemic, and millions of these men (lesbians were unaffected) had to face the reality that they could no longer safely engage in a freewheeling, promiscuous life style. Most homosexual men have realized that to stay healthy they must either confine themselves to a single sexual partner who can be trusted to do the same or exercise greater discretion in their choice of sexual partners and practices (see AIDS in Chapter 15).

PARENTHOOD

The addition of a child to the family unit alters every aspect of married life. Yet the decision to have a child is often made with less thought than the decision to buy a house. Our society lays down more rules for driving a car than for becoming a parent. Many couples stumble into parenthood because they have accepted it as a natural consequence of marriage. Others have children because of pressures from their own parents, or because they regard a child as a confirmation of the husband's masculinity or the wife's femininity. Perhaps the poorest motive for having a child is the belief that a child will hold together a shaky marriage. The one adequate reason for entering parenthood is the desire of two emotionally mature people to produce and raise between them another independent human being in the conviction that a child will be a joyful addition to the life they share, regardless of the difficulties involved.

Disadvantages and Advantages of Having a Child

The birth of a child requires major changes in a couple's life. The pleasures of one-to-one intimacy and privacy can never again exclude some measure of awareness of a third person's welfare. Sexual activity, suspended for a number of weeks before and after childbirth, will be reestablished under wholly new circumstances, handicapped by the fatigue of the new mother and the demands of the infant's routine. There are shifts in the roles of both husband and wife. If the mother gives up her career, she may periodically feel resentful. The father may feel increased pressure to earn a living as head of a household. Adjustment to this situation is made difficult by the great financial cost of parenthood. Both parents must also accept the fact that they will be sharing each other's time and affection with the child.

The drives toward self-absorption and self-fulfillment, the availability of birth control and abortion, and the sheer economic strain of raising a child to adulthood accounted for the generally declining U.S. birth rate during the 1970s. For example, many women now postpone having children until they are in their thirties and more are deciding not to have children at all. This tendency is reflected in the country's general fertility rate, which is defined as the number of births for every 1,000 women aged 15 to 44. The rate dropped from 82.3 in 1971 to 66.0 in 1984. Women's new interest in careers instead of housework, the tendency of men and women to choose alternate life styles, and the increasing divorce rate may also have contributed to this drop in the birth rate. More and more, women want to establish their own lives and a separate identity before they have a child.

On the brighter side, most couples look back on raising their children as the most rewarding experience they have shared. To be responsible for the development of another human being, born out of love, can create profound ties of devotion between partners. To share in a child's growing awareness of the world can lend parents a new and creative perspective on life. The openness with which children show emotion, whether love or anger, can promote a freer expression of feeling between parents. Although it is a mistake for parents to expect repayment, either material or nonmaterial, for their contributions to a child's existence and welfare, they should be able to anticipate the lifelong reward of having produced a loving family.

Readiness for Parenthood

A husband and wife who have considered the advantages and disadvantages of children and have examined their motives honestly must still assess their capacity for parenthood. Are they mature enough to make the many decisions involved in directing another human life for some twenty years? Are they responsible enough to maintain a consistent effort and concern when the results are discouraging, as well as when they are a source of pride? Can they meet the financial burdens of parenthood?

Psychological Readiness. Since there is no way to know just what it is like to be a parent before a child is present, psychological readiness is difficult to assess. The arrival of a child turns the married pair into a triangle with complex possibilities for interaction. Both parents must be mature enough to accept restrictions and expand possibilities. It is useful to talk over fears and self-doubts. Perhaps the young wife is afraid she will be overprotective, like her mother. Perhaps she fears her husband will be too strict a disciplinarian. Perhaps the husband is afraid sexual relations will no longer seem important to his wife once the baby is born. Open discussion can help both wife and husband adapt to parenthood or indicate where outside help is needed.

Child Abuse. The recent increase in **child abuse**—the unrestrained use of corporal punishment to the point of physically harming the child—indicates that many people failed to assess their maturity and preparedness before undertaking parenthood. Current official figures show that more than 500,000 cases of child abuse are reported every year and that probably 1.5 million cases go unreported. Thousands of youngsters die each year as a result of abuse received at the hands of their parents, but hitting a child for misbehavior constitutes only one form of child abuse. Neglect and psychological maltreatment can be as harmful as corporal punishment. It has been suggested that parents who were themselves beaten or unloved as children are likely to repeat this pattern with their own offspring. Whatever the reason may be, individuals who sense this lack of control in themselves should seek help before becoming parents. (The general role parents play in their child's psychological development is discussed in Chapter 1.)

Parents Anonymous is an organization that was founded to help parents who tend to abuse their children, either physically, verbally, or through neglect. The organization's own estimate of child-abuse cases in the United States, reported and unreported, runs to an outside figure of 6 million. By means of telephone calls and meetings of concerned parents, the problem of child abuse is being dealt with very successfully. The organization has set up telephone hot lines for use by parents who feel the urge to abuse their children. Anonymity is carefully observed, and parents who call will be comforted and met with insight and understanding.

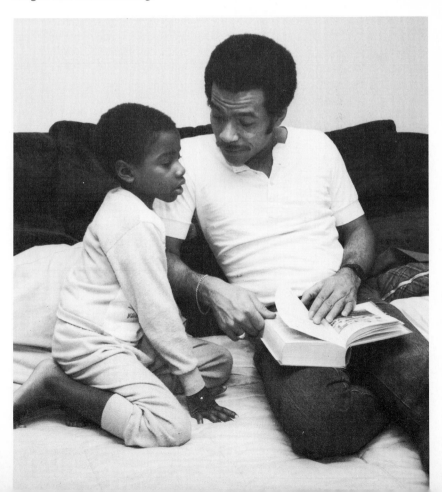

There are more than 10 million single-parent families in the United States.

Economic Preparation. Parenthood today requires economic stability. The initial costs of having a child are inconsequential compared to what lies ahead in the cost of food, clothing, housing, transportation, medicine, and possibly the major expense of higher education. Inflation makes figures obsolete almost as soon as they are printed, but the estimated cost of seeing a child from birth to economic independence, including the loss of a second income that would have been earned by a wife, is almost $200,000. Making sure that the money will be available when the time comes eases many of the worries of early parenthood and enables a couple to enjoy their baby more fully.

Family Planning

Pregnancy and childbirth put a tremendous strain on a woman's body. From a health standpoint alone, pregnancies should be planned and adequate time allowed between them. In a normally fertile group of women who nurse their babies and use no contraceptive techniques, babies are likely to be born about two years apart, given normal sexual activity. This is the medically desirable interval between babies, as reported in a poll of 3,000 doctors by Dr. Alan Guttmacher. The period of fifteen months before the onset of a new pregnancy permits the mother's body to recuperate, gives her a better chance of having another healthy baby, and allows her time to care for the first infant.

Separating the birth of children by about two years seems best from a psychological and financial standpoint as well. The financial burden is less concentrated. Children are close enough in age to share interests and friends, and yet far enough apart to be enjoyed as separate individuals.

There is now evidence of greater health risks to both mother and children as families grow beyond the third child. The mortality rate in childbirth, for example, is about three times higher for mothers bearing more than three children. Many parents are limiting their family size because of financial considerations or because they feel they should not be adding to world overpopulation. The "only child," once the great concern of pediatricians and psychiatrists, is now being viewed in a new light. Though only children are often overpressured or overbabied, they have advantages in terms of parental attention and economic security.

The Single-Parent Family

The rising rates of divorce and illegitimacy have created a new phenomenon on the American family scene—the *single-parent family*. In 1984 such households accounted for 15 million American families, or one in four. Over 7 million contained children under 18, and nine out of ten were headed by a woman. One-parent situations occurred in about 20 percent of white families and 59 percent of black families, the difference being attributable in large part to the greater percentage of black teenage mothers (see box: Unwed Teenage Mothers).

The single-parent household faces many more serious financial problems than do households with two parents. Often when the mother is left alone to support her children, she is unable to earn an adequate living. Her financial dilemma is compounded by the fact that the vast majority of divorced fathers do not continue to pay child support after three years.

Single fathers are becoming less uncommon. Groups such as Fathers United

PROBLEMS AND CONTROVERSIES: Unwed Teenage Mothers

An epidemic of teenage pregnancy is raging out of control in the United States. Our country has the highest rate of teenage pregnancy in the industrialized world, with over 1 million teenage girls becoming pregnant each year and half of them deciding to have the baby, even if they are unmarried. Unwed teenage motherhood is creating untold social problems in the U.S. and becoming a major financial burden. In fact, the present generation of unwed teenage mothers is producing what is on its way to becoming a large underclass of functionally illiterate, unemployed, and unemployable adults.

There are a number of reasons for this development, some of them having to do with society's attitude toward sexuality and others with economic inequality. Contradictory American attitudes toward sex are partly responsible. Sexual activity became more socially accepted during the 1970s sexual revolution, and the message was not lost on the generation then in grade school. A 1982 study found that 20 percent of all 15-year-olds, 33 percent of all 16-year-olds, and 43 percent of all 17-year-olds had had sexual intercourse.

Poverty is another major factor. Though teenage pregnancy occurs among all races and social classes, the problem is most severe in the poor black urban ghetto. Twenty-five percent of all black children are born to teenage mothers, 90 percent of whom are unmarried. With no job skills and no expectations for the future, many poor teenage girls, of all races, become pregnant to give meaning to their lives and raise their sense of self-esteem. In their world, becoming a teenage mother makes them the focus of attention. The medical and welfare costs for caring for these child-mothers and their children amount to $8.6 billion a year.

Unwed teenage motherhood is a self-perpetuating problem that has been said to lie "at the very hub of the U.S. poverty cycle." Because many pregnant teenagers do not seek medical care and neglect their diet, their children are more likely to be born premature, to come down with infectious diseases, and to develop learning disabilities. Many of these children also have to be put in foster homes because their mothers lose interest in them after a year or so, or physically abuse them. As they grow older, many children of unwed teenage mothers are prone to drop out of school, become delinquent, commit crimes—or get pregnant and become teenage mothers themselves.

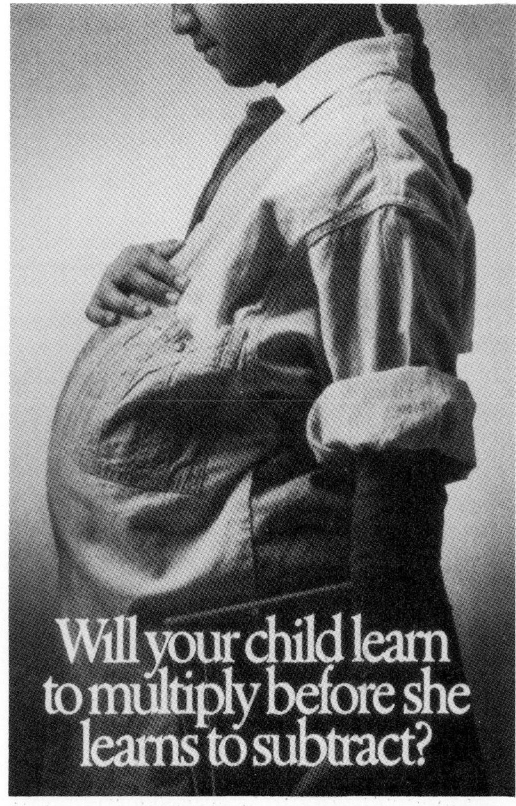
Will your child learn to multiply before she learns to subtract?

Sources: Adapted from "Children Having Children," *Time*, December 9, 1985, pp. 78–90; Sharon Johnson, "Clinics Taking Birth-Control Help and Advice to Teen-Agers," *New York Times*, March 12, 1986, pp. C1, C12.

The Children of Single Parents

Children who grow up in single-parent families have often lost more than a parent: They have lost a childhood. Many single parents, most of them women, cannot cope with the responsibilities of raising a child alone; as a group, they tend to be depressed and to have drinking and drug-abuse problems. Many have no network of friends or relatives to rely upon during difficulties; instead, they turn to their children for solace, support, and advice on matters ranging from finances to sexual relationships. In effect, they abdicate their responsibilities as parents and put their children in charge of their own upbringing.

The burden of acting as parental confidant and counselor forces a great many children to grow up too soon. For example, a 10-year-old may have to forgo afterschool play in order to go home to do housework and care for younger siblings; even 5-year-olds have been expected to shoulder the full-time responsibility of looking after younger brothers and sisters.

Such children are far more likely than those raised in two-parent families to experience social and emotional problems in school and in later years. Because they spend so much time worrying about a parent's depression or drinking problem, many children have trouble concentrating at school and making friends. Their grades often slide, they are frequently absent, and they tend to have behavioral problems. According to psychologist Judith Wallerstein, some children "whose parents are busy working or re-establishing their social lives become depressed and anxious because they feel they have been abandoned."

Problems continue to plague these children in adulthood. According to Alfred Messer, a psychiatrist, a child who has been forced to become an adviser to a parent "always suffers in life from a lack of self-esteem because so much was expected by the parent consciously or subconsciously." Unable to meet such demands, many of these children grow to adulthood with a permanent sense of inadequacy.

Sources: Adapted from John Lee, "Single Parent, Double Trouble," *Time*, January 4, 1982, p. 81; Sharon Johnson, "A Child's Role After Divorce," *New York Times*, January 7, 1985, p. B8.

are providing support and legal advice for single fathers who are challenging the traditional American legal practices of regularly granting custody of children to mothers.

Adoption

Legal adoption of a child is often the happy solution—for both the parents and the child—in cases where a couple is infertile or where a pregnancy is medically inadvisable. In addition, some families satisfy their own needs, as well as those of the children involved, by adopting multiracial, handicapped, or other "hard-to-place" children, even though they are capable of having, or already have, children of their own. Recently, many states have begun to allow qualified single people of either sex, including divorced persons, to adopt children, thus increasing the existing adoption possibilities.

Despite the difficulty in placing some children, the demand for babies is so great that the processing of an adoption application may take years, and more couples are turned down than succeed in obtaining a baby.

As a general rule, it is better to apply for adoption through a private state-licensed agency or a state-operated agency. These agencies are careful to check on the background of both child and prospective parents. They also obtain the child in a legal and proper manner. Agencies try to match the physical characteristics of the child to the parents and take into account intellectual and emotional compatibility. Prospective parents are informed of the child's known physical defects; the child is then placed in their home, often under probation for up to a year before it is legally adopted.

Parents who adopt are naturally apprehensive about their relationship with the child. But many studies have shown that the relationship between adopted children and their parents is usually very close and intimate. Most experts feel that children should be told they are adopted, lest they learn the truth in a shocking manner. They should also be told as young as possible, so the fact of adoption will be taken for granted as they are growing up.

Many of America's adoptees feel a need to know who their real parents are, not merely out of curiosity, but for emotional and medical reasons. It has recently become somewhat easier for adoptees to gain access to their adoption records. In the past very little information or cooperation was available to these seekers. Now the Adoptees' Liberty Movement Association (P.O. Box 154, New York, N.Y. 10033) is involved in class-action lawsuits aimed at opening impounded birth and adoption records to adoptees 18 years old and over. ALMA, as the association is known, also offers individual adoptees help in locating their natural parents through a computerized international registry that cross-indexes vital statistics of persons separated by adoption.

SUMMARY

1. Members of the modern *nuclear family* often look to outside sources for emotional support, entertainment, and even social status—functions that used to be served entirely within the *extended family*.

2. The contemporary stress on personal freedom and self-fulfillment and the changing roles of women have led to later marriages, fewer children, and the *two-earner* and *two-career marriage*. Because so many mothers now work, finding affordable, reliable day-care facilities for children has become a major priority.

3. There is no formula for a successful marriage, but emotional maturity, adequate preparation, and realistic expectations and attitudes before marriage are important predictors of marital success. One's choice of marriage partner is generally based on feelings of love, physical attraction, personality traits, intellectual compatibility, and similarity in background. Each factor must be examined in the light of reality. Aspects of oneself or one's partner that may affect the future relationship should be candidly aired before marriage. Practical matters, such as finances, should be part of marital planning. They can impose hardships on any marriage, but particularly on college marriages.

4. Conflicts in marriage are best handled by communication and compromise. When problems become too difficult to handle, a marriage counselor can help the couple to adjust or, failing that, to decide on *divorce*.

5. Liberalized divorce laws in some states now permit divorce without protracted legal battles, but child custody is still an agonizing issue. The concept of *joint custody* is gaining in popularity, but in most divorces it is the mother who receives sole custody and the father who is supposed to pay child support. The high rate of remarriage of divorced parents has resulted in many *blended families*.

6. Today there are many alternatives to traditional marriage, including the single life lived alone or with roommates and *nonmarital cohabitation*. *Homosexual relationships* range from strictly monogamous arrangements to casual brief encounters, although fear of contracting AIDS has made the latter much less popular in recent years.

7. The availability of contraception and the widely recognized need to limit family size have made it easier for couples to decide to have children because they want the rewards of raising an independent human being in a loving atmosphere, rather than, for example, because of parental pressure or the desire to hold together a shaky marriage. When deciding whether to have a child, couples should take into consideration the new burdens a child would bring.

8. *Child abuse*, the unrestrained use of physical or psychological punishment or severe neglect, is a problem of crisis proportions. Many abusive parents were themselves abused as children; others, particularly teenage parents, are too emotionally immature to deal with the burden of caring for a child.

9. The *single-parent family*, usually headed by a woman, is becoming more common. Children in these families are often forced to grow up too soon and later in life suffer from a lack of self-esteem.

10. Couples who cannot have children may decide to adopt them. The relationship between adopted children and their parents is usually close.

CONSUMER CONCERNS

1. Schools in many areas have adopted excellent courses of study in marriage preparation. Do the schools in your community present such courses?
2. Obviously this is a matter of personal values, but weddings often appear to be unnecessarily lavish. What are some considerations that couples, and their families, might wish to keep in mind before spending money for a wedding?
3. Programs in marriage preparation are available in several religious groups. Have you considered the value of such programs?
4. Marriage counseling might be more beneficial before rather than after serious marital problems arise. Do you agree?
5. There are many illegal operations that function in the area of child adoption. Are you aware that it is safer to adopt through a state agency or a state-licensed agency?
6. What advice would you give a person seeking to place a child in a day-care center?

10

Aging, Dying, and Death

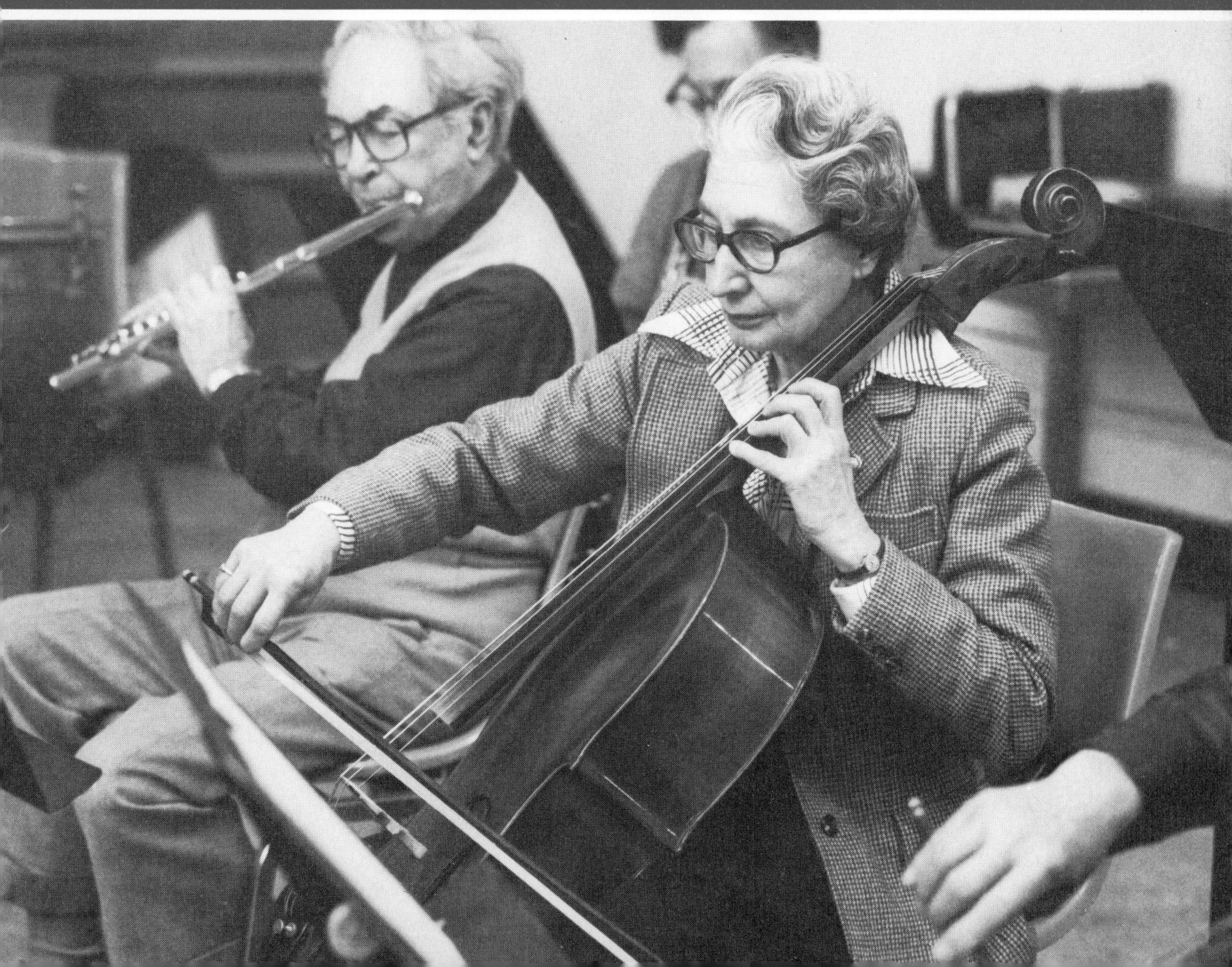

Americans regard old age with a curious ambivalence. On the one hand, the elderly are frequently depicted in fiction and the media as being wise, gentle, and understanding. On the other hand, old age itself is deplored and ridiculed; and old people are dismissed as being incompetent, weak, and a drain on society. The first attitude probably stems from a traditional view of age, a leftover from a time when it was truly extraordinary for an individual to live to be 40 years old. The elderly of two centuries ago were venerated because they were so rare. If one of our colonial ancestors were transported from the eighteenth century to the present, he would be as astonished by the number of 60-, 70-, and 80-year-old people on the streets as he would be by telephones, television, and astronauts.

TABLE 10-1
U.S. Life Expectancy at Various Ages, 1984

Age in 1984	Average Years Life Remaining
At birth	74.7
1	74.5
5	70.7
10	65.8
15	60.8
20	56.1
25	51.4
30	46.7
35	42.0
40	37.3
45	32.7
50	28.4
55	24.2
60	20.4
65	16.8
70	13.6
75	10.7
80	8.2
85	6.2

Source: National Center for Health Statistics, 1985.

The second attitude, that of distaste and ridicule, is more common and has been spawned by our youth-oriented society, which places a premium on youthful good looks and activity. The current denigration of age is so marked, in fact, that it has given rise to the term *ageism*, which is rapidly taking its place beside *racism* and *sexism* to indicate bigotry and prejudice.

The dramatic increase in life expectancy of recent times has produced a rather sudden burgeoning in the number of elderly people. Three thousand years ago a newborn child could expect to live only to age 18; in 1984, a newborn American could expect to live almost 75 years (see Table 10-1). The greatest increase in longevity has occurred during this century, as a result of advances in medical knowledge. From 1900 to 1984, life expectancy in the United States climbed by 27.4 years—from 47.3 years to 74.7 years.

The 65-and-over age group has grown slightly more than 10 percent of the population. This is an increase of 20 percent in just ten years. In the same period the general population rose only 11.4 percent. At this rate, the 65-and-over age group will be almost 30 million strong by the year 2000, and it will constitute more than 12 percent of our total population (see Table 10-2).

The elderly, therefore, are becoming an ever more important social and political group. Aging is, furthermore, a process that will touch most of us personally—both indirectly, through closeness to an aging parent or relative, and directly, through our own inevitable growth and development. In this chapter we shall explore the phenomenon of aging and discuss some of the problems that it raises. We shall also discuss dying and some recent research on the effects of death on friends and family of the deceased, including burial rites, grief, and mourning.

CHARACTERISTICS OF AGING

One of the difficulties of discussing aging is arriving at a definition of old age. Who, exactly, is old? The 75-year-old who jogs every day and plays tennis twice a week? Or the 40-year-old with a paunch and jowls and flabby muscles? We shall consider the chronology of aging later; for the moment, let us look at some of its physical aspects.

Physiological Aging

There are certain universally recognized physical signs of aging: The skin loses its suppleness and wrinkles begin to form; the hair begins to turn gray and thin out, sometimes disappearing entirely; the teeth loosen and drop out. Old people begin to shrink in size because of a decrease in muscle elasticity and changes in the bones and ligaments. But these changes do not occur all at once. As Congressman Claude Pepper, a spokesman for the elderly, has stated, "The aging process is so slow, so gradual, that all you notice is a slight diminishing of some of your faculties." Not everyone ages in the same way, nor at the same rate. In the last few decades it has become apparent that we have more control over the aging process than was formerly thought: A good diet and regular exercise, for example, can retard aging and blunt some of its more debilitating features. Yet some changes will inevitably take place in the body regardless of the care lavished upon it by the most conscientious owner.

TABLE 10-2
The United States Is Growing Older

Year	Median Age
1790	16
1970	28
1981	30
2000	35
2030	40

The Senses. The five senses usually become less efficient as a person ages. Hearing especially is affected—particularly the ability to hear higher-frequency tones. Eyesight is also likely to become impaired. Both hearing and visual deficits have an important effect on the individual because they hinder the ability to communicate. The sense of smell also declines with age, as does the sense of taste. This is one reason why older people sometimes appear indifferent to food and consequently fall into unhealthy dietary habits. Many of the elderly find that it takes longer to perceive something through any of their senses, including touch. While every old person does not necessarily experience all these problems, about 50 percent of the elderly undergo some degree of sensory loss.

Muscles, Bones, Heart, and Lungs. Muscle function slows down as an individual grows older, and muscle weight decreases. The muscles also begin to function less efficiently if the cardiovascular system fails to deliver enough nutrients or if it does not remove all toxic waste products. In addition, poor lung functioning may reduce the supply of oxygen to the muscles. Muscle function is also affected by the changing structure and composition of the skeleton. The bones become hollow, brittle, and weak; because they are more porous, they are more likely to fracture and take longer to mend.

The heart—a highly specialized muscle—suffers some of the same problems as other muscles. Generally, the heart is strained by a decreased maximum blood flow to and from it, and an increased recovery time after each contraction.

The lungs' capacity to take in oxygen is often reduced in old age. Much lung trouble may be attributable to a series of prolonged "insults" such as a lifetime of smoking or continuous exposure to air pollution.

Illness and Disease. As people age, the immune system functions less efficiently. The production of antibodies peaks during adolescence and then begins a lifelong decline. Old people thus have less protection than they had earlier against infections and disease. They are also more likely to suffer from **chronic conditions**—illnesses that occur repeatedly or never go away. The most common

It's Never Too Late

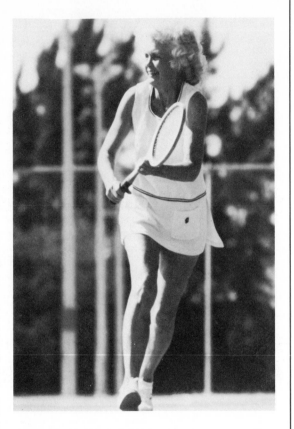

In a series of new studies prompted by the geriatric population explosion, researchers are finding that moderate exercise can not only retard the effects of aging but can actually reverse them.

Furthermore, the findings show that no matter when in life a person starts to exercise, improvements in function can occur.

Dr. Roy J. Shephard, an expert on exercise and aging at the University of Toronto, concluded: "You'd have to go a long way to find something as good as exercise as a fountain of youth. And you don't have to run marathons to reap the benefits. For the average older person who does little more than rapid walking for 30 minutes at a time three or four times a week, it can provide 10 years of rejuvenation."

"Older people, even those over 70 or 80, can make as great a percentage gain as the young," said Dr. Herbert A. deVries, who recently retired as director of the Andrus Gerontology Center at the University of Southern California.

In one of Dr. deVries's earliest studies, more than 200 men and women aged 56 to 87 who lived in a California retirement community participated in a fitness program that included a walk-jog routine, calisthenics, and stretching for one hour a day three to five times a week. After just six weeks, "dramatic changes" were seen, Dr. deVries said: Blood pressure dropped, percentage of body fat decreased, maximum oxygen capacity increased, arm strength improved, and muscular signs of nervous tension diminished. Peak fitness occurred after 18 to 42 weeks.

"Men and women of 60 and 70 became as fit and energetic as those 20 to 30 years younger," Dr. deVries noted in his book *Fitness after 50.* "The ones who improved the most were the ones who had been least active and most out of shape."

However, even one of activity's staunchest advocates, Dr. Everett L. Smith, director of the Biogerontology Laboratory at the University of Wisconsin, readily concedes: "Exercise is not an unending fountain of youth. Eventually we all decline. But the quality of life is so much higher for the elderly who are physically active than for people who sit in a rocking chair waiting for the Grim Reaper."

Source: Jane E. Brody, "Aging: Studies Point Toward Ways to Slow It," *The New York Times*, June 10, 1986, pp. C1, C3.

chronic conditions are arthritis, heart conditions, and high blood pressure; heart disease, cancer, and stroke are the three leading causes of death.

An increase in health problems among the elderly reflects, to a great extent, the body's decreased ability to cope with stress (see Chapter 2). A disease that may be shaken off by a younger person might linger or recur in an elderly one. Unhappily, just as the ability to cope with stress declines, an elderly individual may be exposed to increasingly stressful events such as health problems, loss of sight or hearing, retirement, or widowhood.

Psychological Aging

Just as important as the physical changes of old age is the psychological impact on one's self-image. Stiff joints, shortness of breath, longer reaction times—all alter our ideas about who we are and what we can do. Some old people feel compelled to give up driving a car, for example, while others become cautious about going down a flight of stairs or crossing a street.

The change in appearance that comes with age affects men and women somewhat differently. Men may be concerned about their loss of strength and stature, since these traits are often essential to a man's self-image. Women may be concerned about lessened sexual attractiveness, particularly those who have long been accustomed to measuring their self-worth in terms of physical beauty. Other women, however, find the change in appearance liberating because now that they are no longer treated as sex objects, they feel free to develop and express themselves.

An individual's personality continues to grow and develop throughout life, and the personality changes that are perceived in the elderly are a result of this process. The world looks very different to 60-year-olds than to 20-year-olds. The latter are likely to view life as a challenge, a series of adventures that can be turned to their advantage if they behave in a sufficiently daring and aggressive manner. The elderly, on the other hand, may well view the world as a dangerous and complicated place.

Intelligence. Intelligence does not decline with age, though many believe it does. Although losses of speed and memory begin in late middle age, they are frequently offset by gains in reasoning and understanding.

The single most reliable indicator in predicting intellectual functioning in old age is educational level. Increased education stimulates a desire to stay mentally active. Educated people generally enjoy such activities as reading, analyzing, and discussing. These functions remain at a high level throughout old age.

When there does appear to be a lessening of intellectual ability in the elderly, it is nearly always attributable to failing health, social isolation, or poor formal education; it is never intrinsic to the aging process itself.

Memory. There is some disagreement among experts about the mechanisms governing memory in old age. Some believe that the *ability* to retrieve information from long- and short-term memory does not decrease in old age; older people may need more time to retrieve the information, however. Others suggest that older people may have trouble recalling information once it is stored.

One researcher found that older subjects performed relatively well in recognizing and labeling objects, but poorly on remembering such things as vocabulary lists committed to memory for testing purposes. Others have pointed out, however, that people of all ages tend to remember only what is useful and important

Alzheimer's Disease

It begins with minor memory lapses that are common to many people in late middle age. A man in his 50s or early 60s may forget words, telephone numbers, and familiar faces, but otherwise appear well and normal, with no signs of serious disease such as stroke or brain tumor. Within three to six years, however, he is lying in a hospital bed curled up into a fetal position, unable to utter anything more complicated than "Yes" or "no."

The condition is called Alzheimer's disease, and it is 100 percent fatal. It afflicts almost 3 million people in the United States; 120,000 people die from it each year, making it the fourth leading cause of death among the old. It strikes rich and poor, men and women alike; its famous victims include Rita Hayworth, Otto Preminger, and Norman Rockwell. While those aged 65 and older are its most common victims, it can also strike people in their 40s.

The most telling symptom is a profound memory loss that affects a person's work performance and social life. An elderly but otherwise healthy physician may forget how to set a broken bone, for example, or a 50-year-old woman may head for the kitchen for a drink of water and end up in the basement instead, not knowing how she got there. Victims also forget how to perform routine tasks such as combing their hair, threading a needle, or shuffling a deck of cards. Their judgment is also affected: They may burn themselves in the shower by turning on the hot instead of the cold water, or go outdoors in a swimming suit in midwinter. Behavioral problems are also common. Alzheimer patients are often depressed, suspicious, anxious, and prone to violent outbursts. Personality and judgment may deteriorate to the point where they urinate in public, walk into stores and take things off shelves, or suddenly attack a spouse or close friend. By this stage of the disease, most victims have trouble identifying the season of the year or recognizing the names of family members. Finally, they lose control over their body functions and must be hospitalized; at this point many become comatose and die.

Alzheimer's disease can progress slowly or rapidly. In either case, victims become increasingly dependent on others to perform routine tasks such as bathing and dressing. Their erratic behavior also requires round-the-clock monitoring. The disease imposes a great burden on family members, who have to be custodians and at the same time "experience the anguish of seeing a loved one turn into a witless stranger who no longer even remembers who they are." The medical costs can be ruinous: Lifetime savings can vanish in a few years because "neither Medicare nor private insurance programs will pay for the custodial care its victims need."

So far, the cause of Alzheimer's disease is unknown, and no effective treatment exists. Autopsies show a characteristic pattern of brain damage involving the loss of nerve cells responsible for memory and thought processes. Researchers are optimistic about finding the causes and developing an effective treatment for the disease. They hope to do for Alzheimer's what they did for poliomyelitis many years ago.

Sources: Richard J. Wurtman, "Alzheimer's Disease," *Scientific American*, January 1985, pp. 62–74; "A Slow Death of the Mind," *Newsweek*, December 3, 1984, pp. 56–62; Robert Berkow, ed., *The Merck Manual*, 14th ed. (Rahway, N.J.: Merck, Sharp, & Dohme, 1982), pp. 1305–1306 ("Dementia"). Quotations are from *Newsweek*.

in their lives, and older people may be more selective about what they want to retain. Consequently, they may balk at memorizing useless word lists.

In general, most people over 60 can learn and utilize completely new material. Though they may not be as efficient learners as younger students, they absorb new material against the backdrop of a lifetime of experience and thus may have a greater understanding of it than the young, who tend to see only unrelated facts.

Chronological Aging

Our society groups people by age. Between the years of 6 and 18 we attend school. We cannot vote until we are 18. In many states we cannot legally buy alcoholic beverages until we are 21. At age 65 we are officially designated "old."

This last arbitrary yardstick was created in 1935 by the Social Security Act, which provided stipends for those over 65. People were therefore classified as being aged at 65 years, even if they were active, healthy, and had many more years of productive life left. They were withdrawn from the work force and deprived of a major way of occupying their time and energies.

As a result of a more sophisticated view of the aging process, researchers have begun to distinguish between the "young-old" and the "old-old." The classification is not based on chronological age but rather on physical and psychological abilities. The "young-old" are usually retired and hence have a great deal of leisure. As a rule, they are healthy, vigorous, and well educated. They use their leisure for self-enhancement or community activities. They require far less counseling and assistance in adapting successfully to their aging than the "old-old." The "young-old," moreover, are a growing political force.

The "old-old" are those who, because of poor health or psychological or social problems, cannot perform the basic activities of life without help. They may need assistance that ranges from full-time nursing care and daily delivery of hot meals to help with shopping or cleaning.

REASONS FOR AGING

There is no simple explanation of why we age, but there are many theories. Environment affects the rate at which we age—stress and pollution are two examples—but different people exposed to the same environment will age at different rates. If we understood the process of aging, theoretically we could retard it. Although all the following theories have scientific merit, none is conclusive.

Heredity

Every form of life appears to age according to some genetic code. Among plants there are annuals and there are perennials. Some trees may live for a thousand years—most others, far less. There are differences in the life span of animals: Compare the dog with the elephant. And there are unique life cycles such as those of the frog and the butterfly.

In humans the genetic influence is particularly striking in studies of identical twins, who age at the same rate even if separated and nearly always die at about the same age. Fraternal twins, on the other hand, frequently have dissimilar life spans, even when brought up together. And so there is some validity to genetic theories of aging, although they are not sufficient to explain how people age.

The Wear-and-Tear Theory

According to the wear-and-tear theory, the human body is like a machine that simply wears out as a result of constant use. This theory also takes into account all the injuries and insults to the body that occur over a lifetime, such as radiation, accidents, smoking, and pollution. Critics of the theory point out that many body systems are self-repairing. Skin and red blood cells, for example, constantly repair themselves, as do nerve and muscle cells.

Test Your Aging IQ

T or F

_______ 1. The majority of old people (defined as those over 65) are senile.

_______ 2. All five senses tend to decline in old age.

_______ 3. Most old people have no interest in, or capacity for, sexual relations.

_______ 4. Lung capacity tends to decline in old age.

_______ 5. The majority of old people feel miserable all of the time.

_______ 6. Physical strength tends to decline in old age.

_______ 7. At least 1/10th of the aged live in extended care institutions (nursing homes, mental hospitals, etc.).

_______ 8. Aged drivers have fewer accidents per person than drivers under age 65.

_______ 9. Most older workers cannot work as effectively as younger workers.

_______ 10. About 80 per cent of the aged are healthy enough to carry out their normal activities.

_______ 11. Most old people are set in their ways and unable to change.

_______ 12. Old people usually take longer to learn something new.

_______ 13. It is almost impossible for most old people to learn new things.

_______ 14. The reaction time of most old people tends to be slower than the reaction time of young people.

_______ 15. In general, most old people are pretty much alike.

_______ 16. The majority of old people are seldom bored.

_______ 17. The majority of old people are socially isolated and lonely.

_______ 18. Older workers have fewer accidents than younger workers.

_______ 19. More than 15 per cent of the U.S. population is now Age 65 or over.

_______ 20. Most medical practitioners tend to give low priority to the aged.

_______ 21. The majority of older people have incomes below the poverty level (as defined by the federal government).

_______ 22. The majority of older people are working or would like to have some kind of work to do (including housework or volunteer work).

_______ 23. Older people tend to become more religious as they age.

_______ 24. The majority of old people are seldom irritated or angry.

_______ 25. The health and socioeconomic status of older people (compared to younger people) in the year 2000 will probably be about the same as that of today's older people.

Scoring: Odd-numbered statements are false; even-numbered statements are true.

Source: Dr. Erdman Palmore, Duke University Center for the Study of Aging and Human Development, Durham, N.C. Reprinted by permission of *The Gerontologist*, Vol. 20, No. 6, 1980.

The Homeostatic Theory

The homeostatic theory postulates that, over time, body chemistry becomes increasingly inefficient at maintaining stable levels of its chemical elements. Since the body's chemical processes are delicately interrelated, deterioration in one area can have a cumulative impact on the body as a whole. Some of these mechanisms include the acid-alkaline balance in the cells, blood sugar levels, body temperature regulation, and the excretion of toxins by the kidneys.

Under rest conditions, these self-regulating processes in older people operate at a level similar to those observed in younger people. Older people, however, are less able to return to homeostasis, or normal balance, after physical and emotional stresses, such as anger, high sugar intake, exercise, or great changes in temperature. A stressful event easily tolerated by a young person may therefore damage an older one.

The Cellular Aging Theories

Several theories focus on cellular change in aging bodies. Cellular aging theories take into account that all body cells divide and reproduce only a finite number of times. Some scientists also believe that certain cells begin to reproduce imperfectly. Still others believe that some cells deteriorate as a result of accumulated insults and injuries.

These are just a few of the many theories on the subject of how we age. However, while charts and graphs show statistical reductions in the ability to function as one ages, they cannot predict exactly how any particular individual will grow old. Two 70-year-olds may look and act as if they were 30 years apart in age. Good nutrition and adequate health care over the whole span of life strongly influence the rate and quality of aging in any individual.

SOCIAL PROBLEMS AND THE AGED

Along with the rest of the population the elderly share concerns about crime, health care, housing, and so on, but their age brings a unique slant to the way they cope with them. In addition, the elderly face the question of retirement, and it can be traumatic.

Retirement

For many, old age is almost synonymous with retirement. Retirement in our society is a rite of passage that marks the transition from a working to a nonworking life, from being active and productive to being passive and nonproductive. Retirement has different meanings for different people, depending on how they regarded their work. Because they have spent so much time at their jobs, many people have derived their entire sense of worth and self-esteem from their work. Their leisure activities have tended to be superficial and lacking in meaning. Retirement for these people thus means stepping out of the stream of life. The problem is particularly serious for the less educated and the financially strained, but it can also trouble professional people and executives.

One very important factor that determines what effects retirement will have is a person's health status. Not surprisingly, those who are in good health upon retirement fare the best. Those in ill health fare poorly, regardless of their feelings about leaving the work force.

No matter how a person regards retirement, the change is always stressful and requires a period of adjustment.

Crime

Polls have shown that fear of crime is one of the major concerns of the elderly; older people frequently rank it in importance above sickness, poverty, loneliness, and many of the other problems commonly associated with old age. Studies show, however, that most purported crime waves against the elderly are media-

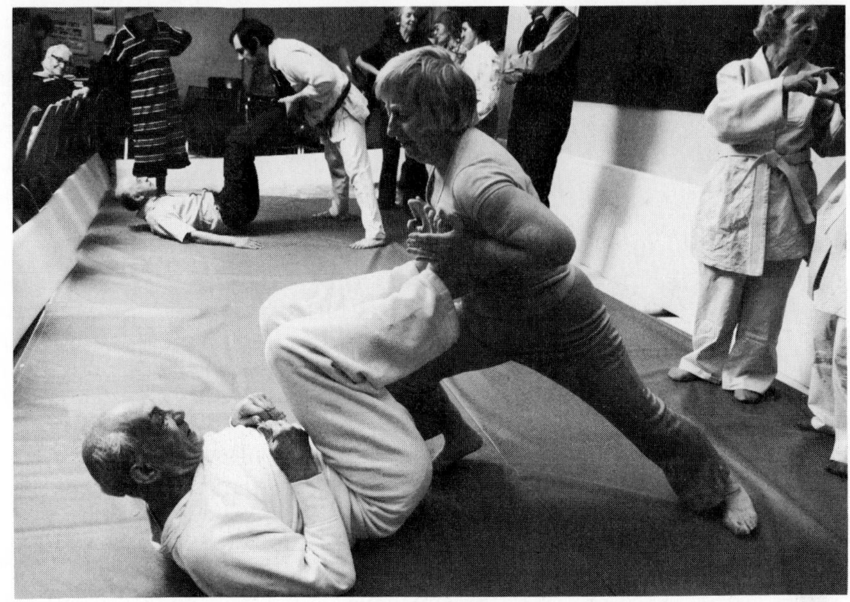
In their concern to be safe from crime, some older people are taking lessons in self-defense.

created events, and that old people are no more liable than the general population to be crime victims.

Older people who live in high-crime areas run a risk, of course, but it is not much greater than that run by their younger neighbors. But because the old are generally less robust, they are more likely to sustain a serious injury during a physical assault and to recover from the injury more slowly.

Health Care

It was assumed that the passage of Medicare and Medicaid legislation would eliminate health-care problems for older people (see Chapter 16). Although these programs have alleviated some health-related problems for older people, they have not been completely successful. Medicaid and Medicare programs are inadequate to overcome financial barriers to health services. As a result, thousands of older people don't get proper medical attention.

Another geriatric health concern is institutionalization. There are about a million people over age 65 in long-term care facilities, and many of them are there because no alternative services are available. Unnecessary institutionalization of the elderly is costly, not only in terms of money, but also in terms of the negative psychological effects on the institutionalized. An alternative that is gaining wider acceptance is home services. These include visiting-nurse programs, some therapy, home health aides, and personal-care services.

Housing

Older people spend much of their time at home, usually because their mobility is reduced. And since their income is nearly always limited, they do not have as much money to spend on housing as they once did. People who plan housing for the elderly rarely take these factors into account. One out of every five older persons lives in substandard housing that is difficult to get to and is inadequately served by transportation facilities. About two-thirds of older people live in cities, quite often in neighborhoods that offer outmoded rental units such as single-room occupancy hotels.

The most common trends in housing for older people are high-rise, low-rent public housing projects for the poor and special retirement communities for more affluent retirees. Both types of facilities are segregated according to age. Researchers and specialists in aging cannot agree about whether this is desirable or not, since opinion is divided about the benefits and drawbacks of age segregation.

Nursing homes are a highly disputed alternate type of shelter. Though the quality and integrity of nursing homes vary widely, studies have shown that many are rife with fraudulent practices, providing little by way of nursing, as one researcher put it, and virtually nothing by way of a home. (A study by a committee of the U.S. Senate in 1986 found that one-third of the country's skilled nursing homes "failed to fully comply with the most essential health, safety, and quality standards of the federal government.") Many patients in

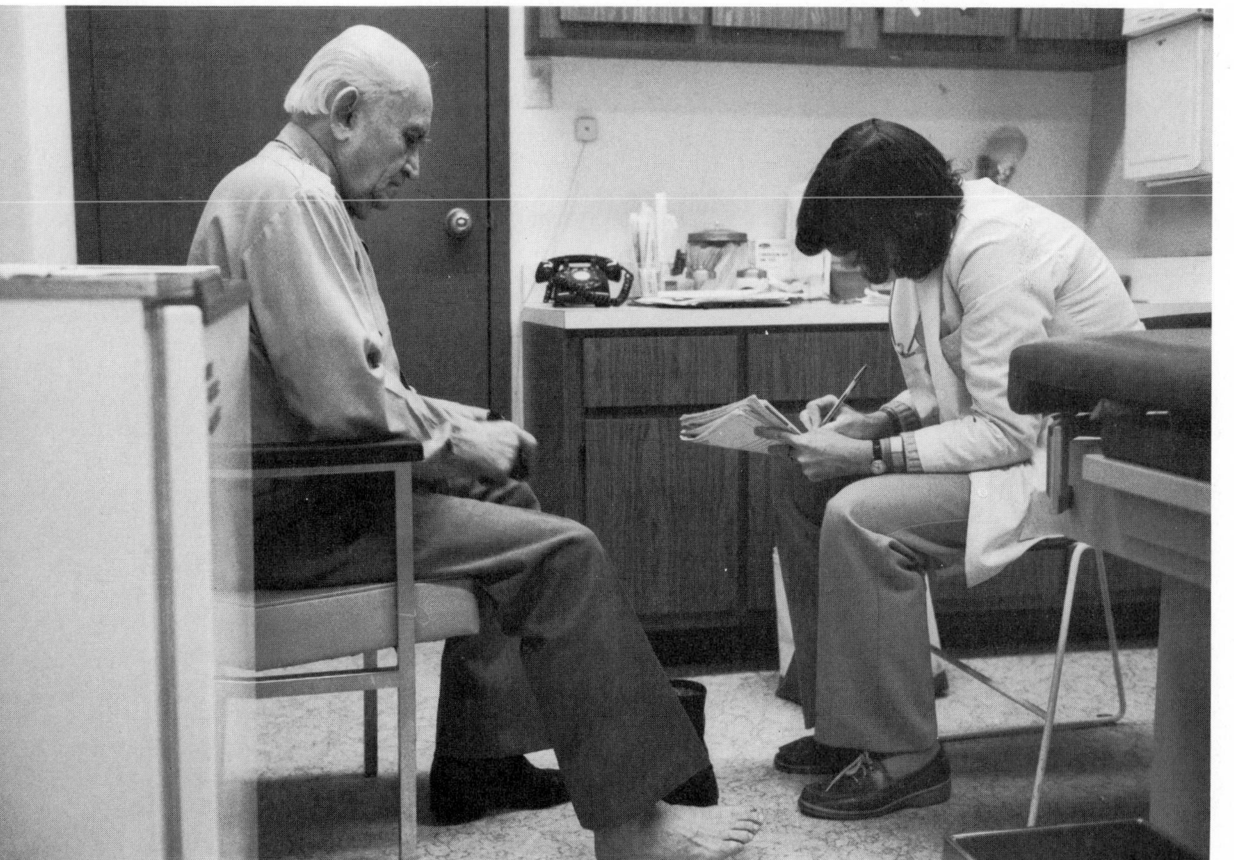

PROBLEMS AND CONTROVERSIES: Abuse of the Elderly

As many as 2½ million Americans over 65 (or 1 out of 25) are physically abused, neglected, or mistreated each year, making abuse of the elderly as common as abuse of children. The problem worsens each year as more and more people live into old age and have to be cared for by families who are not prepared for the task.

The most frequent victims are women aged 75 or older who depend on others for their care. Those most apt to be abusers, in order of frequency, are sons, daughters, spouses, and caretakers. The children of the elderly, perhaps middle-aged themselves, are often angry and resentful over being saddled with the responsibility of caring for a weak, aging parent who is often bedridden, unable to control body functions, and may require being fed. A large number were themselves abused as children by the very parents they are now caring for. In addition, many abusers have their own problems. Some are alcoholics or drug addicts; others are having marital and financial difficulties of their own.

Abuse of the elderly assumes many forms, some of them not obvious to an outsider. For example, sexual abuse often occurs, particularly rape of older women by sons-in-law or caretakers. The most common form, however, is material abuse—that is, denying an elderly person proper nutrition, clean bedding, and adequate toilet facilities. A devastating but hard-to-detect form of abuse is psychological; this ranges in severity from an occasional insult, to threats, to long-term efforts at intimidation.

Besides physical and psychological abuse, a great many elderly persons suffer financial exploitation by family members. Relatives may institutionalize an elderly person in order to confiscate his or her property. Nursing home managements are notorious for capitalizing on the financial resources of the elderly, often through the misappropriation of Social Security, Medicare, or Medicaid funds.

Abuse of the elderly is reported far less often than child abuse, and most of the reports come from third parties. When it is their own children who are the abusers, the elderly may be too embarrassed to tell. They are also afraid that if they cause trouble, their children will put them in a nursing home or some other institution, even when that might be the best solution for all concerned.

The potential for abuse of the elderly is bound to increase as the aging population swells in size. Half of the states have no laws protecting the rights of the elderly, and the laws that exist in the other half are often not enforced or are ineffective. But the same increase in numbers offers hope for improvement of the situation as the aging population becomes an increasingly potent political force in our society.

Sources: Adapted from Kathleen Doyle and Marilyn J. Morrow, "Elder Abuse Awareness Project," *Health Education*, October–November 1985, pp. 11–13; Donald Robinson, "How Can We Protect the Elderly?" *Parade Magazine*, February 17, 1985, pp. 5–7.

these facilities are not only sick but also indigent. Long-term nursing-home care is not covered by Medicare. Nursing-home operators are reimbursed for their services by Medicaid on a flat per-patient basis, and many find it easy to tamper with the system. One Chicago nursing home, for example, charged the government $14 per day per patient for food that cost only 78 cents.

Efforts to reform nursing-home abuses usually fail because the primary victims—the patients—are rarely able to protest their lot. This is an area that older people will doubtless pay more attention to as they become more politically organized.

Social Security

On average, retirement halves an individual's income. For people in the lower economic ranks, this involves a severe cutback in life style. Many rely totally on the Social Security system. Originally meant only to be a form of insurance against unexpected reductions in income, disability, or the death of a wage-earning spouse, Social Security has become for some the main source of income after retirement. In most cases, it is woefully inadequate. In 1984 the average monthly payment to retired workers was $461—a sum clearly not sufficient to meet basic needs.

Ageism

The aged are sometimes referred to as a minority group, and with some justification. Like members of racial and ethnic minorities, the elderly are victims of prejudice, stereotyping, and discrimination. Unlike many European and Asian countries, the United States upholds a standard of youthful beauty, activity, and productivity and stigmatizes those who do not conform to it. This attitude against the aged is so prevalent that the term **ageism** has been coined to denote it.

Ageism has spread to all levels of our society and is so pervasive that it may be impossible to eradicate it. In government, for example, the aged are frequent targets of spending reductions at both national and local levels. In business and industry forced retirement deprives people of their major means of earning a living.

More subtle, but no less inimical, is the treatment of the aged in the media. Television, which does so much to shape American attitudes, usually portrays the aged as either weak and vulnerable or unnaturally wise and kind. Nor do newspapers and magazines portray the aged any more realistically. News reportage on the aged usually concentrates on crime victims or eccentric "old-timers" who for one bizarre reason or another attract attention. Ignored are the many stable and productive old people who remain active in their communities.

Ageism has isolated the elderly from the mainstream of American life and

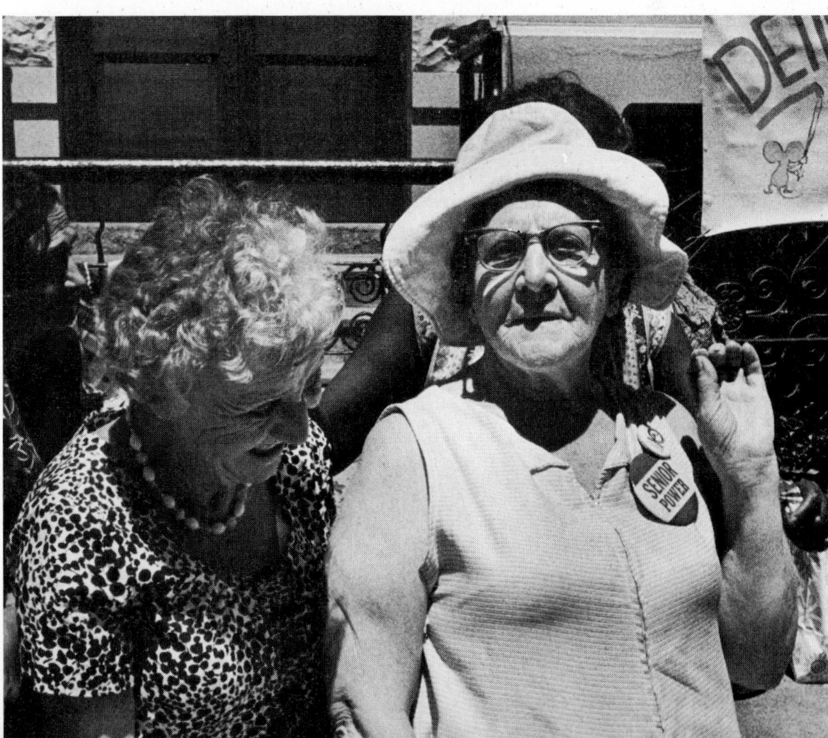

The Companionship of Pets

Psychiatrists, veterinarians, and social workers are just beginning to realize the implications of the fact that in the United States and similar societies, pets can serve as proxy humans. They are rapidly creating a whole industry of pet-assisted therapies based on the principle that animals can provide supportive companionship for people who are deprived of security, warmth, and love in their experiences with real humans. They are bringing pets into psychiatric wards and finding that patients who will not talk to people will talk to dogs, cats, and fish, and that once this breakthrough is achieved, patients become more responsive to their doctors and eventually talk to them, too. Pet-assisted therapies are also making their mark in nursing and retirement homes where loneliness, depression, boredom, and withdrawal are acute problems. After acquiring a pet, nursing home residents interact more with staff and other patients.

As proxy humans, pets can "stir the dead air" of empty apartments, and give countless single people someone to go home to. It is because they are proxy humans that they can stand in for absent or unsatisfactory husbands or wives or children, fill the empty nest, and ease the burden of loneliness which old age so often brings in hyperindustrial cultures. And they can do all this without imposing the suspicions and penalties characteristic of real humans caught up in highly competitive, stratified, and exploitative relationships.

Source: Marvin Harris, *Good to Eat*: *Riddles of Food and Culture* (New York: Simon and Schuster, 1985), pp. 196–97.

reduced their social contacts and income. As older people have grown more numerous, however, they have become a political force to be reckoned with, exerting influence upon legislation in which they have an interest.

Suicide One of the surest indices of the difficulties the aged face in our society is their higher-than-average suicide rate. The suicide rate for men over 65 is twice that for men of all ages. Studies have indicated that though declining health, loss of status, and reduced income are influencing factors in suicides among the aged, the most salient cause is a lack of relationships. It has been found, for example, that widowed males are among the most likely older groups to commit suicide. Among women, the loss of a spouse seems to be less traumatic. Elderly women are more likely to have extended family ties, friends, and club relationships that provide them with social buffers against suicide. Elderly men who have these kinds of contacts are far less likely to commit suicide. The highest suicide rate among the elderly, however, occurs among the socially disadvantaged. Besides being poor, these disadvantaged people are less likely to be married, to be in touch with relatives, or to be involved with social organizations.

If there is one conclusion to be drawn from a study of the aged in America, it is that they are a varied and disparate group. There are too many differences among those in the wide time span that the old age period covers to lump them into a stereotyped mass. There are the active and the ill, the indigent and the solvent, the vibrantly committed and the passively indifferent.

MISCONCEPTIONS ABOUT THE AGED

Many popular myths about the aged have arisen over the centuries, and they are difficult to dislodge, even in the face of contradicting facts. The elderly are often characterized as senile, lacking in individuality, tranquil, unproductive, conservative, and resistant to change. Some of the most distorting myths about the elderly concern older women, who are devalued in our society sooner than men.

Health

The elderly are considered to be more hypochondriacal than the young, and elderly women in particular are thought to have more health problems—real or imaginary—than the rest of the population. Studies show, however, that no substantial difference exists in the health status of older men and women. Sometimes women, many of whom have been rewarded throughout life for appearing delicate, act slightly pessimistic about their health, while men, many of whom have been rewarded for ignoring pain and appearing robust, express more optimism. Elderly women, in fact, are more likely than younger women to avoid seeking necessary medical care; but elderly men are more likely than younger men to go to a physician with a problem. In general, older people who believe they are in good health and have no chronic condition see physicians less often than their younger counterparts.

In general, older people do not neglect themselves as some may think. The fact that more and more people are living into their 70s and 80s is evidence of this. It appears that the older population is adopting healthful living styles just like their younger counterparts.

Widowhood

According to a popular stereotype, a widow continues to base her identity on that of her dead husband. This is generally untrue; older women demonstrate a strong sense of personal identity. Women react not according to their age, but according to their socioeconomic and educational level when confronted with widowhood: Well-educated and working-class women experience less crisis than others.

Nevertheless, women are more likely than men to spend their final years in widowhood. Fifty percent of women over 65 are widowed, 40 percent are married, and only 10 percent are divorced or were never married. Some 79 percent of men over 65 are married, however. This reflects the fact that women as a group outlive men, and the fact that older men who want to remarry after the death of a spouse have more partners in their own and younger age groups to choose from. Marriage between older men and younger women is usually socially accepted, while marriage between older women and younger men rarely is.

Sexual Activity

The most widely held misconception concerning the old is that they are sexually inactive; they are said to lack both the desire and the ability to have sexual relationships. In fact, many studies have found that sex continues to play an important role in most older people's lives, though interest and activity do tend to decline with age. Older men, however, tend to have more sexual interest and to be more sexually active than older women. One reason for this difference

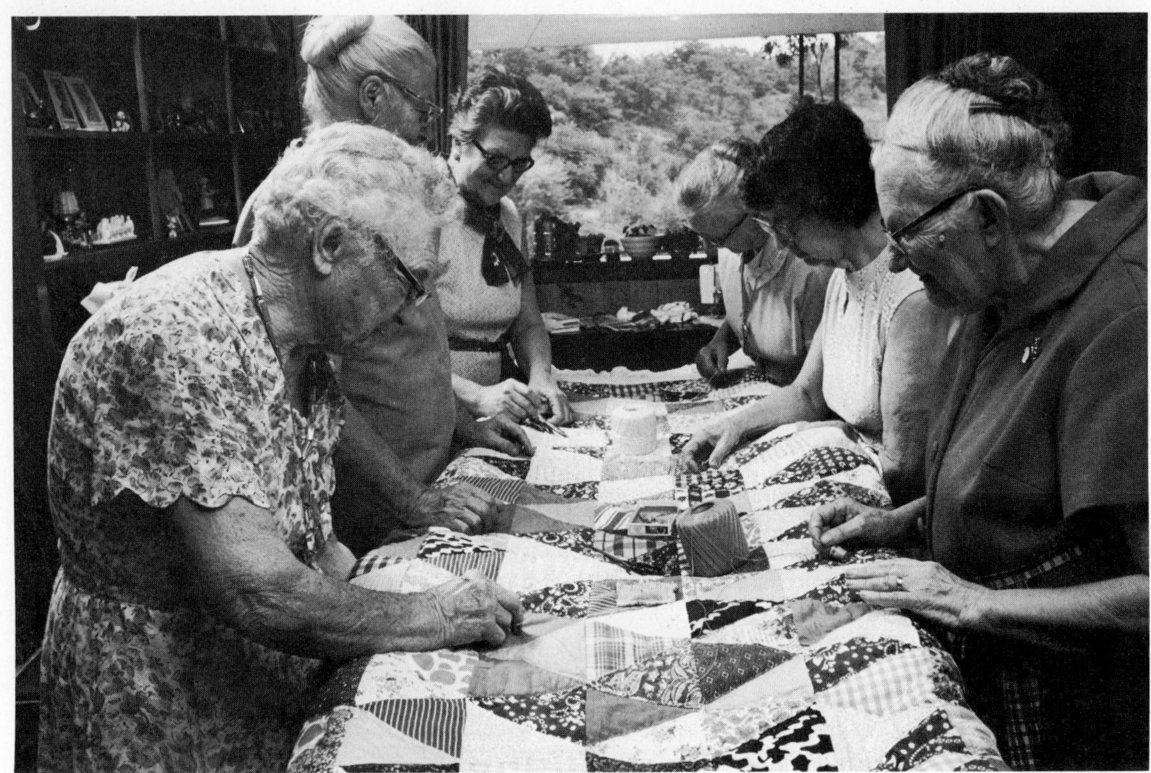

Women outlive men, and there are many more widows than widowers. Those who have led active social lives while married usually continue to do so after the death of their husbands.

may be that older men are more likely to have readily available, socially sanctioned, and sexually capable partners. Many age-related changes in sexual behavior have their antecedents in a person's sexual history. Older people who have been sexually active throughout their adult lives continue to enjoy sexual activity in old age. Those who had less than satisfactory sex lives tend to use age as an excuse for avoiding sex.

Family Ties and the Aged

One of the most persistent myths about the "good old days" is that there was a Golden Age in the United States when most families were composed of several generations, all living happily and supportively together. Studies show, however, that though the extended family was certainly more common in the past than it is today (see Chapter 9), it was never the norm in the United States. Neither is it true, as is often indicated in the press and in fiction, that older persons are usually abandoned by their children. Most old people who live alone today do so voluntarily. About 18 percent of America's aged do live with one of their children. Many others see their children frequently, as often as several times a week. The only safe generalization to make about the aged is that they prefer to be independent.

DYING AND DEATH

Most of us think of dying as something that other people do. We have not been taught to regard death as the inevitable conclusion to the life cycle, the rounding out of a life span. One reason the aged are viewed with distaste is because they are approaching an event that most of us would just as soon not think about. Dying, in our culture, is done out of sight; the terminally ill are segregated from the living in antiseptic cubicles and surrounded by medical paraphernalia. One indication of our society's deep fear of death is the extravagant means our medical technology uses to keep people alive, regardless of the quality of the life that is being so fiercely prolonged. There can be no more explicit statement made about our loathing of death than the sight of a comatose patient hooked up to a "life-support" system that sustains what can only be called a parody of living.

Though people rarely wish to die, the inevitability of death was more easily accepted in past generations. This is because death was not so rigorously hidden from view. In recent years psychiatrists and others have made new efforts to weave death once more into the fabric of life and to remove the apprehension that it generally inspires. We shall discuss some of those efforts in this section and consider some appropriate methods of dealing with grief. But first let us take a look at death itself.

Defining Death

Just as most of us think we know who the aged are, so most of us believe we could recognize death if we saw it. Yet, in the same way that there are different levels of aging, so there are different definitions and degrees of death; medical, legal, and theological experts have disputed exactly when death occurs.

Though death is obviously the cessation of life, its measurement has been subject to debate. Theologians define death as the moment the soul leaves the body. Death occurs in a legal sense when a physician or coroner signs a death certificate.

In the past death was said to take place when the heart stopped beating. It is now known, however, that the brain continues to function for about ten minutes after the cessation of the heartbeat. Consequently, brain activity is the criterion that separates life from death; and when the brain ceases to function, the person is considered to be medically dead. Brain death is most reliably shown on an **electroencephalogram** (EEG), which is a record of brain waves made by a device that detects electrical activity in the brain by means of electrodes attached to the scalp.

Coping with Death

At some point in our lives most of us will be called upon to deal with the death of a parent, relative, or friend. These situations sometimes occur abruptly, making it difficult for us to cope with them. As medical science becomes more sophisticated, however, individuals can be diagnosed as terminal earlier and earlier in the course of their illness. This gives everyone—the dying person as well as family and friends—more time to prepare for death with grace and dignity. Several issues have been raised by this development, as well as by the more enlightened view of dying that is beginning to prevail in our society.

How Long Will You Live?

Start with the number 72.

Personal Facts:

_______ If you are male, subtract 3.
_______ If female, add 4.
_______ If you live in an urban area with a population over 2 million, subtract 2.
_______ If you live in a town under 10,000 or on a farm, add 2.
_______ If any grandparent lived to 85, add 2.
_______ If all four grandparents lived to 80, add 6.
_______ If either parent died of a stroke or heart attack before the age of 50, subtract 4.
_______ If any parent, brother or sister under 50 has (or had) cancer or a heart condition, or has had diabetes since childhood, subtract 3.
_______ Do you earn over $50,000 a year? Subtract 2.
_______ If you finished college, add 1. If you have a graduate or professional degree, add 2 more.
_______ If you are 65 or over and still working, add 3.
_______ If you live with a spouse or friend, add 5. If not, subtract 1 for every ten years alone since age 25.

Life-Style Status:

_______ If you work behind a desk, subtract 3.
_______ If your work requires regular, heavy physical labor, add 3.
_______ If you exercise strenuously (tennis, running, swimming, etc.) five times a week for at least a half-hour, add 4. Two or three times a week, add 2.
_______ Do you sleep more than ten hours each night? Subtract 4.
_______ Are you intense, aggressive, easily angered? Subtract 3.
_______ Are you easygoing and relaxed? Add 3.
_______ Are you happy? Add 1. Unhappy? Subtract 2.
_______ Have you had a speeding ticket in the past year? Subtract 1.
_______ Do you smoke more than two packs a day? Subtract 8. One to two packs? Subtract 6. One-half to one?· Subtract 3.
_______ Do you drink the equivalent of 1½ oz. of liquor a day? Subtract 1.
_______ Are you overweight by 50 lbs. or more? Subtract 8. By 30 to 50 lbs.? Subtract 4 By 10 to 30 pounds? Subtract 2.
_______ If you are a man over 40 and have annual checkups, add 2.
_______ If you are a woman and see a gynecologist once a year, add 2.

Age Adjustment:

_______ If you are between 30 and 40, add 2.
_______ If you are between 40 and 50, add 3.
_______ If you are between 50 and 70, add 4.
_______ If you are over 70, add 5.

_______ **Add up your score to get your life expectancy.**

Source: Robert F. Allen with Shirley Linde, *Lifegain*: *The Exciting New Program That Will Change Your Health and Your Life* (New York: Appleton-Century-Crofts, 1981). Reprinted by permission of Prentice-Hall, Inc.

Informing the Dying. Once an individual is deemed terminal, the question arises whether he or she should be told of the diagnosis. Studies have shown that most physicians prefer not to tell patients of their impending death. Many experts on dying deplore this secrecy and suggest that it robs patients of the opportunity to get their lives in order and to prepare themselves for a dignified death. Still others argue that telling a patient he or she is going to die induces despair and may interfere with the patient's response to a possible cure.

There is no rule of thumb about whether patients should be told of their impending death. Informing the terminally ill of their condition is not, however, as common as one might expect; and this probably reflects the discomfort that most of us feel about death.

Stages of Dying. Most terminal patients are still treated brusquely and fatalistically by medical personnel, as though there is nothing more to be done for them since they are fated to die anyway. Recently, however, attitudes toward dying have become more enlightened, and we are learning that the experience of dying can be enhanced by intelligent and caring assistance. The pioneer in the psychiatric work that has helped professionals deal with the terminally ill is Dr. Elisabeth Kübler-Ross. After working with many terminal patients. Kübler-Ross identified five stages, or phases, that many of the dying pass through. An understanding and acceptance of the normalcy of the dying process enables us to prepare for and be more comfortable with the stages as they occur. It is important to note, however, that not everyone goes through all five of the stages, nor do they occur in any particular order. That is, some patients may go directly to stage 4; other may never leave stage 2.

Stage 1: Denial. "No, not me," is the reaction of many patients immediately after they learn they are terminally ill. They do not believe that such a thing could happen to them, and they search for other, more optimistic, opinions.

Stage 2: Anger. Anger, rage, envy, and resentment replace denial as a defense mechanism against the realization of death. Patients may direct these feelings at doctors, nurses, family, or friends. They feel frustrated that their life plans will not be completed.

Stage 3: Bargaining. At this stage people try to bargain with God, doctors, nurses, clergymen, or anyone they feel can help them live just a little bit longer, or who can help them overcome their pain and suffering.

Stage 4: Depression. When people realize that their time is running out, hopelessness and depression set in. They mourn for things they lost in the past, and for what they will miss in the future. Note that this is a potentially positive stage of dying; it helps people to accept their death.

Stage 5: Acceptance. At this stage people wait quietly for their death. A less fulfilling variation is resignation, in which people simply give up, saying "What's the use?" Kübler-Ross tried to help her patients experience acceptance instead of resignation.

We must realize, however, that people face death in individual ways; we should not try to force anyone into a particular pattern.

Life Expectancy at Birth, Selected Countries

Hong Kong	76
Iceland	76
Japan	76
The Netherlands	75
Norway	75
Sweden	75
Switzerland	75
Canada	74
Denmark	74
Puerto Rico	74
United States	74
Australia	73
Belgium	73
Cuba	73
Finland	73
Greece	73
Ireland	73
Israel	73
Italy	73
New Zealand	73
Spain	73
United Kingdom	73

Source: Population Reference Bureau (with UNICEF), *1982 World's Children Data Sheet* (Washington, D.C., 1982).

Assisting the Dying. If you are put in a position to aid the dying, you should keep in mind these three points:

First, you must accept your own mortality. If you cannot do this, and cannot tolerate the idea of death to any degree, then it will be impossible for you to help someone else arrive at the stage of acceptance.

Second, you cannot appoint yourself to help the dying—you must be chosen

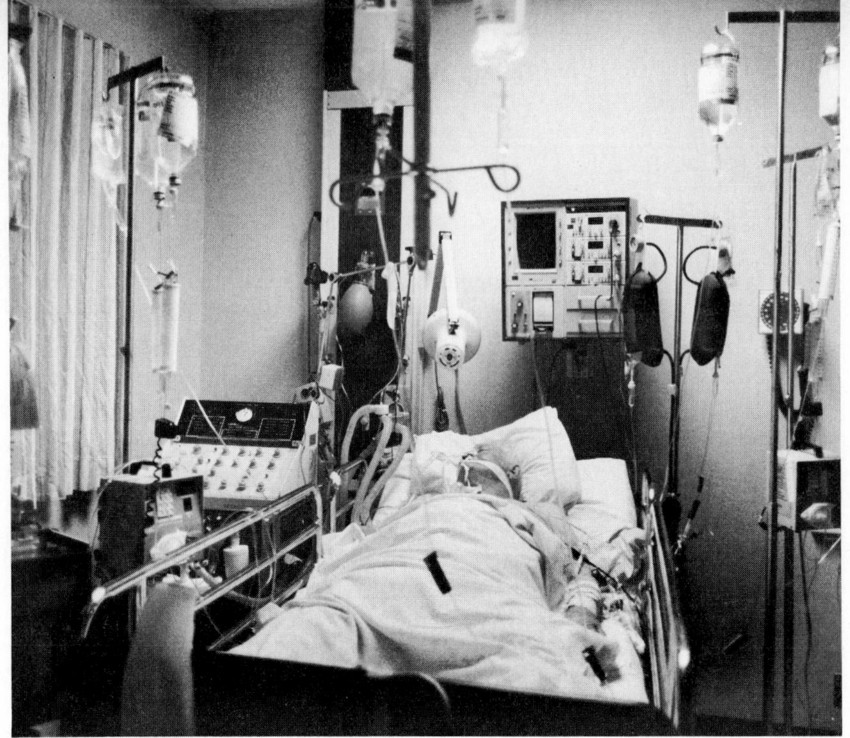

Whether we like it or not, most of us will die away from home, perhaps in the intensive care ward of a hospital.

by them. No matter how strong your feelings of responsibility toward the dying person are, if he or she does not select you for help, your only recourse is to step aside.

Third, if you are selected, your major obligation is to listen. It is a mistake to be aggressively cheerful or relentlessly positive in the face of death. Just let the dying person tell you what he or she is going through.

Rights of the Dying. The act of dying should not deprive anyone of the rights he or she has always had. These include the following:

1. The right to continue to grow and function in all dimensions: physical, mental, emotional, social, and spiritual.
2. The right to receive honest answers to questions.
3. The right to request or refuse medication.
4. The right to be included in any decisions about prolonging life artificially.
5. The right to be treated as a human being, not as a medical exhibit.
6. The right to die in a state of acceptance and peace.

Where We Die

In the past people died at home surrounded by family, friends, and familiar objects; today only about 20 percent of all deaths occur at home. Death has been relegated instead to special premises such as bleak hospital wards and nursing homes. There are signs, however, that such insensitivity to the needs of the dying are changing—although very slowly.

Hospital. Life, not death, is the business of hospitals. Cure, not comfort, is their primary concern. The terminally ill patient in a hospital is often treated like a dehumanized biological specimen, not like a person. In the attempt to

Where to Find Help for the Elderly

American Geriatric Society
10 Columbus Circle
New York, N.Y. 10019
(212) 582-1333

Association for Alzheimer's and Related Diseases
360 North Michigan Avenue
Chicago, Ill. 60601
(800) 621-0379

National Council on the Aging
1828 L Street, N.W., Suite 504
Washington, D.C. 20036
(202) 223-6250

National Hospice Organization
1901 North Fort Myer Drive, Suite 902
Arlington, Va. 22209
(703) 243-5900

For adults who may need protection:

Contact your local department of social services or write to:

Project Focus
Department P, FAS, Room 9438
60 Hudson Street
New York, N.Y. 10013

For information on nursing homes, write to:

American Health Care Association
1200 15th Street N.W.
Washington, D.C. 20005

cure illness and conquer death, hospitals sometimes keep patients alive against all reason. Ironically, physicians and medical staff are often the last ones to accept the inevitability of death. A dying patient often recognizes his or her condition before others do and may wish to let go of life with a measure of dignity. But medical staffs are committed to the philosophy of preserving life and feel it their obligation to employ every available means to forestall death. This attitude has come under intense criticism lately.

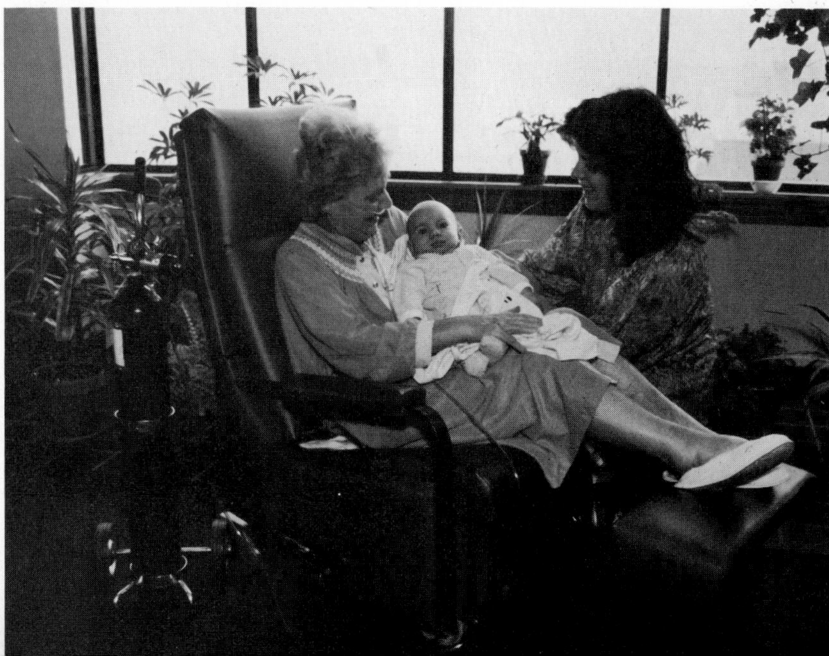

In this dayroom of a hospice, a patient enjoys a visit from her daughter and grandchild while receiving the oxygen she requires.

Hospice Care. It is possible, however, to offer the terminally ill—usually cancer patients—a humanized environment in which to pass their final days and die with dignity. Such an environment can be provided by **hospice** services either in the patient's own home or in a homelike hospice facility.

There are a number of major differences between hospice and hospital care. Unlike hospital care, hospice care is not structured to promote a cure but to make the last days of the terminally ill as painfree and comfortable as possible. For that reason, hospice care is not concerned about a dying patient's becoming addicted to painkilling drugs, so it does not strictly control the dosage of such drugs, as hospitals do. Equally important, hospice care does not include lifesaving measures such as respirators and mechanical support systems. By the time a patient needs hospice care, it is assumed that he or she does not want to be kept alive by artificial means.

Most hospice care takes place in the home, and is provided by the patient's relatives and friends, not by nurses. Nursing care that may be required can be tailored to the patient's situation; it can range from round-the-clock nursing shifts to occasional visits to on-call service. Backup arrangements can be made with a nearby hospital for emergency situations.

Hospice care gives family and friends an opportunity to comfort the dying person and to share time with him or her. While hospitals usually limit the number of visitors a dying person may have, the hospice arrangement encourages them. And while hospitals often put dying patients on a restricted diet, hospice care allows visitors to bring special food. After a patient dies, the hospital

FIGURE 10-1

The living will

TO MY FAMILY, MY PHYSICIAN, MY LAWYER, MY CLERGYMAN
TO ANY MEDICAL FACILITY IN WHOSE CARE I HAPPEN TO BE
TO ANY INDIVIDUAL WHO MAY BECOME RESPONSIBLE FOR MY HEALTH, WELFARE OR AFFAIRS

Death is as much a reality as birth, growth, maturity and old age—it is the one certainty of life. If the time comes when I, ______________________ can no longer take part in decisions for my own future, let this statement stand as an expression of my wishes, while I am still of sound mind.

If the situation should arise in which there is no reasonable expectation of my recovery from physical or mental disability, I request that I be allowed to die and not be kept alive by artificial means or "heroic measures." I do not fear death itself as much as the indignities of deterioration, dependence and hopeless pain. I, therefore, ask that medication be mercifully administered to me to alleviate suffering even though this may hasten the moment of death.

This request is made after careful consideration. I hope you who care for me will feel morally bound to follow its mandate. I recognize that this appears to place a heavy responsibility upon you, but it is with the intention of relieving you of such responsibility and of placing it upon myself in accordance with my strong convictions, that this statement is made.

Signed ______________________

Date ______________________

Witness ______________________

Witness ______________________

Copies of this request have been given to ______________________
____
____
____

closes its file on the case; hospice services, by contrast, maintain contact with family and friends and help them through the mourning process.

At present there are about 1,700 hospice services in the United States. Some are associated with hospitals, while others are independent or are part of the services offered by health-care agencies. Now that new rules make it possible for hospitals to be reimbursed by Medicare for hospice service, such arrangements should become even more widespread. In addition, some private insurance companies are beginning to offer hospice-care coverage.

Terminating Medical Support

Medical technology has made it possible to substitute artificial devices for human body systems. Tubes can deliver nutrition into the gastrointestinal tract and eliminate waste from the body. An artificial respirator can breathe for a patient, and electronic devices can keep the heart going. The body can be kept alive almost indefinitely. For the individual patient, however, the question arises whether such heroic measures are prolonging life or only prolonging dying. For society as a whole, there is the additional question of whether we can afford to use the expensive technology we are capable of producing. When, we must ask, should a terminally ill individual be allowed to die?

Euthanasia. The term *euthanasia* is derived from the Greek words *eu*, meaning "well" or "good," and *thanatos*, meaning "death." Although euthanasia sometimes refers to "mercy killing," or the practice of administering a painless death to the hopelessly ill or injured, in current usage it refers to withdrawing life support from the dying and allowing death to occur naturally.

There are two forms of euthanasia, voluntary and involuntary. *Voluntary euthanasia* occurs when a patient cooperates in allowing his or her death, usually by asking not to be attached to life-sustaining machinery or to have such machinery removed if already attached. Physicians, it must be noted, are under no legal obligation to do as a patient requests. Some physicians, in fact, have been tried for murder after removing life-sustaining machinery.

An organization called Concern for Dying (formerly the Euthanasia Educational Council) has written a contract for dying people that exonerates physicians in the event of voluntary euthanasia. It is called a *living will* (see Figure 10-1), and it states, in essence, that the patient who has signed it does not wish to prolong his or her own life artificially. Thirty-five states and the District of Columbia have laws making the living will a valid representation of its maker's wishes. Surveys show that the overwhelming majority of physicians support voluntary euthanasia. The medical community, however, has avoided going on record as doing so.

Involuntary euthanasia occurs when a patient is in a coma or is otherwise incapable of making a decision. At some point the relatives and the physician may decide that death is preferable to the quality of life that is being sustained. The most celebrated case in recent times is that of Karen Ann Quinlin, who went into a deep coma after allegedly ingesting drugs. She was able to breathe only with the help of a respirator. After three months she showed no sign of improvement, and there was no hope of a cure. When her parents learned that she would not live without the respirator, they decided that their only recourse was to allow her to die, and insisted it be disconnected. Her physicians refused, stating that their goal was to save her life. After a seven-month court battle the parents won the suit, and the respirator was ordered removed. In essence, this decision meant that involuntary euthanasia was now supported by the legal system. (Contrary to the physicians' predictions, Karen Ann Quinlin continued to breathe after the respirator was removed, and remained in a coma but alive for 10 years.)

FUNERALS

Almost every culture in history has employed some kind of formal ceremony or ritual by which to honor the recently dead. Though such ceremonies are performed ostensibly to show respect for the dead, they also undoubtedly benefit the living.

In the United States funeral rites are more lavish and expensive than in most other countries. The average American funeral costs between $1,500 and $2,500, which is about ten times the cost of a funeral in, for example, Great Britain. The major reason for the disparity is that we demand more elaborate burial preparations than do most other countries and feel obliged to put on a greater ceremonial display.

Burial

In the United States formal burial is the most common kind of funeral, and there is usually a specific sequence of events in preparing the body for the ceremony. A funeral director is called in to take the corpse to the funeral home. Then whoever is making the arrangements for the funeral is consulted

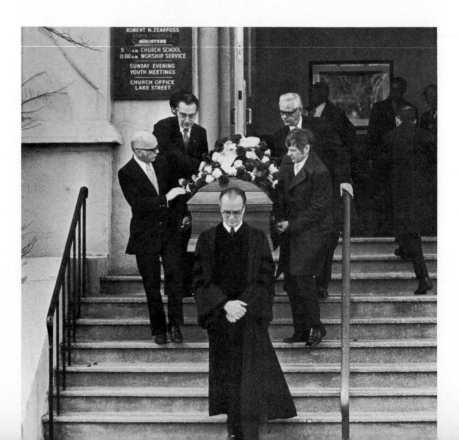

about the type of casket and the details of the service; required forms are filled out.

The body is almost always embalmed. This is not legally required in the United States, although many people think it is. If the funeral service and burial are to take place within twenty-four hours after death, embalming is unnecessary. Beyond that span of time, particularly in warmer climates, the body begins to deteriorate visibly unless it has been embalmed.

After embalming, the corpse is dressed and cosmetics are applied to make it appear lifelike. Often the body is put on view in an open casket for a period of time before the actual service and burial.

Cremation

Funeral expenses can be vastly reduced and the services of a funeral director eliminated by having the body *cremated*—that is, reduced to ashes by the use of fire. Although cremation is one of the oldest forms of disposing of the dead (it was used by the Greeks 3,000 years ago) and one of the most prevalent in modern societies (75 percent of the Japanese dead, for example, are cremated), it is comparatively recent and rare in the United States. The first crematory was constructed in this country in 1876, and today only about 5 percent of all American dead are cremated.

Cremation does not necessarily entail the elimination of funeral practices such as viewing the body, however. The body can be cremated after the service. The savings in cost come about because no casket is required (though most funeral directors urge the use of one); no burial plot is necessary; and if there is no viewing, or if the cremation is held within twenty-four hours of death, embalming can be dispensed with.

The funeral rite plays a significant role in the mourning process because it brings together family and friends and melds them into a support system, pays tribute to the deceased, and soothes the survivors.

MOURNING

Though the experience of grief and mourning varies from person to person, it assumes a fairly predictable pattern for most survivors. Regardless of the degree of intimacy between the survivor and the dead person, death always takes a toll on those left behind. You may recall from our discussion of stress (Chapter 2) that on a scale of 1 to 43, the death of a close friend ranks 17, of a family member, 5, and of a spouse, 1. The death of a spouse is obviously the most stressful event most people ever experience.

Several behavioral and emotional disturbances are common in mourning; these may include difficulty in sleeping, over- or undereating, being easily angered or irritated, feeling guilty, feeling sad, and crying. Such behavior following a death should not be considered abnormal or critical unless it continues beyond a year or so.

Many people go through five stages of mourning that are similar to the stages of dying described by Elisabeth Kübler-Ross. The stages of mourning also resemble the stages of dying in that they vary from person to person in intensity and duration. Many people require two or three years to work through the stages of mourning following the death of a beloved spouse.

Stage 1. When a loved one is ill for an extended time before dying, the

Donation of Body Parts

Medical science can transplant about two dozen different tissues and organs from one person (donor) to another (recipient). In 1968 the Uniform Anatomical Gift Act was introduced federally and passed in each state. The result is a uniform donor card available from your local chapter of the American Medical Association or possibly from your physician. The card may be signed by anyone over 18 and allows one to donate any part or all of his or her body for purposes of transplantation, medical research, or anatomical study. Money cannot legally be paid for the donation. It is a gift. Over 200,000 people are known to have signed such cards, and the number is growing steadily. In fact, there is no reliable way to determine how many have donated part or all of their bodies since many states are now printing an anatomical gift statement (donor card) on the back of their state driver's license. All you need to do is fill it out and sign it in the presence of two witnesses. The gift you give upon your death may indeed help someone else to live a full and productive life.

UNIFORM DONOR CARD

OF________________________

Print or type name of donor

In the hope that I may help others, I hereby make this anatomical gift, if medically acceptable, to take effect upon my death. The words and marks below indicate my desires.

I give: (a) _____ any needed organs or parts

(b) _____ only the following organs or parts

____

Specify the organ(s) or part(s)

for the purposes of transplantation, therapy, medical research or education;

(c) _____ my body for anatomical study if needed.

Limitations or special wishes, if any:____________________

08-21-81 100M/82

Signed by the donor and the following two witnesses in the presence of each other:

Signature of Donor __________ Date of Birth of Donor __________

Date Signed __________ City & State __________

Witness __________ Witness __________

This is a legal document under the Uniform Anatomical Gift Act or similar laws.

For further information consult your physician or

National Kidney Foundation, Inc.
2 Park Avenue, New York, N.Y. 10016

first stage of mourning often begins before death occurs. Most of the time, however, it begins at the time of death and typically lasts about a month. It is characterized by shock and denial of the death of the loved one.

Stage 2. Stage 2 consists of a short period of false acceptance and generally lasts only until the beginning of the second month following the death. The mourner may appear to accept the death but is actually still shocked, numb, and in a state of disbelief.

Stage 3. Stage 3 can best be called pseudo-reorganization. It typically lasts until about the beginning of the third month. In this stage the mourner seems to have adjusted to the death and appears to be on the road to recovery. The appearance is false, however, although it is more convincing than stage 2.

Stage 4. Stage 4 is a period of depression that typically lasts about five months. On the surface the mourner may appear to have recovered, but inside the realization of the finality of death has caused a depression.

Stage 5. Stage 5 is a recovery period, which can begin as early as the eighth month. In this period the death has been accepted by the mourner, who can now take up his or her life where it left off.

Obviously, the times given for these stages can vary greatly, depending upon the personality of the mourner and his or her closeness to the deceased.

Abnormal Grief

Some abnormal psychological reactions to grief may require counseling.

Morbid Grief Reaction. This is a condition in which the mourner postpones the mourning process for days, weeks, months, or even years after the death. Outwardly, the mourner might appear indifferent and become absorbed in work or other involvements. Generally, however, he or she will eventually succumb to the mourning process and work through the five stages.

Pathological Mourning. In this condition the mourner collects, saves, and honors everything the deceased owned or touched. He or she might build a shrine to the deceased, sometimes secretly. The mourner may withdraw from society in order to live in the world he or she has built to commemorate the deceased. In extreme cases, mourners are unable to restructure their lives and must seek professional help.

SUMMARY

1. The aged in the United States are both sentimentalized and disparaged. As the number of elderly continues to grow, however (they will number 30 million by the year 2000), they will constitute an ever more powerful political force.

2. Although everyone does not age at the same rate, certain physical signs can generally be recognized in the skin, hair, body size, and senses. Older people are also more susceptible to illness—particularly *chronic illness*. Although intelligence does not diminish with age, there is some loss in memory ability.

3. Sixty-five has become the generally accepted age at which people are declared senior citizens, or old. This, however, is an arbitrary yardstick that was created by the Social Security Act. It conceals the fact that there are great differences in ability among people in the same age group. For this reason, researchers have begun to group older people into the "young-old" and the "old-old"—categories that are based not on chronological age but on physical and psychological abilities.

4. No one understands exactly why the human body ages, but there are many theories: some believe that heredity controls the aging process; some that the body simply wears out; others believe that the body chemistry degenerates; and still others think that the cells become incapable of reproducing.

5. Old age is practically synonymous with retirement in our society. Retirement can be especially traumatic for those who derived their sense of self-worth entirely from work and for those whose retirement incomes are meager or whose health is poor.

6. Certain social problems take on a special significance for the elderly. Health care, for example, in spite of Medicaid and Medicare, is still inadequate. Housing for the elderly is frequently substandard. Social Security, which constitutes a main source of income for the majority of old people and the sole source for a very significant number, is not enough to meet basic needs. The aged are targets of prejudice so marked that it has given rise to the term *ageism*.

7. Many common beliefs regarding the elderly are being disproved. The most widely held misconception is that the aged lose interest in sexual activity. On the contrary, sex continues to play an important part in most older people's lives.

8. Just as we distort the idea of age, so we try to disguise the reality of death. Death is now said to occur when the brain ceases to function. One of the current disputes about dying is whether to inform a terminal patient that he or she is dying; generally, physicians do not like to do so. A pioneer in the field of dying. Dr. Elizabeth Kübler-Ross, has found that a terminal patient may pass through five stages: denial, anger, bargaining, depression, and acceptance. These stages are not necessarily negotiated in any particular order. Anyone who wishes to aid the dying does best to simply listen to the patient.

9. Traditionally, people died at home. Today they are more likely to die in hospitals or hospices. The *hospice* is a recent institution that is designed especially to aid the dying. Hospice care is also available for patients who wish to die at home.

10. *Euthanasia*, or allowing a terminal patient to die without trying to prolong life artificially, is a controversial social and moral problem. Most physicians favor voluntary euthanasia, though not officially; involuntary euthanasia has been sanctioned by the legal decision in the Karen Ann Quinlin case.

11. The most common type of funeral in America is the burial, which is chosen for 95 percent of the nation's dead. Cremation is an option that costs considerably less.

12. The intensity and duration of mourning vary from individual to individual depending on the degree of closeness to the deceased. Most survivors complete the process of mourning within a year.

CONSUMER CONCERNS

1. A possibility that should receive consideration in respect to caring for the aged is home care. Bringing a service to the elderly rather than taking the elderly to a service has many advantages. Are you aware of them?
2. On retirement the elderly often seek relocation. What might be some sound reasons for moving to a new area at this stage of life? What might be equally valid reasons for not moving?
3. From what sources can a person planning relocation get accurate information on the desirability of different areas? Are you aware of the assistance provided by the American Association of Retired Persons (AARP)?
4. A concern for the elderly upon retirement may be health insurance coverage. A job-based insurance plan may be discontinued. Medicare may prove inadequate. What might be special aspects of a health insurance policy that an older person might require?
5. Preparing a will may prevent much dispute and preclude many legal expenditures out of one's estate. Are you aware of the advantages of having a will and do you know how to go about making one?

11

Alcohol

What Is Alcohol?
Processing Alcohol
Effects of Alcohol on the Body
Alcohol and Our Society
Alcohol and Youth
Women and Alcohol
The Problem of Alcoholism
How Alcoholism Begins and Develops
Effects of Alcoholism on the Individual
Effects of Alcohol on Society
Treatment of Alcoholism
Conquering Alcohol Abuse

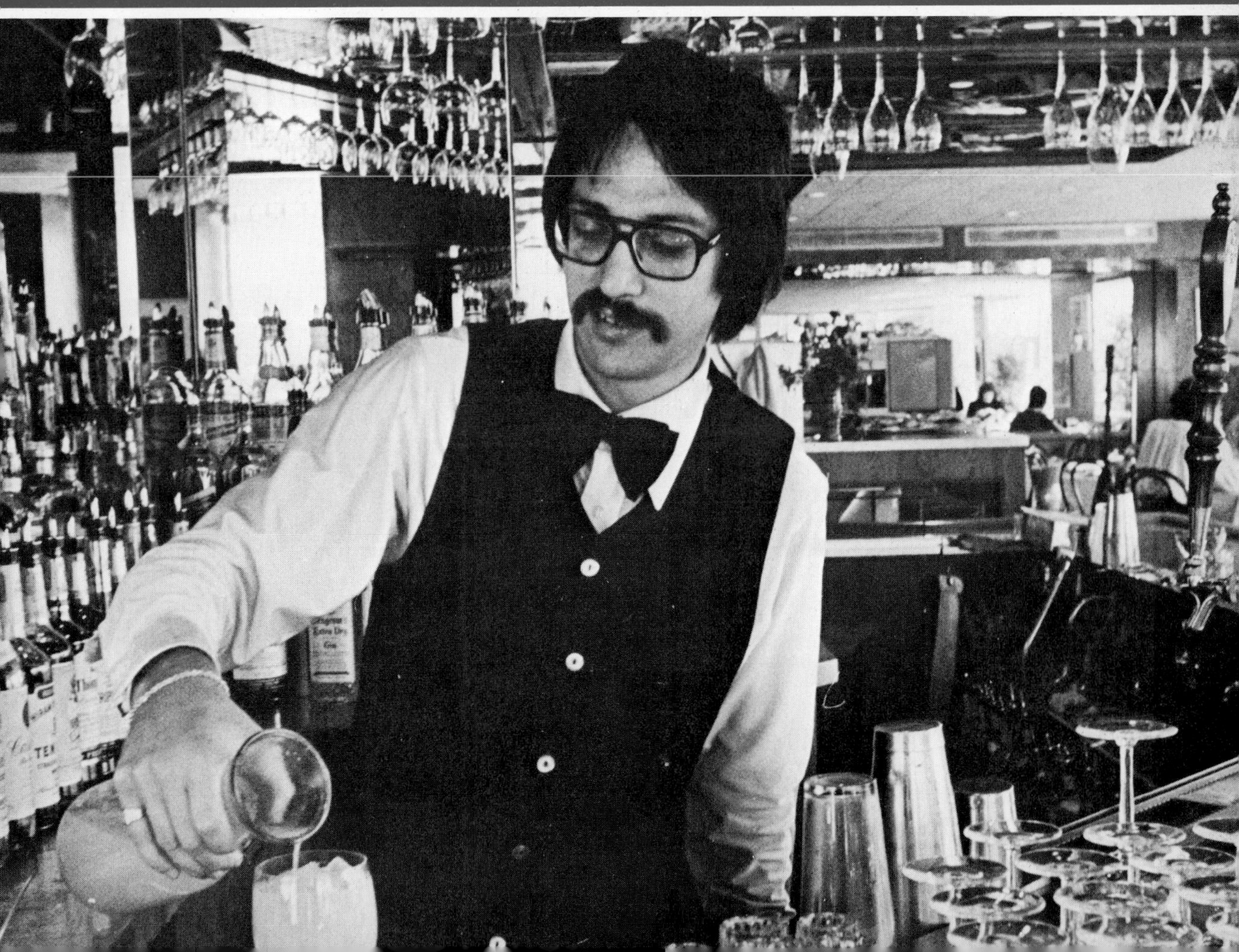

With nearly 14 million problem drinkers in the United States, alcoholism is a growing social and medical problem. Yet alcohol abuse has seldom been considered the serious—indeed, life-threatening—problem that it is. Because alcohol abuse is sheltered by our approval of drinking—and our belief in the individual's right to drink—it has taken us a long time to realize the seriousness of alcohol's effects. But we can no longer ignore the facts. Alcoholism and alcohol abuse costs the nation $117 billion each year in lost production, medical costs, traffic accidents, and judicial, rehabilitative, and social services. Intoxicated drivers are responsible for half of the deaths in automobile accidents each year. Alcohol abuse plays a big role in many of the violent crimes that plague our society, including manslaughter, robbery, and assault. Alcohol has been estimated to be associated with 65 percent of murders, 55 percent of domestic fights, 40 percent of assaults, 35 percent of rapes, 30 percent of suicides, and 60 percent of child abuse cases. In addition, alcoholism tears families apart through domestic violence and divorce, and creates major problems in industry by causing absenteeism and inefficiency.

Alcohol abuse has also filtered down to the young. A significant number of high-school and college students have already developed drinking habits that interfere with their desire and ability to perform academic work and to face the challenges of young adulthood.

Why has alcohol abuse become such a major problem in our society? To find the answer to this question, we must look at the reasons why people drink, the characteristics and capacities of alcohol itself, the nature of alcoholism, and the problems faced by alcoholics and those around them.

WHAT IS ALCOHOL?

In terms of its physiological and psychological effects, **alcohol** is a drug. As far as body cells are concerned, alcohol is also a food: Although it contains no essential nutrients, it has a high caloric content—about seven calories per gram. In its pure state *ethyl alcohol*, the type of alcohol found in alcoholic beverages, is a clear liquid that is lighter than water and has a strong burning taste.

Alcohol occurs naturally through the process of **fermentation**—the growth of yeast in a solution of water and sugar. Since tiny yeast particles are usually floating in the air, it is a simple matter for these particles to settle in any substance containing sugar and water—such as fruit juice—and gradually begin the production of alcohol. In fact, prehistoric humans probably discovered alcohol as a result of this natural occurrence. They might have stored fruit for a time and then consumed the fruit after fermentation had begun.

In modern times we have learned to make many types of alcoholic beverages by fermenting various types of foods and combining alcohol with other chemical substances. Some alcoholic beverages are derived from fruits; others are produced by the fermentation of grains, vegetables, and even cactus.

PROCESSING ALCOHOL

The various types of alcoholic beverages can be divided into two general categories according to the process by which they are made. The first category includes beverages made by natural fermentation, such as wines and beers. The second group consists of beverages made through a process called **distillation.** Examples of this latter type of alcoholic beverage are whiskey, gin, and vodka.

Fermentation

Wines, one of the oldest known alcoholic beverages, are produced from the action of yeast on fruit juices. Though the term *wine* usually refers to fermented grape juice, wines can be made from plums, apples, apricots, and many other fruits. Since natural fermentation stops when the alcohol content of a solution reaches about 14 percent, no wine contains more than that amount of alcohol unless it has been artificially **fortified** with additional alcohol or brandy. (Sherry is an example of a fortified wine.) If the sugar content of the original fruit juice is high, the resulting wine will be "sweet." If the sugar content of the juice is lower, the wine is classified as "light" or "dry."

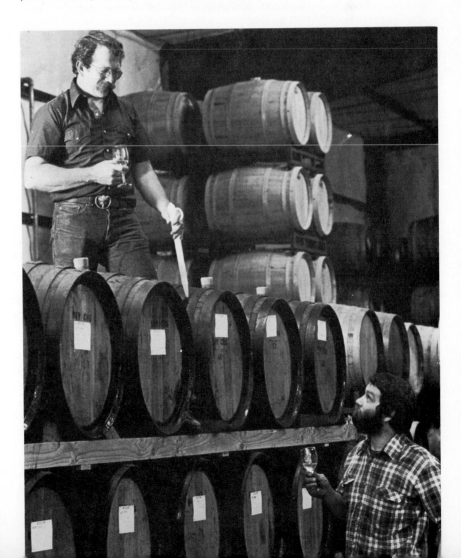

Wine-making in California.

Like wine, **beers** and ales are ancient alcoholic beverages made by a process of natural fermentation. They are derived from grains rather than from fruit juices, however. The process of making beers and ales is called **brewing.** First, **malt** (a grain, usually barley, that has been steeped in water and allowed to germinate) is added to other grains to convert the starch in the grain to sugar. Once sugar has been formed, fermentation can begin.

Distillation

Distilled spirits are actually wines and beers that have been subjected to a process designed to increase their alcoholic content. In distillation the wine or beer is heated to the boiling point. As the alcohol contained in the mixture evaporates, it is collected and condensed back into a liquid. This liquid is the distilled spirit. Distilled spirits are made and consumed all over the world. They include whiskeys, brandy, gin, rum, vodka, and liqueurs.

The term **proof** refers to the percentage of alcohol in a distilled beverage. It is equivalent to twice the liquor's alcohol content. Thus a vodka of 100 proof contains 50 percent alcohol, and one of 80 proof contains 40 percent alcohol.

Distilled spirits differ from wines and beers in several important ways. First, wines and beers contain nutritious elements—vitimins, minerals, and some solids—that can be used by body cells. These elements slow the absorption of these beverages into the body, so they are not as quickly intoxicating as distilled spirits. Second, distilled spirits have a higher alcohol content than wines and beers. In this country most table wines contain 12 to 14 percent alcohol; fortified wines, from 18 to 21 percent alcohol. Beers contain about 4.5 percent alcohol by volume. Alcoholic beverages that have been distilled, on the other hand, average about 45 percent alcohol by volume. California vintners have recently produced and promoted new wine products lower in alcohol content (and calories).

EFFECTS OF ALCOHOL ON THE BODY

There are many myths about drinking and about the effects of alcohol on the body. Mixing the types of drinks consumed in one evening is believed to cause a greater degree of intoxication. Coffee is supposed to "sober up" an intoxicated person. People think that "drinking someone under the table" proves manliness. All of these ideas are seen to be essentially false when the effects of alcohol on the body and its manner of absorption into, and elimination from, the bloodstream are carefully examined.

Absorption of Alcohol

Unlike other foods, alcohol is absorbed directly into the bloodstream from the stomach or the small intestine without being digested. The speed with which alcohol passes from the stomach or small intestine into the blood is governed by a number of factors:

1. *Amount of food in the stomach*. When food is present in the stomach, the effects of alcoholic beverages are substantially delayed. Food can slow the absorption of alcohol into the bloodstream by as much as 50 percent. Fatty foods such as oil and certain proteins like milk reduce the speed of alcohol absorption, and thus help protect the drinker from becoming intoxicated quickly.

2. *Other substances in the beverage*. Wines and beers, which contain larger

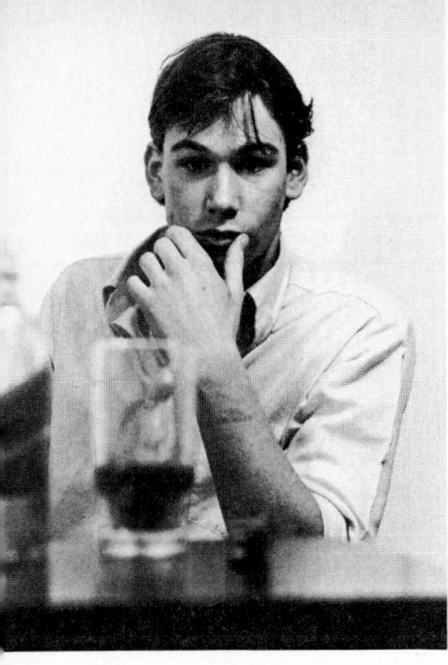

amounts of nonalcoholic elements than distilled spirits, are absorbed much more slowly into the system than distilled spirits. Liquors like vodka and gin, which contain almost no substances other than alcohol, water, and flavoring, are absorbed almost immediately. **Carbonation** can influence absorption, too. The presence of carbon dioxide in an alcoholic beverage causes alcohol to pass more quickly from the stomach into the small intestine and then into the blood. Contrary to popular belief, mixing drinks—that is, drinking alcohol in several different forms during the course of an evening—will not increase the speed of alcohol absorption. It is the total amount of alcohol ingested that determines intoxication—not the form of drink.

3. *Alcohol concentration in the beverage*. The concentration of alcohol in any given beverage will determine how fast alcohol passes into the bloodstream. Tests have shown that beverages with high concentrations of alcohol, such as rum and whiskey, are absorbed more quickly than beverages in which the alcohol is more diluted, such as wine. Thus half an hour after drinking two shots of scotch, the alcohol level in the blood will be higher than after drinking two glasses of wine or two 12-ounce beers, which contain about the same amount of alcohol.

4. *How quickly the alcohol is consumed*. It is in the liver that alcohol is broken down into compounds such as water and carbon dioxide. As long as the liver can keep pace with the amount of alcohol consumed, intoxication will not take place. The average person can absorb approximately one to one and one-half ounces of liquor or one beer or one glass of wine an hour with negligible effect. The level of alcohol in the blood will remain low if one drinks slowly and leisurely.

5. *The body weight of the drinker*. The greater a person's weight, the more alcohol he or she can absorb without showing signs of intoxication. A 140-pound person will not "hold liquor" as well as one who weighs 200 pounds. The lighter person has less blood and fewer tissues where the alcohol can be distributed and diluted, so that alcohol levels in the bloodstream will rise more quickly than they would in a heavier individual. The fact that a lighter person tolerates less alcohol than a heavier person has to do with body weight, not lack of self-control.

6. *The alcohol habituation of the drinker*. Habitually heavy drinkers have a greater **tolerance** for alcohol than do people who drink only occasionally; that is, they must drink greater quantities of alcohol in order to become intoxicated. This pattern reverses as heavy drinking continues. Individuals long addicted to alcohol frequently develop a lower tolerance to it; they can become intoxicated after drinking smaller amounts of alcohol than would affect the average drinker.

7. *Activity of the stomach*. Fear, nervousness, and anger can affect the speed at which alcohol passes from the stomach into the bloodstream. These emotions often increase the acid content of the stomach, which causes alcohol to be absorbed more quickly. Thus the emotional state of the drinker can affect alcohol absorption and cause the rate of intoxication to differ each time the individual drinks.

8. *Chemical makeup of the body*. Two people who weigh the same and drink the same amounts under the same conditions may react quite differently to alcohol. It is believed that individual differences in body chemistry account for these variations in alcohol absorption.

Keeping Your Guests Sober: What You Can Do

Knowing the dangers of excessive drinking does not necessarily lead to responsible drinking—especially at cocktail parties and other social gatherings. To help avoid intoxication at such gatherings, the National Institute on Alcohol Abuse and Alcoholism makes the following suggestions:

- Nonalcoholic beverages should be offered in addition to alcoholic drinks.
- Food with high salt content—potato chips, peanuts, and pretzels, for example—should be avoided.
- Low-calorie snacks that do not go well with alcohol, such as celery sticks, should be served.
- Carbonated mixers should be avoided.
- The host and hostess should make a special effort to introduce people to one another. When people know each other, they are more likely to feel relaxed and less likely to focus their entire attention on drinking.

Intoxication

Once alcohol passes into the bloodstream from the stomach or small intestine, it becomes distributed uniformly in the fluids throughout the body. Tissues that contain a great deal of fluid absorb more alcohol than do bone or fat tissues, which do not have a high fluid content. The circulatory system spreads the drug through the body, eventually carrying it to the brain. It is alcohol's effect on the brain that brings about **intoxication,** a condition of diminished control over physical and mental powers.

Although alcohol is commonly thought of as a stimulant, it is classified by scientists as a depressant. In anything more than minor amounts, alcohol will inhibit the functioning of the central nervous system. For this reason, alcohol was employed as a general anesthetic until the discovery of ether in the middle of the nineteenth century.

The first part of the brain to be affected by alcohol is the cerebral cortex. Here behavior, memory, and reasoning—the higher brain functions—are controlled. The animation associated with beginning intoxication gives the impression that the brain has been stimulated. In fact, just the opposite has happened. The behavior change caused by drinking is due to the depression of the higher brain centers, which normally control behavior.

As the amount of alcohol is increased, its effects spread to the motor centers of the brain and those areas become depressed; loss of coordination and slowing of reflexes follow. Next to be affected by alcohol is the midbrain, which controls speech muscles and eye motion. After this point respiration and circulation—lower brain activities—are threatened. Severe intoxication, therefore, can lead to coma. If the alcoholic depression of the lower brain is strong enough to stop breathing, death will result.

Although alcohol becomes greatly diluted once it enters the circulatory system, the amount of alcohol in the bloodstream, or **blood alcohol level,** necessary to cause mild intoxication is extremely low. The average person will begin to show the effects of drinking when the blood alcohol level is somewhere around 0.02 and 0.03 percent (see Figure 11-1).

Other Effects

Alcohol affects parts of the body other than the brain. The drug irritates the tissues lining the stomach and throat, causing a burning sensation. In small amounts alcohol causes the stomach to secrete digestive juices and create the sensation of hunger. Larger amounts of alcohol over a period of time cause chronic irritation of the stomach lining. Too large a quantity of alcohol on an empty stomach can be irritating enough to cause vomiting.

The heart and circulation are notably affected by drinking. A moderate amount of alcohol will cause blood vessels in the arms, legs, and skin to relax and dilate, increasing circulation. At the same time, there is a slight increase in the heart rate and a slight lowering of blood pressure. More blood is brought to the body surface, creating a momentary sensation of warmth but actually a slight loss of body heat. (One cannot therefore "warm up" with a drink.) Bloodshot eyes are a sign of increased blood flow to the surface of the body.

Not all of these effects are harmful. The relaxing effects of small amounts of alcohol are pleasant and are, indeed, one of the main reasons that people drink. Small amounts of alcohol are sometimes used for medicinal purposes to treat hardening of the arteries, arthritis, and digestive diseases in the elderly.

FIGURE 11-1

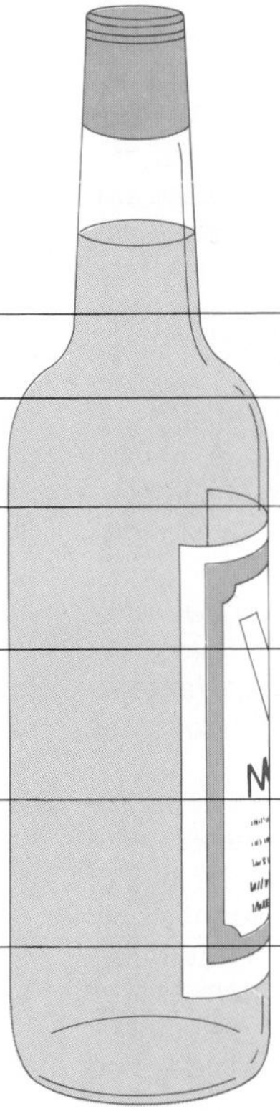

No. of drinks in an hour	Blood alcohol level (in percent)	Effects
1 drink = 1 12-oz bottle beer 1 5-oz glass table wine 1 shot (1½ oz) 80 proof vodka or whiskey.		**Time to sober up: About 1 hr per .02 percent blood alcohol concentration, or per drink on an empty stomach.**
1	.02	Negligible
2-3	.05	Changes in mood and behavior. Judgment and restraint are somewhat impaired, thinking dulled. Maximum level considered safe for driving.
5	.10	Walking, speech, hand movements clumsy. Blurred, split, or tunnel vision may occur. Legal intoxication.
10	.20	Behavior greatly affected; person may become loud, easily angered, tearful.
15	.30	Brain responses very slow and dulled. Disorientation and confusion, visually and aurally.
20	.40+	Unconsciousness, depressed breathing, heartbeat. Sometimes death.

Alcohol can also be used as a sedative, and in rare cases it is prescribed in the diet of diabetic patients because it is a food that can be metabolized without insulin. In addition, according to some studies, moderate drinkers have the lowest mortality rate of any group—including total abstainers. Whether light drinking reduces the rate of coronary artery disease is a matter of controversy (see box: Alcohol and Coronary Artery Disease).

"Sobering Up"

Once alcohol is absorbed into the system, from 2 to 5 percent of it is eliminated in the urine, perspiration, and breath. A far greater amount of alcohol is metabolized in the body, primarily through the action of the liver. This conversion, or **oxidation,** of alcohol yields approximately seven calories for each gram of alcohol. Oxidation of alcohol takes place at a uniform rate for each individual, regardless of blood alcohol level. Most people can metabolize about half an ounce of alcohol per hour. Investigators have tried, rather unsuccessfully, to

PROBLEMS AND CONTROVERSIES: Alcohol and Coronary Artery Disease

To millions of Americans the news was very comforting: Consuming a moderate amount of alcohol every day is actually good for you. Studies done over the last few decades seemed to prove that light drinkers—that is, those who had one or two drinks a day—had less coronary heart disease and fewer heart attacks than both nondrinkers and heavy drinkers. The studies showed that a moderate daily intake of alcohol raised the level of high-density lipoproteins (HDLs) in the blood—an encouraging sign because a high level of HDLs was believed to lower the risk of heart attack. (HDLs are fatty proteins that remove fatty deposits from artery walls and carry them to the liver, where they can be safely stored and excreted.)

But the news turns out not to be so good after all. Two important flaws have been discovered in the studies, one having to do with the characteristics of the groups studied and the other with the nature of the statistical findings.

First, upon looking more closely, researchers discovered that the groups called nondrinkers were composed not only of lifelong teetotalers but of moderate-to-heavy drinkers who had recently quit. They also found that the category moderate drinkers included people who drank very seldom as well as those who regularly put away two or three drinks a day. Thus the unequal distribution of drinking patterns between the two groups led the earlier researchers to a false conclusion.

The studies also failed to consider differences in drinking behavior between socioeconomic classes. Moderate drinkers tend to come from the middle and upper-middle classes, groups that are generally better educated, and more health conscious, and receive better health care. Nondrinkers and heavy drinkers, on the other hand, tend to come from the lower-middle and lower classes, groups that are generally not as well educated nor as alert to health problems.

The second major flaw in the studies concerns the type of HDL observed. It turns out that there are several kinds of HDL, only one of which is beneficial. Upon reevaluating the studies, researchers discovered that the kind of HDL contained in alcoholic beverages had no effect on the accumulation of fat deposits in the arteries.

Thus it remains to be seen whether moderate amounts of alcohol have any beneficial effect on health. As with so much else, moderation—or maybe even abstention—is the best policy.

Source: "Beer or Skittles?" *The Harvard Medical School Health Letter*, XI, No. 3 (January 1986).

find a way to increase the speed of alcohol metabolism. Substances such as coffee can stimulate drinkers so that they feel more awake, but they cannot sober drinkers up by helping them to eliminate alcohol from their bloodstream. Thus, from a safety viewpoint, it is unwise to try to keep awake someone who has had too much to drink and who is going to drive a car. The person will still be intoxicated.

The one major but inconsistent aftereffect of an excessive drinking bout is the much-dreaded hangover syndrome. A hangover usually occurs the morning after alcohol consumption, when little or no alcohol is present in the body. There is some controversy as to what exactly causes the symptoms of a hangover: heartburn, nausea, vomiting, shakiness, headache, dizziness, dehydration, and weakness. One theory is that the anesthetizing effect of alcohol upon the brain causes drinkers to physically and mentally overexert themselves. The hangover the next morning is the consequence of this overindulgence.

Alcohol causes blood vessels to expand, and expanded blood vessels in the cranium are a cause of headache. The heartburn and nausea of the hangover are brought about by the irritating effect of a large amount of alcohol on the lining of the stomach. Fatty proteins such as milk or cheese ingested before beginning to drink will act as a buffer to reduce the irritation to the mucous membrane lining. Drinking slowly will also lessen gastric tissue irritation.

The type of alcohol consumed may affect the severity of a hangover. **Congeners** are chemical agents that are produced during the aging process of alcoholic beverages, primarily of fine liquors and wines. These by-products are toxic, and their presence in the body may intensify hangover symptoms. Fine whiskies like scotch and bourbon, which are aged for several years, have a high concentration of congeners. Vodka, on the other hand, is just a mixture of water and pure grain alcohol. It contains fewer congeners.

The only sure cure for a hangover is the passage of time.

ALCOHOL AND OUR SOCIETY

The discovery and use of alcohol occurred very early in human history. Beer drinking dates 6,000 years to Mesopotamian cultures, and evidence of beer consumption has also been found among such ancient cultures as the Egyptian, Chinese, and Greek. Throughout the centuries the use of alcohol has been an accepted part of the customs of most cultures. Ceremonial occasions have been traditionally highlighted with drink—for example, the toast to an honored guest. So accepted, and even expected, has been the use of alcohol that many nations have distributed rations of alcohol to their soldiers and seamen.

As people from other countries emigrated to the United States, they brought their traditions regarding the use of alcohol. These traditions were soon absorbed into the American life style. For example, the saloon has become a part of the national scene, and so, too, has the custom of drinking at weddings and other ceremonial occasions. Today these and other drinking customs are thoroughly accepted. Both beer and wine are common mealtime drinks, as they have been in many cultures, past and present.

Whether or not a person drinks should be a matter of personal choice. But the encouragement, even pressure, to drink is great in American society. To many, drinking has a magnetic appeal that is difficult to resist. Drinking is

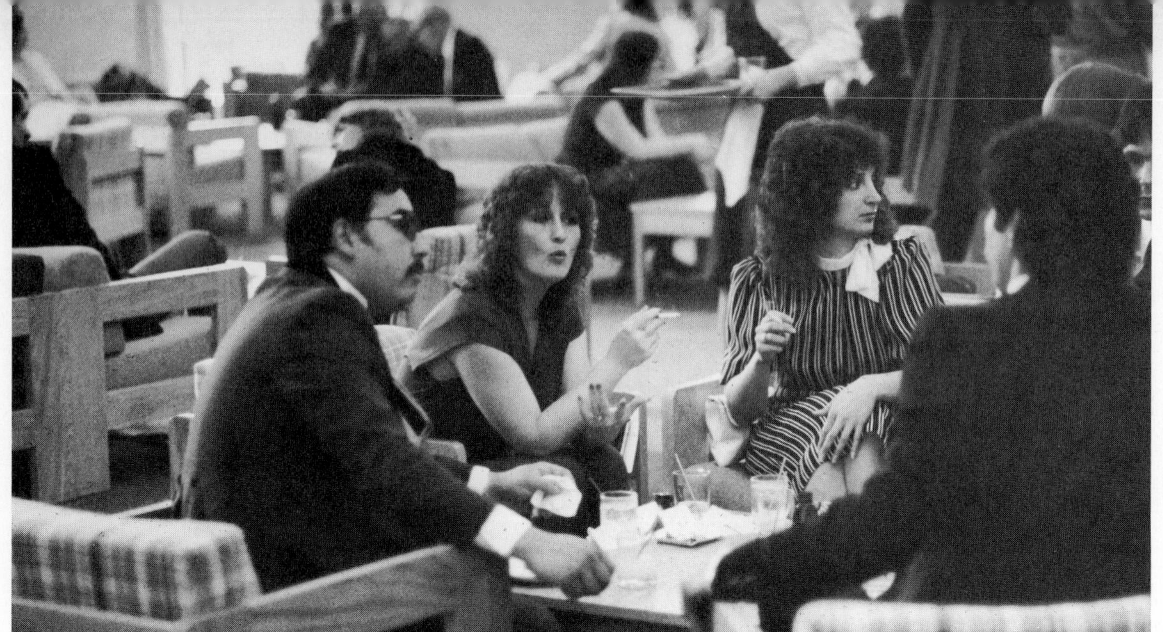

also a symbol of one's status. And, of course, drinking connotes fun and carefree living. As advertisements attempt to perpetuate and reinforce these images, we are exposed to considerable pressure to drink.

About two out of three American adults drink at least occasionally. Our problem is not the number of people who drink, but rather the number of people who drink irresponsibly on occasion. Drinking becomes a problem when it affects, or controls, a person's behavior. Efforts to control abusive drinking by law, however, have not been very successful.

Various attempts have been made in the United States and elsewhere to restrict and even prohibit the drinking of alcohol, usually by controlling its sale. In general, these efforts have failed, and sometimes they have even worsened the situation. It seems that laws passed to regulate drinking are ineffective if people are not willing to abide by them. (An outstanding illustration of this point is the history of Prohibition in this country.) At present some 15 percent of the counties in the United States outlaw the sale of some forms of alcoholic beverage. In the rest of the country there are few restrictive laws other than those regulating the age at which a person can legally purchase alcohol, licensing vendors of alcohol, controlling the hours of sale of alcohol, and penalizing drivers whose blood alcohol level exceeds specified levels.

Given these facts, it is not surprising that alcohol consumption is high in the United States. Drinking patterns vary from year to year. Wine has recently increased in popularity, and "lighter" drinks have found favor among at least that part of the population that is concerned with fitness and weight control. The effect on teenage drinking of recently increased drinking ages in most of the states is not yet clear. Still, we know that about one person in ten who drinks will develop an alcohol problem.

ALCOHOL AND YOUTH

Estimates of the percentage of teens who have sampled alcohol range from 70 to 90 percent. Girls aged 14 to 17 drink just about as much as boys of the same age and, in some cases, more. Although the figures differ, all studies show that most teens are drinking and are beginning to drink at an early age.

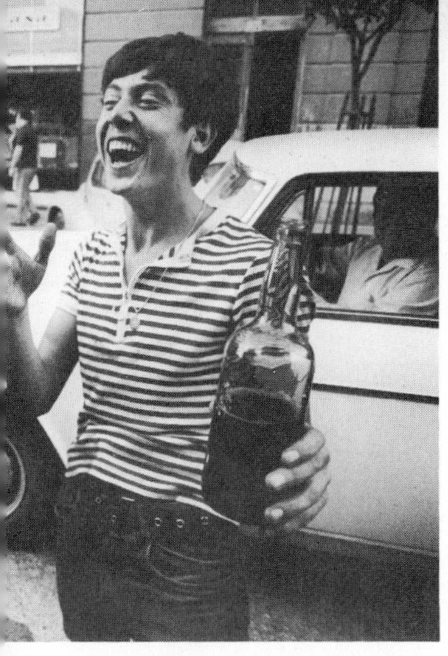

Although the greatest percentage of problem drinkers is in the 18- to 24-year-old group, most of those drinkers began drinking earlier. The average age for having one's first drink is 13. Whether teenagers are drinking more or less than they used to is not clear at this time. The legal drinking age is swiftly being raised to 21 all around the United States as a result of a federal law passed in 1984 that denies some highway funds to states that permit people to drink at younger ages. The response of colleges to the higher drinking age varies. In some, alcohol is now forbidden on campus; in others, students are allowed to do what they like in dormitories so long as their doors are closed; in still others no rules are being changed.

A Gallup poll of college undergraduates taken as long ago as 1984 showed that half of the students surveyed favored raising the legal drinking age to 21. One reason, perhaps, was that nearly one in four students had a friend with a drinking problem and one in five admitted that drinking too much had at least occasionally interfered with his or her academic work.

We can only speculate as to what the actual effect of raising the minimum drinking age will be. Certainly it will be no more difficult for those under 21 to have access to alcohol than it is to obtain marijuana or cocaine, if the person is determined. On the other hand, it is possible that the attention this issue has received may cause sufficient concern among the more responsible to cause a self-imposed control to occur, particularly in respect to the issue of drunken driving.

Mixing Drugs and Alcohol

Alcohol abuse goes hand in hand with drug abuse for many teens. The National Youth Polydrug study found that 80 percent of the adolescents referred for drug abuse treatment were regular drinkers. The typical youth surveyed in the study abused five different drugs. When amphetamines or cocaine were taken as the drug of choice, alcohol was used to lessen the anxiety and agitation produced by frequent use of these stimulants. For users of barbiturates and other depressants, drinking helped alleviate withdrawal symptoms. Alcohol is a depressant and cross-tolerant with other drugs in the group.

Alcohol in combination with certain drugs may boost the power of both drugs and prove fatal; it is especially lethal when taken with Valium and similar tranquilizers. Death usually results from impairment of breathing. Such combinations of alcohol and drugs need not be intentional. A person receiving medication may not have been warned of the hazard of its combination with alcohol. Physicians often fail to mention the danger, and a patient rarely receives printed information with a prescription.

WOMEN AND ALCOHOL

Until recently, reports on alcoholism indicated that the majority of heavy drinkers were men; in fact, the ratio was nearly five to one. That gap is closing. One barometer of the change is the greater amount of alcohol advertising and new products directed to the female consumer. New programs to help alcoholic mothers continue to grow, and research into birth defects resulting from drinking during pregnancy has increased.

Women alcoholics tend to be anxious and depressed and are more likely than men to drink in response to stressful events in their lives. One source of stress that researchers are currently exploring is the conflict over sex roles, which can affect women in either of two ways. On the one hand, women who feel confined or limited by the female role may drink in response to that source of stress. On the other hand, women pursuing careers and experiencing stress in the workplace may also drink in response to conflict. Heavy drinking occurs more often among employed married women than among either single working women or housewives.

Women who drink even moderately during pregnancy risk having a spontaneous abortion or a baby with birth defects and permanent developmental problems. The National Institute on Alcohol Abuse and Alcoholism recommends that women abstain completely from drinking during pregnancy. (see box: Fetal Alcohol Syndrome).

Fetal Alcohol Syndrome

Fetal alcohol syndrome (FAS) is a pattern of physical and mental defects found in the children of some mothers who drink during pregnancy. FAS children are often born physically stunted and are likely to have a number of facial abnormalities and defects of the heart, genitals, urinary tract, and kidneys. Later such children may be mentally retarded, hyperactive, poorly coordinated, and learning disabled.

The problem of FAS has become serious during the last twenty years. There are an estimated 1 million alcoholic women of childbearing age in the United States, and in 1985 alone 50,000 babies were born with some form of damage as a result of being exposed to alcohol before birth.

Since the placenta permits passage of alcohol from the mother's bloodstream to the fetus, "a pregnant woman is literally drinking for two," according to health and science writer Jane Brody; and the more the mother drinks, the more damage the unborn child will suffer. Heavy drinking during pregnancy produces the most severe defects, while lighter drinking may cause less pronounced symptoms. But exposure to even small amounts of alcohol in the womb can cause serious permanent damage. Children born to moderately drinking mothers, for example, are often smaller, less intelligent, hyperactive, and suffer a variety of eye and speech problems. No amount of compensatory nutrition later can undo the damage, and such children remain thin and small.

Doctors warn all prospective mothers not to drink at all from the time they are planning to conceive to the end of the nursing period. Even as little as two drinks a day can harm the fetus, and no form of alcohol is safer than another. The early weeks of pregnancy are the most dangerous because that is when the fetus's central nervous system is undergoing its most crucial growth. And since a nursing mother who drinks can pass alcohol to her child through her breast milk, she is advised not to resume drinking until after the child is weaned.

Source: Jane E. Brody, "Personal Health," *New York Times*, January 15, 1986, p. C6.

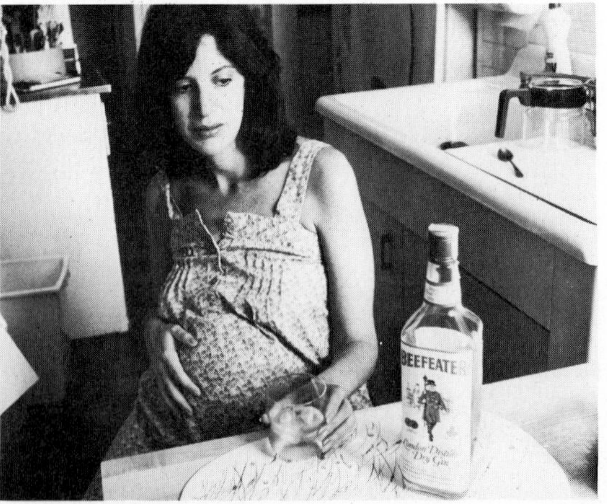

THE PROBLEM OF ALCOHOLISM

Try to conjure up your own image of the average alcoholic. Do you see him or her as dirty, unemployed, a vagrant without family or friends? While this is probably the most common conception of the alcoholic among the American public, it is certainly not borne out by statistics. In fact, only about 3 percent of alcoholics fall into the Skid Row stereotype. The remaining 97 percent of the nearly 14 million problem drinkers and alcoholics in this country appear to be "average" individuals. They are people with jobs and families who live in stable, middle-class communities. They seem to lead respectable lives, pay taxes, educate their children, and function in their occupational roles. Many are young people—high-school and college students under the age of 21; in fact, within the past decade the median age of the alcoholics who fled to New York's Bowery has dropped from 55 to the late 30s (see Figure 11-2).

In a society in which the majority of teenagers and adults drink, and in which there is a great overlap between those who use and those who abuse alcohol, it is often difficult to identify alcoholics. Frequently, it is only when alcohol abusers are in an advanced state of alcoholism that their problems are recognized. In 1982 it was estimated that the amount of *absolute alcohol* consumed averaged 2.73 gallons for every American 14 years or older (see Figure 11-3). This amounts to 331 cans of beer, 12 fifths of table wine, and 11.5 fifths of 86 proof distilled spirits per person, and it includes nondrinkers as well as drinkers. It is estimated by the National Institute on Alcohol Abuse and Alcoholism that 30 percent of the drinking population accounts for 80 percent of the total amount of alcohol consumed, and that 10 percent of all drinkers account for 50 percent of the alcohol consumed in the United States.

Though the distinction between the social drinker, the problem drinker, and the alcoholic may be obscure, the following definitions, while not universally accepted, describe some key symptoms of alcohol abuse:

- *Social Drinker*: The social drinker exercises restraint in respect to the use of alcohol; feels no compulsion to drink; and when he or she indulges in

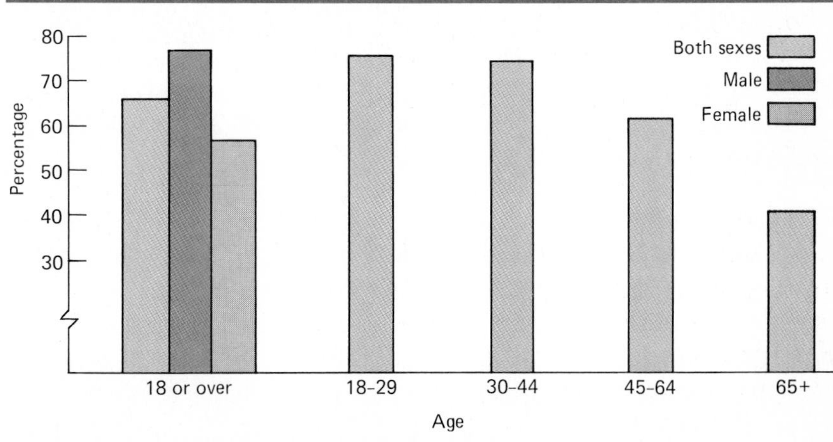

FIGURE 11-2

Percentage of the adult U.S. population that consumes alcohol, by age and sex, 1985

Source: National Center for Health Statistics, *1985 Health Interview Survey*.

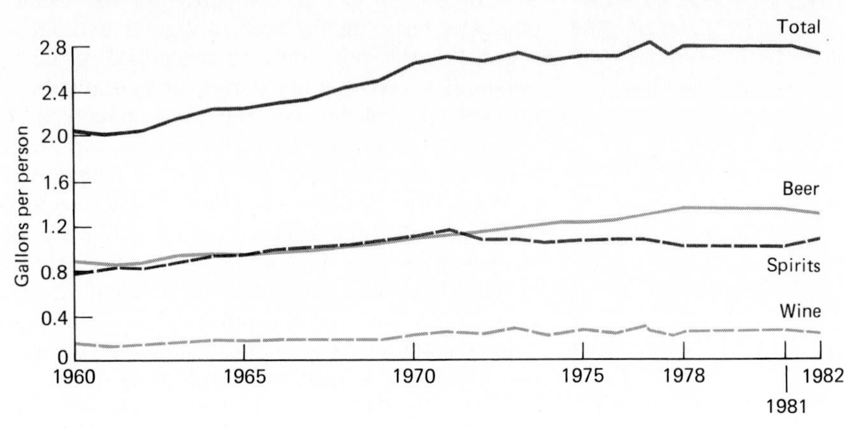

FIGURE 11-3

Average per capita consumption of absolute alcohol in the U.S., 1960–1982*

* Includes nondrinkers. Figures for only the drinking population are approximately 50 percent higher.

Source: Reprinted from "Fifth Special Report to the U.S. Congress on Alcohol and Health, 1983."

alcohol, does it modestly. In essence, the social drinker controls alcohol, instead of the other way around.

- *Problem Drinker*: Anyone who must drink in order to function or to "cope" with life; who gets drunk often; who drinks in the morning or goes to work intoxicated; who requires any medical attention as a result of drinking; who drives while drunk; who is arrested when drunk; who often drinks alone; or who does things drunk he or she would never do when sober.[1]
- *Alcoholic*: A person who is physically dependent upon alcohol and suffers a painful withdrawal when cut off from it; who develops a high tolerance to the effects of alcohol; who suffers brief blackout periods or memory loss for hours, days, or weeks; who contracts alcohol-associated diseases such as cirrhosis, hepatitis, or heart disease; and who is psychologically dependent on alcohol with little control over consumption.[2]

While these definitions may help us identify an alcohol abuser, they do not tell us very much about the nature of the alcohol problem. What makes some people moderate drinkers and other alcoholics? How does alcoholism develop? What are the effects of alcohol abuse on the individual and on society? How is alcoholism treated?

HOW ALCOHOLISM BEGINS AND DEVELOPS

Though it is certain that many factors combine to encourage alcohol addiction, no one knows exactly how alcoholism begins. In seeking to understand the origins of alcoholism, we must consider a variety of physiological, sociological, and psychological factors.

Predisposition Toward Problem Drinking

Both the chemistry of alcohol and the genetic history of alcoholics have been studied to see if there is any physiological basis for alcohol addiction. Some

[1] National Institute of Mental Health and National Institute on Alcohol Abuse and Alcoholism, *Alcohol and Alcoholism*, p. 8.

[2] National Council of Alcoholism Criteria for the Diagnosis of Alcoholism, *American Journal of Psychology*, 129 (August 1972), pp. 127–135.

who treat alcoholism, such as Alcoholics Anonymous, believe in the "allergy" theory: namely, that there is some element in the alcoholic's physical makeup—present even before the person takes up drinking—that both provokes the desire for alcohol and creates the dependence upon it. This theory, however, has not been proved.

Heredity has also been considered a cause of alcoholism, since many children of alcoholics—even those living apart from their natural parents and brought up by nondrinkers—also become alcoholics. However, most children of alcoholics do not become alcoholics themselves, and most alcoholics do not have alcoholic parents. Thus it is unclear to what extent heredity is a factor in causing alcoholism.

Many psychologists have proposed theories concerning personality characteristics that may predispose a person to alcoholism; but it is difficult to ascertain whether the personality characteristics displayed by a majority of alcoholics are the cause or the result of their disease. No one has yet isolated a specific "alcoholic personality." It can, however, be said that many problem drinkers and alcoholics are low in self-esteem and high in dependency needs. They seem unable to cope effectively with life's problems, and so seek in alcohol an escape from anxiety. The sad irony is that alcohol dependence increases feelings of low self-esteem, depression, anxiety, and guilt. Thus alcoholics often

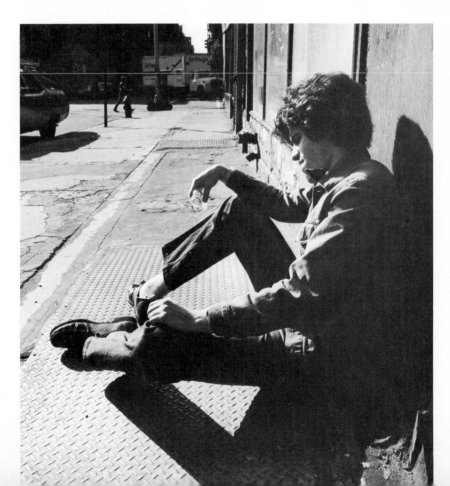

become caught in a vicious cycle, drinking more and more to avoid facing an ever more painful reality.

Some significant insights into the causes of alcohol abuse have come from sociologists. Various national and cultural groups differ widely in their incidence of problem drinking and alcoholism. By comparing the attitudes of these groups toward alcohol use, sociologists have increased our understanding of how alcohol abuse begins. In general, cultures that integrate moderate drinking with eating meals and at the same time view intoxication as a disgrace have a low incidence of problem drinking and alcoholism.

It is important to note that these cultural and religious groups do not necessarily differ in the *amount* of alcohol they consume, but rather in the *way* they consume alcohol. For those groups who use significant amounts of alcohol, a low incidence of alcoholism is usually associated with at least some of the following factors:

1. Parents are moderate drinkers.
2. Children are permitted to drink small quantities of alcohol, but only on social or religious occasions.
3. Drinking is not viewed as proof of adulthood or masculinity. Individuals within the group feel free to turn down a drink.
4. No moral significance is attached to drinking.
5. There is wide agreement within the family or culture about when and how much drinking is appropriate.

The available evidence suggests that children imitate the moderate drinking habits of their parents. (Similarly, parents who are heavy drinkers will tend to have children who are heavy drinkers.) Those parents who insist on abstinence, however, may instill extreme attitudes in their children; some children may remain abstainers, but others may rebel and become problem drinkers.

The Development of Alcoholism

For most people who drink, alcohol never becomes a problem (see Figure 11-4). They ordinarily do not drink enough on any one occasion to become drunk, nor do they ever have a compulsive urge to drink. Even most problem drinkers never become alcoholics. They may continue their unhealthy drinking habits without developing alcohol tolerance—or until they get into a fatal auto accident. The situation is quite different for alcoholics, who generally follow a predictable pattern of drinking that results in alcoholism. In a study based on the case histories of 2,000 alcoholics, E. M. Jellinek found that four stages of alcoholism could be identified. He called these the *prealcoholic symptomatic phase*, the *prodromal phase*, the *crucial phase*, and the *chronic phase*. The four phases provide a framework within which the symptoms and development of alcoholism can be described.

Prealcoholic Symptomatic Phase. Symptoms of the **prealcoholic symptomatic phase** include drinking not merely for enjoyment or sociability, but for relief from tension, depression, or boredom, or to induce positive feelings such as courage, happiness, assertiveness, or relaxation. This type of relief drinking may

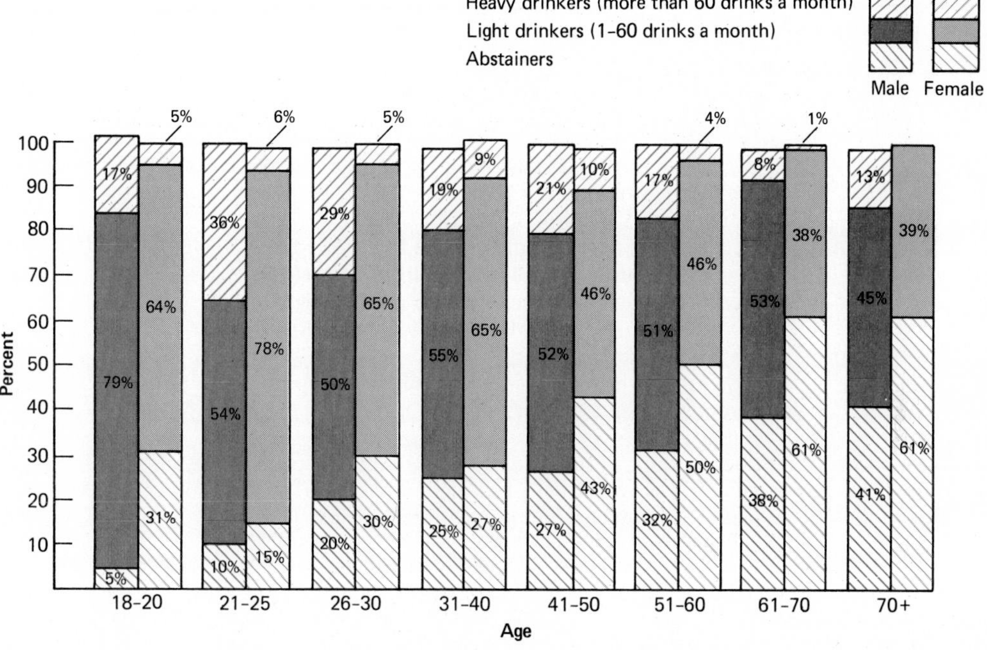

FIGURE 11-4

Drinking patterns in the U.S. adult population

Source: First Statistical Compendium on Alcohol and Health, February 1981.

last for years, during which time an increase in tolerance to alcohol gradually develops.

The Prodromal Phase. Perhaps the most notable symptom of the **prodromal phase** stage is the **blackout,** a loss of memory or amnesia that leaves the drinker unable to recall a recent event. Alcoholics in the prodromal phase become increasingly preoccupied with drinking. They may lie about their drinking, or drink in secret because they are ashamed to have others see their need for the drug. Their lying may cause feelings of guilt so that they eventually refuse even to talk about drinking. The alcoholic is now drinking more frequently and in greater quantity, with an increasing incidence of intoxication.

At this point in the progression toward alcoholism drinking begins to interfere with work and family life. These problems create further guilt about drinking, and the alcoholic commonly seeks solace in still more alcohol.

The Crucial Phase. The third stage of alcoholism, the **crucial phase,** is characterized by total addiction to alcohol and concurrent changes in drinking behavior. Not only are drinkers unable to curb the quantity of alcohol they consume, they cannot control their need to begin drinking in the first place. Drinking sprees may last for days, weeks, and even months.

Test Your Drinking Habits

Yes No

____ ____ 1. Have you been drunk as many as four times in the past year?
____ ____ 2. Do you ever drink in order to work?
____ ____ 3. Do you ever go to school or work intoxicated?
____ ____ 4. Do you ever drive a car while you are intoxicated?
____ ____ 5. Have you ever sustained a bodily injury requiring medical attention as the consequence of drinking?
____ ____ 6. Have you ever come in conflict with legal authority as a consequence of drinking?
____ ____ 7. Do you, under the influence of alcohol, ever do things that you would not otherwise do?

Dr. Morris Chafetz, former director of the National Institute of Alcohol Abuse and Alcoholism, cites the behaviors listed above as symptoms of an alcohol problem. If you answered yes to any of the questions, you may want to reconsider your drinking habits.

Source: *Jane Brody's The New York Times Guide to Personal Health* (New York: Avon, 1983), p. 249. Adapted by permission.

The Chronic Phase. In the last stage of alcoholism, the **chronic phase,** total alcohol addiction is firmly established. The chronic phase is marked by continued deterioration of mental and physical faculties. Without treatment, the chronic alcoholic will die of a disease associated with alcoholism or perhaps of some alcohol-related accident.

EFFECTS OF ALCOHOLISM ON THE INDIVIDUAL

Alcohol does not cause extensive or permanent damage to the mind or body when taken in moderation, even when drunkenness occurs from time to time. But for the alcoholic, drinking poses a serious threat to physical and psychological health and can seriously affect social orientation.

Effects on Health

The long-range health perspective for the alcoholic is certainly not favorable: Alcoholics have a shorter life expectancy (by ten to twelve years) than nonalcoholics. But there also are more immediate effects of alcoholism, including an appearance of poor health, often emphasized by flabbiness; aggravation of physical disorder that already exists, such as a stomach ulcer; the diseases and disorders associated with malnutrition; and neurological impairment.

Since alcohol contains no vitamins or minerals, alcoholics derive sugar energy but no other food value from their drinking. Furthermore, they have a reduced appetite for foods that do contain nutrients, and thus suffer from nutritional deficiences.

Heavy consumption of alcohol can contribute to a wide range of heart diseases. One example is a chronic disease of the heart muscle caused by the alcoholic's poor diet and other unknown factors. In this condition the heart muscle becomes weak and begins to degenerate.

Cirrhosis of the liver—a fatty degeneration and hardening of the liver—is a disorder common to alcoholics, although it also affects nondrinkers. The D.T.'s, or **delirium tremens**, is another disorder that afflicts addicted drinkers. It is the withdrawal syndrome experienced by alcoholics when they are suddenly deprived of alcohol. Delirium tremens is characterized by hallucinations—frequently the victim sees insects or animals ("pink elephants")—and uncontrollable shaking. The D.T.'s may last about a week; then the victim usually recovers, although death can occur in some cases. An advanced and damaging state of mental deterioration known as "wet brain," or **Korsakoff's syndrome,** is often exhibited by long-term alcoholics.

Social Effects

Alcoholism has such a devastating effect on alcoholics' self-respect and self-image that it tends to impel them more desperately to drink. No matter how inebriated they may be, alcoholics are usually aware of how others view them, of how they have let others down, and of the suffering and trouble they have caused others and themselves.

At work alcoholics become increasingly incompetent and unreliable; and by the time they reach the chronic state, they are usually unemployed. Their home life is also visibly affected by their alcoholism. They can no longer provide adequately for the material and emotional needs of their families, who, in turn, can no longer trust them and feel helpless and frustrated in their attempts to relate to them. In seeking to escape from their problems with job and family, alcoholics may turn to fantasies about their own future. And when they begin to base their actions on these fantasies, the consequences are usually self-destructive.

Finally, alcoholics may express their resentment at the disapproval of family and friends in hostile behavior toward the community at large. They may become involved in brawls, be arrested for vagrancy, or in some other way alienate themselves from their social milieu. Sometimes loss of social standing and the resulting sense of disgrace jolt alcoholics into a realization of their problem and may influence them to seek treatment. But often the alcoholic is only forced deeper into alcoholism.

EFFECTS OF ALCOHOLISM ON SOCIETY

While alcoholics themselves are the ones who suffer most from their addiction, many other people, including their families, friends, employers, and communities, are also affected.

The high rate of automobile accidents involving drunken drivers is a serious problem in all communities. It has been estimated that alcohol is implicated in half of all fatal traffic accidents. Recent studies indicate that the figure may be even higher. Concerned groups, such as MADD (Mothers Against Drunk Driving), have been influential in getting stronger legislation passed to deter the drunk driver and save lives (see box: Drunk Drunken in Chapter 3). As public awareness grows through the efforts of such groups, new citizens' action groups are formed.

In most states in this country blood alcohol levels of 0.10 percent can bring conviction for drunken driving. However, impairment of judgment and reflexes frequently occurs at a much lower alcohol concentration, and most authorities agree that any level over 0.05 percent—approximately three drinks for the average person—brings a serious decrease in driving ability (see Figure 11-1). People who attend a function where alcoholic beverages are served, or who plan to spend an evening drinking, should make plans for ways to get home without driving if they have too much to drink. Even comparatively low blood alcohol levels can make the difference between a near miss and a fatal accident.

Although some states have passed tough laws to discourage drunken driving—New Jersey suspends the driver's license of a first offender for six months—the laws are not enforced as rigorously as they should be. In Norway, by contrast,

Test Your Alcohol IQ

T or F

_______ 1. Ethyl alcohol is the ingredient that makes alcoholic beverages intoxicating.

_______ 2. Ethyl alcohol depresses the central nervous system.

_______ 3. Distilled liquors are 100 percent alcohol.

_______ 4. Two ounces of a 100-proof beverage contain one ounce of alcohol.

_______ 5. Wine is commonly 10 to 15 percent alcohol by volume.

_______ 6. A twelve-ounce can of beer at a level of 4 percent alcohol contains more alcohol than one ounce of an 86-proof liquor.

_______ 7. Alcohol is absorbed into the bloodstream more rapidly than most foods.

_______ 8. Some alcohol is absorbed through the walls of the stomach, but most is absorbed through the small intestine.

_______ 9. We behave the way we do when we are drunk because of the effect of alcohol on the brain.

_______ 10. Taking a cold shower or drinking hot coffee speeds up the process of burning up the alcohol in one's body.

_______ 11. Some alcohol escapes from the body when a person exhales.

_______ 12. The amount of alcohol a person has consumed may be measured by taking samples of blood, urine, or breath.

_______ 13. Intoxication results from drinking alcohol at a rate faster than it can be metabolized by the body.

_______ 14. A person cannot get as drunk on wine or beer as on whiskey or vodka.

_______ 15. The rate of absorption of an alcoholic drink such as beer, which has other nutrients, is slower than the absorption of alcoholic drinks that are mostly alcohol and water.

_______ 16. Food in the stomach decreases the rate of alcohol absorption.

_______ 17. The concentration of alcohol in a glass of wine is greater than that in a glass of beer.

_______ 18. The alcohol in champagne and other sparkling wines is absorbed faster than that in still wines.

_______ 19. There is the same amount of alcohol in one ounce of beer, wine, and whiskey.

_______ 20. Generally a large person has an advantage over a smaller person in resisting the effect of alcohol upon the brain.

_______ 21. The accepted standard for avoiding intoxication when drinking is to have no more than one highball or bottle of beer per hour.

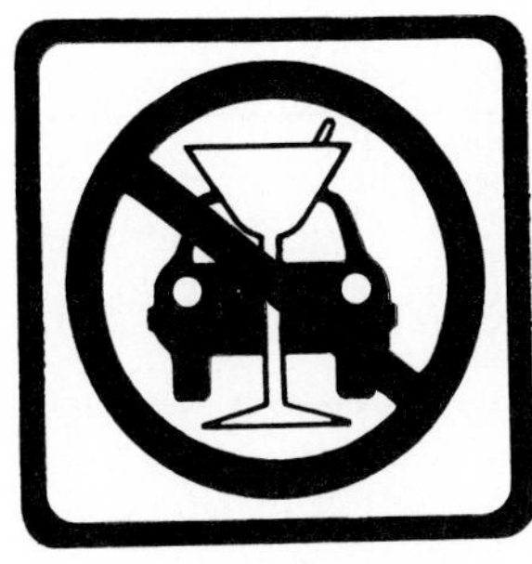

first offenders are sent to labor camp for twenty-one days and lose their licenses for two years. The Norwegian law is effective because it is strictly enforced.

Drunk pedestrians are also involved in a significant proportion of traffic accidents. It has been estimated that about a third of fatally injured adult pedestrians are intoxicated.

Employers, too, are affected by the problems of the alcoholic. Employees with a drinking problem often have been at their jobs for many years. They possess training and experience that are valuable to their company. When such employees abuse alcohol, not only is this expertise lost to their employer, but other negative consequences of their addiction are also felt. Their drinking

_______ 22. Intoxication affects a person's driving skills mostly because it impairs judgment.
_______ 23. Alcoholic drinks are a good source of nutrition.
_______ 24. *Tolerance* is a term that means that a person is no longer affected to the same degree by the same amount of a substance such as alcohol.
_______ 25. Chronic drinkers may become addicted to alcohol and suffer severe withdrawal symptoms when they stop drinking.
_______ 26. Cirrhosis of the liver is a common ailment among alcoholics.
_______ 27. It is advisable for women to restrict their drinking of alcohol during pregnancy.
_______ 28. A person's mood can influence the way alcohol affects him or her.
_______ 29. Alcohol tends to release inhibitions.
_______ 30. The fundamental principle of the Alcoholics Anonymous program is that alcoholics must abstain totally from alcohol.

Scoring: All statements except the following are true.

3. False. Most distilled liquors are between 40 and 50 percent alcohol.
10. False. Only the liver influences the rate of alcohol metabolism.
14. False. Alcohol is alcohol.
19. False. They range from about 3 to about 50 percent alcohol.
23. False. Most alcoholic drinks provide little beyond calories.

Now go back and figure your total number of correct answers.

26–30 right: Right on! You can drive the others home.
21–25 right: Cheers! But don't let it go to your head.
16–20 right: Better than most: What about a return to Prohibition?
11–15 right: You lost. The next round is on you.
6–10 right: You'll never be a bartender.
0–5 right: Stick to milk.

Source: Adapted from *An Ounce of Prevention* (1977), DHEW Publication No. (ADM) 77–454A. National Center for Alcohol Education.

interferes with their job performance and causes them to lose many work hours each year. Alcoholics affect the morale of their co-workers and the efficiency of their company by making poor decisions on the job, losing customers for the firm, and damaging the company's image with the public. Fortunately, many companies have realized that personnel policies aimed at reaching addicted drinkers and helping them get treatment can prevent the loss of valuable employees.

The problem of alcoholism seriously affects the lives of relatives, children, and spouses of addicted drinkers. Alcoholism has been shown to be the cause of spouse abuse, broken homes, brutality to children, divorce, and abandonment. The innocent members of many families are involved. The public is affected too, for it often must assume the cost of maintaining and counseling the dependents of alcoholics who can no longer support their families.

The problem of alcoholism cost this nation $117 billion in 1983, according to estimates by the North Carolina Research Triangle Institute. This amount represents lost production of goods because of the poor functioning of alcoholic workers; health and medical costs; costs due to automobile accidents; costs of alcohol programs and research; and expenditures by the criminal justice and social welfare systems. And it has been estimated that alcohol abuse may be to blame for more than 200,000 deaths annually from disease, accidents, suicides, and homicides. More than half of all homicides and some 30 percent of all suicides are alcohol related. Lesser crimes are also associated with alcohol. These include drunkenness and disorderly conduct, driving under the influence of alcohol, and vagrancy.

Lastly, alcoholism is a waste of human potential. Many talented, capable people are lost to alcoholism each year. Community leaders, heads of families, teachers, and artists destroy their lives through addiction to this drug. It is therefore not only concern about the injury that alcoholics inflict on themselves and society that motivates people who work with them, but also a desire to restore these addicted drinkers to a useful place in the community.

TREATMENT OF ALCOHOLISM

No matter how severe their addiction, most alcoholics can be treated effectively. Naturally, the attitude of the alcoholic is the most important factor in the cure. The essential prerequisites to successful treatment are the alcoholic's desire for treatment and recovery, as well as his or her determination to continue treatment as long as necessary to achieve success. Without such motivation, addicted drinkers will return to drinking, either during treatment or as soon as they leave it.

Alcoholics do not necessarily manifest any single personality pattern; even their drinking patterns are not exactly alike. Therefore the form of treatment selected to rehabilitate the alcoholic must be appropriate for that particular individual.

The treatment of the alcoholic has two aspects: (1) treating the damage to physical health brought about by chronic alcoholism; and (2) changing the behavior pattern of the alcoholic so that addiction will not be resumed.

Hospital Treatment

It is usually recommended that **detoxification** be conducted under medical supervision to guard against the possibility of death in cases of acute intoxication. Furthermore, the symptoms of withdrawal—including delirium, hallucinations, and tremors—are best attended to by professionally trained people. In hospitals the alcoholic is administered tranquilizers and sedatives to ease the discomfort of withdrawal, provided with a special diet designed to combat nutritional deficiences, treated for any wounds or contusions resulting from extreme intoxication, and generally returned to good health, except in cases where advanced alcoholism has led to brain or other irreversible organic damage.

Until the late 1950s most hospitals in the United States were reluctant to accept alcoholic patients for detoxification. The normal procedure was to treat addicted drinkers for their cuts and bruises and then release them. Alcoholics were often considered more criminal than sick. Unfortunately, many institutions still do not treat alcoholics. Consequently, physicians may be forced to enter their patients into a hospital with falsified complaints. A further complication of hospital treatment is that many health insurance companies do not provide coverage for alcoholism treatment in their policies.

Psychotherapy

The nature of psychotherapy for alcoholism varies with the individual and can take any of a number of forms. The alcoholic can be counseled individually or as a member of a group; therapy may be limited to the patient or it may extend to treatment of the addicted drinker's family as well.

Family therapy is a recent approach that has been instituted in rehabilitation centers across the nation. The programs are expected to raise the recovery rates of alcoholics by improving patterns of family interaction that may have

Alcoholism: Where to Go for Help

Here is a list of resources for those seeking professional help for alcoholism. Many of these services have national offices that, if contacted, will provide you with local branches and the appropriate people to contact in your area.

- Alcoholics Anonymous
  See local phone book or write
  175 Fifth Avenue
  New York, N.Y. 10010
- National Clearinghouse for Alcohol Information
  P.O. Box 2345
  Rockville, Maryland 20852
- Veterans Administration
  Alcohol and Drug Dependency Services
  810 Vermont Ave. N.W.
  Washington, D.C. 20420

For those with a friend or relative who has an alcohol problem:

- Al-Anon Family Group Headquarters, Inc.
  P.O. Box 182
  Madison Square Station
  New York, N.Y. 10159

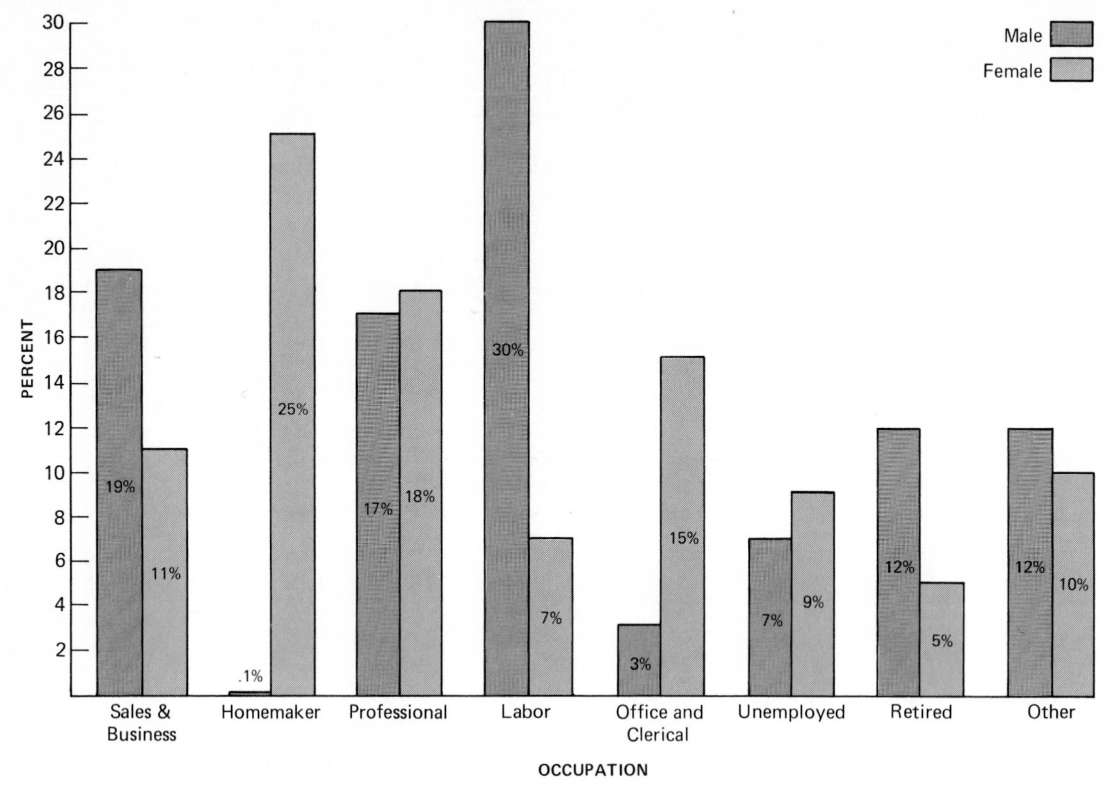

FIGURE 11-5

Occupations represented in Alcoholics Anonymous

Source: Adapted from Alcoholics Anonymous World Services, Inc., *The A.A. Member*, 1978, with permission.

encouraged drinking. Family members who have undergone therapy typically report that they initially agreed to participate in the program to help an alcoholic child, parent, sibling, or spouse, but that therapy gave them an unexpected awareness of their own behavior patterns. Alcoholics undergoing therapy also report satisfaction with their families' involvement. Family therapy helps to address issues that the alcoholic formerly avoided through drinking.

Most psychotherapeutic methods involve the same basic goals: acceptance by patients that they need help; recognition that, although they are sick, there is nothing morally evil about them; understanding by patients of the forces or conflicts that led to alcoholism; and the examination of means other than alcohol addiction that will help patients either resolve their problems or learn to live with them.

One British study, however, found a single session of professional counseling for alcoholism to be roughly as effective as long-term intensive care. This result calls into question the orthodox concepts of intensive counseling for alcoholics. New research must consider the prospect of efficiently utilizing the advantages of less intensive treatment.

Alcoholics Anonymous

Alcoholics Anonymous (*AA*), founded in 1934, is a widely known organization that was established for the treatment of alcoholics. It is an informal society of alcoholics who meet in local community groups to help each other combat the problem of alcoholism. Anyone can join AA, but he or she must do so voluntarily and openly state a need for help and a sincere desire to conquer alcoholism.

Currently, there are about 600,000 members of Alcoholics Anonymous in over 24,000 groups throughout the United States. Worldwide, AA has more than 1 million members in 116 countries. As you can see from Figure 11-5, members of AA come from a wide variety of occupations—a fact that is further proof, if any were needed, of the falsity of the stereotype of the alcoholic as Skid Row bum.

An increasing number of AA groups are composed entirely of teenagers and young adult alcoholics. Alcoholics Anonymous also has groups in hospitals and prisons, as well as special derivative organizations designed to help the families of alcoholics: *Al-Anon* for husbands and wives of alcoholics and *Alateen* for their adolescent children.

There are two types of AA meetings: open meetings, attended by members of AA and their families and friends, where alcoholics speak frankly about their experiences; and closed meetings, designed only for members of AA and usually centered around intensive discussions of the problems that members of the group encounter in staying sober. Through the friendship and encouragement of other alcoholics who have succeeded in remaining sober, it is hoped that the alcoholic who attends AA meetings will gain the confidence and determination to resist the urge to drink.

The philosophy of AA is that the alcoholic is a compulsive drinker who cannot drink moderately and who therefore must abstain from alcohol completely. If a member slips and takes a drink, the response of AA is not punitive; many members continue to come back until (and usually long after) they learn to abstain from drinking alcohol. Alcoholics Anonymous does not aim at correcting the causes that underlie the addicted drinker's problem. Rather, the organization tries to control the problem itself: the alcoholic's self-destructive drinking habit. Of all forms of therapy that have been devised thus far, AA has proven to be the most effective. A resolution to remain in the AA program and to follow its principles can enable an alcoholic to pursue an alcohol-free life.

Drug Therapy

Both hospital treatment and psychotherapy sometimes involve the use of drug therapy to help alcoholics conquer their addiction. One type of drug treatment is called **aversion therapy.** In this form of treatment consenting patients are given a nausea-inducing drug at the same time that they are given an alcoholic beverage. Patients become ill from the drug, but they associate the illness with alcohol. This type of conditioning frequently instills in patients a dislike for alcoholic beverages. Another type of drug therapy involves the use of deterrent agents such as *Antabuse*, which brings uncomfortable physical reactions when alcohol is consumed. Because control of alcoholism ultimately requires a change in the alcoholic's attitude, drug therapy is really effective only when used in conjunction with psychotherapy or programs like AA.

Company Programs

Estimates are that while only 5 to 10 percent of alcoholics in Skid Row situations can be expected to abstain, 80 to 90 percent of other alcoholics or problem drinkers can be rehabilitated. One of the factors contributing to the effectiveness of rehabilitation for this latter group is the emergence of corporate therapy programs. In 1947 Consolidated Edison in New York became the first company to try to rehabilitate its alcoholic employees rather than dismiss them. Since then, government and industrial programs have proliferated to treat alcoholism, which affects about 6 percent of the work force. Instead of stigmatizing alcoholic workers, the companies offer support and positive reinforcement. The already frail self-esteem of alcoholic employees is not threatened. Rather, the companies provide an atmosphere of concern in which alcoholics can feel that they are respected and that people care about their problems.

CONQUERING ALCOHOL ABUSE

If alcohol abuse is to be successfully combated, three major areas must receive attention. First, *better treatment facilities* must be developed for people who already suffer from alcoholism, since the "revolving door" treatment of alcoholics in most American hospitals and criminal justice systems is futile and expensive. While much valuable research has been done in the field of alcoholism, still more research into the causes and nature of alcoholism and possible cures for the disease is needed.

Second, since public attitude is a key factor in appropriating funds for improved treatment and further research, a program of *public education* must be implemented. Public education is necessary, too, in a preventive sense: If Americans learn about responsible drinking rather than merely being exposed to fright campaigns about the dangers of alcoholism, potential problems with alcohol might be avoided.

A program of public education might also ease some of the social pressures attached to drinking. Contrary to the image perpetuated by advertising agencies, drinking is not a necessary part of sexuality or sociability. Anyone should be able to drink moderately—or not at all—without being made to feel guilty. And when alcoholics have discontinued drinking, they should be accepted back into society without discrimination. Laws protecting the rights of nondrinking alcoholics have been passed in places like New York City and are part of the federal regulations affecting firms doing business with the Department of Health and Human Services.

Third, the problem of alcohol abuse would be reduced if states would pass more restrictive laws on the availability of alcohol. While it is clear that Prohibition-style laws are unrealistic and unworkable, laws aimed at specific abuses might prove helpful. For example, it should be illegal everywhere to sell alcoholic beverages to anyone who is obviously intoxicated or to sell more than a certain number of alcoholic drinks to one individual. Charges should be brought against persons serving alcohol to minors without their parents' consent. In addition, licenses of drunk drivers should be revoked. Where such laws already exist, they should be more rigidly enforced. Rather than impose prison terms, some states have required persons repeatedly guilty of drunken driving violations to join AA.

SUMMARY

1. Alcohol use is widespread in our society, a fact that has made detection of the problem drinker difficult and has hindered public understanding of the dangers and prevalence of alcoholism.

2. The type of alcohol found in alcoholic beverages is *ethyl alcohol*. It is produced through the process of *fermentation*—the growth of yeast in a solution of water and sugar. Different types of drinks have different quantities of alcohol. *Fermented beverages*, like wines or beers, have a low percentage of alcohol, unless they are *fortified*. *Distilled beverages*, such as whiskey, vodka, and brandy, have a high alcohol content.

3. Once ingested, alcohol passes directly from the stomach and small intestine into the bloodstream. Some of the factors affecting the speed with which alcohol leaves the stomach are: the amount of food in the stomach, the alcohol concentration in the drink, how quickly the alcohol is consumed, the body weight of the drinker, and the individual's tolerance to alcohol. Once in the bloodstream, alcohol travels throughout the body. It is alcohol's effect on the brain that causes intoxication.

4. Alcoholism among teenagers is a serious problem. It is too early to tell whether the recent change in the legal drinking age to 21 in most states will have much of an effect on adolescent drinking habits.

5. The overwhelming majority of problem drinkers and alcoholics are not the Skid Row type, but are "average" individuals. Precisely what makes alcoholics different from other people is a matter of some controversey. Physical, psychological, and sociological factors have been cited as causes of alcoholism, but none has been conclusively proved. It does appear that the example set by parents, as well as cultural factors, helps determine whether or not an individual will become an alcoholic. Four stages in the development of alcoholism have been described: the *prealcoholic symptomatic phase*, the *prodromal phase*, the *crucial phase*, and the *chronic phase*.

6. Many harmful physical effects have been associated with alcoholism. These include *shorter life expectancy*, *malnutrition*, *heart disease*, and *cirrhosis of the liver*. Alcoholics also suffer many negative social effects from their habit, such as loss of self-esteem and family and work problems.

7. The effects of alcoholism on society are also severe. Over half of all highway fatalities are alcohol related. The job performance of alcoholics suffers and the lives of their families are often shattered. Over half of all homicides and 30 percent of all suicides are alcohol related. Finally, each alcoholic represents a loss of human potential to the community.

8. Treatment of alcoholism usually begins with *hospitalization*. Alcoholics are detoxified under medical supervision. Once treated for their physical ailments, alcoholics must be cured of their need to drink. Rehabilitative treatment can take the form of *psychotherapy*, group support with organizations like *Alcoholics Anonymous*, and deterrent drug treatment, including *aversion therapy*.

9. These forms of treatment are reaching only a fraction of the nearly 14 million problem drinkers and alcoholics in the United States. Better treatment facilities must be developed, and more research into the causes of alcoholism is needed. Perhaps most important, a program of public education must be implemented, so that people understand the consequences of irresponsible drinking. Alcohol abuse would be reduced if there were more restrictive laws concerning the availability of alcohol.

CONSUMER CONCERNS

1. Advertising is a very significant factor in our lives and influences our decisions. In view of this should there be greater restrictions on the advertising of alcoholic beverages?
2. Is there a movement in your state urging the police to be more watchful for drunken drivers and to increase the penalties for drunken driving? Do you agree that these things should be done?
3. Did you have an alcohol program in high school? Was it effective? Why or why not?
4. There is agreement that parents have a responsibility in the alcohol education of their children, but how is this achieved? What are your recommendations?

12
Tobacco

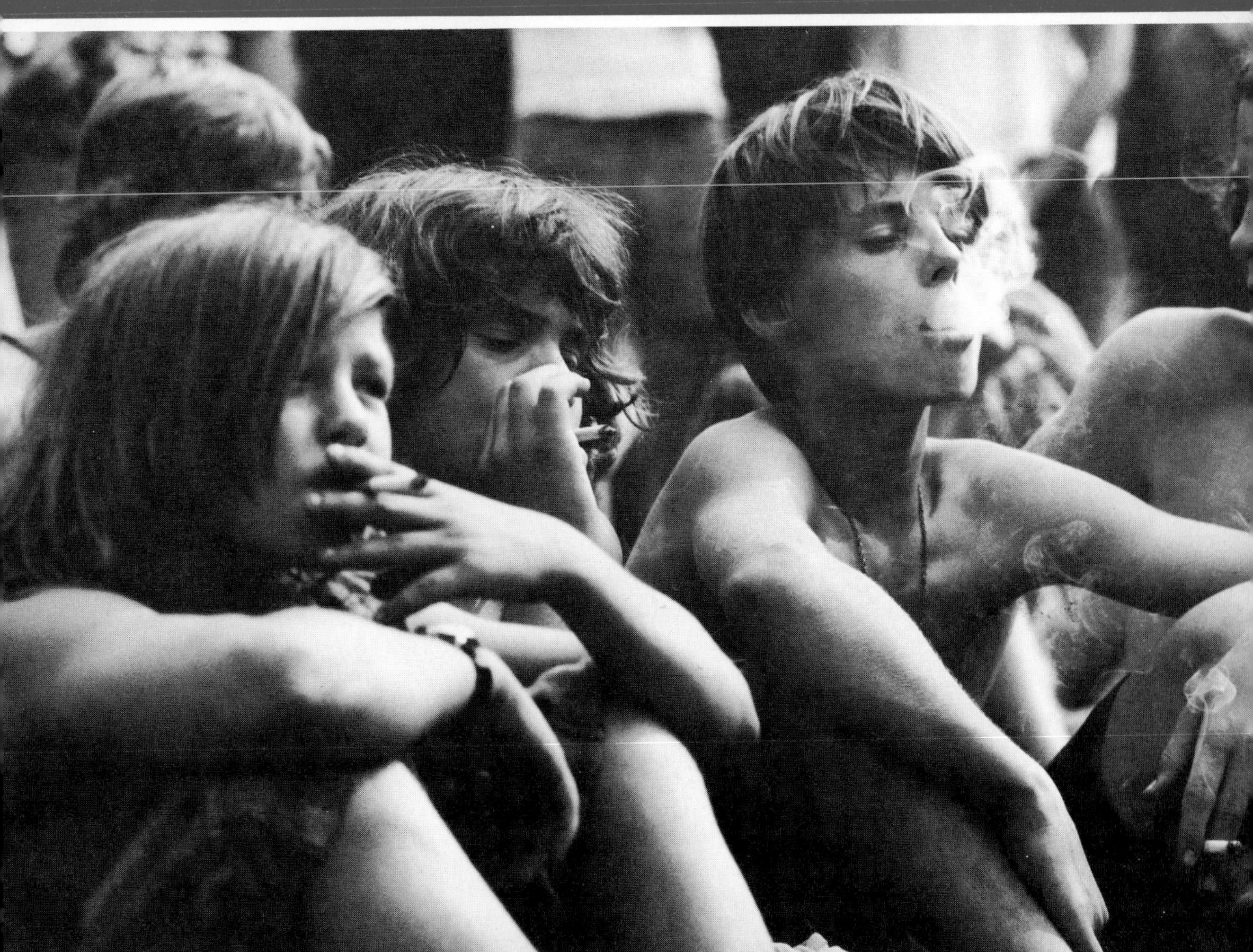

The cigarette has enjoyed a huge popular acceptance in American culture. Its high point of per capita consumption occurred during the 1960s. The then Department of Health, Education, and Welfare estimated that in 1964, 53 percent of men and 30 percent of women in this country had smoked regularly. Twenty years later 33 percent of males and 28 percent of females were smoking regularly. (See Figure 12-1.) These figures prove that a significant change in smoking patterns and attitudes toward cigarettes has taken place. Though advertisements continue to attempt to seduce us into believing that we must inhale cigarette smoke to get the most out of life, our response to this propaganda is no longer the same. Forty-three million Americans had quit smoking by 1985, and the per capita consumption of cigarettes was at its lowest point in forty years. In addition, nonsmokers are now insisting upon their right to breathe air free of tobacco smoke.

The myth of the joy of smoking received its first serious challenge in the 1950s, when researchers revealed a relationship between smoking and a number of physical ailments. But not until 1964, when an advisory committee appointed by the Surgeon General issued its report on the relationship between smoking and health, did the truth about the effects of cigarette smoking become known to the public. The conclusions of the *Surgeon General's Report* were summed up in the sentence, "Cigarette smoking is a health hazard of sufficient importance in the United States to warrant appropriate remedial action." Research since 1964 has strengthened these conclusions and has expanded, in several important respects, our knowledge of the health consequences of smoking. In his annual reports on smoking and health the Surgeon General has extended the list of types of cancer related to smoking. The 1982 report was notable in concluding that "Cigarette smoking is clearly identified as the chief preventable cause of death in our society and the most important public health issue of our time." In 1984 Congress stiffened the warning messages required to be printed on cigarette packages and in ads.

The public response to the 1964 report was by no means immediate. The first group to respond was composed of those who suffered most from the effects of years of smoking—adult males. Ironically, as men gradually discontinued the practice of smoking, women began to take it up in increasing numbers. The result of this trend was that females' rates of smoking-related illness soon began to approximate those of males. More women than men in the 17-to-24 age group now smoke, and lung cancer now takes more women's lives than breast cancer.

In 1985 there were some 52 million Americans who smoked. The figure remained this high, despite the large number who quit, for several reasons. First, tobacco smoking is considered by many researchers to be a physically addicting habit and is therefore difficult to stop; second, many adult women continue to smoke; and third, many teenagers continue to take up smoking.

For all smokers, the effects of waiting too long before quitting are reflected in increased costs. Statistics reveal that $13 billion in medical bills and a loss of $25 billion in productivity are related to smoking. Annually, the number of deaths attributed to smoking keeps increasing as evidence grows connecting smoking to cardiovascular impairment and to various forms of cancer and pulmonary disease.

FIGURE 12-1

Smoking status of persons in the U.S., aged 18 years and over

Source: National Center for Health Statistics, *Advance Data*, November 15, 1985, No. 113.

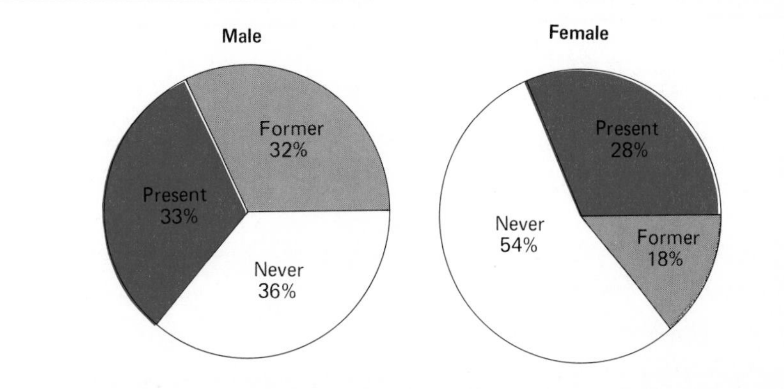

Snuff and Chewing Tobacco

In TV ads and by their own example, major sports figures have glamorized the use of snuff and chewing tobacco in recent years. As a result, the sales of smokeless tobacco products have soared, particularly among adolescents and older children. Of the 10 million Americans who use snuff and chewing tobacco, 3 million are under age 21 and many are under age 13. In some parts of the country half the male teenagers have tried some form of smokeless tobacco; and on campuses 12 percent of the students are now regular users of the products, with an additional 8 percent planning to become users in the future.

Chewing tobacco (such as Red Man and Mail Pouch) is composed of roughly cut stemless tobacco leaves and comes in a variety of plain and flavored forms. The user bites off a portion and holds it in the mouth or chews it. *Snuff* (such as Copenhagen and Skoal) is powdered tobacco that is often toasted and flavored with sweeteners and scents. While English users sniff it through the nose, Americans "dip" it—that is, put it in the mouth and hold it between the lip and gum or cheek and gum. It is an unsightly habit, for both snuff and chewing tobacco must be expectorated. In the absence of cuspidors, users befoul the sidewalks or else carry little paper cups in which to spit.

Many youngsters take up smokeless tobacco in the belief that it is safer than cigarette smoking and less addictive. While snuff and chewing tobacco users do have less lower respiratory tract disease than cigarette smokers, they develop equally serious health problems and are every bit as addicted to nicotine as any three-pack-a-day smoker. In fact, people who chew or dip receive more nicotine than cigarette smokers.

Researchers have discovered a significant relationship between smokeless tobacco use and cancer of the mouth and throat; in fact, snuff and chewing tobacco users are fifty times more likely than nonusers to develop oral cancer. Smokeless tobacco products also cause several other health problems; after three months of dipping or chewing, many users develop receding gums, loose teeth, high blood pressure, and leukoplakia—thick white patches on the tongue and inside the mouth that can turn malignant.

Ignoring the usual protests from the tobacco industry, the major U.S. medical organizations have demanded a ban on television commercials for all smokeless tobacco products and labels on these products such as "Warning: Use of snuff can be addictive and can cause mouth cancer and other mouth disorders."

Sources: "Smokeless Tobacco," *Backgrounder* (July 1985), National Cancer Institute, Office of Cancer Communications; "Into the Mouths of Babes," *Time*, July 15, 1985, p. 68.

Testing Your Attitudes Toward Smoking

Circle the number that corresponds to how you feel about each lettered statement. Then look at the scoring key below.

	Strongly agree	Mildly agree	Mildly disagree	Strongly disagree
A. Cigarette smoking is not nearly as dangerous as many other health hazards.	1	2	3	4
B. I don't smoke enough to get any of the diseases that cigarette smoking is supposed to cause.	1	2	3	4
C. If a person has already smoked for many years, it probably won't do much good to stop.	1	2	3	4
D. It would be hard for me to give up smoking cigarettes.	1	2	3	4
E. Cigarette smoking is enough of a health hazard for something to be done about it.	4	3	2	1
F. The kind of cigarette I smoke is much less likely than other kinds to give me any of the diseases that smoking is supposed to cause.	1	2	3	4
G. As soon as a person quits smoking cigarettes he or she begins to recover from much of the damage that smoking has caused.	4	3	2	1
H. It would be hard for me to cut down to half the number of cigarettes I now smoke.	1	2	3	4
I. The whole problem of cigarette smoking and health is a very minor one.	1	2	3	4

WHY PEOPLE SMOKE

Let us look at some of the forces that encourage us to smoke, the effects of smoking on our health, and some recommended approaches for those who wish to discontinue the habit.

Starting to Smoke

Most beginning smokers are young people. Experimentation with cigarettes can begin as early as the age of 8 and increases during the junior-high-school years. According to recent estimates, 22 percent of all teenagers (one out of five) smoke, and 75 percent of all smokers begin smoking before the age of 20.

J. I haven't smoked long enough to worry about the diseases that cigarette smoking is supposed to cause.	1	2	3	4
K. Quitting smoking helps a person to live longer.	4	3	2	1
L. It would be difficult for me to make any substantial change in my smoking habits.	1	2	3	4

Scoring:

1. Write the number you have circled after each statement in the test in the corresponding space below.

2. Add the scores down each column to get your totals. For example, the sum of your scores A, E, and I gives you your score for the first column, "Importance."

A ______	B ______	C ______	D ______
E ______	F ______	G ______	H ______
I ______	J ______	K ______	L ______
(1) ______	(2) ______	(3) ______	(4) ______
Importance	Personal Relevance	Value of Stopping	Capability of Stopping

Four factors are involved in any effort to stop smoking. If you scored 9 or more for any factor in the test, then that factor is important to you in any attempt you may make to stop smoking. If you scored 6 or less, the factor will not help you, but your score may also indicate that you lack correct information.

Source: National Clearinghouse for Smoking and Health.

With so many adult smokers to observe, it is not surprising that young people experiment with smoking—in a sense, it would be remarkable if they didn't try it at some time. Studies show that parents have an important influence on whether or not their children begin smoking. Children learn about adult behavior through their parents, using them as role models, and may come to associate smoking with being mature. An admired older brother or sister may have a similar effect on a child. Thus many teenagers see cigarette smoking as a symbol of adulthood.

Of course, many young people start smoking even though their parents and relatives do not; in many cases, smoking becomes the teenager's gesture of independence from parents and family. Peer influence is extremely important in the development of the smoking habit during the teenage and college years. Young people often try their first cigarette at the urging of friends, and they may continue to smoke if it is an accepted and admired habit within their social group. One Gallup survey showed that 38 percent of teenagers who start to smoke do so because of peer pressure. Health education is therefore a critical need for students in this age group.

In our society cigarette smoking used to be strongly associated with freedom, independence, urbanity, glamour, and sophistication. Advertising campaigns, now restricted to the print media, still represent cigarette smokers as mature, sophisticated, and attractive. The male smoker is portrayed as tough, the female as liberated; party goers still smoke, and so do people in love. Yet public awareness of the dangers of smoking, combined with the recent physical fitness movement, has helped many people to see such ads as ridiculous. Advertising is losing its power to persuade because antismoking campaigns have portrayed a truer image of smokers, depicting them as unhealthy victims of a powerful habit and sadly out of step with the times.

The Four Types of Smokers

Smoking is widespread throughout the United States among all groups, cutting across the lines of race and socioeconomic background; seemingly, no major personality characteristics differentiate smokers from nonsmokers. Most persons who smoke are at some stage of becoming habituated—or perhaps addicted—to nicotine, or are in transition from one stage to another.

1. **The Pleasure Smoker.** Pleasure smokers love their cigarettes and are not habituated to **nicotine.** They reach for a cigarette because they enjoy its taste and experience either relaxation or stimulation from smoking. They also enjoy the ritual of smoking; for example, they may like to watch the smoke as they exhale. Pleasure smokers usually have little trouble giving up cigarettes, since they have not yet developed a physical or psychological dependence on nicotine; it is relatively easy for them to substitute another enjoyable experience.

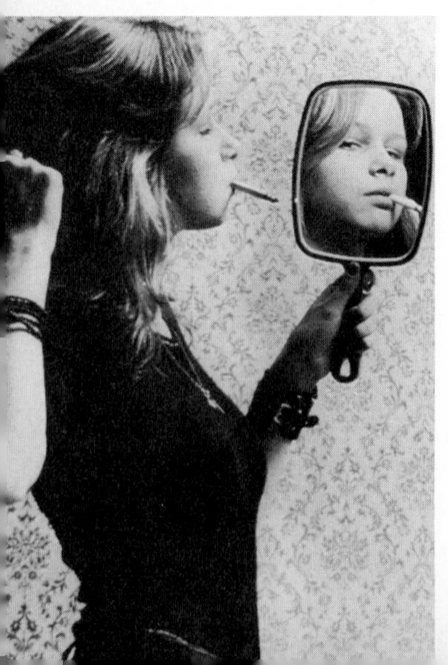

2. **The Negative-Affect Smoker.** Negative-affect smokers are beginning to become habituated to nicotine and use cigarettes as a crutch; they reach for a cigarette in times of crisis. The nicotine in tobacco smoke produces a sedative effect that relieves negative feelings of nervousness, anger, worry, shame, or disgust. The negative-affect smoker is closely related to the pleasure smoker, since relief from stress is also a pleasurable experience. The best help for negative-affect smokers lies in giving up cigarettes before they develop a stronger habit and in learning to deal with problems in more direct and less harmful ways.

3. **The Habitual Smoker.** Habitual smokers frequently crave a cigarette and smoke automatically; in fact, they do not feel at peace with themselves unless they have a lighted cigarette nearby. Because they have developed a strong habit, habitual smokers must make a concerted effort to give up cigarettes.

4. **The Heavy Smoker.** Heavy smokers have become strongly habituated to nicotine. They are the "chain smokers" who live for cigarettes, already lighting the next as they near the end of the one they are smoking. According to many psychologists, heavy smokers feel acutely uncomfortable unless they maintain a certain level of nicotine in their systems at all times. They reach for a cigarette even before getting out of bed in the morning and continue to smoke cigarettes at the rate of one every ten or fifteen minutes during the day. They often do not sleep well at night, perhaps because they are experiencing a mild form of nicotine withdrawal. More than any other type of smoker, heavy smokers need outside help to give up cigarettes.

SMOKING AND HEALTH

In addition to its habit-forming properties, tobacco smoke contains over 2,000 chemical compounds, many of which are known **carcinogens,** or cancer-causing agents. The smoke is made up of gases, organic vapors, and particulate matter, which includes **tar** and nicotine. Cigarette, pipe, or cigar smoke varies in chemical composition with the type of tobacco and the temperature of the smoke during puffing.

Particulate matter, which forms about 8 percent of tobacco smoke, contains the greater part of the known cancer-producing agents found in tobacco smoke. There are about 5 billion particles per milliliter of smoke from a nonfilter cigarette—more than 50,000 times as many particles as in an equal amount of polluted air. The remainder of tobacco smoke consists of gases such as nitrogen, carbon dioxide, oxygen, and carbon monoxide.

SURGEON GENERAL'S WARNING: Cigarette Smoke Contains Carbon Monoxide.

Considering the chemical composition of tobacco smoke, the physical effects of smoking on the body are not surprising. Evidence shows that life expectancy is reduced an average of eight years in heavy smokers (two packs a day or more) and four years in light smokers (one-half pack a day). In a recent publication the Public Health Service stated, "At every age from 35 on, death rates are higher for cigarette smokers than for nonsmokers. This is true of women as well as men. . . . Compared to the nonsmoker, the two-pack-a-day smoker has more than twice the chance of dying of heart disease and 20 times the chance of dying of lung cancer."

Lung Cancer

Cigarette smoking has been causally related to many forms of cancer. (Cancer is an uncontrolled growth of cells that invades neighboring tissue and spreads to other parts of the body, destroying healthy cells in the process; see Chapter 14.) Perhaps the most dangerous form of cancer that has been directly linked to smoking is lung cancer.

Lung cancer took approximately 130,000 lives in 1986. It is the major cause of cancer death among Americans. Eighty-five percent of all cases of lung cancer in men and 75 percent in women develop among smokers. The death rate for this disease is about eight times higher for smokers than for nonsmokers and about twenty times higher for two-pack-a-day smokers.

Just sixty years ago lung cancer was relatively uncommon. The majority of tobacco users before World War I were men who smoked cigars or pipes or chewed tobacco. Relatively few of these smokers inhaled because of the harshness of the tobacco used in cigars and pipes. Gradually, cigarettes became more popular, and in the 1930s women began to smoke too. With the increase in cigarette usage came an increase in the number of smokers who inhaled, a change in practice that has undoubtedly led to the increase in lung cancer and other respiratory diseases over the past four decades.

When smokers inhale, they draw the smoke through the mouth and throat and down into the lungs. The gases and particles of the smoke pass into the **bronchi,** two large tubes through which air travels to the lungs, and where most cases of lung cancer originate. Over a period of time the tissue of the bronchial lining begins to react to the irritating presence of smoking residue.

First, the number of cells immediately below those lining the surface of the bronchi increases and the manner in which tissues react to irritation is altered. Next, the fine, hairlike growths, or cilia, along the surface of the lining, whose function is to clean the lungs of foreign particles, begin to slow or stop their movement. In time, the cilia may disappear altogether, and as a consequence carcinogenic substances remain in contact with sensitive cells in the lining of the bronchi instead of being removed in the mucous. This contact over long periods of time is believed to cause the development of cancer. At this stage a *smoker's cough* may develop. It is a feeble attempt by the body to clear the lungs of foreign particles in the absence of functioning cilia. Symptoms of lung cancer are a persistent and nagging cough, shortness of breath, chest pains, increased coughing up of phlegm, occasionally blood-streaked sputum, and eventually loss of strength and body weight.

> SURGEON GENERAL'S WARNING: Smoking Causes Lung Cancer, Heart Disease, Emphysema, And May Complicate Pregnancy.

Because some of these symptoms are also caused by other types of illness, very few lung cancer patients consult their doctors during these early stages while their disease can still be successfully treated. The death rate from lung cancer is therefore very high, with only about 13 percent of its victims surviving more than five years after diagnosis and treatment. If cancer of the lung is discovered in time, its spread can sometimes be halted by surgical removal of the cancerous growth, a process that often involves removal of a lung.

Other Types of Cancer

Not only is there an important causal link between smoking and lung cancer, but there is also every reason to believe that smoking causes tens of thousands of deaths each year from cancer of the mouth, esophagus, prostate, bladder, and stomach. As the mortality chart for smokers shows (Figure 12-2), smokers run at least twice the risk of developing these types of cancer as nonsmokers.

FIGURE 12-2

Mortality ratio of smokers to nonsmokers for several diseases

Source: "Cigarette Smoking or Your Health," *Medical Times*, 110, No. 6 (June 1982), pp. 37–43.

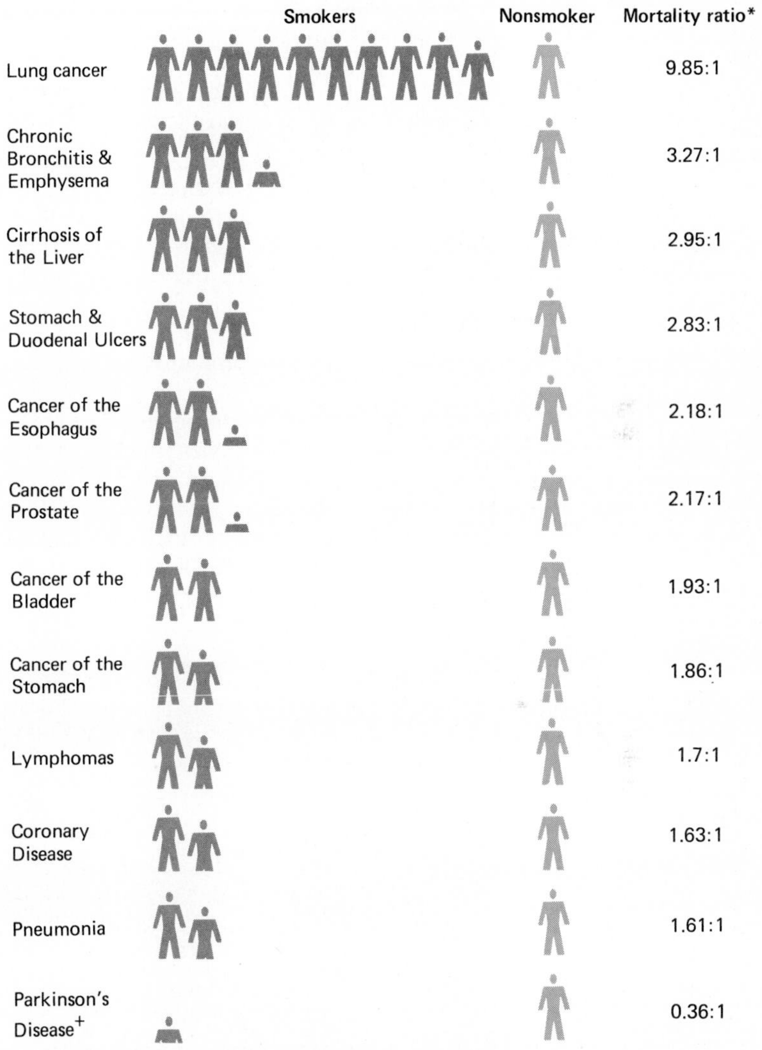

	Smokers	Nonsmoker	Mortality ratio*
Lung cancer			9.85:1
Chronic Bronchitis & Emphysema			3.27:1
Cirrhosis of the Liver			2.95:1
Stomach & Duodenal Ulcers			2.83:1
Cancer of the Esophagus			2.18:1
Cancer of the Prostate			2.17:1
Cancer of the Bladder			1.93:1
Cancer of the Stomach			1.86:1
Lymphomas			1.7:1
Coronary Disease			1.63:1
Pneumonia			1.61:1
Parkinson's Disease+			0.36:1

*A mortality ratio of 1:1 means that the death rate for smokers is the same as that for nonsmokers.

+This is the only condition with a clearly lowered death rate in cigarette smokers

In some of these forms of cancer the relationship between smoking and the disease seems fairly direct. For example, pipe smokers who usually hold their pipes in the same position in their mouth frequently develop cancer of the lip in that area. The association between smoking and other forms of cancer seems less direct.

Smoking and Other Diseases

The effects of smoking are not limited to cancer. Statistics also clearly demonstrate a greater probability that smokers will suffer from heart disease, a number of respiratory disorders, and peptic ulcers, as well as other diseases.

Diseases of the Heart and Circulatory System. The nicotine and carbon monoxide present in cigarette smoke are believed to be major contributors to the development of coronary disease. Approximately 225,000 people die each year from the effects of smoking-related heart disease. If everyone in the country stopped smoking, the heart attack rate would drop by 20 percent. Diseases affecting the coronary arteries are three times more common among smokers than nonsmokers, and the risk of suffering from these disorders increases with age and duration of smoking. Studies reveal that smoking can cause cardiovascular malfunction, and there is also evidence that arteriosclerosis, or hardening of the arteries, may be promoted by smoking.

Chronic Diseases of the Lung and Bronchi. Each year approximately 19,000 people die from the effects of smoking on their lungs and bronchi. The severe changes in the lungs brought about by tobacco smoke make them susceptible to respiratory diseases as well as cancer. Pulmonary **emphysema** is one such disease. Emphysema results from obstruction of the small bronchial tubes (the bronchioles), brought about by the effect of smoking on the cilia. The function of exhaling becomes especially impaired. Symptoms of pulmonary emphysema

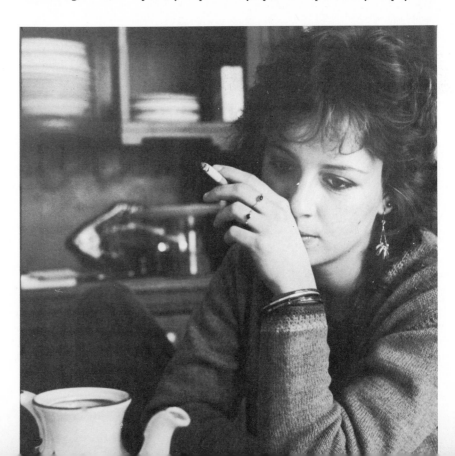

include breathlessness, coughing, attacks of bronchitis, wheezing, and, in the later stages, bloating and distortion of the chest cavity.

Chronic bronchitis, another respiratory disease most frequently caused by cigarette smoking, is an inflammation of the mucous membranes of the bronchial tubes. Chronic bronchitis begins as a cough appearing in the cold months of the year, often called the "winter cough." Symptoms include congestion of the lungs, coughing up of phlegm, and difficulty in breathing. If the disease is not treated, it can lead to more serious disorders of the lungs and eventually result in death. Treatment of either emphysema or chronic bronchitis always includes cessation of smoking. These are incapacitating diseases, forcing many relatively young people into premature retirement.

Peptic Ulcers. Recent studies have shown that men who smoke have a 50 percent greater chance of suffering from *peptic ulcers*—especially gastric ulcers—than men who have never smoked. Although it is not known whether smoking causes ulcers, a strong correlation between smoking and the delayed healing of ulcers has been found.

Problems Found in Infants Born of Mothers Who Smoke. Mothers who smoke increase their chances of giving birth to babies with a variety of problems. Babies born to mothers who smoke weigh an average of half a pound less than other babies. Low-birth-weight babies often have serious physical and mental problems, whether or not they are born prematurely. They are also more likely to be victims of sudden infant death syndrome. Studies have shown that smoking may take its toll even before the baby is born. Mothers who smoke nearly double their risk of losing their babies through spontaneous abortion. They also increase their chances of having *placenta previa*—a condition in which the placenta is attached abnormally low in the uterus—which can lead to serious problems during labor and birth. Infant prematurity, stillbirth, neonatal death, and malformations of the heart and other organs are linked to maternal smoking. All physicians clearly warn pregnant women that they must stop smoking for the health of their unborn child. Recent evidence suggests that in order to avoid birth complications, prospective mothers should discontinue smoking at some point before pregnancy.

SURGEON GENERAL'S WARNING: Smoking By Pregnant Women May Result in Fetal Injury, Premature Birth, And Low Birth Weight.

Noncancerous Oral Diseases. Diseases of the mouth affecting the gums, bones, and tissue around the teeth are more common among smokers than nonsmokers. Research indicates that smokers suffer more from *gingivitis*, an inflammation of the gums; from deterioration of the jawbone around the sockets of the teeth; and from inflammation of the palate. Loss of teeth and delayed healing after tooth extraction may also be associated with smoking.

Smoking and the Pill. Women over age 30 who smoke and use birth control pills increase their chances of dying from heart attack and circulatory disease. They are three times as likely as nonsmokers who take the Pill and ten times as likely as women who neither smoke nor use the Pill to suffer from heart disease. Furthermore, women between the ages of 40 and 44 who take the Pill but do not smoke have a death rate from heart attack of 11 per 100,000. When they combine smoking with the Pill, their death rate skyrockets to 62 per 100,000 a year. To warn women against these serious dangers, package inserts are included in all birth control packages. The insert tells Pill users in no uncertain terms not to smoke.

Poor General Health. Smokers tend to suffer more than nonsmokers from many types of illness. For example, heavy smokers are more susceptible to influenza and pneumonia and to various parasitic diseases than those who have never smoked. The National Health Survey indicates that males between the ages of 45 and 64 who smoke experience a 28 percent higher incidence of disability from illness than do nonsmoking males of the same age. Workers who smoke lose some 77 million workdays annually in excess of the normal rate of loss from worker disability. And because smoking decreases the body's efficient use of oxygen ("wind") and increases the heart rate, smokers perform less well than nonsmokers in physical work and exercise. Studies of college students indicate that smokers perform less proficiently than nonsmokers in a variety of exercises and athletic events because of reduced lung and heart efficiency.

SMOKING VARIABLES AND HEALTH

Not all smokers are physically affected to the same degree by smoking. Research into the morbidity and mortality rates of smokers versus those of nonsmokers has shown that several important factors govern the health dangers of smoking. As might be expected, the *number of cigarettes consumed* has an important effect on health: The more cigarettes a person smokes, the more harmful the impact on the body. A man of 25 who has never smoked can expect to live 4.6 years longer than a man who smokes one to nine cigarettes a day; 6.2 years longer than a man who smokes twenty to thirty cigarettes a day; and 8.3 years longer than a man who smokes over two packs a day. A boy who starts smoking before the age of 15 and continues to smoke has only half the chance of living to age 75 as a boy who never took up the habit (see Figure 12-3).

The *extent of inhalation* is also reflected in health statistics. Individuals who inhale deeply and fill their lungs with smoke are more likely to suffer harmful health effects than those who do not inhale. Another important factor is the *duration of smoking*. People who have smoked for many years have a greater chance of developing diseases associated with smoking than those who have smoked for a shorter time.

Damage to the body from smoking also varies with the type of cigarette smoked. Filter cigarettes are less dangerous than nonfilters. Cigarettes with large quantities of nicotine and tar—the "strong" cigarettes—are more harmful

FIGURE 12-3

Death rates of smokers by age smoking began, per 100,000 population.

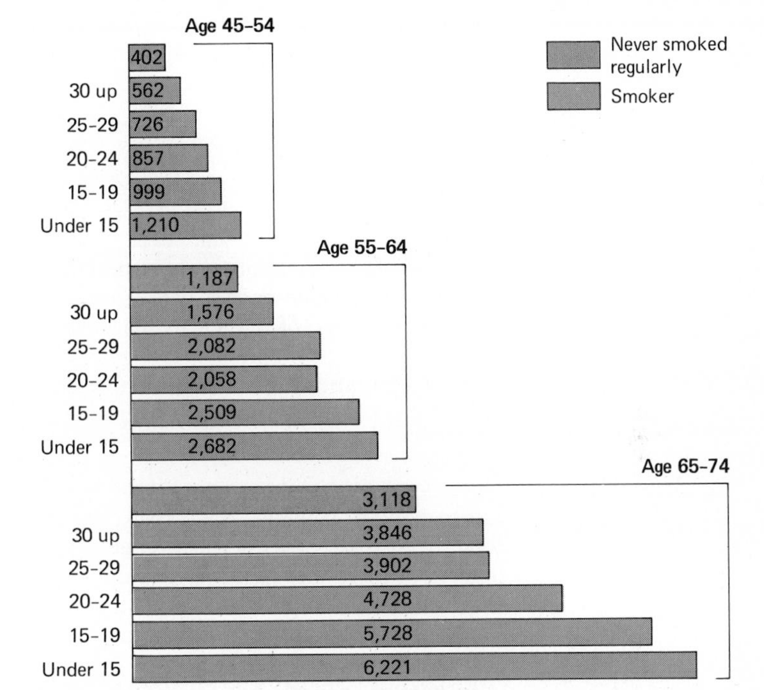

than milder brands. The American Cancer Society cautions that low-tar brands should be smoked by people who refuse to quit altogether.

How close to the end a cigarette is smoked also influences its harmful effects. Tests have shown that the last half of the cigarette contains 60 percent of the tars and nicotine; the last few puffs are even worse and contain an inordinately high level of tar and nicotine.

Until a few years ago women suffered far less than men from lung cancer because their smoking habits differed. Investigators found that not only had women been smoking for a shorter time than men but also that their smoking habits were less dangerous. They smoked less, they inhaled less, and they more often smoked filter-tip and low-tar and low-nicotine cigarettes.

Statistics comparing male and female population groups are significant because environmental factors are constant for the two groups: Women and men have the same diets, breathe the same air, live under the same stresses, and are exposed to the same viruses. Yet, until recently, the rate of lung cancer among women was always much lower than the rate among men. Now an increasing number of women are smoking. They are starting at a younger age, and they are smoking more heavily. Thus within the last generation the lung cancer rate for women has more than tripled.

Many people are unaware of the positive side of quitting smoking, believing that they have already damaged themselves beyond repair. However, the effects of smoking on the lungs and bronchi are usually reversible if an individual "kicks the habit" before invasive cancer occurs. Gradually, the nuclei of the cells lining the bronchi return to normal, and the lung-cleansing cilia are restored. Chances of incurring respiratory disease also greatly diminish with the cessation

SURGEON GENERAL'S WARNING: Quitting Smoking Now Greatly Reduces Serious Risks to Your Health.

of smoking. Breathing becomes easier, "wind" improves, and the smoker's cough disappears. Even some of the harmful effects of smoking on the cardiovascular system are reversible once a person ceases to smoke. Circulation improves, as does the exchange of oxygen in the lungs. And since the heart does not have to work as hard as before, the incidence of coronary disease among ex-smokers is lower. Conditions such as peptic ulcers and oral diseases are also more likely to heal if a person quits smoking cigarettes.

DECIDING TO QUIT

Once smoking has become an established part of people's life styles, what can be done to convince them that they should give up smoking, or to protect them from some of its negative effects in the event that they cannot quit? In order to muster the willpower to stop, confirmed smokers must become aware that smoking is a powerful habit and a serious hazard to their health; they must see the dangers of smoking as relevant to them; and they must admit that they can and should quit.

In spite of uncomfortable withdrawal symptoms, smokers who desire strongly enough to quit smoking can stop the practice on their own, perhaps with the help of pamphlets and brochures distributed by health organizations. Even many habitual and heavy smokers fall into this category. They simply decide to stop and never smoke again. Quitting outright, or "cold turkey," as this is called, is the method used by 95 percent of smokers who are successful in breaking the habit. Over 43 million Americans have successfully quit smoking. They were motivated and able to quit for many reasons: concern about their health; desire to be free of a physically habituating drug; disgust with unpleasant aspects of smoking such as odor, falling ashes, and burned clothing; unwillingness to set a bad example for others, such as their children or spouse; or simply wanting to be rid of the daily expense.

Factors That Affect Quitting

Many smokers have a difficult time overcoming their nicotine habit. In order to break it, they should ask themselves why they smoke. When are they likely to reach for a cigarette? This kind of self-analysis is necessary for a change in behavior to take place. The specific answers to these questions also will help the smoker select the best way to kick the habit.

Those who are quitting smoking might consider a temporary substitute—gum, candy, or the like. The fear of weight gain is not unfounded, but only a third of those who quit gain weight; the second third stay the same; and the last third actually lose weight. A temporary weight gain is far less harmful than continued smoking. Someone who smokes during a particular activity—while having coffee, for example—might concentrate particularly hard on not smoking during that activity. Those who see giving up cigarettes as a terrible self-denial can remind themselves frequently of the consequences of smoking—or take up exercise as an outlet for their irritation.

Remembering the positive aspects of not smoking is also helpful. Food tastes better; you have more energy; your sense of smell improves; the bad taste in your mouth disappears; you breathe more easily; you sleep more soundly; and you no longer carry an odor offensive to nonsmokers. Most important, people who quit have the satisfaction of knowing that they are mature enough to understand the future consequences of their present acts and that they are capable of controlling their own lives.

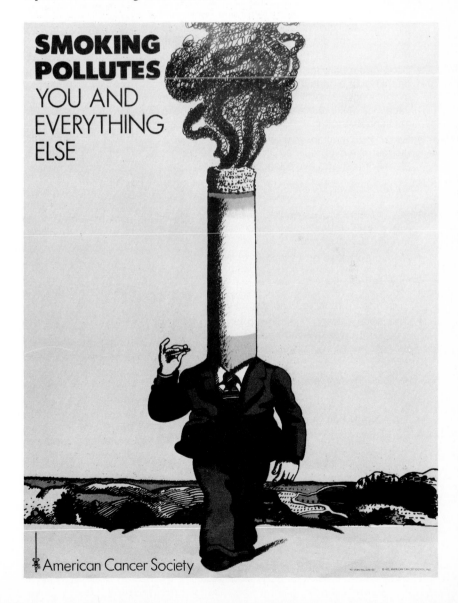

Clearing the Air: A Guide to Quitting Smoking

When Thinking about Quitting . . .

- List all the reasons why you want to quit.
- Every night before going to bed, repeat one of the reasons 10 times.
- Decide positively that you want to quit. Try to avoid negative thoughts about how difficult it might be.
- Develop strong personal reasons in addition to your health and obligations to others. For example, think of all the time you waste taking cigarette breaks, rushing out to buy a pack, hunting a light, etc.
- Set a target date for quitting—perhaps a special day like your birthday, your anniversary, a holiday. If you smoke heavily at work, quit during your vacation. Make the date sacred, and don't let anything change it.
- Begin to condition yourself physically: start a modest exercise regimen; drink more fluids; get plenty of rest and avoid fatigue.

Involve Someone Else . . .

- Bet a friend you can quit on your target date. Put your cigarette money aside every day, and forfeit it if you smoke.
- Ask your spouse or a friend to quit with you.

Switch Brands . . .

- Switch to a brand you find distasteful.
- Change to a brand that's low in tar and nicotine a couple of weeks before your target date. This will help lessen your physical dependence on cigarettes.

Cut Down the Number of Cigarettes You Smoke . . .

- Smoke only half of each cigarette.
- Each day, postpone lighting your first cigarette one hour.
- Decide you will smoke only during odd or even hours of the day.
- Decide beforehand how many cigarettes you'll smoke during the day. For each additional smoke, give a dollar to your favorite charity.
- Don't smoke when you first experience a craving. Wait several minutes; and during this time, change your activity or talk to someone.
- Stop buying cigarettes by the carton. Wait until one pack is empty before buying another.
- Stop carrying cigarettes with you at home and at work. Make them difficult to get to.
- Smoke only under circumstances which are not especially pleasurable for you. If you like to smoke with others, smoke alone.
- Make yourself aware of each cigarette by using the opposite hand, or putting cigarettes in an unfamiliar location or different pocket to break the automatic reach.
- If you light up many times during the day without even thinking about it, try to look in a mirror each time you put a match to your cigarette—you may decide you don't need it.
- Don't smoke "automatically." Smoke only those you *really* want.
- Reward yourself in some way other than smoking.
- Reach for a glass of juice instead of a cigarette for a "pick-me-up."
- Change your eating habits to aid in cutting down. For example, drink milk, which is frequently considered incompatible with smoking. End meals or snacks with something that won't lead to a cigarette.
- Don't empty your ashtrays. This will not only remind you of how many cigarettes you have smoked each day, the sight and smell of stale butts will be very unpleasant.

Just before Quitting . . .

- Smoke more heavily than usual so the experience becomes distasteful.
- Collect all your cigarette butts in one large glass container as a visual reminder of the filth smoking represents.
- Practice going without cigarettes. Don't think of *never* smoking again. Think of quitting in terms of one day at a time. Tell yourself you won't smoke today and then don't.

On the Day You Quit . . .

- Throw away all cigarettes and matches. Hide lighters and ashtrays.
- Visit the dentist, and have your teeth cleaned to get rid of tobacco stains. Notice how nice they look, and resolve to keep them that way.

- Make a list of things you'd like to buy yourself or someone else. Estimate the cost in terms of packs of cigarettes, and put the money aside to buy these presents.
- Keep very busy on the big day. Go to the movies, exercise, take long walks, go bike riding.
- Buy yourself a treat, or do something special to celebrate.

Immediately after Quitting . . .

- The first few days after you quit, spend as much free time as possible in places where smoking is prohibited.
- Drink large quantities of water and fruit juice.
- Try to avoid alcohol, coffee, and other beverages with which you associate cigarette smoking.
- Strike up a conversation with someone instead of a match for a cigarette.
- If you miss the sensation of having a cigarette in your hand, play with something else—a pencil, a paper clip, a marble.
- If you miss having something in your mouth, try toothpicks or a fake cigarette.

Avoid Temptation . . .

- Instead of smoking after meals, get up from the table and brush your teeth or go for a walk.
- If you always smoke while driving, take public transportation for a while.
- Temporarily avoid situations you strongly associate with the pleasurable aspects of smoking, e.g., watching your favorite TV program, sitting in your favorite chair, having a cocktail before dinner, etc.
- Until you are confident of your ability to stay off cigarettes, limit your socializing to healthful outdoor activities or situations where smoking is prohibited.
- If you must be in a situation where you'll be tempted to smoke (such as a cocktail or dinner party), try to associate with the nonsmokers there.

Find New Habits . . .

- Change your habits to make smoking difficult, impossible, or unnecessary. Try activities such as swimming, jogging, tennis, or handball.
- Do things to maintain a clean mouth taste, such as brushing your teeth frequently, and using a mouthwash.
- Do things that require you to use your hands. Try crossword puzzles, needlework, gardening, or household chores. Go bike riding; take the dog for a walk; give yourself a manicure; write letters; try new recipes.
- Stretch a lot.
- Get plenty of rest.
- Pay attention to your appearance. Look and feel sharp.

When You Get the "Crazies". . .

- Keep oral substitutes handy—things like carrots, pickles, sunflower seeds, apples, celery, raisins, sugarless gum, and so on.
- Take 10 deep breaths, and hold the last one while lighting a match. Exhale slowly, and blow out the match. Pretend it is a cigarette, and crush it out in an ashtray.
- Take a shower or bath if possible.
- Learn to relax quickly and deeply. Make yourself limp, visualize a soothing, pleasing situation, and get away from it all for a moment. Concentrate on that peaceful image and nothing else.
- Light incense or a candle instead of a cigarette.
- Never allow yourself to think that "one won't hurt"—it will.

Marking Progress . . .

- Each month, on the anniversary of your quit date, plan a special celebration.
- Periodically, write down new reasons why you are glad you quit, and post these reasons where you'll be sure to see them.
- Make up a calendar for the first 90 days. Cross off each day and indicate the money saved by not smoking.
- Set other intermediate target dates, and do something special with the money you've saved.

Source: Abridged from DHEW Publication No. (NIH) 78–1647, U.S. Dept of HEW, Public Health Service, National Institute of Health.

Quitting Smoking: Where to Go for Help

American Cancer Society*
777 Third Avenue
New York, N.Y. 10017

American Heart Association*
7320 Greenville Avenue
Dallas, Tex. 75231

Office on Smoking and Health
U.S. Department of Health and Human Services
Park Building, Room 110
5600 Fishers Lane
Rockville, Md. 20857

American Lung Association*
1740 Broadway
New York, N.Y. 10019

Office of Cancer Communication
National Cancer Institute
National Institutes of Health
Bethesda, Md. 20205
(800) 4-CANCER

* Consult your local telephone directory for listing of local chapters.

Where to Find Help

Some smokers may want to consult their private physician to work out a plan for stopping. In fact, many smokers try to stop in the first place because they have been advised to do so by their doctors. Some heavy smokers may need intensive programs in order to give up the habit. To aid this type of smoker, *antismoking clinics* have been developed. Most of these clinics are patterned after organizations such as Alcoholics Anonymous and Weight Watchers; smokers who are trying to break their habit meet to offer each other support and encouragement in abstaining from cigarette use. Other clinics use forms of aversion therapy—such as giving the smokers a mild shock every time they reach for a cigarette—to implant negative associations with cigarettes in smokers' minds. Be sure to check the validity of any program before joining. Your consumer protection agency and heart, lung, or cancer association may be able to assist you in your selection.

If you are successful at quitting, you may be in for even greater rewards than improved health. Some insurance companies have begun to reduce their rates for certain kinds of life and fire insurance policies for people who have discontinued smoking. Their rationale is that nonsmokers should not have to pay a penalty for smokers' shorter life spans.

PROTECTION AGAINST SMOKING

As our experience with alcohol and Prohibition suggests, a worldwide ban on the marketing of cigarettes and tobacco would not be effective. More viable alternatives are to control the advertising and promotion of cigarettes by the tobacco industry, expand antismoking advertising campaigns, and provide public instruction concerning the dangers of smoking.

The Tobacco Industry and Economics

Controls over the amount and type of advertising conducted by the cigarette industry depend primarily upon the attitudes and concern of our national legislators. But legislators generally have been unwilling to exercise rigid controls over an industry that is so important to the economy and that pours such large sums of money into its lobbying efforts in Washington. The federal govern-

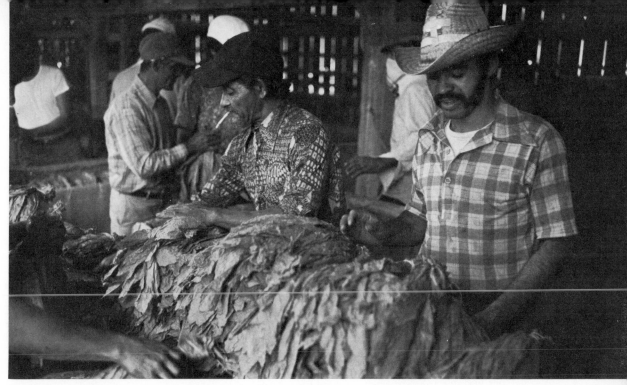

The tobacco industry supports migrant workers as well as farmers, manufacturers, advertisers, and small shopkeepers. It brings in more than $8 billion a year in taxes. Nonetheless, public pressure to restrict smoking continues to grow.

ment collects over $4.1 billion in tobacco taxes annually, and under the Reagan administration a law was passed to double the tax on cigarettes. State and local taxes account for another $4.2 billion. The tobacco industry employs thousands of people, and of course cigarettes are an important revenue source for small shopowners and vending machine companies. Furthermore, tobacco products are an important export item. In fact, they are so crucial to the United States' balance of payments that the government provides subsidies to the tobacco industry to enable tobacco farmers to sell their goods abroad competitively. Paradoxically, the government also subsidizes research that proves the health danger of cigarettes.

Antismoking Campaigns

Despite the fiscal importance of tobacco products, public pressure following issuance of the Surgeon General's Report on cigarettes led Congress to ban broadcast advertising of cigarettes starting in 1972. However, cigarette companies sharply increased their advertising in other media and, according to recent estimates, are spending over $600 million a year for newspaper and magazine ads. Public pressure to ban all tobacco advertising has gained some momentum—the American Medical Association called for such a ban in 1986—but there is little evidence that it will result in legislation in the near future.

Another effective measure to reduce cigarette consumption has been to change the image of the smoker. Antismoking organizations are trying to do just that. In the belief that well-planned "counteradvertisements" can help people stop smoking or help prevent the younger generation from starting to smoke, they are using the mass media to get their message across: that smokers are harming themselves and their children and that, far from presenting an image of glamour or sophistication, they look sad and rather seedy. However, the amount of

PROBLEMS AND CONTROVERSIES: Passive Smoking

Does the right to life, liberty, and the pursuit of happiness suggest there is a right to smoke? Does anyone have a right to smoke in your living room, near your desk or your table? Or is smoking a privilege that must be extended by others because by its very nature it encompasses others? When the question arises—in offices, in some college classrooms, in restaurants, at dinner parties—tempers flare quickly. Nonsmokers who complain appear arrogant, intolerant, and pious to the smoker. To the nonsmoker, the man or woman lighting a cigarette seems selfish, boorish, and even dirty.

Nonsmokers who hate the smell of smoke and suspect the hazards of sidestream smoke blowing their way used to have to grin and bear it. Over the past decade, however, antismoking propaganda has effectively destroyed the image of the debonair smoker. More and more people have quit—some of them becoming intolerant of smoke and openly disdainful of friends and family members too weak to follow their example. Four out of five states and many localities have passed laws limiting smoking in public places. And some research confirms the belief that *passive* smoking—exposure to tobacco smoke—is harmful to those who do not smoke.

What is the evidence? While controversy still surrounds the effects of sidestream smoke on the health of nonsmoking adults, the 1984 Surgeon General's Report presents strong evidence that it poses a danger to children. Children whose parents smoke were found to have significantly more respiratory symptoms and severe illnesses such as bronchitis and pneumonia than those raised in nonsmoking households. They were also out sick from school and hospitalized more often.

For those adults who have allergies, or are already ill with heart disease and respiratory problems, the dangers of passive smoking have been established. The effects of sidestream smoke upon healthy adults who do not smoke are not quite so certain. Studies in Japan and Greece showed that the nonsmoking wives of heavy smokers are more likely to develop lung cancer than wives of nonsmokers. But a twelve-year study by the National Cancer Institute of over 175,000 nonsmoking women showed that wives of heavy smokers are at no higher risk than wives of nonsmokers.

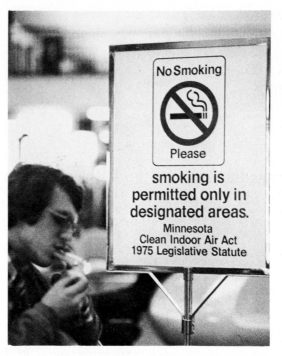

The 1984 Surgeon General's Report sums up the most serious claims that can be made so far about the negative effects of sidestream smoke. 1) It significantly pollutes indoor environments. 2) Nonsmokers absorb a certain amount of nicotine from environmental tobacco smoke. 3) Sidestream smoke irritates the eyes and may cause small changes in the pulmonary functioning of nonsmokers. And 4) exposure to sidestream smoke at home clearly damages the health of children.

Regardless of the mixed results from research on passive smoking, few would argue that polluted air is as good as clean air. And as the number of protesting nonsmokers increases, more and more laws are sure to be passed outlawing smoking in enclosed spaces.

Source: U.S. Surgeon General, *Summary of the Health Consequences of Smoking*: *Chronic Obstructive Lung Disease*, U.S. Department of Health and Human Services, National Institutes of Health (Washington, D.C.: U.S. Government Printing Office, 1985).

money available for these antismoking commercials is limited and broadcasters have been reluctant to donate free time.

Concerns of Nonsmokers

One positive trend in recent years has been the increased willingness of nonsmokers to speak out against smoking. Many nonsmokers are annoyed by others' tobacco smoke and are aware that **passive smoking**—being exposed to tobacco smoke in the environment—can be harmful (see box: Passive Smoking). They have made their feelings known to legislators; as a result, many agencies and municipalities have recently made smoking in public places illegal. In addition, about forty states have banned smoking, at least to some degree, in public places.

Perhaps the most important step to be taken to reduce cigarette consumption is the implementation of a nationwide public education program. Such a program could be effective for those who are already habituated. But it would be even more important as a preventive measure if it were instituted in elementary schools, for it is here that the image of the cigarette smoker as a cool sophisticate begins to take hold and that cigarettes become an outlet for rebellion. Such a program of education should stress not only the hazards of smoking but also the artificiality of the smoking image and the foolishness of associating cigarettes with independence. Only by creating a negative image of smoking in the minds of the young can the use of cigarettes finally be curtailed.

SUMMARY

1. Despite the fact that cigarette smoking has been proven injurious to health, 52 million Americans still smoke. Most people begin smoking during the teenage years, generally because their parents smoke, their friends smoke, or they identify smoking with being grown up.

2. Most regular smokers fall into one of the following four categories: the *pleasure smoker*, who is gratified both by cigarettes and the process of smoking but is not yet habituated; the *negative-affect smoker*, who is beginning to become habituated to nicotine and uses cigarettes as a crutch when tense, nervous, or angry; the *habitual smoker*, who has become habituated without realizing it and smokes automatically; and the *heavy smoker*, who is strongly habituated to nicotine.

3. Some of the particulate matter in cigarettes includes *tar* and *nicotine*. These particles are known *carcinogens*, or cancer-causing substances. *Lung cancer* is the most dangerous form of cancer that has been directly linked to cigarettes. Inhaled tar is deposited in the *bronchi* and lungs, leading to a condition in which the cells below the bronchial lining increase in number. Gradually, the *cilia*, hairlike projections that cleanse the lungs, may disappear. A smoker's cough may develop as the body attempts to dislodge tar particles. Finally, physical changes in the bronchial cells may lead to the formation of a localized cancer. This cancer can eventually spread throughout the lung, especially if smoking continues.

4. Other diseases associated with smoking are cancer of the esophagus, prostate, bladder, and stomach; diseases of the heart and circulatory system; *pulmonary emphysema*; and *chronic bronchitis*. In addition, peptic ulcers and poor general health are associated with smoking. Low birth weight, prematurity, and other serious problems in infants are more likely to occur when the mother smokes. Women who smoke and take the Pill are greatly increasing their chance of heart attack.

5. As might be expected, the number, type, and length of cigarettes smoked, the duration of smoking, and the extent of inhalation influence the amount of physical harm caused by smoking.

6. Since many of the physiological effects of smoking are reversible before the onset of disease, it is important that smokers give up the cigarette habit. In order to stop, smokers must come to realize that smoking is a very powerful physical habit that must be overcome; they must critically examine their reasons for smoking; and they must learn to adapt themselves to life without cigarettes. Those smokers who can't quit should cut down on cigarette consumption, inhale less, smoke less of each cigarette, and switch to filter and low-tar and low-nicotine cigarettes.

7. Protection against cigarette smoking has been hindered by the economic importance of the tobacco industry and the continued desire of great numbers of people to smoke. The tobacco industry tries to portray the smoker as popular, virile, and independent, an image that antismoking advertising continues to counter, showing smokers as immature, unhealthy slaves to a habit. More nonsmokers have become aware of the dangers of *passive smoking*—being exposed to other people's tobacco smoke—and have been instrumental in passing laws against smoking in public. What is needed is a total ban on cigarette advertising and an expanded program of public education about the dangers of smoking.

CONSUMER CONCERNS

1. The fact that 75 percent of all smokers begin to smoke before the age of 20 suggests that school antismoking programs could be improved. What would you suggest?
2. Government subsidization of the tobacco industry has been criticized frequently. What is your opinion on this issue?
3. Several cigarette companies base their advertising campaign on the low-tar factor. What is your reaction?
4. Do you believe that the Surgeon General's warning statements that appear on all packages of cigarettes and in all advertising have any effect? Do you believe that even more strongly worded statements would be more effective?

13
Drugs

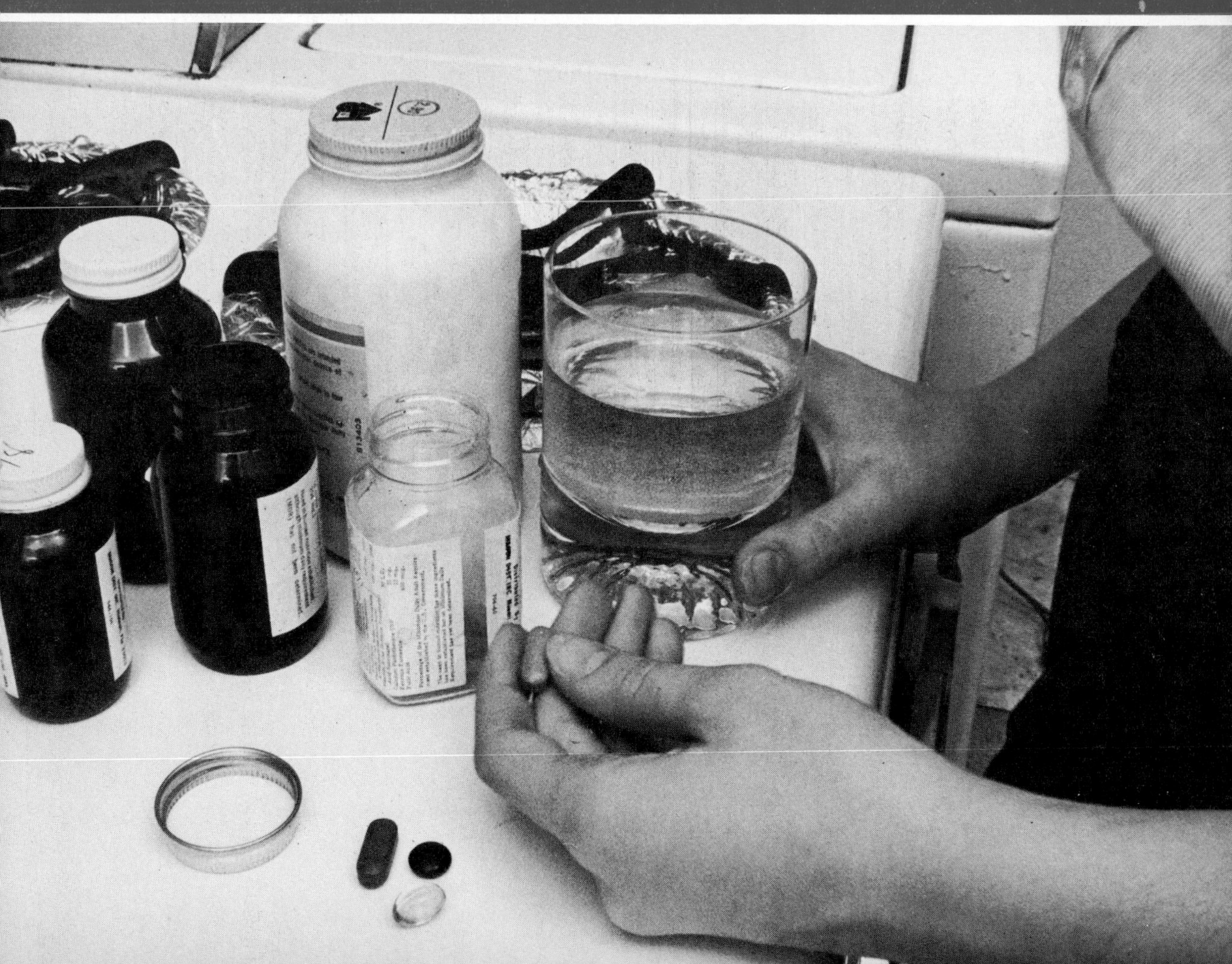

Ours is a drug-oriented society. We are urged constantly to buy the magic formula that will provide relief from our ailments, imagined or real. And we respond by swallowing billions of pills each year that will put us to sleep, keep us awake, reduce our tensions, and ease our headaches and backaches. Some of us also find refuge in alcohol or tobacco when we wish to calm ourselves at a moment of crisis. Yet despite the dependence upon, and the abuse of, these various substances, many of us believe that the drug problem in our society is restricted to the use of heroin, LSD, "angel dust," cocaine, or marijuana—in essence, to the use of illegal drugs by a deviant subculture.

The distinction our society makes between so-called therapeutic drugs and illegal drugs ignores the fact that in many ways the two are linked. Studies have shown, for example, that the children of parents who use legal drugs such as sleeping pills and alcohol are more likely than other children to use illegal drugs. The widespread availability of thousands of drugs, the pervasive advertising of drugs as a solution to all problems, and perhaps our own fondness for instant cures for our symptoms and difficulties all create an atmosphere in which both legal and illegal drugs are likely to be abused.

It is also important to recognize that our society's acceptance of some drugs and rejection of others is often a reflection of cultural bias rather than logic or fact. There is no denying, for example, the physical, psychological, and social consequences of narcotics abuse. However, the extent of the harm caused by some legal drugs far exceeds the harm caused by narcotics such as heroin. In the United States there are fewer than half a million heroin addicts, compared with nearly 14 million problem drinkers and alcoholics and about the same number of heavy smokers. Cigarettes and alcohol are directly responsible for hundreds of thousands of deaths each year. Most heavy drinkers are also heavy smokers, and nearly half of all alcoholics who seek treatment also abuse tranquilizers. We have become a nation of polydrug abusers. Yet our drug laws are designed almost exclusively to discourage the use of narcotics and hallucinogens purchased on "the street."

In this chapter we shall try to look at the problem of drug abuse objectively. We shall examine both licit and illicit drugs and their effects, see where our knowledge is lacking, and note where our society's approach to the drug problem can be improved.

SOURCES AND TYPES OF DRUGS

Drugs are chemicals, natural or synthetic, that alter the functioning of the body in some way. Most drugs are designed to relieve pain or to prevent or cure disease. Aspirin, a simple, relatively mild **analgesic** (painkiller), is a drug; heroin, a dangerous and illegal narcotic, is a drug. Between these two extremes are thousands of other drugs, all of which alter body functions to various degrees.

Drugs come from many and varied sources. They are extracted from plants, animal tissues, and minerals. Morphine, for example, a powerful (and addictive) painkiller, is derived from opium poppy seedpods. Insulin, used to treat diabetes, is extracted from the tissues of sheep. Common drugs such as iron and Epsom salts (magnesium sulfate) are simple minerals. Antibiotics such as penicillin, used to fight bacterial infections, are produced in cultures of bacteria, yeast, molds, and other live microorganisms. In addition, entirely new synthetic drugs have been developed, such as the sulfa drugs, which are used to fight infection.

Psychoactive Drugs

The word *drug* is commonly used to describe **psychoactive substances**—that is, substances that affect the central nervous system. Psychoactive drugs produce altered states of mind and include narcotics, sedatives, painkillers, stimulants, and hallucinogens.

Psychoactive substances, whether obtained illegally, by prescription, or over-the-counter in a store, are the most frequently abused drugs. Not all of them are physically addicting, but all produce a craving among those who abuse the drugs. Very broadly, psychoactive drugs fall into three categories: stimulants, depressants, and hallucinogens.

Stimulants are chemicals that produce hyperactivity. They include the amphetamines, cocaine, and caffeine. (Nicotine is sometimes classified as a stimulant, although its effects are more like those of a depressant.) Generally, stimulants are craved for their euphoric and energizing effects. High doses dangerously increase heart rate and can produce convulsions.

Depressants, or **sedatives,** work on the body and brain chemistry in the opposite way. They slow down metabolism and relax the system. Depressants include alcohol, the barbiturates, the minor tranquilizers, and the opiates, or narcotics.

Because these two categories of psychoactive drugs work on the central nervous system in opposite ways, symptoms produced by taking a stimulant may also be produced by withdrawing from a depressant. For example, a large dose of cocaine can cause convulsions; abrupt withdrawal from Valium, a sedative, also produces convulsions.

Hallucinogens, a third broad category of psychoactive drugs, have effects that are mainly psychological and therefore vary from user to user, according to expectations, setting, and other factors. Hallucinogens include LSD, peyote and mescaline, psilocybin, and the extremely dangerous compound PCP. Marijuana and hashish are no longer classified as hallucinogens because the hallucinations they sometimes produce, like alcohol-induced hallucinations, are neither common nor, usually, desired, but rather the result of overdose.

Over-the-Counter and Prescription Drugs

Nonprescription, or over-the-counter (OTC), drugs are those that can be bought in drugstores and supermarkets without restriction. This is true of a great many drugs, including aspirin compounds, cold capsules and tablets, cough syrups and cough drops, laxatives, vitamins and mineral supplements, and liniments, ointments, and lotions. Some are psychoactive. These drugs generally have the recommended dosage stated on the label or container, but they can be purchased in unlimited quantities and have a high potential for abuse.

Easily acquired, ordinary household products such as coffee, tea, tobacco, glue, cleaners, and solvents frequently contain chemicals that affect body functioning (see box: Caffeine: The Benefits and the Risks). We often interpret such easy availability as meaning that the substance involved is thought to be relatively harmless, that the amount of the chemical involved is considered inconsequential, or that abuse of the chemical is not yet seen as a social problem. However, some substances are harmful even though they are easily available;

Caffeine: The Benefits and the Risks

One of the oldest stimulants known (drinks containing it are thought to have been made in the Stone Age), caffeine has long been appreciated for its ability to excite the mind and the senses. Caffeine relieves drowsiness, quickens reaction time, and enables us to work faster and more alertly. Caffeine agitates the body. The amount in two cups of coffee or three cans of cola (150–300 milligrams) is enough to raise the heart rate, metabolism, body temperature, blood pressure, and blood sugar level.

While the amount of caffeine in two cups of morning coffee is not likely to harm anyone, larger amounts create habituation and have potentially damaging effects on the body. A regular daily intake of 500 to 600 milligrams (the amount in about four cups of coffee) is thought by some researchers to produce tolerance; and heavy coffee drinkers sometimes experience withdrawal headaches, cravings, and depression. Because of caffeine's effect on the heart, moderate-to-heavy coffee drinkers were found in one study to be at a 60 to 120 percent greater risk of heart attack than nondrinkers. Caffeine is also believed to contribute to heart problems by raising the levels of fatty acids in the blood.

Women who consume a lot of caffeine should be aware that it may promote the growth of benign lumps in breast tissue, and those who have benign lumps are at a greater risk of developing breast cancer. Equally important, pregnant women who consume a lot of caffeine may be at greater risk of having an abnormal baby.

Because so much caffeine is added to soft drinks (some clear ones contain even more caffeine than the colas), medical authorities worry about its effect on children. Owing to their small body size, children are more susceptible than adults to the average amount of caffeine in many products, but the only effects reported so far are insomnia and rapid heart beat. Still, some doctors recommend that children not be given caffeinated soft drinks.

Because of all the warnings about the possible effects of caffeine, many people have switched to decaffeinated products, especially decaffeinated coffee. But even here there may be a health risk. The food industry stopped using one chemical in the decaffeination process when it was found to cause cancer. It then began to use another one, but this chemical may also be carcinogenic. Nevertheless, most doctors say that pregnant women are better off drinking decaffeinated coffee than the pure product.

Source: Richard G. Schlaadt and Peter T. Shannon, *Drugs of Choice: Current Perspectives on Drug Use*, 2nd ed. (Englewood Cliffs, N.J.: Prentice-Hall, 1986), pp. 87–94.

the main reason for this is that the production and sale of many substances are not sufficiently controlled by the federal government. Certain commonly used drugs do not really do what their labels or advertising promise; others can do far too much. We shall discuss over-the-counter drugs in Chapter 16.

A great many drugs can be legally acquired only by written order, or **prescription,** from a physician. Almost all drugs that are addictive or habit-forming require a prescription, as do drugs that are not safe for use except under the supervision of a physician. A prescription must be written on a form containing the physician's name, address, and license number, as well as the name and quantity of the drug to be used, instructions to the pharmacist on how it is to be prepared, and explicit directions for its use by the patient. The *dosage*, or amount of the drug to be used during a specified period of time, is also noted.

Unfortunately, both the spirit and the letter of these laws are sometimes violated. Many prescriptions are illegally obtained, and some physicians are lax in weighing the side effects of the drugs they prescribe. And many people pay no attention to the warnings of side effects listed on drug containers, just as they ignore the warnings on cigarette packages. Thus many drugs are overprescribed and overused.

Some physicians and pharmacists illegally supply dealers and addicts with hundreds of thousands of prescription drugs. Only a handful of such professionals do this, but they are considered by law enforcement officials to constitute a major source of illicit prescription drugs.

DRUG EFFECTS

The method by which a drug is administered or applied is related to the way in which the drug works. To achieve a localized effect, a drug is administered topically to the specific area under treatment. The application of an antihistaminic spray to the swollen mucous membranes of the nose and throat in the case of a cold is an example of **topical administration.**

General, or systemic, **effects** are achieved when a drug is absorbed by the blood and circulated throughout the body. Depending upon the drug, either the entire body or a single internal system or organ may be affected. The most effective method of administering a drug for general effect is **intravenous injection,** or injection into a vein. But drugs for this purpose may also be given by **intramuscular injection** (into a muscle) or **subcutaneous injection** (under the skin). Drugs taken by mouth (oral administration) usually have a much slower effect, since they must first pass through part of the digestive tract.

Primary and Secondary Effects

The **primary effect** of a drug is the desired effect for which the drug is introduced into the body. Medical research has learned relatively little about how drugs act to produce their effects, but by and large the effects themselves are well known. Central nervous system (CNS) stimulants, as we have seen, excite the body cells into increased activity; CNS depressants decrease body cell activity. This action is often selective, and a particular drug may affect the cells of only one type of body tissue. A general analgesic, such as morphine, when injected intravenously, depresses cell activity in the central nervous system. It deadens the brain's response of pain to the signal it is receiving through the nervous system from the injured portion of the body.

The desired or primary effect of a drug may be accompanied by **secondary,** or side, **effects;** and these may be either harmful or beneficial. These effects vary in intensity with the dosage and the physical condition of the patient. Some people are *hyposensitive* and require extra amounts of a drug to gain the desired effects. Some people experience dangerous reactions to relatively harmless drugs because of **hypersensitivity** to the compounds. For example, many people have strong allergic reactions to tetanus vaccine and to penicillin.

Such hypersensitive reactions range from mild upsets—diarrhea, nausea, constipation, drowsiness—to more severe reactions such as skin rash, fever, blood clots, and convulsions. In some cases, the intravenous administration of a drug may produce **anaphylactic shock,** a severe and rapidly occurring condition marked by collapse of the circulatory system and heart arrest. A physician who prescribes any drug must first make sure the patient is not allergic to it.

Tolerance

The body is said to develop **tolerance** to a drug when the original dosage no longer produces the desired results. To counteract tolerance, the dosage may be increased or a stronger drug may be prescribed. An important example of tolerance occurs in the use of antibiotics, where the infecting microorganism itself may develop a tolerance to the drug—or even a liking for it.

Regular users of narcotic depressants develop a tolerance so great that the desired effect of the drug can be achieved only by a dose far larger than would normally be considered fatal. The usual dose of morphine is 8 to 20 milligrams for relief of severe pain; 200 milligrams is thought to be a fatal dose for most people. Regular users of morphine, however, have been known to take as much as 5,000 milligrams a day.

Drugs that are chemically similar often cause **cross-tolerance.** That is, tolerance, or resistance, to one drug in the group produces tolerance to all drugs in the group. Similarly, a craving for one drug in the group can be physically, if not psychologically, satisfied by other drugs in the group.

Dependence: Habituation and Addiction

You have undoubtedly heard people say that they cannot get started in the morning without coffee and cigarettes. Perhaps you know someone who absolutely must have a martini before dinner. It may have occurred to you that these people are, in some way, dependent upon these substances. Certain drugs, when used repeatedly over an extended period of time, can induce a state of **dependence.**

Precise degrees of dependence are extremely difficult to define in practical terms because so little is known about the phenomenon of drug dependence. In an effort to clarify the situation, the World Health Organization has distinguished between physical and psychological dependence.

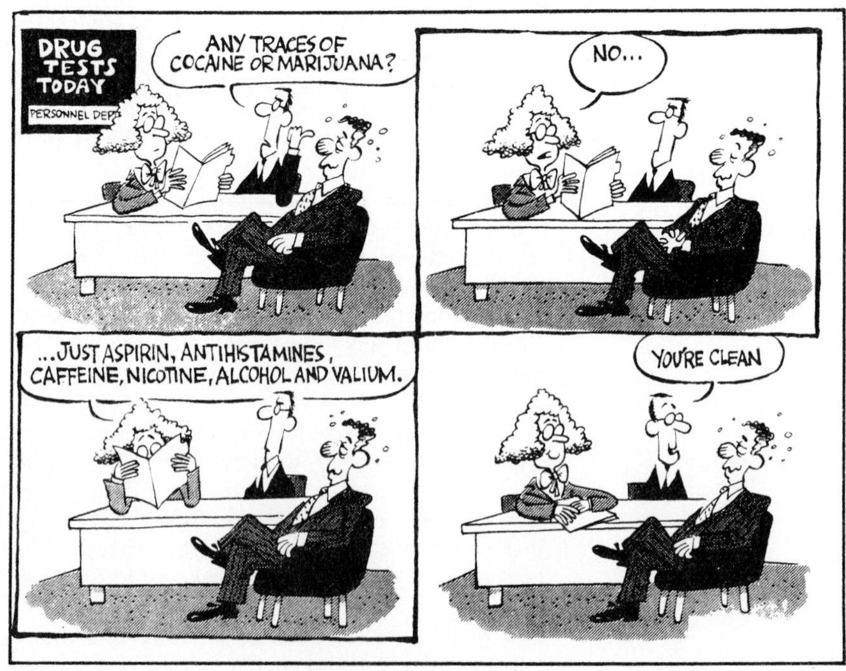
DRUG TESTS TODAY
PERSONNEL DEPT
ANY TRACES OF COCAINE OR MARIJUANA?
NO...
...JUST ASPIRIN, ANTIHISTAMINES, CAFFEINE, NICOTINE, ALCOHOL AND VALIUM.
YOU'RE CLEAN

Are You in Control?

Check the degree to which you use the items in the categories at the left. Should your use of them fall in the shaded boxes, you may wish to reconsider your drug habits.

Category of Substance	Frequency of Use			
	Never	*Occasional*	*Frequent*	*Extreme*
I *Beverages containing caffeine*				
II *Over-the-counter drugs*				
III *Prescription drugs*				
IV *Illegal drugs*				

Scoring:

I Caffeine-containing beverages (coffee, tea, colas). The abuse of these beverages can produce restlessness, irritability, and interference with sleep. Caution should be exercised during pregnancy in particular. Habituation may occur.

II Over-the-counter drugs (sleeping aids, digestive aids, vitamin supplements, laxatives, painkillers, etc.). As nonprescription items these drugs can be purchased at the discretion of the user. Therefore they are easily and frequently abused. Abuse can cause impairment of bodily functions, and habituation may occur.

III Prescription drugs (amphetamines, barbiturates, tranquilizers). Though these are legal drugs prescribed by physicians for medical reasons, they are among our most frequently abused drugs. They are all capable of producing drug dependence.

IV Illegal drugs (heroin, cocaine, LSD, PCP, marijuana). These drugs have virtually no medical use in the United States, and each is capable of some adverse side effect, ranging from mild to fatal. It is possible that all may produce dependence, and most have been proven to do so.

Physical dependence is a condition in which the body has adjusted to the presence of a drug. If individuals cease to use the drug, they will suffer discomfort and illness, or **withdrawal symptoms.** The word **addiction,** then, is used to mean physical dependence.

Psychological dependence is a condition that arises when individuals who receive satisfaction from their initial use of a drug continue to take it for the feeling of well-being it produces. Through the repeated use of the substance, they may come to rely on it to help them adjust to life. Removal of the substance may cause psychological discomfort, but no physical withdrawal symptoms. We use the word **habituation** to mean psychological dependence.

The problem of definition is compounded because many experts disagree about the addictive properties of certain substances. Nicotine, for example, is considered by many psychologists to be addictive because cigarette smokers find it so difficult to stop smoking and often experience severe withdrawal symptoms when they do. But pipe smokers ingest little nicotine, and yet they do not seem to find it any easier to give up tobacco than cigarette smokers do. On the basis of this evidence, some psychologists have concluded that smokers are only habituated. Quitting smoking almost always produces some degree of psychological upheaval, especially symptoms of nervousness and irritability. Ex-smokers will often overeat at first because their appetites are no longer suppressed by the deadening effects of nicotine on the central nervous system.

Obviously, any substance can be used habitually, and given the complexity and unpredictability of the human mind, many substances can induce a state of psychological dependence. But only a few substances are known to be physically addictive. Compulsive use of these addictive substances, however, can easily produce psychological as well as physiological dependence. Whereas individuals may have used an addictive drug at first to achieve a sense of pleasure or escape, they will continue to use it later to avoid the pain of physical withdrawal. Therefore they have become psychologically dependent on a substance that has also caused physiological changes.

While the word *addiction* has a simple definition, the process of addiction is a complex phenomenon that involves the drug user's physical and psychological condition, the particular drug and how it is used, the amount taken, the frequency with which it is taken, and the social setting in which it is used. *Alcohol* is the most widely used addictive substance in the United States and the most widely sold drug in the world. Yet some people can use alcohol regularly without ever becoming addicts or even problem drinkers. They are able to control their alcohol consumption. For reasons that are not entirely clear, other people consume alcohol compulsively and are addicts. (The problem of alcohol abuse is discussed in Chapter 11.)

Similarly, the addictive effects of narcotics or barbiturates are not always predictable. For example, it is the popular belief that one dose of heroin, a narcotic, will turn a person into an addict. In fact, large doses taken daily over a period of two or more weeks are usually required. It is obvious that not everyone who tries heroin will do so frequently enough to become an addict. It is equally obvious that not everyone who tries heroin will be able to avoid becoming an addict. Some of the factors that might predispose an individual to addiction are discussed later in this chapter.

DRUG ABUSE*

Drug abuse is the taking of any substance for any purpose other than that for which it is intended, and in any way that could damage the user's health or ability to function. Legal as well as illegal drugs are abused by Americans.

Legal Drugs

The most widely used drugs are the most widely abused. Several billion aspirin and aspirin compound tablets are consumed every year in the United States. Some people boast of eating aspirin like candy, even though the recommended

* Some of the material in this section is based on information contained in Richard G. Schlaadt and Peter T. Shannon's *Drugs of Choice: Current Perspectives on Drug Use*, 2nd ed. (Englewood Cliffs, N.J.: Prentice-Hall, 1986).

dosage, shown on every bottle sold anywhere in the United States, is two tablets every four hours and no more than eight in twenty-four hours. (Considerably larger doses than this are often recommended for arthritis sufferers, however.) If taken habitually and excessively, aspirin can cause gastric ulcers with gastrointestinal bleeding and can interfere with the clotting of the blood. Aspirin is also suspected of increasing the risk of a rare liver disorder known as Reye's syndrome in children who take it when they have flu or chicken pox.

Prescription drugs are also frequently abused. Indeed, a 1982 report of the General Accounting Office compiled from national drug-abuse statistics stated unequivocally that more Americans die or suffer medical emergencies from using prescription drugs improperly than from the use of "all illegal drugs combined." The study reported that people who abuse legal drugs obtain them from doctors who unintentionally misprescribe them, from unscrupulous doctors who write prescriptions for profit, from forged prescriptions, and from thefts from pharmacies and illegal sales by druggists. Chief among these prescribed drugs are mild analgesics and narcotics for the relief of pain and mild tranquilizers for calming nerves. Amphetamines, which were once widely prescribed as weight-reducing aids, are less frequently prescribed today because physicians have been alerted to their abuse as well as to their harmful side effects, which include increased blood pressure and heart rate while the drug is working and depression and fatigue when the drug's effects wear off.

Overprescription by physicians of legal drugs, for convenience or as placebos, constitutes a wide area of potential abuse. The abuse of a class of drugs called the **minor tranquilizers,** especially Valium and Librium, deserves special attention. Valium use probably peaked in 1981, when some 60 million prescriptions were written for it and nearly 15 percent of the U.S. population had used it at least once, mostly for relief of anxiety. Currently the drug is prescribed at less than half that level, but its potential for abuse remains great. It is prescribed for women about two and a half times as often as for men, and many of its users are from the middle or upper class.

Among the many dangers of Valium and similar drugs, two should be remembered by anyone contemplating their use. First, the minor tranquilizers are highly addictive. One can become physically addicted by taking as little as 5 milligrams of Valium a day. One of the biggest dangers of addiction is abrupt withdrawal, which may, and very often does, result in fatal seizures or convulsions, in many cases several days after ceasing to take the drugs. Second, alcohol and Valium boost each other's effects on the central nervous system. They are both CNS depressants that impair the body's ability to perform such survival functions as breathing after consciousness has been lost. In a **synergistic reaction,** wherein two substances interact powerfully and with unpredictable results, the central nervous system may be seriously impaired. Alcohol acts as a **potentiator,** boosting the effects of other depressants. Most people think they know how many drinks or how many milligrams of Valium they can safely take without passing out. The tricky interaction of these two drugs, however, makes such forecasts a gamble at best. Barbiturates and narcotics combined with alcohol pose the same problem. Death usually results when the user has fallen asleep and critical "involuntary" mechanisms such as coughing and respiration are too depressed by the drugs to function.

PROBLEMS AND CONTROVERSIES: Drugs in the Workplace

On-the-job drug abuse has soared in the United States over the last twenty years. Some authorities claim that between 10 and 25 percent of the nation's workers either take illegal drugs on the job or are already high when they arrive. And the problem is bound to get worse. Surveys have estimated that as many as two-thirds of the young adults entering their first jobs have used illegal drugs.

The economic and human costs of employee drug abuse are enormous. In terms of time lost from work, on-the-job injuries, thefts of cash and products, and property damage, the illegal drug epidemic is costing the U.S. economy $60 billion a year. In the railroad industry alone drug-addicted and alcoholic workers have caused at least fifty train accidents in which thirty-seven people have died and $34 million worth of property has been destroyed over the last ten years. And government authorities are worried that addicted workers in the space and defense industries may be tempted to sell secrets to support their expensive drug habits.

On-the-job drug abuse also takes its toll in work performance. Stoned employees generally perform about a third below their normal ability. Marijuana, for example, slows a person's reaction time and impairs short-term memory for as long as twenty-four hours; and the bizarre delusions of cocaine users may lead them to make disastrous business decisions.

To maintain safe working conditions and ensure product reliability, many companies are making prospective and current employees take blood and urine tests to detect the presence of drug by-products in the body. Undercover agents are being used to entrap drug buyers and sellers on company premises, and workers' movements are being monitored through hidden video cameras. Some employers are sending dogs into locker rooms and onto shop floors to sniff out illegal drugs and alcohol. Once they have identified the guilty parties, however, many employers are finding it far more humane and cost-effective to rehabilitate them by means of employee-assistance programs than to fire them and train new personnel.

The use of drug tests and surveillance methods has raised a number of ethical problems. First, the tests themselves are said to produce a significant number of false positives, thus causing innocent people to be stigmatized or fired. Second, even reliable tests do not pinpoint when or how often a person has used a drug. Thus someone may be fired for having smoked a joint of marijuana on a weekend several days before. Third, employees' rights groups claim that the tests and surveillance methods violate constitutional rights to privacy—including privacy of the body—and due process. Furthermore, they turn the traditional legal presumption of innocence upside down. Employers counter that the civil rights amendments apply only to issues between citizens and the states, not to private transactions between employers and employees. The problem for the courts now is to weigh these conflicting values.

Sources: "Battling the Enemy Within," *Time*, March 17, 1986, pp. 52–61; "Taking Drugs on the Job," *Newsweek*, August 22, 1983, pp. 52–60.

Who is to blame? Some blame the drug companies; some, the doctors who overprescribe the minor tranquilizers; and some, the moral degeneration of a nation of pill poppers. In fact, all three—manufacturer, dispenser, and consumer—are responsible, according to the authors of a popular book *The Tranquilizing of America*. There is no supply without demand, yet promises of a cure for anxiety create demand. The physicians are caught in between, perhaps because of the traditional focus of American medicine on the reduction of discomfort rather than prevention.

Illegal Drugs

The use of illegal drugs, or of drugs acquired illegally, is another kind of abuse of particular concern. Illegal drugs such as LSD, heroin, and PCP have almost no medically accepted application; their importation into the United States and the manufacture, sale, or possession of any of them within the country are prohibited by law. Penalties for violations of the law include stringent fines and lengthy prison terms. But there are estimated to be close to half a million heroin addicts in the United States, and the use of marijuana is extremely widespread; these facts indicate that the law is not particularly effective. (Drug laws and their limitations will be examined in greater detail later in this chapter.)

Legal drugs that produce a "high"—morphine, codeine, barbiturates, amphetamines, and tranquilizers—are frequently obtained illegally. They reach the market by various means: from illegal laboratories operating clandestinely; through use of forged prescription blanks; through the collusion of unscrupulous physicians and pharmacists; and through thefts from pharmaceutical companies. (The major companies all report thefts running into millions of dollars' worth of drugs each year.)

CLASSIFICATION OF ABUSED DRUGS

As we have seen, all drugs have the potential for abuse, and many ordinary drugs are overused. But there may be more cause for concern over the abuse of psychoactive drugs that affect the central nervous system and the mind than over the abuse of less potent substances. This is because such drugs can cause psychological aberrations or changes, not all of which may be temporary or desirable. A number of the drugs described on the following pages are also addictive; and many of them, by adversely affecting some part of the nervous system, can cause physical harm and even death (see Table 13-1).

Opium and Opiates

Opium, its derivatives, and a number of synthetic drugs that have similar effects upon the nervous system are the drugs classically connected with illegal drug use and drug addiction. All are depressants of the central nervous system; all are analgesics, or painkillers; and all are **narcotics** with the power to induce drowsiness and sleep. An addict who tries to stop using any of these substances is likely to suffer restlessness and anxiety, diarrhea, nausea, increased respiratory rate, alternating chills and fevers, cramps, severe weight loss, runny nose, and watery eyes. These symptoms are caused by withdrawal of the drug from the body system. Physiologically, withdrawal symptoms occur because of the biochemical changes the drug has produced in the individual. If the human nervous system is confronted with opiates frequently and intensely, it gradually becomes both used to them and dependent on them. When these substances are no longer present, the nervous system will be in distress until it can readjust to its preopiated state.

Opium. **Opium** is an extract of the poppy plant (see Figure 13-1), which is cultivated extensively in Turkey, India, Egypt, Mexico, and Southeast Asia. The thick, milky fluid obtained from the unripe seedpods of the plant is dried to a gummy brown substance that is then roasted or shredded. In this form it is either smoked or pounded into a powder that can be diluted or treated to extract one or more derivative substances, particularly morphine.

Both the analgesic and euphoric effects of opium were known to the ancient Egyptians and Persians, and the use of opium to relieve pain was practiced in

TABLE 13-1

Drugs: Medical Uses, Symptoms produced, and Dependence Potentials

Name	Slang name	Chemical or trade name	Source	Classification	Medical use	How taken
Heroin	H., horse, scat, junk, smack, scag, stuff, Harry	Diacetyl morphine	Semisynthetic (from morphine)	Narcotic	None in U.S.	Injected or sniffed
Morphine	White stuff, M.	Morphine sulphate	Natural (from opium)	Narcotic	Pain relief	Swallowed or injected
Codeine	Schoolboy	Methylmorphine	Natural (from opium), semi-synthetic (from morphine)	Narcotic	Ease pain and coughing	Swallowed
Methadone	Dolly	Dolophine, Amidone	Synthetic	Narcotic	Pain relief	Swallowed or injected
Cocaine	Corrine, blow, coke, Bernice, flake, star dust, snow	Methylester of benzoylecgonine	Natural (from coca, *not* cocao)	Stimulant, local anesthetic	Local anesthesia	Sniffed, injected, or swallowed
Marijuana	Pot, grass, tea, gage, reefers, weed	*Cannabis sativa*	Natural	Relaxant, euphoriant, in high doses hallucinogen	In glaucoma; as treatment for nausea after cancer chemotherapy	Smoked, swallowed, or sniffed
Barbiturates	Barbs, blue devils, candy, yellow jackets, phennies, peanuts, blue heavens	Phenobarbital, Nembutal, Seconal, Amytal	Synthetic	Sedative-hypnotic	Sedation, relieve high blood pressure, epilepsy, hyper-thyroidism	Swallowed or injected
Amphetamines	Bennies, Dexies, speed, wakeups, lid proppers, hearts, pep pills	Benzedrine, Dexedrine, Desoxyn, Methedrine	Synthetic	Sympatho mimetic	Relieve mild depression, con-trol appetite and narcolepsy	Swallowed or injected
LSD	Acid, sugar, big D, cubes, trips	D-lysergic acid diethylamide-25	Semisynthetic (from ergot alkaloids)	Hallucinogen	Experimental study of mental function, alcoholism	Swallowed
PCP	Angel dust, goon, busy bee, hog, crystal, elephant tranquilizer, super joint, heaven and hell	Phencyclidine	Synthetic	Anesthetic, in high doses hallucinogen	Animal tranquilizer	Smoked, swallowed, sniffed or injected.
Mescaline	Mesc.	3,4,5-trimeth-oxyphenethyl-amine	Natural (from peyote)	Hallucinogen	None	Swallowed
Psillocybin	Mushrooms	3-[2-(dimethyl-amino)ethyl]indol-4-ol dehydrogen phosphate ester	Natural (from *Psilocybe mexicana)*	Hallucinogen	None	Swallowed
Methaqualone	Meth, ludes, Quaaludes, soapers	Quaalude, Sopor, Parest, Optimal, Somnafac	Synthetic	Sedative	Sleeping aid	Swallowed

Source: Adapted from *Resource Book for Drug Abuse Education.*

Usual dose	Duration of effect	Effects sought	Long-term symptoms	Physical dependence potential	Mental dependence potential	Organic damage potential
Varies	4 hours	Euphoria, prevent withdrawal discomfort	Addiction, constipation, loss of appetite	Yes	Yes	No
15 mg	6 hours	Euphoria, prevent withdrawal discomfort	Addiction, constipation, loss of appetite	Yes	Yes	No
30 mg	4 hours	Euphoria, prevent withdrawal discomfort	Addiction, constipation. loss of appetite	?	Yes	No
10 mg	4–6 hours	Prevent withdrawal discomfort	Addiction, constipation, loss of appetite	Yes	Yes	No
Varies	Varies, short	Excitation, talkativeness	Depression, convulsions, paranoid delusions	No	Yes	Yes?
1–2 cigarettes	4 hours	Relaxation, increased euphoria, perceptions, sociability	None?	No	Yes	Yes
50–100 mg	4 hours	Anxiety reduction, euphoria	Addiction w/ severe withdrawal symptoms, possible convulsions, toxic psychosis	Yes	Yes	Yes
2.5–5 mg	4 hours	Alertness, activeness	Loss of appetite, delusions, hallucinations, toxic psychosis	No?	Yes	Yes?
100–500 mcg	10 hours	Insightful experiences, exhilaration, distortion of senses	May intensify existing psychosis, panic reactions	No	No?	No?
Varies	Varies	Euphoria, exhilaration, distortion of senses	May intensify existing psychosis, uncontrollable rage, panic, reactions, toxic psychosis	No	No?	Yes?
400 mcg	12 hours	Insightful experiences, exhilaration, distortion of senses	May intensify existing psychosis, panic reactions	No	No?	No?
25 mg	6–8 hours	Insightful experiences, exhilaration, distortion of senses	Paranoid delusions?	No	No?	No?
300–600 mg	4–6 hours	Relaxation, euphoria	Depression, convulsions	Yes	Yes	Yes

China more than ten centuries ago. In Europe during the eighteenth and nineteenth centuries opium smoking was fashionable, and "opium dens" operated legally in London. Opium has long been used to relieve pain and to treat diarrhea; until the early 1900s it was a frequent ingredient of home remedies and patent medicines.

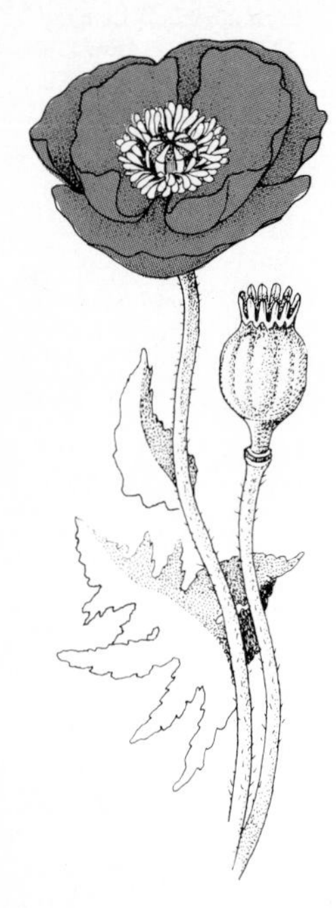

FIGURE 13-1

The opium poppy flower.

Opium derivatives share with opium certain distinct characteristics: All act as depressants on the nervous system, particularly on respiration and sensory perception. In practical terms, they lower the rate of breathing and the action of the heart, reducing the amount of oxygen to the blood cells. The results are a feeling of well-being, or a **high,** and drowsiness. As side effects, all will cause constipation, perspiration, lowered body temperature, and constriction of the pupils of the eyes, as well as a reduction of mental aptitude, physical coordination, appetite, sexual drive, and ability to concentrate. Body tolerance to all opium derivatives develops rapidly with regular use.

Of all the opium derivatives, only a few figure prominently in our society in drug abuse: morphine, heroin, and codeine.

Morphine. **Morphine,** first isolated from opium in 1804, contains about 10 percent opium by weight and is employed medically for the relief of severe pain. It was widely used in the United States in army hospitals during the Civil War. The drug's addictive potential was not well understood, with the result that some 400,000 soldiers became addicted to it, and morphine addiction became known as the "army disease."

Morphine was just as carelessly used in civilian hospitals during the latter part of the nineteenth century; as a consequence, by 1912 one person in every 400 in the United States was addicted either to morphine, opium, or laudanum (a wine and opium mixture). Morphine is at present a distant third on the list of abused narcotics, after heroin and methadone. It is most widely abused where and when heroin is scarce. Morphine generally becomes addictive when the therapeutic dose of 8 to 20 milligrams a day is taken for three weeks. Derivatives of morphine such as Percodan and other opiates in pill form have become increasingly popular on the black market among narcotics abusers who do not inject.

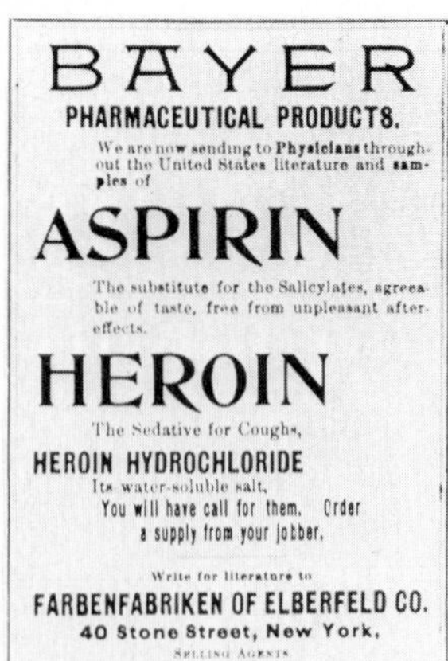

The manufacture of heroin was legal in the United States until 1924.

Heroin. **Heroin** is a derivative of morphine, a partially synthetic substance that is created by the action of chemical agents on morphine. Produced and marketed starting in 1898, it was believed to be a powerful but nonaddictive painkiller and, ironically, was first introduced into this country as a substance useful in the treatment of morphine addiction. Unfortunately, heroin proved addictive, and morphine users simply switched to it. The drug has no accepted medical application in the United States today, though because it is such an effective painkiller—stronger than morphine—there have been proposals to legalize it for terminally ill cancer patients in severe pain. Its manufacture and possession are illegal in the United States but legal in Great Britain.

No other opiate is as widely abused as heroin, as is evidenced by the large number of heroin addicts in this country. The drug may be used in a variety of ways to produce mild or strong highs. It is sometimes inhaled or smoked in a pipe for a slow high of long duration, or injected subcutaneously for much the same result. But heroin addicts usually inject a solution of the drug intravenously to achieve an instant "rush."

Heroin is sold in small glassine envelopes, or "bags," at prices that vary with the strength of the drug and the market supply. The average heroin addict uses about four bags daily, but many use more. The average heroin addict may need $35,000 annually to support a habit, and this is the primary cause of drug-related crimes.

The heroin available in the United States is cut, or adulterated, with quinine, milk sugar, or other white crystalline powders. In most instances, heroin makes up only 2 to 5 percent of the total ingredients of a bag. When the market is glutted, prices fall and the strength per bag increases. Although this variation in strength can sometimes lead an addict accustomed to a weak concentration of heroin to overdose, overdosing is generally a result of other factors, such as contamination or the concurrent use of other substances.

The late 1960s and early 1970s were the time of the greatest number of drug-related deaths in the United States. Since the mid-1970s heroin-related deaths have declined, partly as a result of more effective international controls and a greater coordination of intelligence among the nations concerned with the problem of heroin. More effective controls, however, have not eliminated the heroin market. As the supply dwindles, addicts switch temporarily to other drugs, only to go back to heroin when the supply is plentiful again.

Babies born of heroin-addicted mothers suffer from many serious problems

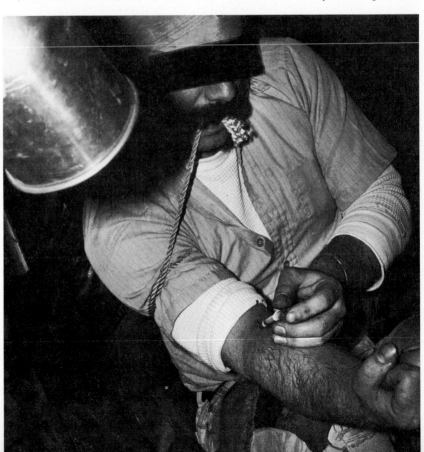

Shooting heroin.

and deficiencies. Because their mothers usually do not eat properly or receive adequate medical care during pregnancy, many are born underweight and malnourished. And although they may not experience withdrawal symptoms, a great many are born with some degree of heroin addiction and have to be given special care during their first weeks of life. In addition, heroin-addicted newborns may have poorly developed muscular and nervous systems, be mentally retarded, and develop behavioral abnormalities. Unfortunately, these symptoms also appear in babies of mothers who are taking methadone and other heroin substitutes.

Codeine. **Codeine** is a natural derivative of opium, but it is usually prepared from morphine. It is not as powerful as either morphine or heroin, but its effects are similar. Because it depresses the part of the nervous system that controls the cough reflex, it is sometimes an ingredient of cough medicines. Codeine is occasionally used by heroin addicts when heroin is scarce.

Synthetic Opiates. Several synthetic opiates have the same primary effects as opiates, but not their heavy sedative side effects. The most widely used of these drugs is Demerol, a brand name for meperidine hydrochloride. Although its chemical structure differs markedly from that of morphine, its analgesic effects are similar. And although Demerol is an addictive drug, addiction to it is rare. Since it does not appear to have cross-tolerance with morphine, it is frequently used as an alternative pain reliever in postoperative care.

By far the most controversial of the synthetic opiates is the drug **methadone.** It is now being widely used to counteract heroin addiction; but methadone itself is addictive, a fact that has spurred the controversy. (A discussion of methadone treatment of heroin addicts appears later in this chapter.) It is a strong analgesic and causes marked depression of the respiratory system.

Barbiturates

All **barbiturates** are derivatives of barbituric acid, or malonyl urea. They are depressants of the central nervous system. Barbiturates are frequently called sedatives (as opposed to narcotics) because a moderate dose relaxes the user without inducing sleep. But some stronger barbiturates are termed **hypnotics.** These hypnotics will induce euphoria, drowsiness, and sleep. Much doubt, however, has been cast upon the ability of barbiturates to induce sleep when used beyond a period of two weeks. In total, some 2,500 barbiturate compounds have been synthesized; and about 50 are available on the market. Many of them simply duplicate one another's effects. It has been estimated that, for medical purposes, six different barbiturates would suffice.

Barbiturates (known in slang as *downers*) are usually classified according to the duration of their effect upon the body. *Phenobarbital*, sometimes sold under the trade name Luminal, is a long-lasting barbiturate; *Nembutal* (pentobarbital) and *Seconal* (secobarbital) are intermediate- to short-acting; and *Pentothal* (thiopental) is an ultra-short-acting barbiturate. All are usually given orally to induce relaxation and bring about sleep for various periods of time. Use of long-lasting barbiturates often results in a drug hangover or grogginess upon arising. Heavy barbiturate users frequently resemble those intoxicated with alcohol; like drunk persons, they are unable to coordinate muscle action.

Heavy, prolonged use of barbiturates will lead to addiction. The body develops tolerance for the drug, and the dosage has to be increased to produce the desired effect. The lethal dose is difficult to determine, for many bodily factors are involved. But one study estimated that 5,000 deaths associated with the use of barbiturates occur each year in the United States. More than ten times the normal dose will usually produce severe poisoning.

Withdrawal from barbiturate addiction is very nearly as dangerous as the taking of the drug itself—in fact, it may lead to death. The symptoms of withdrawal include anxiety, tremors, rapid pulse, increased temperature, and convulsions that bear a striking resemblance to epileptic seizures. In a later stage, which may last up to fourteen days, withdrawal may produce hallucinations, paranoid delusions, and symptoms of schizophrenia. Treatment involves administering barbiturates in gradually decreasing dosages.

Methaqualone (Quaaludes) and related hypnotics are nonbarbiturates that nevertheless produce a "barbiturate high" and cause similar withdrawal symptoms. They had wide popularity as a black market drug in the 1970s and early 1980s, especially among young people. Mixing with alcohol boosts the sedative effects of Quaalude just as it does with the barbiturates.

Minor Tranquilizers

The **minor tranquilizers** are nonbarbiturate, nonopiate depressants. They were first developed in the early 1950s for use as sedatives and for the relief of neurotic anxiety, and were believed originally to be free of the dangers common to barbiturates. Time has indicated, however, that these tranquilizers also reduce muscle coordination and mental alertness, cause drowsiness, and are addictive.

Minor tranquilizers are popular, and their trade names are well known. These include Miltown, Equanil (meprobamate), Librium (chlordiazepoxide), and Valium (diazepam). They depress the central nervous system, relax muscles, relieve emotional tension and anxiety, and induce light sleep. All are anticonvulsants whose sudden withdrawal can cause convulsions in the abuser who is addicted to them. One research study has indicated that Librium, Equanil, and Miltown may cause serious birth defects if used in the early stages of pregnancy. The dangers of Valium abuse have already been discussed.

Major Tranquilizers

Except by name, the **major tranquilizers** bear no similarities to the minor tranquilizers. Their use is by and large restricted to hospital wards and prescriptions for psychiatric patients. The reason why the major tranquilizers, or *phenothiazines*, are not popular on the street is that they produce no desirable high. Drugs such as Mellaril, Thorazine, Compazine, and Taractan in fact often cause a feeling of ill-being and itchy skin in most people who are not suffering truly psychotic symptoms such as those manifested by schizophrenics or the clinically depressed. Similarly, *lithium salts*, a natural compound successfully used for the treatment of manic-depressive psychosis, cause unpleasant sensations in normal people. The drugs are called *major* because they are used to treat psychoses rather than neuroses.

Amphetamines

Amphetamines are synthetic stimulants of the central nervous system. They are classified into three distinct chemical groups but all have roughly the same effects upon the body.

Amphetamines, which have been in clinical use since the middle 1930s, act in ways not yet clearly understood, stimulating the central nervous system

Look-Alike Drugs

In the late 1970s new, nontraditional companies started manufacturing and distributing what have come to be called look-alike stimulants. These over-the-counter drugs usually consist of caffeine, ephedrine, and phenylpropanolamine, and have an effect on arousal and alertness similar to that of amphetamines. They are called look-alikes because their manufacturers package them in a variety of pills and capsules whose markings give them the appearance of prescription medications. Heavy use can lead to tolerance and harmful side effects such as high blood pressure and stroke.

Source: Schlaadt and Shannon, *Drugs of Choice*, p. 95.

and suppressing the appetite. They are used to treat *narcolepsy*, a condition characterized by involuntary attacks of sleep, and hyperkinetic disorders in children. Amphetamines have also been widely used to aid in weight reduction, but this application is now discouraged by medical authorities. The amphetamine user quickly develops a tolerance for the drug, and its appetite-suppressing effects disappear after a week or two.

Known informally as **pep pills** or *uppers*, amphetamines are often used to overcome fatigue—particularly by those who wish to stay awake for an extended period, such as long-haul truck drivers and college students cramming for final examinations. They produce feelings of euphoria and exhilaration and a sense of increased perceptiveness. A person who stops using amphetamines generally becomes depressed. For these reasons, amphetamines create psychological dependence. A slight overdose of amphetamines may impair judgment; excessive ingestion may lead to exhaustion; and continued use may result in blackouts.

The amphetamines most used are Dexedrine and Benzedrine. Methamphetamine, or Methedrine, another widely used amphetamine, was originally known as *speed*, a term that is now popularly applied to all amphetamines. Most Methedrine is produced in the illicit market and is not used for medical purposes. It is increasing in popularity because it can easily be manufactured in "street labs" and is a very profitable illicit drug. Among drug abusers, methamphetamine is frequently heated and injected intravenously to produce a rapid and excited euphoric effect. Heavy intravenous use may result in paranoia and can lead to the collapse of respiratory functions, coma, and death. In fact, the symptoms of paranoia in heavy amphetamine or cocaine users are indistinguishable from symptoms of paranoid schizophrenia: delusions of grandeur, persecution fears, and even auditory hallucinations.

Many drug abusers take barbiturates in conjunction with amphetamines, hoping to regulate their sleep-wake cycle chemically. This effort invariably fails. The two drugs have a combined mood-elevating effect, and the user becomes progressively more dependent on both.

Cocaine

Cocaine, or *coke*, once an expensive, stylish drug used mostly by movie and rock stars and celebrity athletes, has now been taken up by people at every level of society. Steep price declines in the last few years have made it the

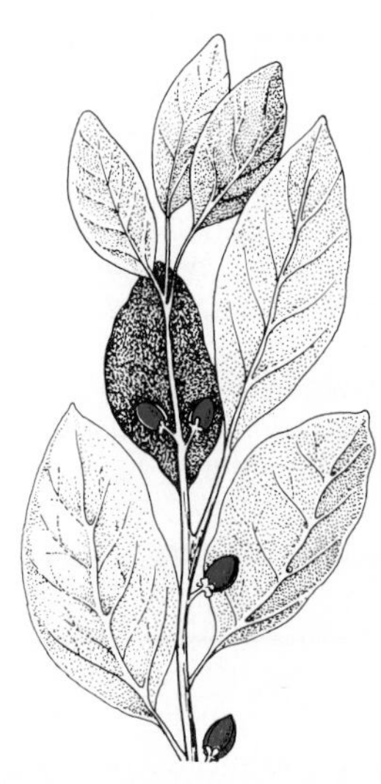

FIGURE 13-2

The fruiting branch of the coca plant.

most popular illegal stimulant in the United States; more than 25 million people have used it, and each day 5,000 more try it for the first time. Between 4 and 5 million Americans use cocaine regularly, and 5 to 20 percent of them are profoundly dependent on it.

Cocaine is a white, odorless, bitter-tasting powder extracted from the leaves of a coca bush (*Erythoxylon coca*) that grows in the highlands of the Andes Mountains in South America (see Figure 13-2). For centuries the Indians of Peru and Bolivia have chewed the leaves to reduce hunger pangs and to help them endure the cold. In the nineteenth century Sir Arthur Conan Doyle's famous detective Sherlock Holmes sang the praises of cocaine in *The Sign of the Four*, touting its ability to increase physical and mental prowess and mask fatigue and hunger; and Sigmund Freud, a confirmed user, extolled its virtues as early as 1884. Today it is used legitimately as a local anesthetic by eye, ear, nose, and throat specialists.

Cocaine is usually taken in one of three ways. The most common method—called *snorting*—is to swiftly inhale the powder through the nose by means of a thin tube or from a small coke spoon. It can also be swallowed, injected, or smoked.

The effects of moderate quantities of cocaine are stimulating and euphoric. For twenty to thirty minutes after taking the drug, users feel extra alert and buoyantly in charge of their lives: They become talkative and feel surges of muscular strength and sexual energy. An indescribable optimism flows through the psyche. Many compare the rush of cocaine to sexual orgasm and rate it higher on the scale of human pleasures. Other primates seem to agree: In laboratory tests apes prefer cocaine to both sexual pleasure and food. A powerful distilled form of cocaine called *free base* produces even more intense highs. When injected or inhaled from the vapors of a heated water pipe, free base gives the user a dramatic, exhilarating rush and an overpowering desire to continue using it. A highly potent, easily manufactured, and inexpensive form of free base called *crack* or *rock* began to be produced in the mid-1980s. Smoked through a glass pipe, crack produces an almost instantaneous rush, followed a few minutes later by a crash. An intense compulsion to use the drug develops

Sudden Death

On Tuesday, June 19, 1986, Len Bias, "the best college basketball player in America," was drafted No. 1 by the Boston Celtics of the National Basketball Association. Two days later he was dead. The medical examiner reported that he had been "in superb athletic condition, with no evidence of any heart damage or disease." His blood showed, though, that he had ingested a moderate amount of cocaine, apparently by sniffing it. There was no evidence that he had used the drug previously, that he was allergic to it, or that it was adulterated. There was no evidence of alcohol or other drugs in his body. What happened was that the cocaine interrupted the electrical activity in his brain, causing his heart to beat irregularly. "This resulted in the sudden onset of seizures and cardiac arrest," according to the autopsy report.

"Nothing but the cocaine killed him," concluded the state's attorney investigating the death. "The reason he died was cocaine."

Cocaine Babies

Now that powerful, cheap "crack" cocaine has become available to millions of teenagers and young adults, a new generation of cocaine-damaged babies has begun to appear. Many are stillborn or premature. Those who survive suffer from a variety of mental and physical defects. Because cocaine induces sharp changes in the mother's blood pressure, alternately cutting off the blood supply to the infant's brain and sending in surges of blood that cause a strokelike condition, a great many babies are born brain-damaged. In addition, they will have to spend two or three weeks undergoing the slow torture of withdrawal—longer than it takes for heroin-addicted infants. Finally, they are in for a difficult childhood: Doctors predict that many will be mentally retarded, while others will suffer from learning disabilities and severe problems in motor coordination.

One researcher warns women who may be tempted to take cocaine that during pregnancy, "There is no such thing as 'recreational' drug use."

Source: "Cocaine Babies: Addicts Bear Ailing Infants," *Time*, January 1, 1986, p. 50.

within only a few weeks, in contrast to the three to four years that the National Institute on Drug Abuse estimates is typical of regular cocaine. Crack is by far the most dangerous form of cocaine.

While not physically addictive in the same manner as heroin, cocaine overstimulates the brain, releasing chemicals called neurotransmitters that probably cause the euphoria experienced by the user, and then blocking their return to the nerve cells, creating a chemical deficiency that may be responsible for a craving for more of the drug. The result is a psychological dependence and a physical tolerance, meaning that larger and larger doses are needed to achieve the same effect. And while abruptly stopping its use usually causes no severe physical withdrawal symptoms, it can bring on depression and, after heavy usage, an irritability and jumpiness that may force the user to seek relief in alcohol, strong sedatives, and even heroin.

Cocaine is not a harmless drug—in fact, even recreational use can be deadly. Cases have been reported in which *moderate* users of unadulterated cocaine have experienced no dangerous symptoms for a period of one to five hours after sniffing it and then have suddenly gone into convulsions and died (see box: Sudden Death). Morever, it is not a drug that invites moderation; a user rarely gets what he or she considers to be enough. Excessive quantities can produce tactile, olfactory, and auditory hallucinations in which users may feel insects crawling over their skin, smell smoke and foul odors, and hear voices whispering in their ears.

Cocaine damages the body in a number of ways. Free-basers who inhale the drug can do irreparable damage to their lungs. Snorting the drug often causes *rhinitis*, an inflammation of the nasal passages and sinus membranes; in addition, it makes the user prone to frequent upper respiratory tract infections. Cocaine sniffers are also apt to develop "coke nose," a condition in which the septum (the wall that separates the nostrils) becomes perforated. Chronic use can also destroy liver cells and suppress the appetite to such an extent that some users experience serious weight loss. Injecting the drug puts street users at risk of contracting AIDS from contaminated needles. And an increasing

Snorting cocaine.

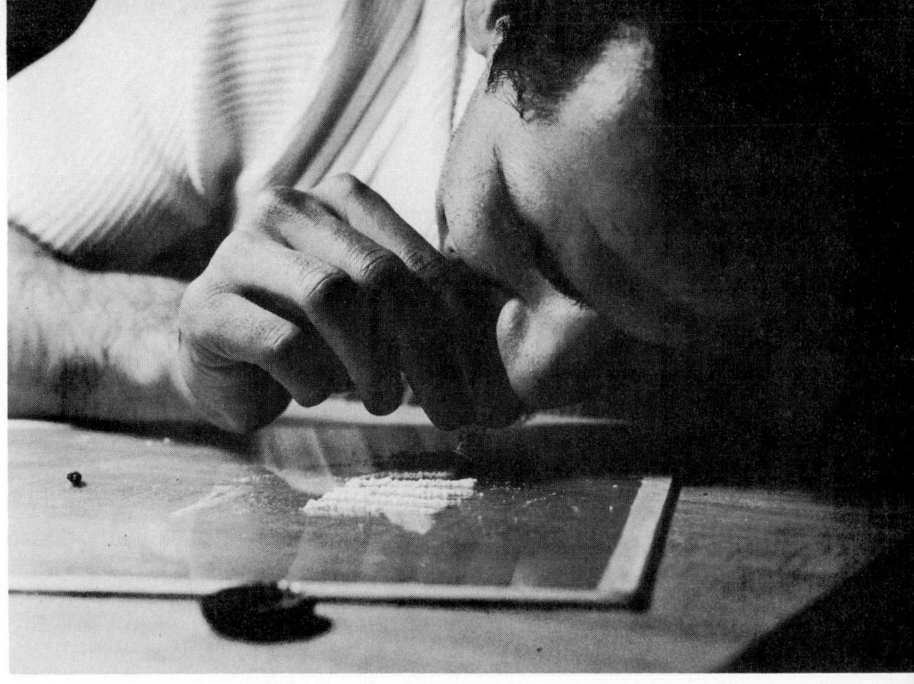

number of damaged babies are being born to mothers who use the drug (see box: Cocaine Babies).

Hallucinogens

The term **hallucinogen** refers to a group of substances that alter consciousness and produce hallucinations. These compounds are found in many plants, and several have been isolated in laboratories. One of the most potent and widely used hallucinogens is the chemical synthetic *d-lysergic acid diethylamide-25*, or LSD-25. Among other hallucinogens are PCP, mescaline, and peyote. The exact action of the hallucinogens is not well understood; that they have a powerful effect on the brain is evident, but researchers are still studying their primary and secondary effects.

LSD. **LSD,** a colorless, odorless liquid, was developed in the late 1930s but was not discovered to be a hallucinogen until 1943. It was first widely used by counterculture groups in the 1960s and early 1970s; it then declined in popularity during the next decade but seems to have made a comeback in the mid-1980s. It has been taken in a variety of forms, ranging from the sugar cubes and animal crackers of twenty years ago to the gelatin chips called *windowpanes* of the 1970s to what is called *blotter* today. In the last form a piece of blotting paper is first saturated with the drug and then cut up into pieces about a quarter the size of a postage stamp which are then chewed and swallowed. The average dose today is much smaller than it was ten or fifteen years ago. At that time it ranged between 150 to 200 micrograms, whereas now it is between 40 and 60 micrograms, probably because most users do not want an intense "trip."

Researchers believe that LSD heightens the sensitivity of the region of the brain that is responsible for sensory information and emotion. Thus users often experience distortions in depth, touch, color, and sound perception. Some senses may become blended—that is, a user might "see" a sound. In general, LSD

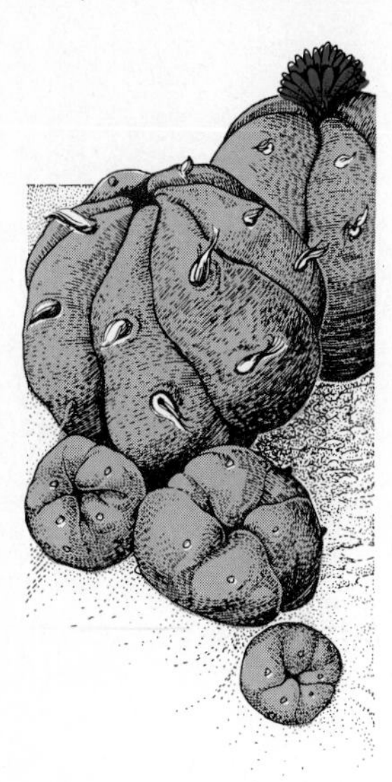

FIGURE 13-3

The peyote cactus plant.

overloads the senses, making it difficult or impossible for the user to think clearly. Tolerance to the drug, but not addiction, develops with regular use.

The quality of an LSD trip varies with the conditions under which it is taken and the personality of the user. Those who plan ahead of time to take it are more apt to have a "good trip," while those who take it unsuspectingly or on the spur of the moment often have a "bad trip," the effects of which can be frightening, disorienting, long-lasting, and dangerous.

PCP. **PCP,** or phenycyclidine, is a hallucinogenic drug abused especially by teenagers in the United States, who use it as a substitute for mescaline and LSD. Informally known as *angel dust*, it was originally developed as a tranquilizer in the 1950s, but was banned when tests revealed its undesirable side effects. Today PCP's only legal use is as an animal tranquilizer.

The effects of the drug are highly unpredictable, ranging from euphoria to hallucinations to depression to uncontrollable rages. When large dosages have been taken, death has resulted. PCP can be sniffed, swallowed as a pill, injected as a fluid, or dusted over parsley or marijuana and smoked. Its manufacturer requires only the most basic equipment, and even a person who has had no training in chemistry can produce the drug. The National Institute on Drug Abuse reported that 2.3 percent of high-school seniors were using PCP in 1984.

Peyote. **Peyote** is the button of the peyote cactus (see Figure 13-3). The button is dried and chewed, or boiled to make tea. The initial sensation is usually nausea, which quickly subsides, to be replaced by effects similar to those described for mescaline use below. Peyote has been used in religious ceremonies among the Indians of the southwestern United States and Mexico for many centuries. Its only legal use in the United States today is in the ceremonies of the Native American Church.

Mescaline. **Mescaline** is the active agent in the peyote cactus. It is usually taken in capsule form in fairly large doses, about 400 milligrams. Like LSD (with which it is cross-tolerant), mescaline produces hallucinations and changes in sensory perception. Laboratory studies of the psychological effects of mescaline have proved difficult because subjects under the drug's influence often break into prolonged fits of laughter when asked to perform routine tasks. The effects may last up to twelve hours.

Psilocybin. **Psilocybin** is the active ingredient in certain mushrooms, including *Psilocybe mexicana*. Hallucinations resemble those of mescaline. Psilocybin was used by the Aztecs in religious rituals and has been successfully synthesized.

Marijuana

Marijuana has been classified in various ways, but chemically it acts as a hallucinogen (though it is not potent enough to cause hallucinations). Marijuana is the leaves, stems, and flowering tops of the female Indian hemp plant *Cannabis sativa*. It is dried, shredded, and smoked, either in pipes or in cigarettes, or eaten in various foods and beverages. The active ingredient in marijuana, **THC**

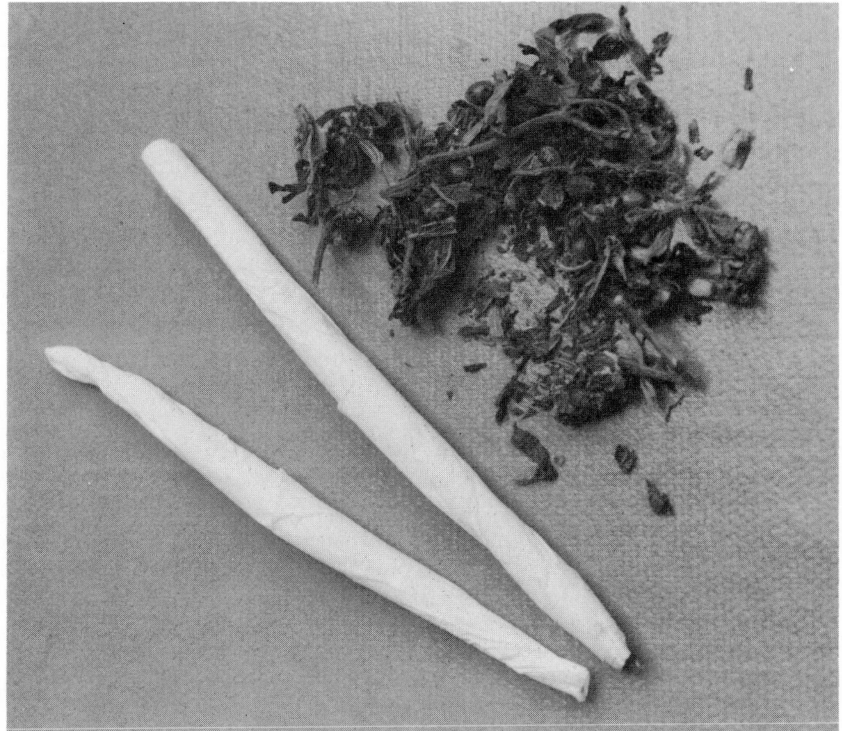

Marijuana cigarettes and the dried plant.

(tetrahydrocannabinol), is found in other forms of the same drug, such as *hashish* and *khif*, commonly smoked in North Africa, Turkey, and Iran, and *bhang*, a tea popular in Asia.

Marijuana smoking gives the user a pleasant, relaxed, and mildly euphoric feeling, as well as changed perceptions of space and time. For many users, it also induces a feeling of hunger. In psychiatric research it has been found that marijuana, like other hallucinogens, may, with regular use, emphasize an individual's neurotic or psychotic symptoms. In the past there was no indication that the effect was permanent, and little evidence that marijuana, or any other form of *Cannabis*, posed any permanent danger to the occasional user, although it was known that the drug generated psychological dependence. But according to the 1977 federal government report *Marijuana and Health*, it is now well substantiated that tolerance to marijuana does occur. There is also firm evidence that heavy users develop withdrawal symptoms when they stop taking the drug. Some of these are irritability, tremors, nausea, vomiting, and diarrhea.

According to current public opinion samplings, marijuana has become widely accepted throughout American society. The home growing of billions of dollars' worth of marijuana, including powerful botanical hybrids such as *sinsemilla*, on United States soil has contributed to this trend. Estimates of its market value in the mid-1980s established it as the nation's second leading cash crop, if not the first.

Young adults use marijuana as their parents use liquor. Organizations no less influential than the American Medical Association and the American Bar Association have called for the elimination of criminal penalties for marijuana use. A sizable number of states have already decriminalized possession of small quantities of the substance. The experience of Oregon, where decriminalization has been in effect since 1973, appears to demonstrate that this measure does not stimulate an appreciable increase in users. Nor do the latest figures on marijuana use bear out the claim that the substance is a stepping-stone on the path to harder drugs. However, new varieties of the plant are being grown that are ten times as powerful as those that were common in the early 1980s, and the effects of this new high-potency marijuana are not yet clear.

The Institute of Medicine of the National Academy of Sciences has expressed concern over the widespread use of marijuana and its possible health hazards, calling for continued research. The findings of the committee appointed to study the subject are important to users. THC impairs both motor coordination and perception, making driving dangerous. These effects last several hours after the initial high from smoking has passed. Because marijuana is known to impair short-term memory and learning, its effect on education is seen as a social problem, even though a 1984 survey of high-school seniors showed that the percentage of daily users had dropped to 5 percent from a high of 11 percent in 1978. Marijuana raises the heart rate and therefore may have a deleterious effect on people with heart conditions. Smoking may also harm the lungs. While marijuana use does not cause infertility, regular use does lower sperm count in men and decrease ovulation in female laboratory animals. The positive medical effects of marijuana, however, were bolstered by research findings: THC was shown to be beneficial in treating glaucoma and asthma and in mitigating some of the bad side effects of chemotherapy for cancer patients, including vomiting and nausea.

Polydrug Abuse

In the world of drug abuse it is difficult nowadays to find a pure alcoholic, pot smoker, or cocaine sniffer: Most drug abusers rely on more than one drug to get through the day. The last several years have seen the rise of **polydrug abuse**—the addiction to, or dependency on, two or more drugs at the same time. Most common is some combination of alcohol, marijuana, and cocaine. Amphetamines, PCP, or heroin may also be included, however.

Polydrug abuse occurs in all age groups and social classes. While many people take a number of "recreational drugs" simply to enjoy the compound effect, a great many others do so for more expedient reasons. People who start out drinking on the job, for example, may resort to cocaine or amphetamines in order to "sober up" and improve their work performance. Cocaine users, on the other hand, may need depressants to eliminate the jittery, irritable feeling that cocaine often produces; they look especially to alcohol and sedatives for their calming effect—and a growing number are relying on heroin.

Far from restoring efficiency and equilibrium, however, the ingestion of several addictive drugs at the same time imposes frightful, even tragic, costs on the abusers themselves, those they work for, and those close to them. Polydrug abusers are prone to distorted judgment, false perceptions of reality, and a propensity for dangerous, risk-taking behavior. They cost their employers hundreds of millions of dollars every year because they are less productive, more accident prone, and less healthy than other employees. The typical polydrug-abusing employee, for instance, is late more often, misses twice as many days of work, is sick three times more often, and has three times as many accidents. Polydrug abuse outside the workplace takes a high toll in other ways. California studies of highway fatalities have found that four in ten of the drivers had taken more than one drug. The polydrug users' behavior also increases the misery of those around them, especially their families. Finally, polydrug abuse can have tragic results for newborns: A growing number of women are using a variety of drugs during pregnancy and giving birth to babies with multiple addictions and serious brain damage (see box: Cocaine Babies).

CAUSES OF DRUG ABUSE

We have already suggested some of the factors that contribute to drug abuse: the widespread availability and acceptance of drugs, the advertising of drugs as the answer to every physical and emotional difficulty, and the natural human desire to escape from problems or find immediate solutions to them. These factors do not, however, explain why some individuals are more likely than others to become drug abusers. For the answer to this question, we must look to the community and to some psychological aspects of drug abuse.

Many personal, cultural, and social factors go into the making of a drug abuser (see box: The Addictive Personality). People who feel incapable of controlling their destinies—the poor, the alienated, the unemployed, the mentally ill—have been shown to be more likely than others to turn to drugs as a solution to their problems. For these people, the temporary tranquility or excitement drugs provide make life tolerable. We can begin to solve the problem of drug abuse only when we come to understand its social and psychological causes. In this way, we might be able to design effective programs of prevention and rehabilitation, rather than concentrate our efforts on punishment. In general, however, until we solve the problems that plague our society as a whole, our ability to deal with the problem of drug abuse will be limited.

Community Factors

Many but by no means all drug abusers are found in communities filled with poverty, gloom, and despair. This is not surprising: The goal-oriented constructive behavior valued by our society is likely to be perceived as irrelevant in a community where opportunities are severely limited. In fact, the values most likely to be admired, especially by the young, are those that emphasize one's ability to survive in a hostile world: instant gratification, defiance, rebellion, and lawlessness. Drug abuse, with its attendant risks, combines all these qualities. People who wish to achieve status in their community or group can therefore do so conveniently by abusing drugs.

Poor communities are also likely to contain an excessive number of alienated individuals who are denied a positive relationship to the larger culture that surrounds them. They may turn to drugs to escape their own feelings of hopelessness or the despair they see around them. Of course, alienation is not restricted to poverty areas. Any community in which parents are absorbed in their own interests and neglect their children, in which schools are indifferent to the needs of their students, in which employment opportunities are unavailable, and in which wholesome diversions and social services are not provided will produce large numbers of alienated individuals who may become drug abusers. Therefore wealthy suburban communities also have serious drug problems that affect their young people.

Personal Factors

It would be inaccurate to attribute drug abuse to social factors alone. Many people who live in good communities and enjoy great opportunities become drug abusers, and others who live in the direst poverty manage to work their way steadily to achievement and success. Personal and psychological factors play an important role in determining whether an individual will become a drug abuser.

Many who have achieved the highest levels of success also seem prone to abuse. Does this represent an insatiable appetite for self-fulfillment or self-indulgence? Is it the price of remaining at the top of the pile?

The Addictive Personality

Social scientists have begun to isolate traits that are unique to the addictive personality and that make an individual prone to compulsive, self-destructive behavior. Though mental health experts have not devised a uniform personality profile that covers all addictions, they have identified a number of traits common to people who are addicted to a variety of things, including heroin, food, gambling—even work. The personality traits that contribute most heavily to addiction are the following:

- Rebelliousness
- Impulsiveness
- A desire for instant gratification
- Sensation seeking
- Noncomformity
- Disregard for generally approval goals of achievement
- Sense of alienation
- Acceptance of deviance
- Greater than usual stress
- Tendencies toward depression
- Dependent behavior
- Focusing on short-term instead of long-term goals
- Lack of self-esteem
- Heightened anxiety

Many addicts appear to have been abused as children by their parents, who were themselves frequently dependent on alcohol or other drugs. Addicts have often undergone childhoods in which they were lied to, humiliated, or shamed by parents who behaved in an inconsistent manner. A mother, for example, might have instructed the child to behave in a way that the father strongly disapproved of, or she might have lavishly praised the child one moment and criticized him or her in a destructive way the next.

The availability of drugs and society's attitudes toward them also help determine whether drug addiction will develop and continue. Ninety-two percent of the Vietnam veterans who were addicted to heroin, for example, discontinued using it when they returned to the United States. (However, many of those who stopped then became addicted to alcohol and other widely available drugs.) Physicians, who have ready access to all sorts of drugs, also have the highest rate of drug addiction of any group studied.

Most people, however, do not become addicts. According to some experts, the background of the nonaddict usually includes strong family ties, some kind of religious involvement, and good social relations.

Source: Bryce Nelson, "The Addictive Personality: Common Traits Are Found," *The New York Times*, January 18, 1983, pp. C1, C8. © 1983 by The New York Times Company. Used by permission.

Self-assured people who are motivated to work hard and who derive satisfaction from tangible accomplishment are unlikely to need the status or escape provided by drugs. Studies have shown that many drug abusers are unhappy individuals who come from troubled homes. They might be persons with strong feelings of inadequacy or anxiety who seek the solace of drugs; or they might be dependent individuals who are afraid of their own aggressive feelings and use drugs to induce passivity. In either case, the abuse of drugs is literally self-destructive.

It is clear the drug abuse is the result of a complex interrelationship between psychological and environmental forces. The drug abuser is likely to be someone with emotional problems who lives in a community that reinforces drug abuse and in a society that encourages drug use. It is in this light that the effectiveness of our drug laws and treatment programs must be evaluated.

TREATMENT OF DRUG ADDICTION

Drug addiction is a physiological phenomenon. As a result, research for drug-addiction treatment has often focused on *chemical therapy*—the discovery of a substance, such as methadone for opiate addiction, that can placate addicts' craving for drugs or limit their sensitivity to them. In recent years, however, it has become clear that although actual addiction is physical, it is almost always caused by social and psychological factors. Hence psychotherapeutic anti-drug efforts have come into wide use. Both chemical therapy and psychotherapy have advantages and disadvantages, but neither has proved to be the final answer to the drug-abuse problem.

Both treatment concepts share one common problem: how to motivate drug addicts to stop using drugs. Addicts are motivated to continue using drugs partly by the fear of painful withdrawal symptoms: stomach cramps, fever and chills, nausea, and general physical discomfort. They are also driven to continue using drugs because of the high and the release from tension and anxiety. Addicts who continue to crave a high, no matter what the cost in health and money, are unlikely to seek treatment that will deny them this release. And regardless of society's value judgments on their life style, addicts are often convinced that this is the best choice. Therefore the thinking and life goals of drug addicts must be totally reoriented before they can be cured. But even if addicts are motivated to change and are cured, a return to the environment where they first learned to use drugs is likely to lead them directly back into addiction. Obviously, then, there is no quick, easy treatment for addiction.

Methadone Programs

Methadone programs take a chemical-therapy approach to the treatment of heroin addiction. They center on the application of the drug methadone, which has cross-tolerance with heroin and other opiates but not with barbiturates, tranquilizers, or amphetamines. When methadone is taken in relatively small doses, it can block the high normally achieved with the use of heroin, morphine, or codeine.

Methadone is usually administered orally. The dose is large enough to produce a cross-tolerance effect with other opiates but too small to give the regular user a high. Dosage is gradually adjusted until a **maintenance dose** is achieved—an amount the user must take every day or two or else suffer the withdrawal symptoms common to all opiates. The main advantages of methadone are that

A methadone maintenance clinic.

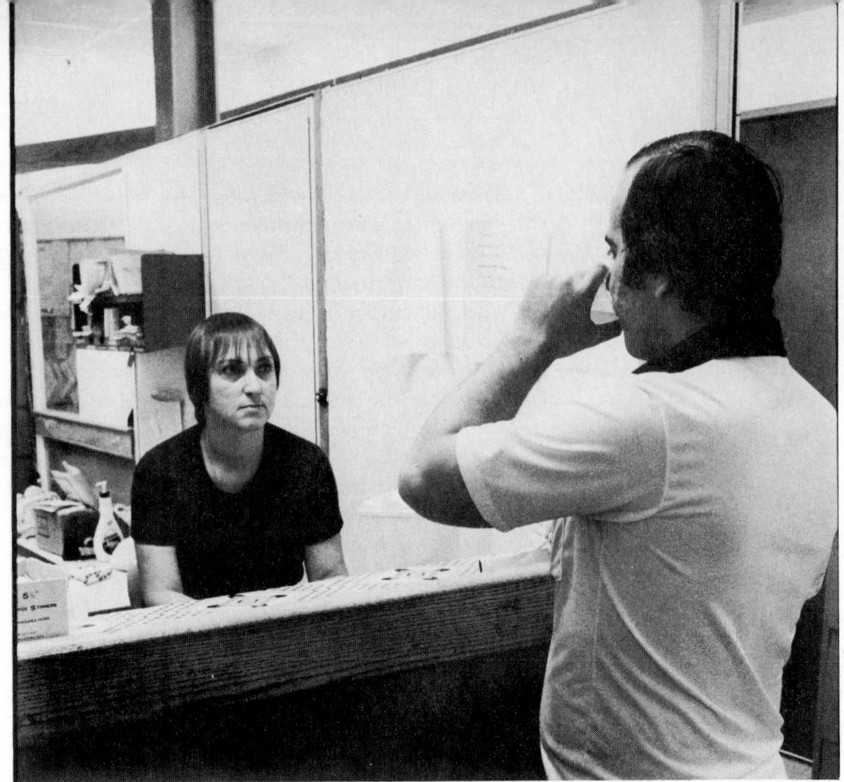

it is long-acting—thus producing more stability for use in treatment—and, unlike heroin, it does not have a soporific (sleep-inducing) effect. Thus the normal everyday functioning of the methadone user is not impaired.

Methadone maintenance programs have been criticized on the grounds what they substitute one addictive substance for another. Scandals involving clinic operators and physicians, and the militancy of neighborhood groups protesting local clinics, have further weakened the U.S. methadone program. Some critics contend that our society makes methadone freely available because it wishes to cut down on drug-related crimes and that the interest in curing the addicts is secondary. One problem is the illegal market in methadone, which continues to thrive. Methadone has become a street drug whose abuse takes hundreds of lives each year.

Drug Abuse: Where to Go for Help

Cocaine Abuse Hotline
(800) COCAINE

Do It Now Foundation
P.O. Box 5115
Phoenix, Ariz. 85010-5115
(602) 257-0797

Drug Crisis Hotline
(800) 522-5353

Drug Abuse Clearinghouse
Room 10A53
5600 Fishers Lane
Rockville, Md. 20857
(301) 443-6500

Source: *The Columbia University College of Physicians and Surgeons Complete Home Medical Guide* (New York: Crown Publishers, 1986). Reprinted by permission.

Therapeutic Communities

Psychotherapeutic programs, called *therapeutic communities*, have been used to treat drug addiction in a number of U.S. cities. Unlike methadone programs, they treat all forms of drug addiction. Perhaps the best-known therapeutic community is Phoenix House in New York City, which was set up in 1967.

The psychotherapeutic approach is based on the view that most addicts are under severe emotional strain and are unable to assume responsibility for their lives. The program, which lasts from six to twenty-four months, is essentially a condensed life experience in which residents are held increasingly responsible for their own actions; in the process they are expected to gain self-confidence and thereby become mature adults.

The heart of the treatment is a form of group therapy called an *encounter session*. Several sessions are held every week, and attendance is mandatory. In them, participants air their grievances toward one another and, in turn, are questioned about their own attitudes and behavior. The object is to help addicts recognize their own faults and virtues and change the self-defeating aspects of their behavior. Upon successful treatment, the participants are expected to take up normal lives in the larger society.

Therapeutic communities have not proven to be very successful—especially with opiate addicts—for a number of reasons. Because of space limitations, only a small number of addicts can be treated at a time. The length and cost of treatment are also drawbacks. But the major problem with this system of treatment is that because of its supportive, unthreatening nature, it shields participants from the harsh reality of the world they have left and to which they must ultimately return. Furthermore, many addicts are unable to assimilate the middle-class values of self-discipline and achievement these programs try to instill. Many others cannot withstand the emotional strains generated by the course of therapy. Most of those who leave before completing treatment return to drug abuse.

Other Treatment Programs

Until recently, most drug-treatment programs in the United States were directed toward lower-class heroin addicts. However, with the recognition of the epidemic of cocaine use and polydrug addiction among middle-class whites, new approaches and treatments have emerged. These new programs, like their predecessors, begin with detoxification. Most follow the basic principles of Alcoholics Anonymous, which stress the importance of self-examination and mutual support. But whereas older treatment programs like AA held that the addict must "hit bottom" before being ready for rehabilitation, the new philosophy advocates direct confrontation and early intervention by employers, family members, and friends before drug abusers make a shambles of their lives.

Several social factors are responsible for this new treatment focus and its acceptance. One of the most important has been the courage of a few public figures. For example, in 1978 Betty Ford, wife of former President Gerald R. Ford, publicly stated that she was an alcoholic and a pill abuser and was going to seek treatment for her condition. In the years following, well-known entertainers such as Elizabeth Taylor and Richard Pryor made similar announcements, thus removing some of the stigma of polydrug abuse.

There had also been a considerable stigma attached to being a woman drug

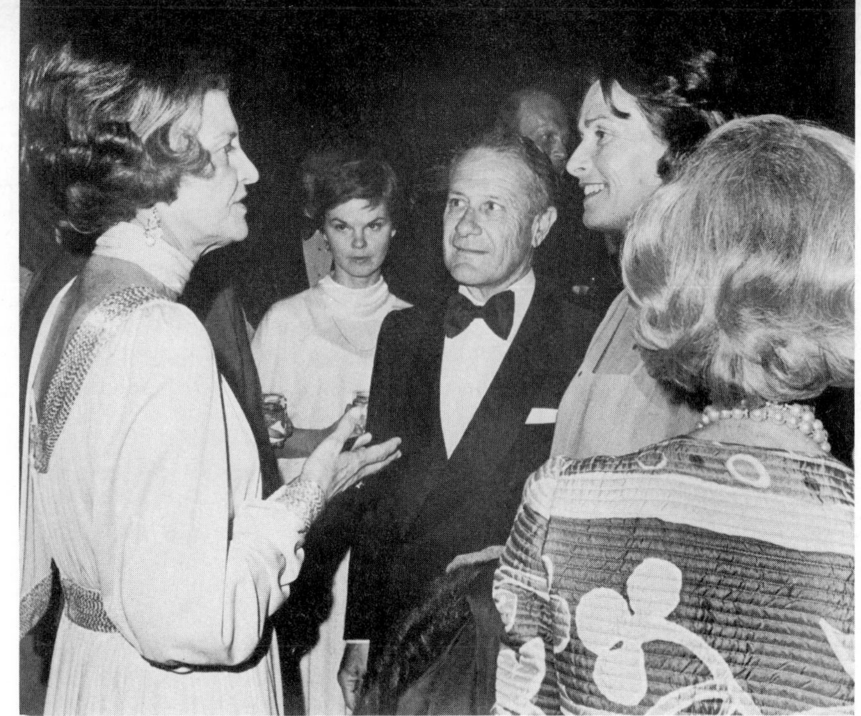

The public acknowledgment of addiction to alcohol and drugs of people like Mrs. Betty Ford has helped to remove the stigma from polydrug abuse.

abuser. Chauvinistic attitudes toward women's drug and alcohol problems had prevented many women from seeking treatment. Whereas society traditionally tolerated male alcoholism and addiction, it considered addicted women to be particularly immoral and self-indulgent. But because of the example of Mrs. Ford and others in recent years, women now make up 30 to 40 percent of all those seeking rehabilitation.

Private Treatment Programs. Private treatment programs are offered in various settings ranging from private hospitals to outpatient clinics. Besides detoxification and family counseling, many new programs stress group activities. Since most heavy drug abusers lead solitary, isolated lives, a major goal of treatment is to get them involved with others. Programs geared to teenagers and young adults, such as Outward Bound, conduct activities that often involve risk-taking or represent a challenge, such as sailing or rock climbing. The purpose is to expose the participants to situations that stress responsibility, self-reliance, and in some cases mutual cooperation.

Employee Assistance Programs. More than 5,000 companies and public agencies have set up **employee-assistance programs** (EAPs) to rehabilitate workers whose skill, training, and expertise would be difficult to replace. Some companies run in-house programs, while others use the services of outside contractors. EAPs elicit employee trust by pledging strict confidentiality and by guaranteeing that their treatment for any drug-abuse problem will be kept out of their personnel files. Employees may voluntarily drop in to the company medical department, or they may be referred by supervisors who have noticed behavioral peculiarities or poor work performance. After a medical exam and a series of counseling sessions, employees may then receive treatment at an outside drug clinic. They are given sick leave, and the costs of treatment are often covered by company health-insurance benefits. (Blue Cross has recently expanded its coverage to include drug abusers.) After returning to work, employees are expected to attend follow-up counseling sessions.

Hotlines. Several private hospitals and public agencies have established toll-free 800 telephone hotlines to give confidential advice on drug problems to workers who may be reluctant to see a company adviser. Volunteers at these numbers also provide medical advice, treatment referrals, and, most important, a sympathetic ear.

Success Rate. Such policies seem to be paying off. Most participating companies report lower absenteeism, fewer medical claims, and fewer accidents among their employees. If the number of people seeking treatment is any indication, Americans are at least more aware of the dangers of drug and alcohol abuse than they were even a few years ago. But the problem is not one that is going to go away (see box: Preventing Drug Abuse).

DRUG ABUSE AND THE LAW

Our experience with Prohibition suggests that it is almost impossible to ban a substance that is in great demand and has a high profit potential. This is confirmed by our present experience with the drug problem. People who obtain illegal drugs are quite single-minded in their determination to abuse them for the sake of euphoric pleasures. They are stopped neither by the physical and psychological dangers such drugs pose nor by the legal penalties for their possession. Paradoxically, the large profits that motivate people to become drug dealers are possible only because these drugs are illegal.

The ineffectiveness of our drug laws is compounded by the fact that they are somewhat hypocritical. There is not a great deal of difference between the street heroin user and the middle-class abuser of minor tranquilizers, barbiturates, and amphetamines. The former may have to resort to burglary to support his or her habit, while the latter can obtain drugs through prescriptions; but in terms of psychological and physical dependence, they are both abusers. So is the alcoholic.

Our drug laws also reflect a certain cultural bias. Alcohol and tobacco have been in use for centuries. They are an accepted part of daily life and are legally available. Yet these substances harm more individuals in our society than drugs such as heroin or cocaine. In part, the reason narcotics have been declared illegal is that these drugs have always been outside the mainstream of our culture.

Finally, it should be noted that some government officials have fabricated or exaggerated the effects of certain substances (particularly marijuana) or have used scare tactics in order to discourage their use. This has caused some people to question all government information about drugs (no matter how well verified elsewhere) and to violate drug laws.

The Trend in Drug Laws

For many years the sale of most drugs, including those with the greatest potential for abuse, was unregulated. This lack of regulation existed because neither the extent to which these drugs were misused nor the dangers of abuse were recog-

Preventing Drug Abuse

Drugs will always be available. Fighting drug abuse by eradicating drugs or making them inaccessible is like fighting a disease by treating its symptoms instead of destroying the virus that is causing it.

Our society combats drug abuse by arresting and imprisoning traffickers, prohibiting imports of abusable substances, and issuing dire warnings in the media. The federal government spends billions of dollars tracking down drug-law violators, prosecuting owners of "head shops" that sell drug paraphernalia, and negotiating with foreign governments to put a stop to the ever-growing international drug trade. Such measures have their place, but they do not get at the root of the problem of drug abuse.

People use drugs because they are dissatisfied with their lives in some way. They turn to chemicals to simulate the success, love, relationships, rewards, and satisfactions they feel are lacking in their lives. It is futile to tell unhappy, frustrated people that the high they crave in order to escape such feelings is self-destructive or morally wrong. Most will grasp the intellectual content of the message, but remain emotionally unmoved. In such circumstances feelings are infinitely more powerful than rational arguments. Most people will choose any method they can to avoid stress and anxiety—and drugs, in the short run at least, offer just such a method.

In the long run, of course, the extensive use of drugs to escape life's disappointments will lead to social disaster. Yet nothing substantial can be accomplished by threats of fines and prison terms; even warning people of the dreadful physical consequences of drug abuse has had little effect. Instead, the solution to the problem is to mend the social fabric—to bring people into harmony with their families, schools, and communities. Drug abuse will not be overcome by eliminating addicting drugs, but by creating social conditions that will give people a sense of control over their lives, of continuity with the past, and of responsibility for future generations.

Drug abuse is a thorny and complex problem that does not lend itself to easy solutions. Even so, the only effective approach is to help potential drug abusers—and this includes just about everyone—look inside themselves, rather than outside, for sources of well-being. Not an easy solution, certainly, but a goal worth striving toward.

nized. However, when cocaine and morphine and, later, heroin dependence became widespread, the need was felt for legal restrictions on the manufacture and sale of these drugs.

Beginning in 1906, the Pure Food and Drug Act required the accurate labeling of patent medicines containing opium and certain other drugs. Next, a series of federal and state laws was passed in 1914 to control the use of narcotic drugs and their derivatives. The Treasury Department began to expand its domain with the passage of the Harrison Act during the same year. Drug abuse, once seen as a medical problem that required a medical solution, became a criminal problem. Just as the psychiatric and legal definitions of mental illness have been historically out of step, so have the medical and legal perspectives on drug problems since 1914.

Some of these early laws required only that a tax be paid by anyone possessing narcotics. The development of new drugs and the ever-mounting problem of drug abuse caused the scope of the laws to be broadened. Both new and old drugs came under stringent regulation, and penalties for violations were sharply increased. The epidemic of drug abuse during the 1960s led to the passage of even stricter laws covering a wide variety of drugs. These laws are in a state of flux, however, subject to constantly developing new information about drugs and to changes in public attitudes.

Federal Laws

A new schedule of federal drug penalties designed to update former narcotics statutes took effect in 1970. This law, the Comprehensive Drug Abuse Prevention and Control Act, created five classes of drugs over which the federal government has jurisdiction. Illegal possession of any of these drugs is punishable by up to a year in prison and/or a $5,000 fine (for a first offense). The law also covers the manufacture, distribution, use, and sale of these drugs.

Class 1 drugs are considered to have the greatest potential for abuse. They include such drugs as heroin, marijuana, LSD, and mescaline. Manufacture and sale of these drugs is punishable by a prison sentence of up to fifteen years and/or a $25,000 fine. Penalties for subsequent offenses are higher. Even more stringent penalties are prescribed for persons over 18 who distribute these drugs to a minor.

Class 2 drugs include morphine, cocaine, methadone, Quaaludes, and amphetamines. These drugs have a high potential for abuse, but also have some limited medical application. Class 3 drugs are those with some therapeutic value, such as barbiturates. Class 4 drugs are mild depressants (such as a mild barbiturate) and tranquilizers (such as Valium). Class 5 drugs are low-strength narcotic derivatives (like codeine). The penalties for violations associated with Class 2, 3, 4, and 5 drugs are progressively lower than the penalties for Class 1 violations.

The 1970 law further extends the penalties for illegal distribution and possession of barbiturates and stimulants to include manufacturers, wholesale and retail pharmacists, hospitals, clinics, research laboratories, and public health agencies, all of which must now keep accurate records of the drugs they handle and dispense.

State Laws

Because of the great variation among states regarding drug-abuse penalties, whenever both state and federal agencies are involved in prosecution of an individual on drug charges the federal government usually bows to the state's action. In states that have less stringent laws, a drug abuser may try to plead guilty to a state offense in order to avoid stiffer federal prosecution. It is possible, however, for an individual to be prosecuted under both state and federal statutes.

SUMMARY

1. Both legal and illegal drugs are widely abused in our society. In part, this is so because drugs are easily obtainable, companies advertise drugs as the solution to all problems, and many people seek instant relief for their physical and psychological ailments.

2. Drugs are natural or synthetic substances that alter the function of the body in some way. Some drugs are *psychoactive*—that is, they act on the central nervous system to produce altered states of consciousness. The three categories of psychoactive drugs are: *stimulants*, which excite body cells to increased activity; *depressants* and *sedatives*, which decrease cell activity; and *hallucinogens*, which have effects that are mainly psychological.

3. The intended effect of a drug is called its *primary effect*; unintended effects are termed *secondary*, or *side*, *effects*. One common side effect of repeated use of a drug is *tolerance*: The body becomes accustomed to the drug and no longer responds to it as it did originally. Many chemically related drugs are

cross-tolerant; meaning one can substitute for the other.

4. Using drugs over a period of time may cause *dependence*. Physical dependence is known as *addiction*; the user will suffer the physical symptoms of *withdrawal* if the drug is removed. Psychological dependence is called *habituation*.

5. Drug abuse is the taking of any substance in any way that can damage the user's health or ability to function. Aspirin, laxatives, tranquilizers, amphetamines, alcohol, and tobacco are commonly abused legal drugs. Heroin, cocaine, LSD, PCP, and marijuana are the most-abused illegal drugs. The drug groups most associated with drug abuse, in addition to alcohol and tobacco, are the *opiates*, *barbiturates*, *tranquilizers*, *amphetamines*, *hallucinogens*, and *cocaine*. It is common for people to be *polydrug abusers*—that is, addicted to two or more drugs at the same time.

6. Treatment of heroin addiction generally involves *methadone maintenance* or *psychotherapy*, or both. In a methadone program the addict is given small oral doses of the drug on a regular schedule. The chief advantages of methadone maintenance are that it is relatively inexpensive and that the drug allows the addict to function normally. The chief disadvantages are that the addict is still drug dependent and that methadone can be used only for opiate addiction. At the present time a controversy is raging over the effectiveness and morality of the entire program. Psychotherapeutic programs in therapeutic communities have tried to treat the emotional problems of addicts, but so far have not been very successful. New treatment programs advocating *detoxification* and mutual help instead of psychotherapy have been much more successful. Company-run *employee-assistance programs* have likewise proved effective at reducing addiction in the workplace.

7. The 1970 Drug Abuse Prevention and Control Act established five classes of drugs over which the federal government has jurisdiction. These range from Class 1 drugs such as heroin, marijuana, and LSD, to Class 5 drugs such as codeine. Penalties are higher for Class 1 violations and become progressively lower for Class 2, 3, 4, and 5 violations. State laws are generally patterned after federal statutes. Many critics believe that our drug laws have been ineffective: They have neither deterred drug abuse nor provided for the rehabilitation of drug offenders.

CONSUMER CONCERNS

1. One abuse that occurs in respect to pharmaceuticals is overuse of the word *relief*. Advertisements suggest the problems from which we should seek relief as well as their solution—the "instant fix" phenomenon. Do you consider this kind of advertising to be a part of the drug problem?
2. Do you feel that sufficient warning accompanies prescription drugs that are addictive? Whose responsibility is this—the physician's, the pharmacist's, the consumer's?
3. If we are losing the drug battle, is it because we emphasize punishment rather than prevention? In this respect what do you see as constructive roles for the various branches of government?
4. Do you believe that school antidrug programs could be more effective, or are the dimensions of this problem too large for the schools to cope with?

14

Cardiovascular Diseases and Cancer

- Cardiovascular Diseases
- The Circulatory System
- Major Cardiovascular Diseases
- Risk Factors and Prevention
- Cancer
- Types of Cancer
- Protection Against Cancer
- Cancer Treatment
- Cancer Prevention

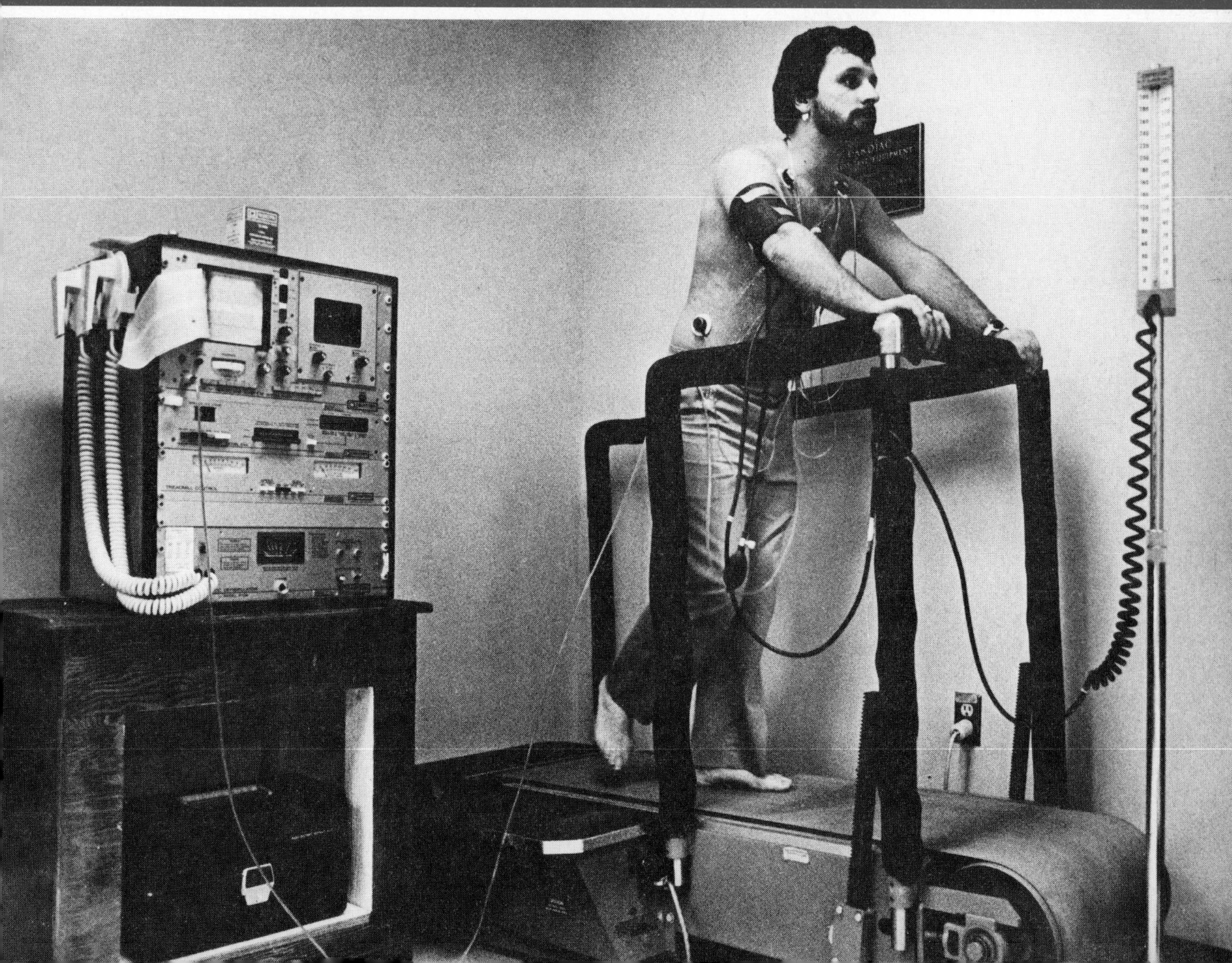

Cardiovascular diseases (diseases of the heart and blood vessels) and cancer are responsible for two out of every three deaths in the United States. This is true despite recent success in lowering the death rate from heart disease and despite the fact that, with the single exception of cancer of the lung, cancer death rates have remained stable. Although we tend to associate both kinds of diseases with the elderly, the truth is that persons of every age are susceptible. This fact and the high death rate associated with them make cardiovascular diseases and cancer our primary health problems.

Cardiovascular diseases and cancer have not always been our leading causes of death. In 1900 influenza and pneumonia, which now account for only 2.9 percent of the mortality rate, were the major causes. The fundamental reason for this reversal is our increasing ability to control communicable diseases. As people contract these diseases less frequently, and still fewer die from them, our **life expectancy** rates continue to increase. The Census Bureau reports that a female child born today can be expected to live beyond the age of 78, and a male, beyond 71. This continual lengthening of life span itself contributes to the frequency of cardiovascular diseases and cancer. If, as is believed, these ailments occur as the result of the long-term existence of certain conditions of the body, or the long-term exposure to certain substances, then the likelihood of their occurring increases as we age.

We shall first review the cardiovascular disorders, our principal cause of death, and follow with a discussion of cancer.

CARDIOVASCULAR DISEASES

Census figures record a steady decline in the American heart disease rate since 1950. After a slow beginning, this decline has accelerated in recent years. And despite an older and larger population, the mortality rate from cardiovascular disease among both elderly and younger groups continues to decline as well. Should the decline continue at its present rate, the heart disease death rate would be halved by the year 2005.

This lowered rate has probably come about because of increased attention to diet and nutrition, increased participation in exercise programs, and the widespread discontinuance of smoking among adults. However, recent cross-cultural studies have shown some puzzling results when life-style changes are considered. In the United States fatal heart attacks have been dropping by 3 percent a year since 1968. In Sweden, however, medical campaigns against smoking, high-cholesterol food intake, and other high-risk factors have been just as zealous as campaigns in the United States. Yet fatal heart attacks have been *increasing* in Sweden. In Switzerland more and more women are smoking and eating fatty foods, yet fatal heart attacks in that country for women are *decreasing*.

The World Health Organization, faced with these unexpected findings, is now launching a more thorough study. Despite the puzzling statistics from this initial study, Americans presumably can continue to lower their mortality rate due to **cardiovascular diseases**—diseases of the heart and blood vessels—by conscientiously avoiding risk factors. Cardiovascular disease is still the number-one health problem in the United States, and is responsible for over 50 percent of all deaths (see Figure 14-1).

FIGURE 14-1

Leading causes of death in the United States, 1984.

Source: National Center for Health Statistics, 1986.

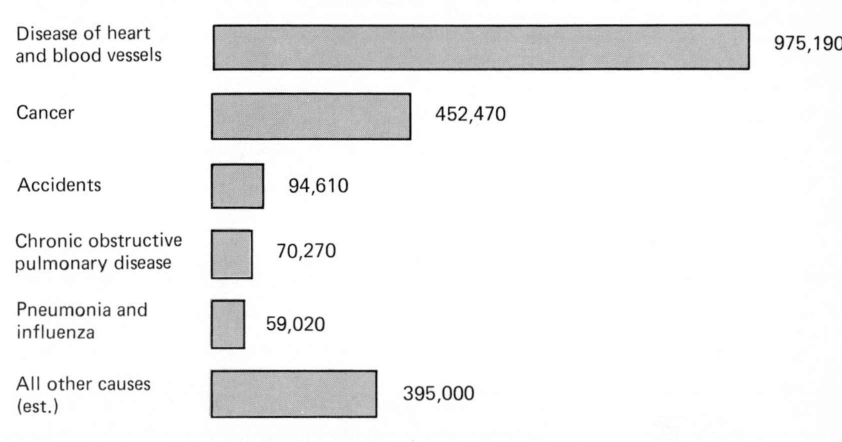

The conditions that precipitate a heart attack are many. High blood pressure, for instance, correlates very highly with heart attacks. Obese persons, as life insurance statistics show, are especially prone to heart attacks, as are smokers. Cholesterol levels in the blood, although it is difficult to distinguish the factors that cause them, are related to the chances of experiencing a heart attack. Other disorders, such as kidney impairment or diabetes, also play a role. The tensions of certain occupations and life styles can make an individual susceptible to heart attack as well. In fact, the personality type called Type A is especially prone to stress and heart disease (see Chapter 2). The activity pattern of the individual is extremely important because of its relationship with blood cholesterol levels. Smoking, ironically a habit that is pursued voluntarily, is one of the most significant causes of heart disease.

Although heart attack and stroke do not generally occur before the middle years, the predisposing conditions exist long before. During childhood and the teenage years certain important habits are established, such as how and what we eat, and whether or not we exercise or smoke, that have a bearing on our health in later years. Some conditions are even present at birth, as in children born with congenital impairments of the heart. Infections in childhood can lead to rheumatic heart disease. Hypertension is being diagnosed in more and more children as well as in adults; and atherosclerosis of the coronary arteries is also much in evidence among young adults. These facts should signal to us the importance of being alert throughout our lives to conditions or behavior patterns that play a role in the development of cardiovascular impairment.

THE CIRCULATORY SYSTEM

The **circulatory system** is the body's transportation network; it conveys the necessary food and oxygen to the cells and carries away the cells' waste products. Materials entering and leaving the cells are transported in the blood through a system of blood vessels—the arteries, veins, and capillaries. The blood is pumped through the body in a continuous circuit by the heart.

The Heart

The **heart** is located in the chest cavity between the lungs, slightly to the left of the center of the body. In an adult the heart is roughly the size of a closed fist and weighs about eleven ounces. The heart of an average adult beats about seventy-five times a minute. The period during which the heart muscle contracts is called **systole;** the period during which it relaxes is called **diastole.** Heartbeat can be measured by counting the pulsations that can be felt at pressure points in the wrist or neck. These pulsations give us the **pulse rate,** which is identical to the rate of the beat of the heart.

The normal heart is strong enough to withstand the demands of the most vigorous physical activities.

Blood Vessels

Arteries. The system of blood vessels that carries blood from the heart to the body is the **arterial system.** The principal artery in the body, the **aorta,** is connected directly to the heart; the left side of the heart discharges blood into the aorta. Arteries lead continually into smaller arteries and **arterioles,** which are no larger than a human hair. The arterioles lead into the capillaries.

Capillaries. **Capillaries** are the primary distributors of blood to the cells of the body. Because the walls of a capillary consist of a single layer of cells, nutrients, oxygen, and other substances carried in the blood can easily diffuse out of a capillary and into the body cells. Similarly, waste products from the cells, such as carbon dioxide, can easily enter the bloodstream through the capillary walls.

Veins. Upon leaving the capillaries, blood drains into very tiny veins called **venules.** The venules join together to form veins, and the veins increase in size as they approach the heart. Veins return blood of reduced oxygen content to the heart.

Blood Pressure

Blood pressure refers to the presure of the blood against the inner walls of the arteries. Like body temperature, it can be determined easily and quickly and is one indication of a person's health.

In a young adult male **systolic pressure** displaces about 120 millimeters of mercury, and **diastolic pressure** about 80 millimeters of mercury. This is usually written 120/80 (one-twenty over eighty). The reading for a young adult female is usually about 110/70. Systolic pressure gradually increases with advancing age, but diastolic pressure normally falls into the 70 to 90 range even in later years. Everyone's normal blood pressure varies, however, at different times during the day, from day to day, and from year to year. Blood pressure increases when a person is involved in strenuous physical activity or is in an aroused emotional state. Blood pressure is normally lowest when a person is sleeping.

Blood

If a sample of blood is drawn from the body, treated to prevent clotting, and left to stand for a while, it will separate into two layers. The bottom layer (about 45 percent of the total quantity of blood) will consist mainly of red blood cells, plus a much smaller number of white blood cells and blood platelets. The upper layer (about 55 percent of the total quantity) will be a clear, slightly yellow liquid called plasma.

Plasma. **Plasma** is about 92 percent water. The remaining 8 percent consists of chemical substances dissolved or suspended in the water: proteins, salts, amino acids, glucose, fats, hormones, antibodies, enzymes, vitamins, dissolved gases such as oxygen and nitrogen, and waste products. These substances help to keep the body alive and functioning normally.

Red Blood Cells. **Red blood cells** are vital to the body because they transport oxygen to the cells and carry away carbon dioxide. Arterial blood is about 20 percent oxygen by volume, whereas blood returning to the heart via the veins is only about 14 percent oxygen by volume. A shortage of red blood cells or hemoglobin results in a condition called **anemia.** Anemic individuals are typically pale, weak, and lethargic, because their body cells are not receiving enough oxygen. **Iron-deficiency anemia** can be caused by an excessive loss of blood due to internal bleeding, as with ulcers, or by a deficiency of iron in the diet. In the latter case, the anemia can usually be alleviated by increasing the intake of iron, preferably through iron-rich foods. **Pernicious anemia,** on the other hand, results from failure of the bone marrow to produce a sufficient number

A person with type O blood can donate blood to anyone else; a person with type AB blood can receive blood from anyone else.

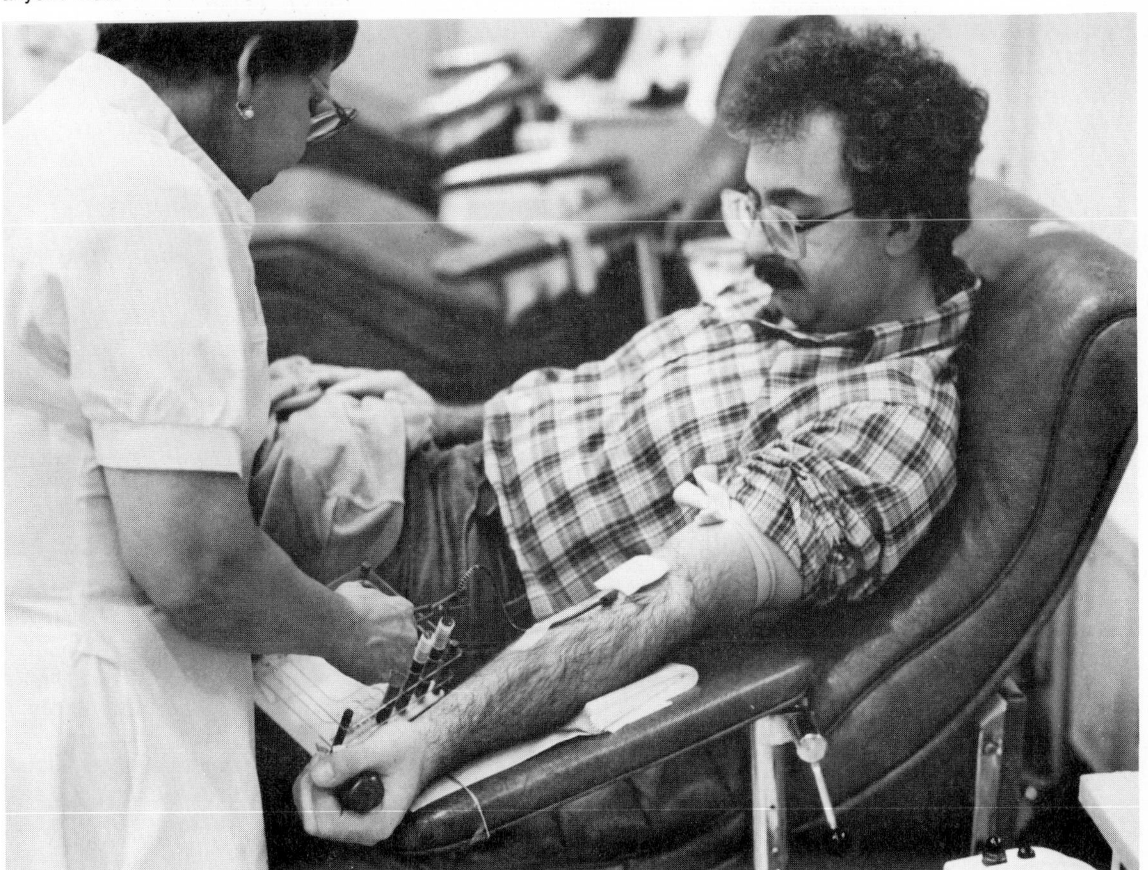

of red blood cells. This disease is generally the result of a vitamin B_{12} deficiency* (B_{12} is necessary for the production of red blood cells) or of exposure to excessive radiation. *Sickle-cell anemia* is a hereditary disease involving the hemoglobin in red blood cells; it affects mainly black people.

White Blood Cells. The primary function of **white blood cells,** or **leukocytes,** is to protect the body against foreign microorganisms. Leukocytes destroy microorganisms by surrounding them, absorbing them into their cell bodies, and digesting them. Because of their role in fighting bacteria, leukocytes increase in number enormously during periods of illness. In fact, a physician can often diagnose a specific disease by noting the number and kind of leukocytes in the body.

Blood Platelets. Blood **platelets** play an essential part in blood clotting. When bleeding occurs, the platelets disintegrate, initiating a series of chemical reactions that check the flow of blood.

Blood Groups

Nearly everyone at some time is given a blood test to determine which blood group he or she belongs to: type A, B, AB, or O. These blood groups have varying degrees of compatibility, and therefore it is essential to know the blood type of both the donor and the recipient before a transfusion is attempted. The mixing of incompatible blood groups produces clotting.

The compatible blood types are as follows:

Recipient	*Donor*
A	A, O
B	B, O
AB	AB, A, B, O
O	O

In addition, the Rh factor is associated with a reaction in the blood. This factor is significant in both blood transfusions and births, and is discussed in Chapter 7.

MAJOR CARDIOVASCULAR DISEASES

We shall divide the major cardiovascular diseases into seven categories and discuss them in order. They are (1) congenital heart disease, (2) rheumatic heart disease, (3) arteriosclerosis, (4) atherosclerosis, (5) hypertension, (6) coronary heart disease, and (7) stroke.

Congenital Heart Disease

According to the American Heart Association, about 25,000 babies are born in the United States each year with **congenital heart disease,** in which the heart develops abnormally before the baby is born. Although the rate of children born with this condition is increasing, afflicted children have a better chance to lead normal lives than ever before because of medical advances in detection and treatment.

Science still does not know in all cases what causes abnormal development of the heart before birth. The most common identifiable cause, but one that accounts for only about 5 percent of all congenital heart disease, is maternal

* See the section on vegetarianism in Chapter 5 for the relationship between B_{12} deficiency and vegetarianism.

viral infection—usually rubella (German measles), although sometimes mumps or influenza. Excessive doses of vitamin D taken during pregnancy can, in certain instances, do serious damage to the brain, kidneys, and the circulatory system of an unborn child.

Recently, it has been learned that women who take oral contraceptives (not realizing they are pregnant) or female hormones during the second and third months of pregnancy are twice as likely to bear children with heart abnormalities. Indeed, there are reasons to be concerned about any drug a woman takes during pregnancy—even aspirin. It is also thought that smoking may cause damage to the fetal heart.

Rheumatic Heart Disease

Rheumatic heart disease is the single most common heart disease in children and young adults. Because the disease usually occurs as a complication of a streptococcal infection, the proper diagnosis and treatment of such infections is imperative.

In 3 cases out of 1,000 a streptococcal infection (such as strep throat, scarlet fever, or strep ear) is followed in two to four weeks by rheumatic fever. The symptoms of rheumatic fever include fever, sore joints, and profuse sweating. A very rapid pulse and the presence of a **heart murmur,** an unusual rushing sound heard through a stethoscope when the heart valves open or close, indicates that the heart has become involved. The murmur results from the failure of the valves to function properly, causing an interference with the normal flow of blood in the heart.

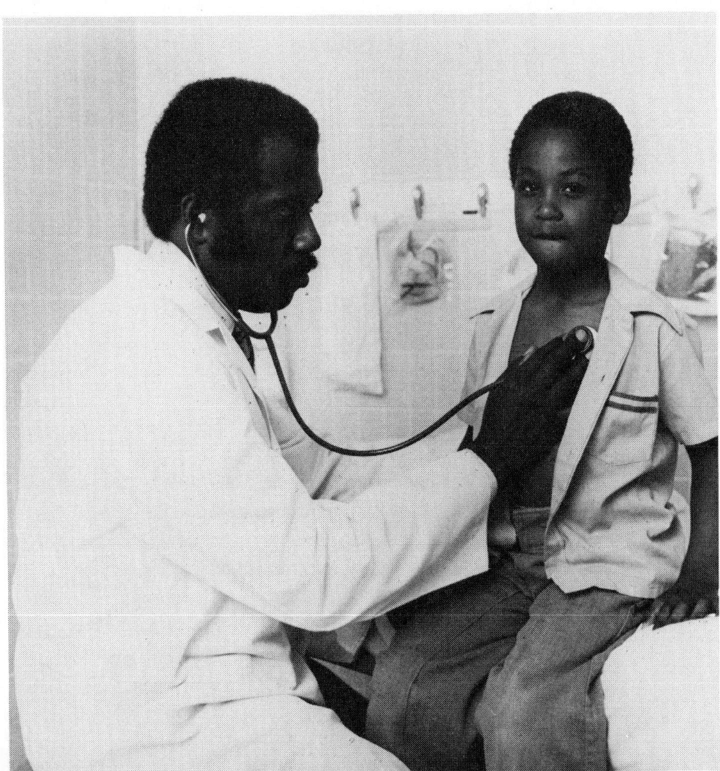

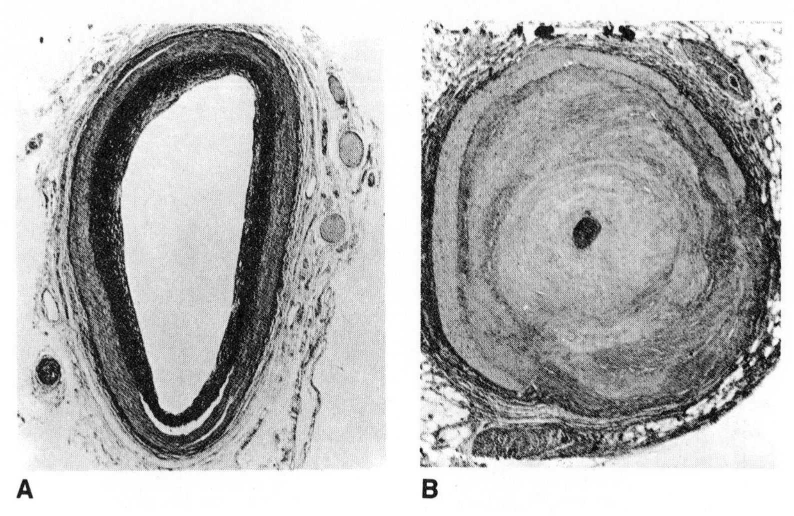

A. Cross section of a near normal artery through which blood can easily flow. B. An artery totally blocked by atherosclerosis.

In rheumatic heart disease the **endocardium**, the inner lining of the heart, becomes inflamed. This inflammation, called **endocarditis**, results in the formation of scar tissue around the heart valves, which prevents their opening or closing properly. As a result, the efficiency of the heart decreases: The heart must work harder to supply the body with blood.

The immediate treatment for rheumatic heart disease is complete bed rest, to avoid any further strain on the heart, and the administration of antibiotics, to prevent the spread of the streptococcal infection. Recuperation from the immediate effects of the disease is lengthy, and the patient must often spend several months in bed until the endocarditis has fully disappeared. A major concern is the susceptibility of the individual to a recurrence of the disease. Unless specific reasons indicate otherwise, however, there is nothing to be gained in denying the postrheumatic fever patient the benefits of physical activity.

Arteriosclerosis

Arteriosclerosis, or hardening of the arteries, is a condition in which the normally flexible connective tissue forming the walls of the arteries gradually degenerates and is replaced by hard, inflexible scar tissue. ("Sclerosis" means hardening of the tissues.)

As the condition progresses, the thickening and growing inelasticity of the walls of the arteries restrict the amount of blood that can flow through these vessels, thus raising the blood pressure. An added danger is that the narrowed arteries may trap a blood clot. This would block the flow of blood to tissues that are fed by the artery. A sclerotic artery may also rupture, as in the case of apoplexy, or stroke.

A number of factors have been linked to arteriosclerosis. One is a high level of cholesterol in the body. Another is heredity. It also appears that individuals who suffer from diabetes mellitus, kidney disease, and hypertension are more likely to develop arteriosclerosis than other people.

Atherosclerosis

Atherosclerosis is a type of arteriosclerosis in which deposits of a fatty substance build up within the arteries. The deposits (called **plaque**) form in the inner wall of the artery and reduce the artery's diameter, restricting blood flow, as in arteriosclerosis. Also, atherosclerosis may narrow an arterial passage so much that a blood clot can seal off the artery entirely, causing extensive damage to the artery and to the organs it supplies.

Atherosclerosis has been linked to several factors. Among these are: the rich and fatty American diet, which may contribute to high levels of cholesterol in the bloodstream (cholesterol is the major substance in plaque); overweight; lack of exercise; cigarette smoking; emotional stress; heredity; diabetes mellitus; and hypertension.

Hypertension

Hypertension, or high blood pressure, is the most common disease of the circulatory system. Over 54 million Americans have this disease and over 31,000 die of it each year. Moderate hypertension occurs among black Americans twice as often as among whites and severe hypertension three times as often. Hypertension affects mainly middle-aged and elderly individuals, but the most recent research shows that high blood pressure can be observed even early in life.

Normal blood pressure for an adult between the ages of 18 and 25 is approximately 120/80 (see the section Blood Pressure, above). When the reading reaches 140/90 or higher and remains there, medical attention is necessary, even though this reading indicates only a mild case of hypertension. Persons with systolic readings of over 160 are in a more dangerous state and must take precautionary measures.

Although high blood pressure does seem to run in families, other factors may be as important as heredity. Nervous tension will cause an increase in

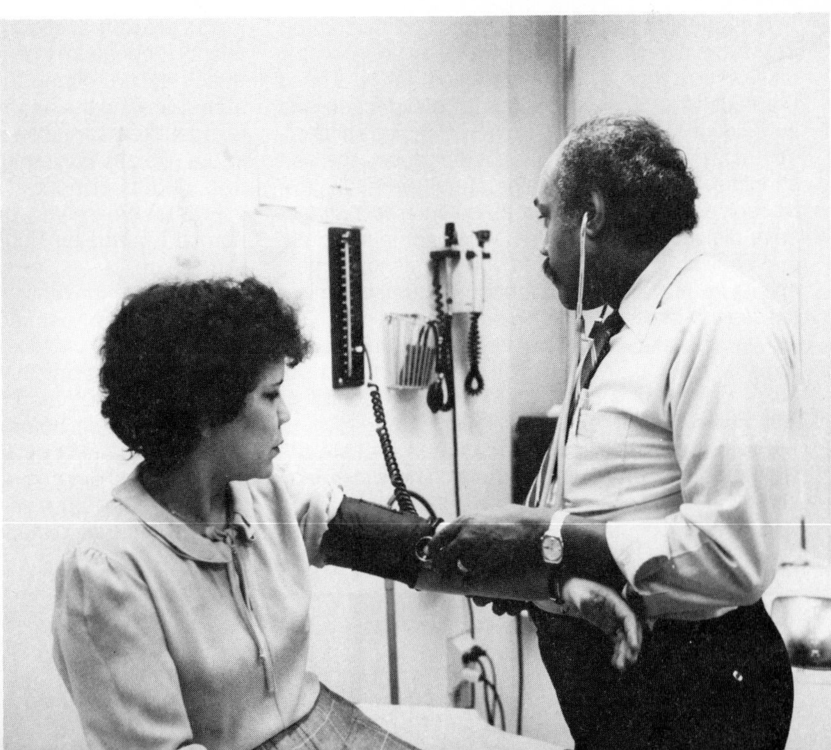

blood pressure—even worrying about blood pressure can cause blood pressure to rise. Overweight is another factor that has been linked to this disorder. Cigarette smoking also appears to be associated with this disease. And a significant curable cause of hypertension is becoming increasingly common: the use of oral contraceptive drugs.

While the death rate for hypertension was once very high (up to 50 percent), it is now quite low. Although the chances of preventing hypertension are rather dim at the moment, recent therapies have proved effective in controlling the disease. But the first step is to identify the illness. Nationally, the aim is to locate unsuspecting victims, usually those who are poor and have little access to medical care. Black people in particular should be alert to their susceptibility to this condition and as a precaution should have their blood pressure checked periodically (see Figure 14-2).

Coronary Heart Disease

Coronary heart disease is the major cause of all cardiovascular deaths: Nearly 550,000 Americans die from this disease each year. Coronary heart disease is almost always caused by a malfunction of the **coronary arteries**—the arteries that deliver blood to the heart muscle itself. Generally, the diseased arteries are unable to supply a part of the heart with sufficient blood, and this, in turn, causes that part of the heart to malfunction.

One symptom of coronary disease is **angina pectoris,** an extremely severe pain over the heart. The pain often radiates over the left side of the chest and along the left arm. Angina pectoris usually follows physical exertion, emo-

When a Heart Attack Happens

A heart attack may begin with a mild discomfort in the chest. It also may begin with an excruciating pain, as if a rope were being pulled tightly around the midchest, causing feelings of constriction and suffocation. The pain, sometimes intermittent, sometimes constant, may radiate down the left shoulder and arm; it may also affect the neck, jaw, or back. The victim may break out in a cold sweat, have difficulty breathing, feel weak and nauseated, and possibly vomit. The face sometimes turns gray, and there may be palpitations. Frequently, the victim feels a sense of doom and hopelessness.

A heart attack may be triggered by unaccustomedly vigorous exercise or an emotional crisis, but it can occur just as often during a period of little stress or activity.

There are also "silent" heart attacks that are accompanied by very few symptoms. The victim may shrug off these initial signs as indigestion. Some people have been known to continue jogging or doing push-ups during one of these mild attacks, just to prove that nothing is wrong. This is a serious mistake because the greatest danger from heart attack occurs during the critical moments immediately following the onset of symptoms. Heart rhythm is most likely to become abnormal and degenerate into a useless quivering or twitching during the first few minutes or hours.

Prompt emergency procedures can help restore normal heartbeat. This may be done by electrical stimulation, drugs, or even chest massage. More and more Americans are learning how to do **cardiopulmonary resuscitation (CPR),** discussed in the Appendix.

To delay seeking help can be fatal. More than half the 550,000 Americans who die of heart attacks each year do so before reaching a hospital.

If a heart attack patient is promptly hospitalized, the chances of recovery are excellent. As many as 85 percent of those who reach the hospital live to tell about their experience. Most return to normal lives.

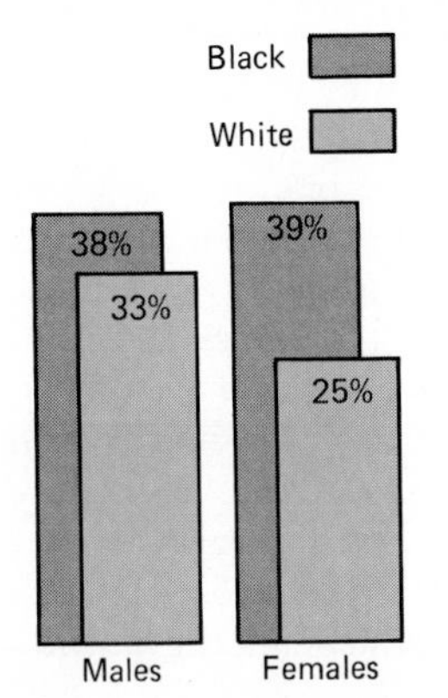

FIGURE 14-2

Hypertension prevalence by sex and race among U.S. adults.

Source: American Heart Association, *Heart Facts*, copyright © *1986*, p. 5. Reprinted with permission.

tional tension, or a heavy meal. The precise cause of the pain is unknown, but in general it results from a shortage of oxygen in a part of the heart muscle. It is therefore similar in nature to a muscle cramp in any other part of the body. This occurs when a muscle cannot receive oxygen fast enough to perform its function.

Most cases of angina pectoris are associated with arteriosclerosis of the coronary arteries. No cure or specific treatment exists, although medicines that dilate the blood vessels bring quick relief from the pain. The great danger of arteriosclerosis or atherosclerosis in the coronary arteries is that these conditions may damage the heart muscle. Because the inner surfaces of a sclerotic artery are rough, blood clots can form on the sclerotic tissues. The clotting is usually initiated by platelets in the blood as they pass over these roughened areas. A blood clot that forms within a blood vessel is known as a *thrombus*; the formation of this clot is called **thrombosis.**

If a clot should form within one of the coronary arteries and grow large enough to restrict severely or cut off blood flow in the artery, the area of the heart dependent on the artery will die. The formation of plaque deposits in an atherosclerotic artery may become so thick they block up the artery, and again, destruction of the heart muscle occurs. This blockage is known as a **coronary occlusion.** The small area of dead heart muscle that results from thrombosis or occlusion is called a **myocardial infarction.**

The symptoms of sudden coronary thrombosis or occlusion are what is commonly known as a *heart attack*. They include a severe pain in the chest that resembles the pain of angina pectoris, except that the pain of a heart attack may last for hours or days. In addition, the victim displays the symptoms of severe shock. The diagnosis of a heart attack is confirmed with the aid of an electrocardiograph (an instrument that measures electrical impulses produced within the heart).

The severity of coronary thrombosis or occlusion depends on the size of the obstruction and the size of the artery that is blocked. Also important is the presence or absence of alternate pathways through which the blood can reach the heart tissue. Exercise can build up these pathways. The consequences of thrombosis or occlusion can therefore be so mild as to be unfelt or so severe as to result in sudden death. Usually, people who exercise regularly suffer milder heart attacks and recover more quickly than those who do not.

Treatment of coronary thrombosis or occlusion includes prolonged bed rest to relieve the heart of as much strain as possible; a light diet, which also helps relieve heart strain; and the administration of oxygen, so that the body can obtain the oxygen it needs without overworking the heart. In addition, special drugs that prevent the formation of blood clots within the circulatory system may be administered; these drugs may be dangerous, however, because they also inhibit the normal clotting of blood. With care, the heart attack victim can usually resume a full, normal, and healthy life. In fact, it is not uncommon for persons who have had a heart attack to become more physically active afterward than before.

Stroke

Stroke is the second major cause of all cardiovascular deaths: Over 156,000 Americans die of it each year. Together, coronary disease and stroke account for over 71 percent of all deaths from cardiovascular disease in the United States.

A **stroke** (or **apoplexy**) is a condition resulting from an insufficient supply of blood to the brain. The blood supply to the brain may be cut off by the formation of a blood clot (thrombus) in an artery of the brain, by a **cerebral hemorrhage** (rupture of an artery in the brain), or by an **embolus** (a blood clot detached from its place of origin) that lodges in an artery and restricts blood flow. Whatever the cause, the result is that a part of the brain loses its blood supply and the brain cells dependent on that supply die. If enough cells are affected, the parts of the body controlled by that area of the brain become paralyzed because they no longer receive nerve impulses.

If the stroke is the result of a cerebral hemorrhage, the paralysis may be caused by the pressure of the blood on specific neurons. As the blood is gradually reabsorbed into the circulation, relieving the pressure on the brain, the individual may gradually regain use of the affected parts of the body.

There is no cure for a stroke and no sure prevention—stroke can occur in a person of any age, and affects the two sexes equally. However, a stroke is much more likely to occur in older individuals suffering from arteriosclerosis or hypertension. Measures to prevent these conditions—such as quitting smoking, maintaining a proper diet, and exercising—will lessen the chances of being afflicted by a stroke.

RISK FACTORS AND PREVENTION

In studies of thousands of persons who have suffered heart attacks, the great majority of victims were found to have one or more of the following habits or conditions: high cholesterol levels in the blood; overweight; hypertension; sedentary habits; cigarette smoking; diabetes mellitus; and a family history of heart disease. There is strong evidence that the presence of any one of these risk factors will increase the chances of a heart attack and that the more risk

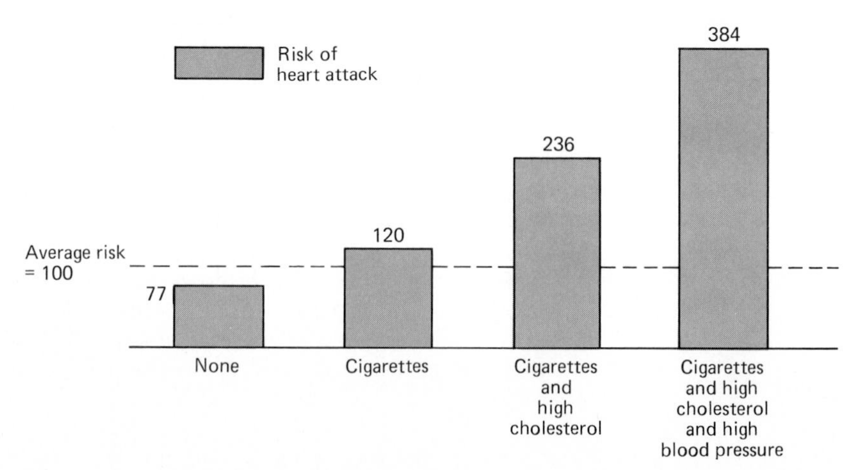

FIGURE 14-3

The danger of heart attack increases as the number of risk factors present increases. (These figures are for a 45-year-old male.)

Source: American Heart Association, *Heart Facts*, copyright © *1986*, p. 5. Reprinted with permission.

The Warning Signs of Stroke

Many fatal strokes can be prevented if high blood pressure is diagnosed and controlled. Many major strokes are preceded by "little strokes" or warning signals experienced days, weeks, or months before the more severe event. Prompt medical or surgical attention to these symptoms may prevent a fatal or disabling stroke from occurring:

- Sudden, temporary weakness or numbness of the face, arm, and leg on one side of the body.
- Temporary loss of speech, or trouble in speaking or understanding speech.
- Temporary dimness or loss of vision, particularly in one eye.
- Unexplained dizziness, unsteadiness, or sudden falls.

factors present, the greater the risk (see Figure 14-3). The millions of Americans who follow the familiar pattern of sedentary living, a high-fat diet, and cigarette smoking are thereby greatly increasing the likelihood of an early death due to heart disease. These detrimental habits are usually well entrenched by the age of 40. To effectively reduce the risk of heart attack, therefore, people should begin to revise these habits in their teens or 20s. This is especially true of diet, for cholesterol levels begin to build up during the teenage years or even earlier.

Cholesterol and Diet

Cholesterol is a fatty substance that is for the most part manufactured by the body. It is also present in most animal foods and products, especially egg yolks, meats, shellfish, and dairy products such as cheese and butter (see Table 14-1). When there is an excess of cholesterol in the body, it is deposited in the arteries and becomes the main component of the plaque that produces atheroschlerosis.

Diets and drugs can lower cholesterol levels by no more than 40 percent—not enough, some experts claim, to affect the rate of heart disease or heart attacks. Furthermore, a generation of clinical trials has not provided conclusive evidence that lowering blood cholesterol through diet reduces the risk of heart attack. Some authorities even doubt that cholesterol is the main culprit, regardless of its origins.

Cholesterol is carried in the blood by fatty proteins called *lipoproteins*. Three kinds of lipoproteins have been distinguished: high-density (HDL), low-density (LDL), and very-low-density (VLDL). The cholesterol carried by HDLs has been referred to as "good cholesterol," and that carried by the LDLs and VLDLs as "bad." The reason for this is that HDLs (actually, only type-2 HDLs) remove cholesterol from the artery walls and transport it to the liver, which either stores it or excretes it. The LDLs and VLDLs, by contrast, keep cholesterol circulating in the bloodstream. HDL levels run highest in newborn babies and decrease with age, but they are also affected by diet and activity. Losing weight, exercising vigorously, and eating a diet low in saturated fats are all effective ways of raising HDL levels and thus lowering cholesterol levels in the blood.

Recommended Cholesterol Levels. The average daily American diet contains 43 percent fat and 485 milligrams of cholesterol. A 1984 report of the National Institutes of Health recommended that this be reduced to 30 percent fat and 250 to 300 milligrams of cholesterol. *Blood levels* of cholesterol higher than 180 milligrams in people under 30 and higher than 200 milligrams in people over 30 are thought to increase the risk of heart disease, and the risk goes up even further with higher levels. *Moderate risk* is defined at 240 milligrams, *high risk* at 260 in persons over 40 years of age.

It has long been assumed that only adults need worry about cholesterol levels, but recent research has shown that the foundations for a heart attack are laid in childhood. In one study autopsies were performed on children, teenagers, and young adults who had died in accidents or as a result of homicide or suicide. Eighty-five percent of them had already developed large streaks of fat in the aorta, a precursor of atherosclerosis. Given this and other evidence, an NIH panel of physicians recommended that children over the age of 2 follow the same low-fat, low-cholesterol diet as adults; teenagers are cautioned to keep their intake of fat-loaded hamburgers and hot dogs to a minimum.

In general, a low-cholesterol diet is one that contains little saturated fat. Adhering to it involves cutting back on fat-streaked red meat, egg yolks, whole-milk dairy products (especially hard cheeses and butter), and shellfish, and substituting lean red meat, skinless poultry, fish, egg whites, and skim-milk dairy products. One should take care to maintain a balanced diet when trying to reduce cholesterol intake. Some nutritionists fear that injudicious attempts to cut dietary cholesterol could produce nutritional deficiencies.

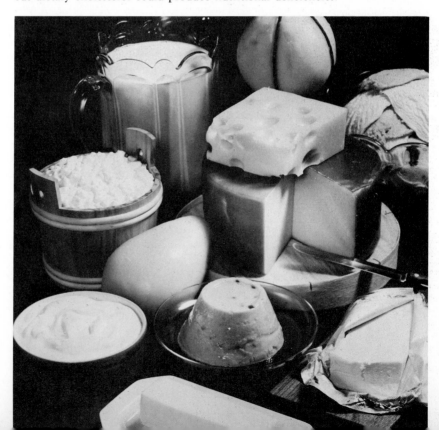

Dairy foods are an important source of calcium, but whole-milk products are high in cholesterol.

TABLE 14-1
Cholesterol Content of Common Measures of Selected Foods (in Ascending Order)

Food	Amount	Cholesterol (mg)
Milk, skim fluid, or reconstituted dry	1 cup	5
Cottage cheese, uncreamed	½ cup	7
Lard	1 tbs	12
Cream, light table	1 fluid oz	20
Cottage cheese, creamed	½ cup	24
Cream, half and half	¼ cup	26
Ice cream, regular, approximately 10% fat	½ cup	27
Cheese, cheddar	1 oz	28
Milk, whole	1 cup	34
Butter	1 tbs	35
Oysters, salmon	3 oz, cooked	40
Clams, halibut, tuna	3 oz, cooked	55
Chicken, turkey (light meat)	3 oz, cooked	67
Beef, pork, lobster, chicken, turkey (dark meat)	3 oz, cooked	75
Lamb, veal, crab	3 oz, cooked	85
Shrimp	3 oz, cooked	130
Heart, beef	3 oz, cooked	230
Egg	1 yolk or 1 egg	250
Liver: beef, calf, hog, lamb	3 oz, cooked	370
Kidney	3 oz, cooked	680
Brains	3 oz, raw	more than 1700

Source: R. M. Feeley, P. E. Criner, and B. K. Watt, "Cholesterol Content of Foods," *Journal of the American Dietary Association*, 61 (1972), p. 134. Reprinted in U.S. Department of Agriculture, *Fats in Food and Diet*, Agriculture Information Bulletin No. 361 (August 1976).

Overweight

According to the American Heart Association, middle-aged men who are more than 20 percent overweight are two or three times more likely to have a fatal heart attack than men of normal weight. It has also been shown that overweight adolescents have higher blood pressure than those whose weight is normal. Excess weight strains the heart and circulatory system. It can also lead to the deposit of fat in the arteries, which can cause atherosclerosis. For most Americans, weight gain begins around the age of 25, when there is a sudden drop in physical activity without a decrease in caloric intake. A sedentary job, lack of exercise, and three full meals a day can be a very harmful combination.

Lack of Exercise

Scientists have found that regular exercise helps to keep the heart healthy. People who lead sedentary lives run a higher risk of heart attack than those who remain active. And those active people who do have heart attacks appear to have a three times higher rate of survival than more sedentary individuals

A study in England revealed that bus conductors, who are constantly on the move, have a lower heart attack rate than bus drivers, who sit behind the wheel all day. The conductors are also more likely to survive heart attacks. Similar comparisons of active and nonactive theater ushers in America yielded the same results.

Risk Factors in Heart Disease

	SCORE
1. Age	
Age 56 or over	1 ____
Age 55 or under	0 ____
2. Sex	
Male	1 ____
Female	0 ____
3. Family History	
If you have:	
Blood relatives who have had a heart attack or stroke before age 60	12 ____
Blood relatives with a known history of heart disease at or before age 60 but no heart attacks or stroke	10 ____
Blood relatives who have had a heart attack or stroke after age 60	6 ____
No blood relatives who have had a heart attack or stroke	0 ____
4. Personal	
50 or under: If you have had a heart attack, a stroke, or heart or blood vessel surgery	20 ____
51 or over: If you have had any of the above	10 ____
None of the above	0 ____
5. Diabetes	
Diabetes before age 40 and now on insulin	10 ____
Diabetes at or after age 40 and now on insulin or pills	5 ____
Diabetes controlled by diet, or diabetes after age 55	3 ____
No diabetes	0 ____
6. Smoking	
Two packs per day	10 ____
Between one and two packs per day or quit smoking less than a year ago	6 ____
If you smoke 6 or more cigars a day or inhale a pipe regularly	6 ____
Less than one pack per day or quit smoking more than one year ago	3 ____
Never smoked	0 ____
7. Cholesterol (If cholesterol count is not known, answer 8)	
Cholesterol level – 276 or above	10 ____
Cholesterol level – between 225 and 275	5 ____
Cholesterol level – 224 or below	0 ____
8. Diet (If you have answered 7, do not answer 8)	
Does your normal eating pattern include:	
One serving of red meat daily, more than seven eggs a week, and daily consumption of butter, whole milk, and cheese	8 ____
Red meat 4–6 times a week, 4–7 eggs a week, margarine, low fat dairy products, and some cheese	4 ____
Poultry, fish, little or no red meat, three or less eggs a week, some margarine, skim milk, and skim milk products	0 ____

	SCORE
9. High Blood Pressure	
If either number is:	
160 over 100 (160/100) or higher 10	_____
140 over 90 (140/90) but less than 160 over 100 (160/100). 5	_____
If both numbers are less than 140 over 90 (140/90) 0	_____
10. Weight	
Ideal Weight Formula:	
Men = 110 lbs. plus 5 lbs. for each inch over 5 feet	
Women = 100 lbs. plus 5 lbs. for each inch over 5 feet	
25 pounds overweight 4	_____
10 to 24 pounds overweight 2	_____
Less than 10 pounds overweight 0	_____
11. Exercise	
Do you engage in any aerobic exercise (brisk walking, jogging, bicycling, racquetball, swimming) for more than 30 minutes:	
Less than once a week 4	_____
1 to 2 times a week 2	_____
3 or more times a week 0	_____
12. Stress	
Are you:	
Frustrated when waiting in line, often in a hurry to complete work or keep appointments, easily angered, irritable 4	_____
Impatient when waiting, occasionally hurried, or occasionally moody 2	_____
Comfortable when waiting, seldom rushed, and easy going 0	_____
TOTAL POINTS	_____

Score Results

Tabulate your points. Compare them with the charts below.

Please note! A high score does not mean you will develop heart disease. It is merely a guide to make you aware of a potential risk. Since no two people are alike, an exact prediction is impossible without further individualized testing.

With Answer to Question 9		Without Answer to Question 9	
High Risk	40 and above	High Risk	36 and above
Medium Risk	20–39	Medium Risk	19–35
Low Risk	19 and below	Low Risk	18 and below

Source: Arizona Heart Institute Foundation, P.O. Box 10,000, Phoenix, AZ 85064, (602) 955-1000, Edward B. Diethrich, M.D., Medical Director.

Cardiovascular Disease: Where to Go for Help

American Heart Association 7320 Greenville Avenue Dallas, Tex. 75231 (214) 750-5300	National Stroke Association 1565 Clarkson Street Denver, Colo. 80218 (303) 839-1992

Exercise aids the circulation of blood in the veins (where blood pressure is lower than in the arteries) and the flow of lymph in the lymph vessels. Exercise also benefits the heart itself. The heart becomes stronger, and the new and enlarged blood vessels that develop to feed the strengthening heart muscle lower the risk of heart attack. Another benefit of exercise is that it helps prevent overweight. Finally, exercise reduces cholesterol levels in the blood.

Anyone who has led a sedentary life and who is considering taking up an exercise program should first have a physical examination (see page 92). For those over the age of 40 such a checkup should include an exercise electrocardiogram, as pictured on page 363.

Cigarette Smoking

In addition to high-fat diets and high blood pressure, cigarette smoking has been singled out as a major risk factor leading to premature coronary deaths. Risk of a fatal coronary disease is two times greater for cigarette smokers than for nonsmokers, and three times as great for heavy smokers. Eighty-five percent of those with hardening of the arteries smoke.

Increased pulse rate and constricted blood vessels result from smoking. Scientists are not certain whether nicotine, carbon monoxide, or something else in cigarettes is responsible for these effects. But they are certain that quitting smoking cuts the incidence of heart attacks by one-third to half the rate found among smokers, and reduces the risk of a fatal heart attack to almost the same level as that for people who have never smoked.

Diabetes Mellitus

Diabetes mellitus is a disease in which the body's ability to metabolize sugar and carbohydrates is impaired because of inadequate secretion of the hormone **insulin.** Since untreated diabetes alters cholesterol and fat metabolism, it greatly increases the chances of a heart attack, even more so when in combination with hypertension. How this occurs is still not understood, and therefore ways of controlling this risk factor are few. Diabetes can be controlled, however, with regular checkups and prompt treatment. Today a diabetic who regularly consults a physician, is careful about diet, exercises, and takes maintenance doses of insulin (if necessary) should enjoy a normal life expectancy.

Stress and Personality Factors

Recent studies have associated certain personality traits and environmental influences with coronary heart disease and hypertension. Factors affecting those diseases include behavior, emotional response, personality, nationality, social status, urbanization, geography, race, and sex (see Chapter 2).

Two types of personality have been identified as behavior models in this area. **Type A** is a person who is characterized as aggressive, competitive, restless, impatient, and mistrustful—and two to three times as prone to heart disease as a **Type B** person, who is more relaxed and unhurried, and who is able to deal with problems and changing life situations in a calmer and more accepting manner. It appears that the stresses of urban life aggravate the tendency to heart disease.

Of course, treating heart disease is not nearly as effective as preventing it. There are still some hazards associated with heart surgery, and the drugs used to treat heart disease often have harmful side effects. Nearly 200,000 Americans a year undergo coronary bypass surgery, in which a vein from the leg replaces a blocked coronary artery. But there is little evidence that most of those who have the surgery live longer than those who do not, although the operation does relieve chest pain. Furthermore, intensive heart care frequently involves enormous financial costs. Finally, not everyone can be treated in time. Of the 550,000 people who die of heart attacks in the United States each year, 350,000 die before they even reach a hospital. Proper diet, exercise, and avoidance of cigarettes will not guarantee freedom from heart disease, but they are still the best prescription available.

CANCER

The National Cancer Institute (NCI) estimated a total of 930,000 new cases of cancer, excluding nonmelanoma skin cancer, in 1986, the greatest annual number yet recorded. Cancer has long been the second leading cause of death in the United States.

About 30 percent of all Americans will be stricken with cancer; three out of four families are affected. Only four out of ten people who have contracted cancer are expected to survive longer than five years after treatment has begun (see Figure 14-4). In 1986, according to NCI estimates, about 164,000 Americans who died of cancer might have been saved by earlier detection and treatment. Over 5 million Americans who have a history of cancer are alive today. Of these, 3 million were diagnosed over five years ago. Most of these 3 million are considered "cured." By "cured," the NCI means the person is free of the disease and currently has the same life expectancy as a person who never had cancer.

As we did with cardiovascular diseases, we will now examine the nature of cancer, its treatment, and how people can protect themselves against cancer.

What Is Cancer?

In simplest terms, **cancer** is a disease of the cells characterized by a change in basic cell behavior and structure and by the unrestricted growth and spread of the diseased cells. Since every living thing is made up of cells, cancer can affect plants and animals as well as human beings. And the discovery by paleontologists of cancerous cell formations in the bones of prehistoric dinosaurs points to the existence of the disease long before human beings ever appeared.

Much has been learned about cell structure through the use of sophisticated instruments such as the electron microscope, which can magnify objects to over 100,000 times their original size. With the aid of such instruments, differences between normal and cancerous cells have been observed in great detail.

The Cancerous Cell

Cancer Cell Structure. Cells in the very early stages of cancer are usually similar in appearance to cells of normal tissue. As cancer progresses, however, cell changes become more apparent. The extent of cell change in an abnormal cell varies according to the type of cancer involved: Highly malignant tissue may appear so different from normal tissue that it is difficult to tell where a cell from such tissue originated.

One striking characteristic of a cancer cell is chromosome abnormality. Instead of containing the normal forty-six chromosomes, a human cancer cell may contain double that number, or even several hundred chromosomes.

Of every seventeen people, five will have cancer

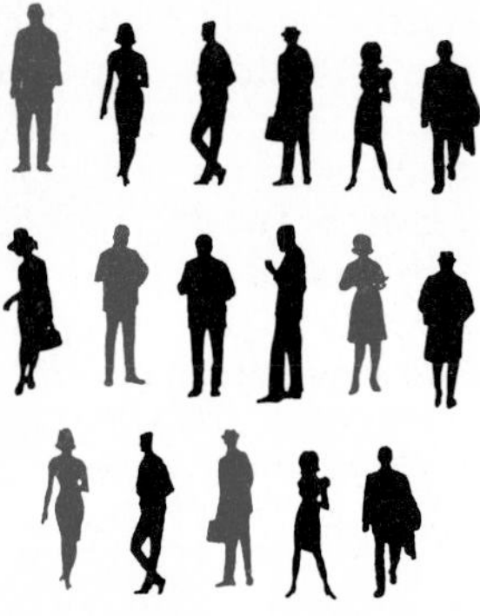

Two will be saved by treatment

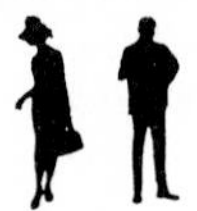

One will die who could have been saved by an earlier diagnosis

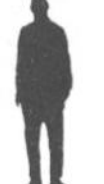

Two will die of types of cancer that future research must control

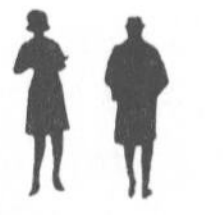

FIGURE 14-4

Cancer Survival Rates

Cancer Cell Division. In the cancer cell the mechanism that regulates cell growth, development, and differentiation breaks down. Cell growth is unregulated: Cells continue to divide even though they are not needed by the body. In most types of cancer this uncontrolled division of cells results in a mass or lump of excess tissue, known as a **tumor.** Not all tumors, however, are cancerous, or **malignant**; noncancerous tumors are said to be **benign.** Benign tumors are localized; they do not spread in the same way that malignant tumors do, and they rarely develop into malignancies. Warts and birthmarks are common benign tumors. Researchers believe that cancer cells develop gradually over a period of time. There is much evidence to indicate that a cancer that might eventually prove fatal can originate in a single malignant cell.

Cancer Cell Movement. Cancer cells multiply at an abnormally high rate and possess the ability to spread to other parts of the body and invade healthy tissue. Cancer cells can travel all over the body, regardless of the tissue of their origin. Furthermore, the mechanism that tells the cell when to cease moving is faulty in a cancerous cell. When a cancer cell encounters other cells, contact inhibition is absent. Instead of attaching itself to a group of cells, the malignant cell invades and eventually overruns neighboring cell masses. Such growth is called **invasion.**

Cancer cells can easily become dislodged from one another and spread through the bloodstream or lymph system to other parts of the body. This spreading process is known as **metastasis,** and the new colonies are called **metastases.**

A third pattern of cancer cell behavior is manifested in cancer involving the body cavities. Malignant tissues may spread by a process called **implantation,** or **diffusion,** in which poorly adhering cancer cells slough off of a tumor and lodge in nearby organs, where new cancerous growths develop.

The two characteristics of cancer cells—their rapid division and their ability to spread throughout the body—account for the high fatality rate of cancer. The multiplying cancer cells demand the nutrients and the space that would otherwise go to normal cells. Normal tissue is starved and squeezed out. Furthermore, the presence of cancer cells throughout the body interferes in some way with the body's blood-producing organs. Red and white blood cells and platelets are produced in insufficient quantities, leading to severe anemia, repeated infection, and internal bleeding.

TYPES OF CANCER

Cancer is actually a name for many diseases, all characterized by abnormal cell growth. Cancers that affect the **epithelial** cells, or skin cells and cells lining many body organs, are known as **carcinomas.** (An epithelial cancer that has not yet penetrated to deeper tissue is known as a **carcinoma in situ.**) Cancers that involve connective tissue such as the bones, muscles, and cartilage are called **sarcomas.** Both carcinomas and sarcomas are classified as **solid tumor cancers,** since they are characterized by the formation of a primary growth that generally spreads by metastasis. Cancers that affect the blood-forming organs are called **leukemias.** Leukemias, along with **lymphomas,** or cancers of the infection-fighting organs, are classified as **generalized cancers,** since they either begin as a widespread condition or diffuse so rapidly throughout the body that they become generalized very soon after their onset. (See Figure 14-5.)

Carcinomas

Cancer of the Skin. **Skin cancer** is the most common form of cancer and, fortunately, the most responsive to treatment. (A tumor of the melanin, or pigment-carrying skin cells, is called a **melanoma** and is a much more serious illness.) Skin cancer develops as a growth or sore on the epidermis, usually on the face or neck. In its early phase the sore has a tendency to bleed easily and is likely to ulcerate, forming a hard crust or scab. If diagnosed at this stage, skin cancer can usually be cured. If the disease remains untreated, it will eventually spread along the surface of the skin and grow inward to form a tumor. Surrounding bone and cartilage may become affected; and the cancer

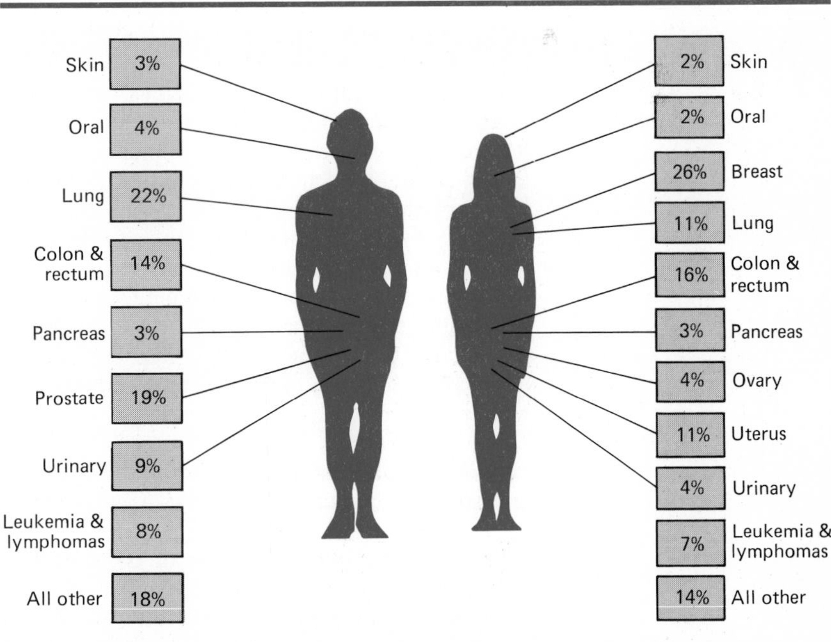

FIGURE 14-5

Cancer incidence by site and sex (excluding superficial skin cancer and carcinoma in situ)

Source: Courtesy: American Cancer Society, *Cancer Facts and Figures*, *1986*.

is likely to metastasize, by way of the local lymph nodes, to other parts of the body. About 95 percent of all cases of skin cancer can be cured completely if sores that do not heal promptly or changes in moles or skin blemishes are brought to the attention of a physician.

A correlation between the incidence of skin cancer and the amount of exposure to sunlight indicates that ultraviolet radiation from the sun may contribute to the development of the disease. Skin cancer occurs with greater frequency in the South than in the North, where solar radiation is less intense. It also tends to affect those whose occupations keep them out of doors a great deal, such as farmers or sailors. People with light skin pigmentation are more prone to skin cancer than darker-skinned individuals because of the greater sensitivity of light skin to sunlight. Other environmental factors can also contribute to the development of skin cancer. Investigations into chemical causes of cancer have uncovered a high incidence of skin cancer among those whose occupations involve contact with X rays, radium, coal, arsenic, creosote, lignite, and petroleum by-products.

Breast Cancer. Carcinoma of the breast accounts for the largest number of cancer cases and the second-largest number of cancer deaths among women. **Breast cancer** usually begins with a small, painless lump in the top outer area of the breast tissue. When the lump or tumor is close to the surface, it is likely to be accompanied by a conspicuous dimpling of the skin in the affected area. When the tumor is more deeply imbedded, there may be a feeling of soreness when the area is pressed, signs of retraction of the nipple, or an abnormal discharge from the nipple. There may also be a conspicuous change in the shape or size of the affected breast.

In 1986 there were an estimated 123,000 new cases of breast cancer and over 40,000 deaths resulted. Although breast cancer occurs in some women in their 20s and early 30s, it usually develops after the age of 35 and is the leading cause of death among women between the ages of 40 and 44. The fact that the incidence of the disease is higher among childless women has led researchers to believe that hormonal factors play a crucial role in its development.

Most abnormalities of the breast that are detected are not malignant: Up to 80 percent prove to be benign tumors. Even when a cancerous condition exists, the five-year survival rate (widely recognized as indicating cure) is 91 percent for patients who are treated early, before the disease spreads to the lymph system. Since early symptoms can be detected by self-examination and women who receive prompt treatment have a high rate of survival, fatalities can be significantly reduced if women practice the simple technique of self-examination and learn to recognize the first signs of breast cancer. (See the section Self-Examination for Breast Cancer on page 390.)

Cancer of the Uterus. Cancer of the uterus is the seventh largest cause of cancer death in women. It occurs primarily among women 40 to 49 years old. There is some evidence that the disease may be viral in origin. The first symptoms of **uterine cancer** are irregular bleeding and unusual discharge. Cancer of the uterus usually begins as a small growth near the opening of the cervix

Testicular Cancer

Testicular cancer occurs most often between the ages of 15 and 34, and is one of the most common cancers seen in young men. Most testicular cancers arise in the sperm-producing cells. The cause is unknown, but the cancers occur more frequently in young men with a history of undescended or late-descended testes. Early signs include a swelling or lump in the testicle, and sometimes pain or discomfort. All young men should learn testicular self-examination (see below) and practice it each month or so. Any suspicious swelling or hard lump should be checked by a doctor.

Treatment of testicular cancer depends upon the stage of the disease. In all cases, the diseased testicle is removed surgically; if the cancer has spread to other organs, as is often the case, additional surgery, radiation, or chemotherapy may be indicated. When treated in its early, localized stage, nearly 100 percent of all patients can expect to be cured. Even when the disease has spread, effective surgery, radiation, or chemotherapy can result in survival rates of 85 percent. Testicular cancer is, indeed, one of the "success stories" in the development of adjunctive cancer treatment principles.

TESTICULAR SELF-EXAMINATION Support the testicles with your left hand and feel each with your right. You will be able to feel the tubular structure (epididymis) which covers the top, back, and bottom of each testicle. (See Figure 7-1 on page 157.) This structure is smooth to the touch. You will be able to gently separate it from the testicle with your finger and examine the testicle itself. If a hard mass is found in either testicle, a doctor should be seen promptly.

Source: The Columbia University College of Physicians and Surgeons *Complete Home Medical Guide* (New York: Crown Publishers, Inc., 1985), p. 416. Reprinted by permission.

(the neck of the uterus), and is known as **cervical cancer.** If left untreated, the growth eventually spreads deeper into the wall of the cervix, farther into the uterus, and into the upper part of the vagina. A second form, **endometrial cancer,** affects the lining of the uterus and is less frequently encountered. Ultimately, uterine cancer can affect the entire pelvic area, spreading to the bladder or rectum as well. Early detection of cancer of the uterus is possible by means of pelvic examinations.

About 50,000 new cases of uterine cancer are reported annually. Though the present death rate is high—almost 10,000 per year—it has actually decreased by more than 70 percent during the last forty years. The death rate could be even further reduced if all women had pelvic examinations at regular intervals. The **Pap smear** is particularly effective in identifying cancers originating in the cervix.

Cancer of the Prostate. Another type of carcinomatous cancer is cancer of the prostate gland. The prostate surrounds the origin of the male urethra at its junction with the urinary bladder. **Prostatic cancer** is the second most common cancer in males. Cancer of the prostate gland first manifests itself through difficulty in urination. A man in the middle stage of the disease may notice blood in the urine and will often feel an urgent need to urinate when, in fact, there is no physiological reason to do so. In the later stages of the disease he will experience considerable pain during urination. If prostate cancer is not treated, it will metastasize through surrounding veins and lymphatic vessels to nearby organs.

Acid phosphatase, an enzyme in the bloodstream, has long been an early warning sign of prostate cancer. There is increased likelihood of cancer of the prostate after the age of 60.

Cancer of the Colon and Rectum. **Colon** and **rectal cancer** ranks second to lung cancer in incidence (excluding common skin cancers). The warning signals symptomatic of colon and rectum cancer should be brought to the immediate attention of a physician. They include: (1) any change in bowel habits that persists over a period of time; (2) any bleeding at the anus or blood present in the stool; and (3) loss of appetite, accompanied by nausea and vomiting. A special examination of the rectum and colon can reveal cancers while they still respond to therapy. During the examination the physician directly inspects the walls of the rectum and lower colon with the aid of a lighted tube called a proctoscope. More than 140,000 new cases of the disease are discovered annually, and over 60,000 Americans die from it each year. While colon and rectal cancer occurs slightly more often in women, the incidence rises sharply in both sexes after age 40. At present, 52 percent of those who get the disease survive longer than five years, but with early detection, 95 percent could do so.

The incidence of colon and rectal cancer has been found to be associated with diets high in fat and low in fiber. (See box in Chapter 5: Dietary Fiber.) One theory explaining the correlation is that fat is broken down by intestinal bacteria into carcinogenic substances that, in the absence of fiber, tend to remain for a longer time in the colon. Fiber, on the other hand, is believed to swell the bulk of the stool, thereby diluting the concentration of carcinogens; equally important, it stimulates bowel action and thus moves the stool out of the colon more rapidly.

Nutrition experts therefore recommend eliminating as much fat as possible from the diet and including foods high in fiber such as whole grains, fruits, and vegetables—especially peas and beans. Furthermore, most physicians recommend that everyone over age 40 have a digital rectal examination every year; and that everyone over 50 have in addition an annual test to detect blood in the stool and a proctoscopic exam every three to five years.

Stomach Cancer. In the United States the incidence of another cancer of the digestive tract, **stomach cancer,** has steadily decreased in both sexes over the past two decades. Although this decrease is so far without explanation, researchers have found a correlation between stomach cancer and a high intake of smoked, fermented, and starchy foods and a below-normal consumption of fresh vegetables and fruits.

As in cancer of the colon and rectum, the first symptoms of stomach cancer may appear similar to those of indigestion. The victim suffers from a lack of appetite, sometimes loses a taste for meat or rich foods, and experiences chronic stomach discomfort. The feces may also appear darker than usual. In later stages the symptoms of anemia, weight loss, and stomach pain may appear. One of the principal problems with early detection of stomach cancer is that its symptoms are not particularly alarming. Most patients consult a physician only after their condition has persisted many months—usually too late for cure.

If the malignancy is not treated in time, it will spread outside the stomach into the lymphatic system and go on to grow within the abdominal walls and other organs.

Lung Cancer. Without a doubt, **lung cancer** is one of the major health problems in the United States today. It is now the primary cancer killer among both men and women. Cancer of the lungs usually affects the lining of the

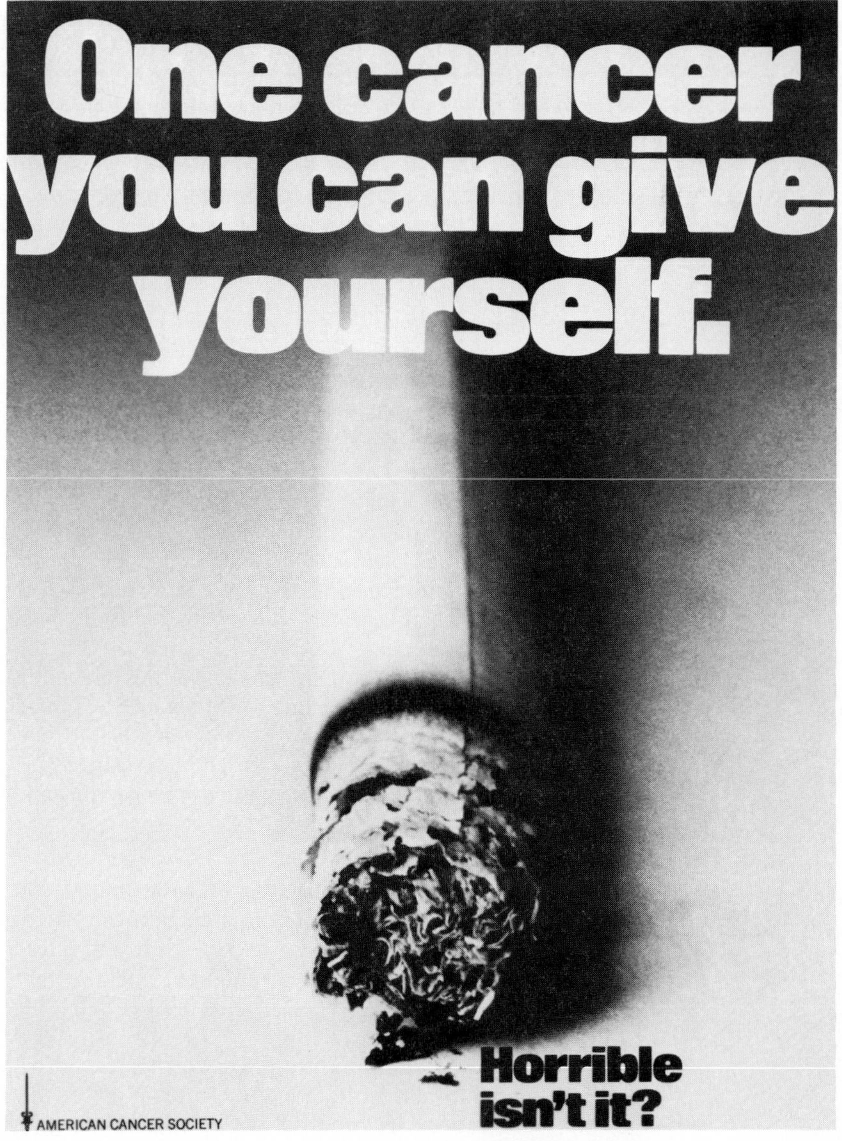
One cancer
you can give
yourself.
Horrible
isn't it?
AMERICAN CANCER SOCIETY

bronchi (the two major branches of the windpipe), which lead to the lungs. Symptoms of lung cancer are: (1) nagging and persistent cough; (2) hoarseness; (3) coughing up of blood; and (4) generalized chest pains. In 1986 approximately 130,000 Americans died from lung cancer, and the disease is still on the increase. Although more than twice as many men as women die from lung cancer, the incidence of the disease has increased sharply among women over the past decades. Since cancer of the lungs is difficult to diagnose before it has passed the stage at which it can be cured, only about 13 percent of its victims are saved.

The most effective preventive measure against lung cancer requires changing one of the most widespread habits of Americans—smoking. Several chemicals in tobacco smoke are known to be carcinogens. In fact, 83 percent of all cases of lung cancer occur among smokers. The sharp rise in the lung cancer rate among women has been attributed to their increased cigarette smoking in the decades that followed World War II. (The nature of tobacco and its effects on the lungs and other parts of the body are discussed in detail in Chapter 12.) Effective control must be exercised over other harmful agents as well, such as air pollutants, asbestos particles, coal-tar fumes, and radioactive ores, all of which contribute to the development of cancer of the lung.

Sarcomas

The second type of solid tumor cancer is known as a *sarcoma*. Sarcomatous cancers affect nonepithelial tissue—bones, muscles, and cartilage.

Bone Cancer. Symptoms of **Ewing's tumor,** a type of **bone cancer** that affects some male children, are pain in the bones (resembling rheumatism), fever, and a gradually developing tumorous structure. **Multiple myeloma,** which occurs primarily in men over 40 years of age, develops within the bone marrow. Bone cancer almost invariably proves fatal, although treatment can slow its progress for a time. Eventually, however, it spreads to the lungs or to other bones and body organs.

Though many bone cancer victims are under 15 years of age, adults are also affected. The occurrence of bone cancer in adults may be related to environmental factors. Individuals who have been frequently exposed to X rays show a comparatively higher rate of bone cancer. Likewise, a higher rate is found among people whose occupations involve the handling of beryllium, a radioactive substance.

Leukemia. Leukemia is considered one of the most tragic cancers because many of its victims are children between the ages of 3 and 14, and because it usually results in death. However, leukemia actually affects almost twelve times as many adults as children, and the rate at which it strikes adults is increasing. Some types of leukemia are fatal, but others can now be cured by chemotherapy.

Briefly, **leukemia** is a disease characterized by aberrations in the production of white blood cells, which eventually lower the number of red blood cells in circulation. Symptoms of both acute and chronic leukemia are anemia, bleeding from the mucous membranes, and weakness. *Acute leukemia* has become increasingly prevalent as a childhood disease; it accounts for 50 percent of cancer mortality among children. Important research advances have lengthened the expected life span of victims of acute childhood leukemias. The disease used to be fatal within a few months; but with chemotherapy some forms are now 65 to 75 percent curable. *Chronic leukemia*, which often strikes adults over the age of 25, is less virulent than acute leukemia, and the expected life span of its victims is generally longer.

A very high incidence of leukemia among X-ray technicians and survivors of the atomic bomb blasts in Japan has led to the conjecture that radiation may be causally related to the disease. There is also a close relationship between the presence of certain viruses and the onset of leukemia in animals. In addition, benzol, a chemical by-product of coal-tar distillation, has been implicated as a possible cause of leukemia.

FIGURE 14-6

Five-year cancer survival rates.

Sources: National Cancer Institute and American Cancer Society

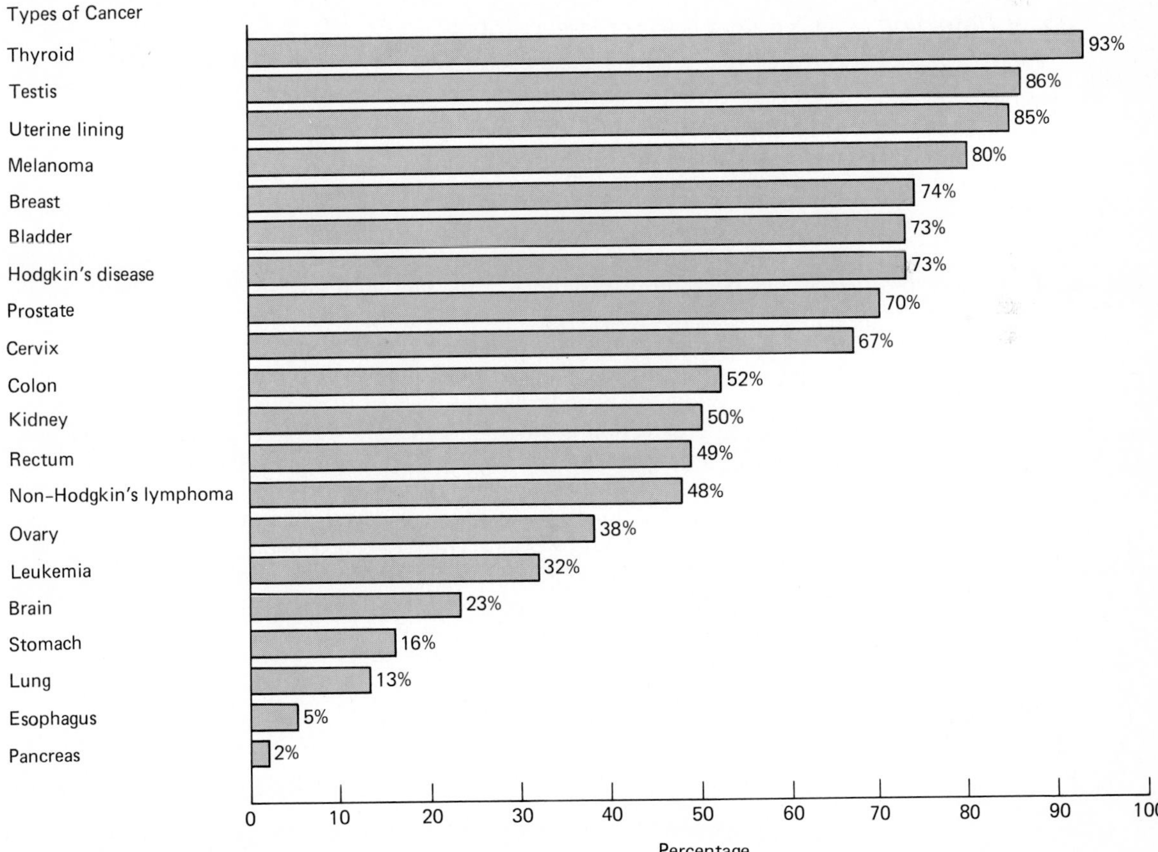

Lymphomas

Some evidence indicates that certain types of lymphomas may be associated with the presence of viruses in the cells. Lymphomas include such diseases as Hodgkin's disease and lymphosarcoma. Warnings of the presence of lymphatic cancer include: (1) enlargement of the lymph nodes; (2) sore throat and difficulty in swallowing; and (3) pain in the back, legs, or abdomen.

Malignant lymphomas have a slightly higher incidence in males than in females, and they are generally confined to persons between the ages of 20 and 40.

Though some patients with lymphosarcomas live five years or longer, most die within one or two years. For patients with Hodgkin's disease, the five-year survival rate is about 73 percent. Some patients with this desease have lived twenty-five years or even longer.

PROTECTION AGAINST CANCER

Early detection and treatment of cancer, as the American Cancer Society has been informing the public for years, can result in a greater rate of survival. There are seven warning signals that everyone should be aware of:

Cancer Detection

- Change in bowel or bladder habits
- A sore that does not heal
- Unusual bleeding or discharge
- Thickening or lump in the breast or elsewhere
- Indigestion or difficulty in swallowing
- Obvious change in a wart or mole
- Nagging cough or hoarseness

It would be a mistake, however, to wait until any of these warning signals appears. Since many forms of cancer do not exhibit noticeable symptoms until they are near the stage where cure is no longer possible, examination of specific cancer sites—the breasts, rectum, lungs, oral cavity, uterus, prostate, and skin—should be conducted periodically.

While early detection is a desired and standard factor in cancer protection, attitudes regarding certain cancer-screening techniques have begun to change. The frequency of Pap tests for cervical cancer is now open to question. Not all women may require Pap tests annually. And **mammography,** a technique for the detection of breast cancer that depends upon the use of radiation, should be performed as seldom as possible. A current alternative to mammography, now recommended as a routine screening measure, is *Graphic Stress Telethermometry* (GST), a heat-measuring technique that meters the increased surface temperature associated with breast cancer.

Self-Examination for Breast Cancer

In addition to checking for general symptoms of cancer, there is a specific technique of self-examination for breast cancer (see Figure 14-7). The American Cancer Society recommends that women follow these three steps:

1. **In the shower:** Examine your breasts during bath or shower; hands glide easier over wet skin. Fingers flat, move gently over every part of each breast. Check for any lump or thickening.

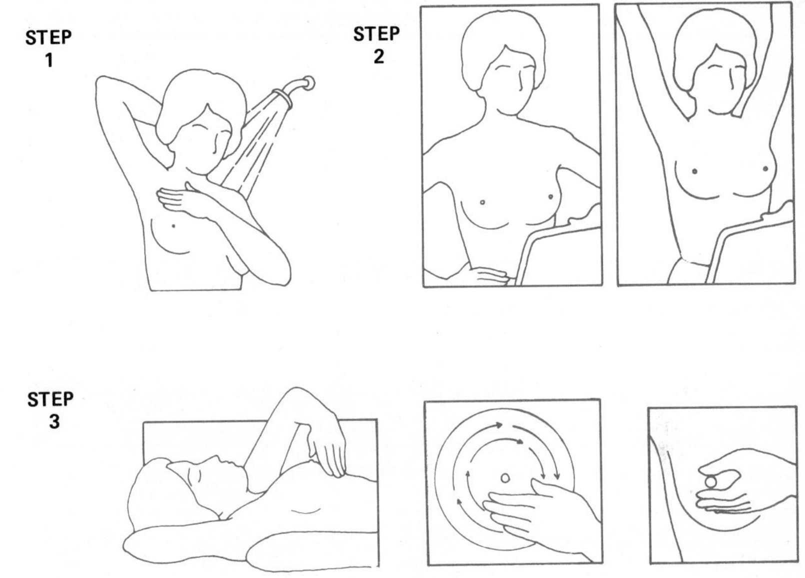

FIGURE 14–7

The three-step procedure for self-examination of the breasts.

Source: Courtesy: American Cancer Society.

2. **Before a mirror:** Inspect your breasts with arms at your sides. Next, raise your arms high overhead. Look for any changes in contour of each breast, a swelling, dimpling of skin, or changes in the nipple. Then rest palms on hips and press down firmly to flex your chest muscles. Left and right breast will probably not exactly match—few women's breasts do. But regular inspection shows what is normal for you and will give you confidence in your examination.
3. **Lying down:** To examine your right breast, put a pillow or folded towel under your right shoulder. Place right hand behind your head—this distributes breast tissue more evenly on the chest. With left hand, fingers flat, press gently in small circular motions around an imaginary clock face. Begin at outermost top of your right breast for 12 o'clock, then move to 1 o'clock, and so on around the circle back to 12. A ridge of firm tissue in the lower curve of each breast is normal. Then move in an inch, toward the nipple; keep circling to examine every part of your breast, including the nipple. (This requires at least three more circles.) Now slowly repeat the procedure on your left breast with a pillow under your left shoulder and left hand behind head. Notice how your breast structure feels. Finally, squeeze the nipple of each breast gently between thumb and index finger. Any discharge, clear or bloody, should be reported to your doctor immediately.

This procedure should be performed at the end of the menstrual cycle for best results. Lumps that are felt before menstruation may simply be small cysts or collections of fluid. More than 90 percent of breast cancers are discovered by women themselves through breast self-examination.

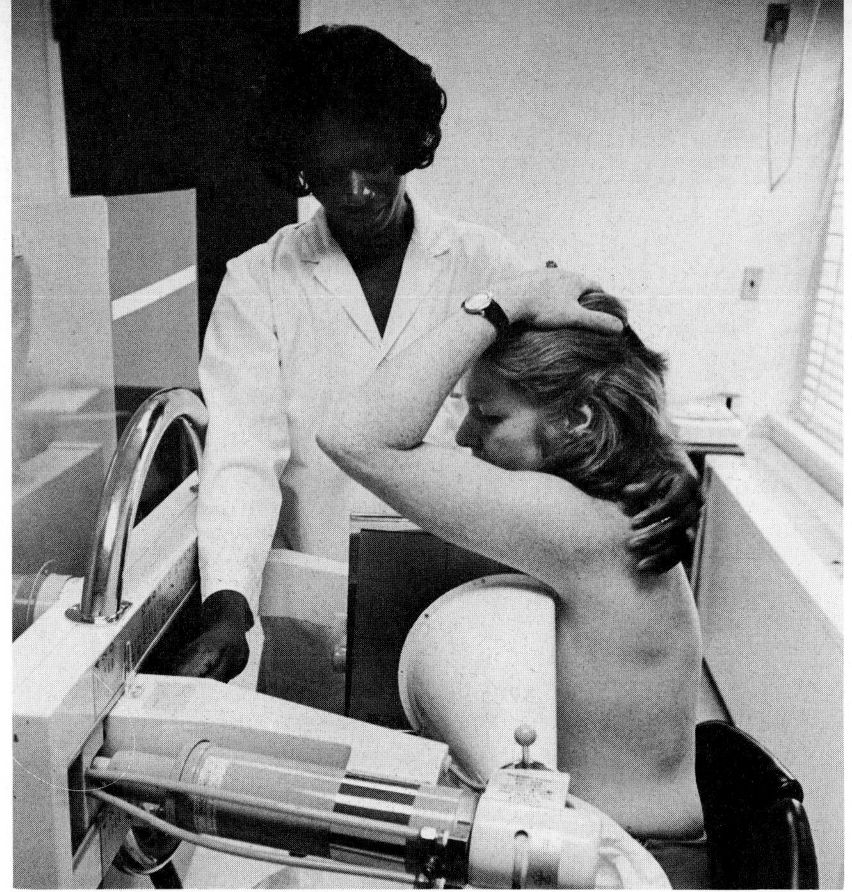

Cancer of the breast can be detected in the hospital by mammography, but most cases are discovered by self-examination in the home.

CANCER TREATMENT

Once detected, cancer can be treated in a variety of ways. Some procedures are successful in bringing about a cure. Others may achieve a temporary **remission** of the disease—that is, the symptoms of cancer may disappear for a time, only to return at a later date. Still other treatment procedures succeed only in slowing the progress of cancer and decreasing, to some degree, the suffering of the patient.

Surgery

The presence of a malignant tumor often necessitates surgery, both as a cure and as a preventive measure. Preventive surgery may involve the removal of hormone-producing glands that are associated with the growth of a cancer in addition to removal of the malignant tumor itself. Often large quantities of tissue surrounding a malignant growth are taken out as a precaution against the possibility that they, too, have become cancerous.

Radiation

One cancer treatment technique that is used in combination with surgery is **radiation therapy.** In fact, radiation is a highly effective form of treatment in its own right. There are several types of radiation treatment: bombardment with X rays, implantation or injection of **radioisotopes** (radioactive chemical elements that release destructive gamma rays and alpha and beta particles), use of laser beams, and cobalt treatment. Essentially, radiation is used to systematically destroy cancerous tissue.

Breast Cancer: Mastectomy vs. Lumpectomy

For almost a century the preferred treatment for breast cancer was *radical mastectomy*, a surgical procedure in which the breast, underlying chest muscles, and the lymph nodes in the armpit were removed. To many women the cure seemed worse than the disease, so they put off seeking treatment when they noticed suspicious lumps in the breast.

Over the last twenty years, however, cancer surgeons have been moving away from the disfiguring radical mastectomy procedure because survival figures have indicated that *total mastectomy*—in which only the breast is removed—is just as effective as radical mastectomy. And a recent three-year study by the National Cancer Institute suggests that the survival figures for *segmental mastectomy*, or *lumpectomy*—in which only the tumor itself and a small amount of surrounding tissue are removed—seem to be the same as for the two earlier procedures. Cancer specialists estimate that half the cases of breast cancer each year can be treated effectively by lumpectomy followed by a course of radiation. They warn, however, that the procedure can only be used when the tumor is less than one and a half inches in diameter. Moreover, not everyone in the medical profession is entirely convinced that lumpectomy results in a permanent cure; some physicians are waiting to see the five- and ten-year survival rates.

Drugs

Researchers have found that the rate at which cells divide greatly influences the effects of drugs upon them, for most drugs are active against cells in the process of division. **Drug-sensitive cancers** are those with many cells in the dividing state. Leukemia, for example, which has a high percentage of cells reproducing at a given time, is much more responsive to drug therapy, or **chemotherapy,** than lung cancer, in which cell division is slow.

At the present stage of development of chemotherapy, two important problems are being faced. First, there is the problem of **toxicity:** The long-term use of cancer drugs may harm healthy body tissue. Second, cancer cells within the body have a tendency to build up an immunity to the effects of cancer

Cancer: Where to Go for Help

Cancer Information Service Hotline
(800) 4-CANCER

American Cancer Society
National Headquarters
90 Park Avenue
New York, N.Y. 10016
(212) 599-8200

Cancer Counseling and Research Center
Suite 140
6060 North Central Expressway
Dallas, Tex. 75206
(214) 692-6311

Leukemia Society of America
800 Second Avenue
New York, N.Y. 10017
(212) 573-8484

National Cancer Institute
Cancer Information Clearinghouse
Office of Cancer Communications
Building 31, Room 10A18
9000 Rockville Pike
Bethesda, Md. 20205
(301) 496-4070

Marijuana and Cancer

Some cancer patients find the side effects of chemotherapy terribly wracking; in a few extreme cases, patients have become so nauseated that they vomit violently enough to risk cracking their ribs. Many of these patients have found that their nausea can be dramatically eased by the therapeutic use of marijuana or THC, a derivative of marijuana. Cancer specialists have urged the federal government to make the drug legally available to them.

drugs. This resistance to drugs results in their decreased effectiveness, which may lead to a recurrence or acceleration of the disease.

Cancer Quackery

An unfortunate consequence of the frustrating war against cancer is that the continued elusiveness of a cure has given rise over the years to much quackery. Medical quackery thrives on one ingredient: hope. As patients who are far advanced in their disease respond less and less to conventional therapies, they frequently turn toward more unorthodox treatment and seek out bizarre cures.

One such recent "cure," and certainly one of the most publicized, was laetrile, a substance made from crushed apricot pits. Thousands of cancer victims in the United States have taken the drug, even though the Food and Drug Administration has declared that it is useless against cancer. Laetrile contains 6 percent

Immunotherapy

Effective cancer treatments are not without drawbacks: Surgery can be mutilating, and chemotherapy and radiation often have toxic side effects. Cancer researchers today, however, are finding that in some cases it may be possible to use the body's own natural line of defense—the immune system—to attack and destroy malignancies. This new form of treatment, called *immunotherapy,* minimizes toxic side effects. Two substances, interferon and interleukin-2 (IL-2), among others, have captured the attention of the media in recent years.

Interferon is an antiviral protein that is produced by cells when they are invaded by a virus. Researchers hoped that interferon would be a potent anticancer tool. At first extremely rare and expensive to produce, interferon began to be made in quantity in 1981 by recombinant DNA techniques, and researchers have had a chance to use it against several kinds of cancer. Unfortunately, interferon therapy has been successful against only two rare forms of leukemia, and has caused some remission of Kaposi's sarcoma, a frequently AIDS-related form of cancer. It is possible that, when combined with other new cancer-fighting agents, interferon will still prove to be useful.

Interleukin-2, another natural substance produced by the body, helps regulate the immune system. When used in immunotherapy, IL-2 transforms the body's white blood cells into "killer cells" that destroy tumors. IL-2 therapy involves withdrawing white cells from the blood of a cancer patient and "incubating" them with IL-2 for three or four days. The newly transformed killer cells are then "infused" back into the patient, along with an extra dose of IL-2. The first trials were promising, but it is too early to say more than that. Since the treatment is extremely expensive, it can be offered to very few people. However, genetic engineering techniques should enable larger amounts of Il-2 to be made fairly soon.

Sources: Harold M. Schmeck, Jr., "Cautious Optimism Is Voiced About Test Cancer Therapy," *New York Times*, December 6, 1985, pp. A1, A22; Gerald V. Quinnan, Jr., "AIDS," in *1985 Medical and Health Annual* (Chicago: Encyclopaedia Britannica, 1984), p. 189; "Search for a Cure," *Newsweek*, December 16, 1985, pp. 60–66.

cyanide, enough to be fatal; and patients have often received doses of the drug contaminated by bacteria. There are three types of laetrile users:

1. Those who have never had cancer but who attribute their "recovery" from a benign tumor to the drug.
2. Those who experience temporary improvement after taking the drug because of the *placebo effect* (they expect to feel better and so actually do feel better). These people will ultimately die of cancer and would be better off taking a safer placebo.
3. Those who take laetrile in conjunction with some other therapy and are convinced that it was laetrile that brought about their cure.

PROBLEMS AND CONTROVERSIES: Carcinogens in the Environment

Millions of Americans believe that they are in danger of developing cancer because of their exposure over a lifetime to the synthetic chemicals that seem to saturate the environment, particularly the pesticides in food. It will come as a surprise to most to learn that in spite of the steady increase in industrial pollution over the last thirty to forty years, the U.S. cancer rate has more or less remained the same—with the single exception of smoking-induced lung cancer. It may come as an even bigger surprise to learn that nature contributes 10,000 times as many carcinogens to the environment as human beings do—a fact that poses problems for an anxious public and government policymakers.

Nature, for example, has created a great swath of danger in an area of the United States called the Reading Prong, a geological belt extending from eastern Pennsylvania into New Jersey and New York State that contains some of the world's highest levels of radioactive radon, a known carcinogen. Radioactive radon, a colorless, odorless gas, causes anywhere from 5,000 to 30,000 deaths a year. While a high incidence of lung cancer has been found among uranium miners and people living in houses built from contaminated material, it may be small in comparison to the number of cases caused by the radon that seeps up from the ground in the Reading Prong. But the problem of eliminating this source of radioactivity is immense.

If some problems of environmental carcinogens are insurmountable, others are absurdly exaggerated. For example, thousands of natural and synthetic chemicals in human food have been found to cause cancer when given in large quantities to laboratory animals. In minute traces, however, they do not cause cancer in human beings. The tannin in tea and red wine, for instance, and the aflatoxins found in molds that grow on peanuts and corn cause cancer in lab animals but pose little danger to human beings. Getting rid of all natural carcinogens in the environment would be both unnecessary and impossible. The FDA, accordingly, has set a reasonable limit on the quantity allowable in food. It has had to do the same with some synthetic chemicals like the pesticides used in agriculture to control insects and plant diseases. Eliminating the use of all pesticides because laboratory animals develop cancer after being given large amounts of them would leave the public vulnerable to a host of new diseases, drastically reduce the food supply, and send food prices soaring.

Finally, another group of environmental carcinogens—a group 10,000 times as large as the natural and synthetic chemicals just discussed—poses risks to health, but these can be controlled or eliminated by everybody. As we saw with colorectal cancer, for example, the fats in meat and dairy products may be broken down into carcinogenic substances in the intestines; these can be reduced by simple changes in the diet. Then there are the *mutagens*—substances that cause the DNA in body cells to change and perhaps turn malignant—and other chemicals that are created when food is burned. The skin of charcoal-broiled, fried, and barbecued meats, burned toast, and even caramelized sugar contain potentially carcinogenic mutagens, and we can easily control our consumption of them.

Protect Yourself Against Cancer

- *Don't use tobacco*. Quitting smoking is the best way to prevent lung cancer as well as several other serious diseases. Avoiding all forms of smokeless tobacco is the best way to prevent cancers of the mouth, throat, larynx, and esophagus.
- *Watch your diet*. Keep the number of high-fat foods to an absolute minimum; instead, increase the amount of foods rich in fiber and in vitamins A and C.
- *Don't oversun*. Sunbathe in small doses, especially if you have a fair complexion. If you have to be out in the sun a lot, cover up sensibly and use sunscreen lotions to help prevent skin cancer.
- *Don't abuse alcohol*. If you are a heavy drinker, you are at risk for cancers of the mouth, throat, larynx, esophagus, and liver; you increase this risk greatly if you also use tobacco.
- If you are a woman, *do a breast self-examination*. By examining your breasts every month, you will be able to spot any developing tumor in time for it to be treated successfully.
- *Have a colorectal examination*. If you are age 40 or over, have a digital rectal exam every year; if you are over 50, have a blood stool test every year in addition, and a full proctoscopic exam every three to five years.
- *Get a Pap test*. Have a Pap test every three years (after two initial negative tests) to protect yourself against cervical cancer.
- *Have an oral exam*. Your dentist or physician can easily recognize the early symptoms of mouth cancer. Schedule visits regularly.
- *Get a complete checkup*. A regular physical examination should include examinations for cancers of the thyroid, testes, prostate, mouth, ovaries, skin, and lymph nodes. Women between 20 and 40 should have a full pelvic exam every three years; women over 40 should have one every year. Men over 40 should have a prostate exam every year.

Source: *1986 Cancer Facts and Figures* (New York: American Cancer Society, Inc., 1986).

Many of the so-called miracle cures are ineffective, but that does not mean that they are harmless. In 1985, for instance, cancer victims who had gone to the Bahamas for "immuno-augmentative therapy" were found to have been given blood-derived drugs thought to be contaminated with AIDS virus. And the use of any unproven cancer therapy discourages the continuation of orthodox therapy that might afford relief, remission, or cure.

Only one thing is sure in the continuing war being waged against cancer: As long as a remedy for the disease continues to escape medical science, there will be a barrage of quack cures aimed at hopeful and uncritical cancer victims.

CANCER PREVENTION

Except for the sharp increase in lung cancer, the cancer rate in the United States has not changed very much over the last few decades, even with the addition of thousands of synthetic chemicals to the environment. And while it is beyond doubt that prolonged exposure to certain chemicals causes cancer, the number of cases arising from such exposure has not been large enough to affect the death rate. This is not to say that federal agencies and citizen groups should stop monitoring the 2,000 or more carcinogenic chemicals currently used by industry. Tolerance levels for only a few of these have been established, and many industrial workers continue to be in danger of developing cancer from their work environment. It is simply to say that the normal amount of exposure of most people to the great majority of synthetic chemicals in the environment has not seemed to result in a higher general incidence of cancer (see box: Carcinogens in the Environment).

Meanwhile, we all can do a number of things to protect ourselves against cancer (see box: Protect Yourself Against Cancer). The first and most obvious step we can take is to stop smoking—or chewing—tobacco. This step alone would eliminate 83 percent of all the lung cancer cases in the United States. The next most important step is to watch what we eat. Perhaps a third of all cancer deaths could be prevented by changes in the diet, especially by cutting down on the amount of animal fat and increasing the intake of fiber-rich foods. We should also avoid prolonged exposure to sunlight, for this has been implicated as the major cause of a variety of skin cancers. Watching our intake of alcohol is another important preventive step. Alcohol—particularly large quantities of it and especially when used in combination with tobacco—markedly increases the risk of mouth, larynx, throat, esophageal, and liver cancer.

Finally, early detection is the next best step. Pap tests, breast and testicular self-exams, and annual colorectal tests for people over 40 can detect cancer or a precursor condition early in its development when it is most curable.

SUMMARY

1. *Cardiovascular diseases* (diseases of the heart and blood vessels) and *cancer* are the leading causes of death in the United States today.

2. The circulatory system is composed of the *blood*, the *heart*, the *arteries*, *capillaries*, and *veins*. It transports food and oxygen to the body's cells and carries away the cells' waste products.

3. The heart pumps blood of reduced oxygen content to the lungs. There carbon dioxide is removed and oxygen diffuses into the blood. The blood then returns to the heart and is pumped throughout the body.

4. The contraction of the heart is called *systole*, and the relaxation of the heart is called *diastole*. *Blood pressure* refers to the pressure of blood against the inner walls of the arteries during systole and diastole. The level of blood pressure is one indication of a person's health. *Pulse rate*, or the arterial flow of blood, can be used as a measure of heart rate.

5. Blood is composed of *red blood cells*, which transport oxygen and carry away carbon dioxide; *white blood cells* or *leukocytes*, which fight infection; *plasma*, a clear liquid containing many chemical substances, including wastes; and *platelets*, fragments of larger cells that play an important role in blood clotting. A deficiency in red blood cells is called *anemia*.

6. Blood is classified into type *A*, *B*, *AB*, or *O*. A person with type AB is a universal recipient; an individual with type O is a universal donor.

7. The major types of cardiovascular disease are: *coronary heart disease* (an impairment of heart function caused by *thrombosis* or *occlusion* of a coronary artery); *stroke* (a condition in which part of the brain fails to receive a sufficient amount of blood); *arteriosclerosis* (hardening of the arteries); *atherosclerosis* (arteriosclerosis characterized by the deposit of *plaque* within the arteries); *hypertension* (high blood pressure); *rheumatic heart disease* (caused by rheumatic fever and resulting *endocarditis*, which impairs the functioning of the heart valves); and *congenital defects* (for example, holes in the walls and chambers of the heart). Two types of vascular disorders are *thrombosis* (formation of a blood clot within a blood vessel) and *embolism* (obstruction of a blood vessel by a blood clot that has detached itself from its point of origin and circulated in the bloodstream).

8. A high-cholesterol diet, lack of exercise, overweight, hypertension, diabetes mellitus, cigarette smoking, nervous tension, and a family history of heart disease appear to be the important risk factors for cardiovascular disease. To reduce the risk of heart attack people should engage in regular vigorous exer-

cise, reduce the amount of cholesterol in their diets, stop smoking, and have regular medical checkups.

9. Psychosocial factors, those concerned with personality and environment, affect one's adjustments to life. It has also been amply demonstrated that the stressful conditions of modern urban life aggravate tendencies toward heart disease.

10. *Cancer* is a disease of the cells characterized by a change in basic cell behavior and appearance and by the unrestricted growth and spread of the affected cells. A mass of cells whose division is unpredictable is known as a *tumor*. Tumors can either be *benign* (noncancerous) or *malignant* (cancerous).

11. Cancer cells differ in structure from normal cells, their cell division is unregulated, and they have the capacity to spread throughout the body. *Invasion* is the movement of cancer cells to adjacent tissue; *metastasis* is the spread of cancer cells through the bloodstream or lymph system; and *implantation* is a condition in which cancer cells slough off of a tumor and lodge in nearby organs.

12. There are many types of cancer. Those that affect the skin cells and the linings of organs are called *carcinomas*; those affecting bones, muscles, and cartilage are known as *sarcomas*. *Leukemias* are cancers of the blood-forming organs, and *lymphomas* are cancers of the infection-fighting organs.

13. The seven warning signals of cancer are: (1) Change in bowel or bladder habits; (2) A sore that does not heal; (3) Unusual bleeding or discharge; (4) Thickening or lump in the breast or elsewhere; (5) Indigestion or difficulty in swallowing; (6) Obvious change in a wart or mole; and (7) Nagging cough or hoarseness. Watching for these signs is by no means the only precaution that should be taken. Women should examine their breasts after each menstrual cycle, and everyone should have periodic cancer checkups. Until major advances in cancer therapy occur, early detection and treatment offer the best chance of survival to victims of cancer.

14. Cancer can be treated by *radiation therapy*, *surgery*, or *chemotherapy*. Each method has advantages and disadvantages, and no one method has proven to be effective for all types of cancer. *Immunotherapy*, which uses the body's own immune system to attack and destroy malignancies, is a more recent form of treatment that looks promising.

15. Carcinogens in the environment—both those naturally occurring and those introduced by human beings—are a serious problem and should continue to be monitored. But the most effective protective measures against cancer are those that are well within the control of the individual: stopping smoking, avoiding overexposure to the sun, watching what we eat and drink, performing self-examinations, and having regular medical checkups.

CONSUMER CONCERNS

1. Since the majority of Americans die from cancer or cardiovascular impairment, it would appear prudent to carry the type of health insurance that is adequate for such costly illnesses. What are some of the actual benefits of a policy of this type—namely, major medical insurance?
2. One of the expensive techniques that has been employed quite frequently with cardiac patients is heart bypass surgery. How successful have these operations been and how does the technique compare with other options?
3. As there are many possibilities and decisions in respect to heart disease and cancer, it is wise to seek advice from more than one source—to get a second opinion. Is a third opinion advisable at times?
4. Cancer patients often reach a stage in which all appears futile. At this point some people feel that it is appropriate to use any technique that has even the remote chance of effecting a cure. Do you agree?

15
Communicable Diseases

Pathogens
The Body's Immune System
Sexually Transmitted Diseases (STDs)
Other Common Communicable Diseases

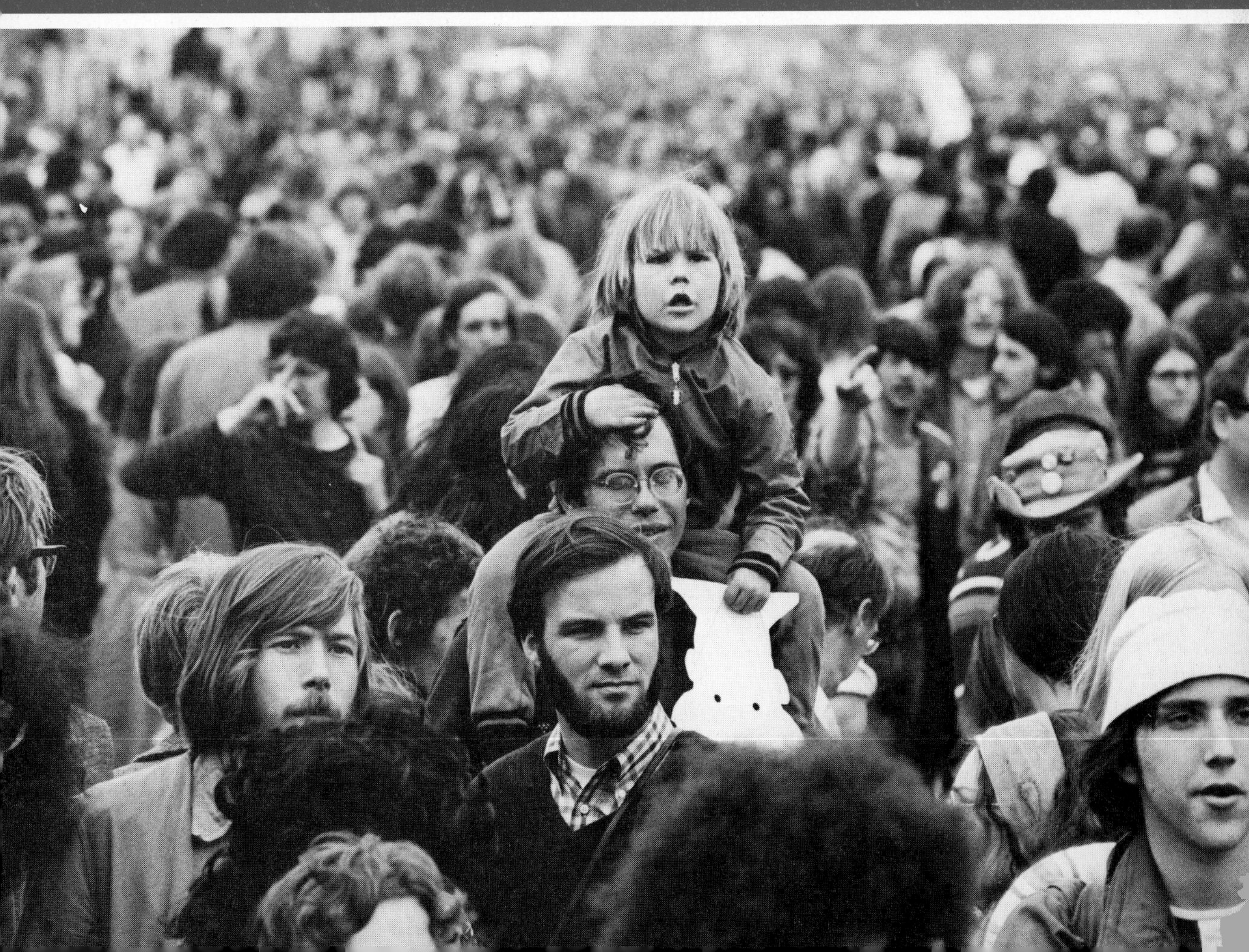

Few if any medical achievements in our history have brought greater human benefit than the ability to cope with the illnesses and death caused by disease-producing microorganisms. Since they can be transmitted from person to person, directly or indirectly, the illnesses these microorganisms produce are called **communicable diseases.**

Communicable diseases can spread among populations so swiftly and thoroughly that great numbers may quickly become stricken and die. There are many examples of such outbreaks, or **epidemics,** in our history. Between the years 1347 and 1351 the infamous bubonic plague claimed an estimated 75 million lives—a staggering figure that amounted to a third of the population of Europe at the time. Even in our own century an eight-month epidemic of influenza caused the deaths of some 10 million people just as World War I was coming to an end. This figure is twice the number who died as a direct result of hostilities during the entire course of the war.

Communicable diseases, however, are not confined to periodic outbreaks; they are an ever-present danger. Pneumonia and influenza were the leading causes of death in the United States at the turn of the century, accounting for 11.8 percent of the total. Though medical advances—notably the discovery of antibiotics and various vaccines—have reduced their frequency, pneumonia and influenza are still among the leading causes of death in this country. The same is true of other communicable diseases. Although the death rate for tuberculosis, for example, and for certain diseases of early infancy continues to decline, their potential risk to human health remains.

Many important steps have been taken to control disease-producing microorganisms. In some cases, we have been able to reduce or eliminate their presence from our food and water supplies. Other approaches have concentrated on the control of insect carriers, such as mosquitoes and ticks, and of disease-bearing animals. Important contributions have been made through isolation of the sick as well as successful methods of therapy with those who become ill. And of utmost significance have been the programs of immunization that enable us to resist infection despite exposure.

Immunization techniques have not been developed for some forms of communicable diseases, however, including the sexually transmitted diseases. Public health agencies attempt to keep the incidence of these diseases under control by providing information and by encouraging infected people to seek treatment immediately. Despite modern medical knowledge that makes syphilis and gonorrhea curable, the rate of new infections for both diseases is significantly higher than during the mid-1950s, when they were at their lowest point. In addition, there has been an upsurge of other less serious but still worrisome and potentially debilitating diseases such as herpes and chlamydial infections. And a new disease, most often sexually transmitted and to date inevitably fatal, is spreading rapidly in many parts of the world. This new infection has been given the name *acquired immune deficiency syndrome,* or *AIDS.* The fight against these diseases requires not only an arsenal of improved drugs and medical care, but also the support of an informed and enlightened public.

In this chapter we shall discuss those communicable diseases that represent the greatest threat to our well-being, the manner in which they are transmitted, and public or personal measures that can be taken to prevent them from occurring.

PATHOGENS

Communicable diseases are produced by some kind of microorganism that has invaded a living person. Such a microorganism is considered a **parasite,** since it lives within or upon another organism, known as the **host.** Many parasites are not dangerous to the host body. Some, however, are **pathogens,** or disease producers, which rob the host's tissues of nutrients and may also produce poisons. This invasion by pathogenic organisms produces the symptoms of an infectious disease.

There are six general types of disease-producing parasitic microorganisms: bacteria, viruses, rickettsias, protozoa, parasitic worms, and fungi. They differ in size, shape, and certain characteristic ways in which they function. Within each of the six general types there are an infinite number of specific examples. Each specific form of microorganism is capable of causing only one type of disease.

Some people are **carriers** of these pathogenic organisms—that is, they themselves are immune to the disease produced by the pathogen but can transmit it to other host bodies. A great many communicable diseases are transferred from one person to another, either by direct contact, by coming into contact with some secretion of the host carrier, or by some object they have touched. These directly or indirectly transmitted diseases are called the **contagious diseases.** Colds, measles, and the sexually transmitted diseases are examples.

Some communicable diseases are transferred from one host body to another via animal or insect **vectors** or by **vehicles** such as food and water. Diseases in this category such as infectious hepatitis and mononucleosis are called **infectious diseases.**

Bacteria

Bacteria are microorganisms that exist in vast numbers all around us. They live in small streams, lakes, large rivers, and the seas; they exist by the billions in every pound of garbage, in cesspools, and in any waste left to rot; they are present in the water vapor floating in the air over our cities; and they live in our mouths, ears, and nasal passages. Bacteria break down dead animal and plant matter into simpler compounds, which other plants and animals utilize to live and grow, and they are responsible for the fertility of the soil. If bacteria were eliminated, all life on earth would end.

A few forms of bacteria have the capacity to convert into spores, and can exist in a state of inactivity when conditions in the environment become unsuitable. A **spore** is a dormant cell surrounded by a hard coat that develops within the bacterium. Spores are highly resistant to extremes of heat or cold, drought, strong acids, and alkalis, and they can remain dormant for years—perhaps, as some believe, for thousands of years. When conditions are again suitable, the spore germinates into a living bacterium identical to the original bacterium. Indeed, some of the most virulent and fatal diseases that human beings can contract—tetanus and botulism, for example—are caused by spores that rapidly develop into their pathogenic state once they gain entrance into the body.

Pathogenic bacteria have two characteristics that endanger the well-being of the host. First, bacterial pathogens grow rapidly in the body. As a result, they interfere with the normal functioning of the host cells, since the bacteria consume the nutrients the cells themselves need for survival. Second, pathogenic bacteria excrete toxic (poisonous) substances that can destroy the host cells or interfere with the normal metabolism of the body. These two modes of action are, in general, responsible for the symptoms of most bacterial infections.

Tuberculosis, pertussis (whooping cough), diphtheria, meningitis, typhoid fever, tetanus, scarlet fever, food poisoning, and some of the sexually transmitted diseases are caused by bacteria.

Viruses

Viruses are the smallest known parasitic organisms. Usually about 1/500 the size of bacteria, viruses enter a bacterium or cell and take control of the metabolic machinery of the host. Viruses consist of long filaments of nucleic acid (DNA or RNA) molecules surrounded by a protein coat or capsule that gives them form. The nucleic acid molecules control the metabolic and genetic characteristics of the viruses. There are innumerable types of viruses; relatively few, however, are pathogenic.

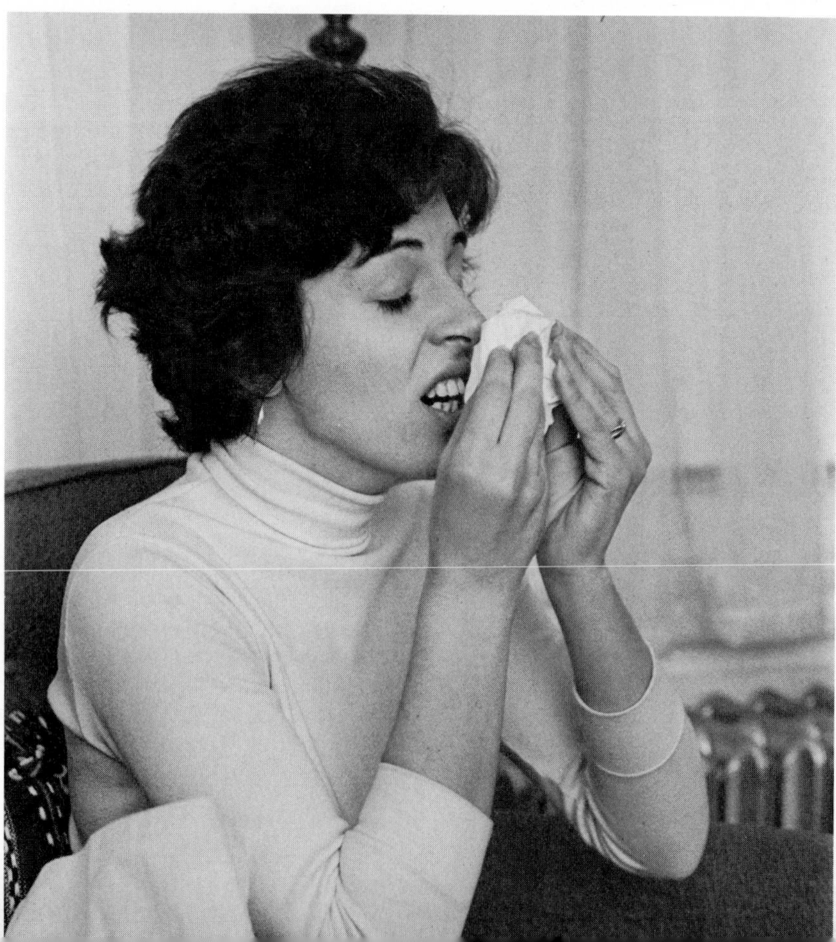

A typical virus lives and reproduces in the following manner. The virus attaches its capsule to the wall of the host cell, opens a passageway through the cell's membrane, and then discharges its content of nucleic acid molecules into the cell. The capsule then disintegrates, and nucleic acid molecules take control of the host cell. The invaded cell abandons its own normal metabolic activities and reproduces quantities of the viral nucleic acid and its protein capsule. From fifteen to twenty-five minutes after the virus has entered the cell, about 200 exact replicas of the original virus have been produced and have escaped from the host cell to infect other cells.

The manner in which the body defends itself against a viral infection is distinctly different from the way in which it fights off a bacterial infection. Unless a vaccine is available for a particular virus (such as the poliomyelitis, rubella, mumps, smallpox, and measles vaccines), there is no way of resisting initial infection by a viral strain. Fortunately, the body does produce antibodies (proteins that neutralize the effects of viruses and other germs) in response to the viral infection. Once certain viral diseases have run their course, a person usually has developed a lasting immunity. For other viral infections, such as the common cold, no immunity is developed.

Influenza, rabies, encephalitis, hepatitis, infectious mononucleosis, herpes, genital warts, and AIDS are among the viral infections.

Rickettsias

Rickettsias are microorganisms intermediate in size between bacteria and viruses. Like the viruses, they can survive only within a living cell. In nature rickettsias are parasitic on insect hosts. They can, however, be transmitted to a human by an insect vector (an insect carrying the pathogen). Rickettsias are named after Howard Taylor Ricketts, an American pathologist who discovered that the microorganisms of Rocky Mountain spotted fever and typhus fever are transmitted to man by ticks and lice, respectively.

Protozoa

Protozoa are single-celled animals (such as the amoeba) found most often in moist soil and bodies of water. They can cause such diseases as amoebic dysentery, malaria, and trichomoniasis. Some protozoa can exist in a dormant stage as cysts for long periods until they once again become infectious and cause a recurrence of the disease.

Parasitic Worms

Parasitic worms are the largest parasites that infest man. They are divided into roundworms, which include hookworms and pinworms, and flatworms, which include tapeworms and flukes. Worm infestations and their diseases are treated by emetics, purgatives, and other drugs.

Fungi

Like bacteria, **fungi** comprise a very large group of organisms that are basically parasitic. Unable to manufacture their own foodstuffs from simple organic compounds as plants do, the fungi (like bacteria) must live off other forms of plant and animal life. Molds, rusts, smuts, and mushrooms are types of parasitic fungi. Only a few are parasitic on man or on other animals, but some of these can cause death. The most common human fungus—ringworm—is, however, more annoying than dangerous.

THE BODY'S IMMUNE SYSTEM

More than 100 communicable diseases are now recognized, some of them highly **virulent**—that is, with a great capacity for producing illness; and undoubtedly there are others that remain unidentified. In view of these facts, we may well wonder how so many millions of us manage to survive childhood—let alone live seventy years and more. The answer is that the body has its own weapons and lines of defense against microscopic invaders. These defenses consist of physical barriers against the entry of pathogenic organisms, chemical agents produced by the body, and specialized body cells that actively fight disease organisms.

Natural Body Defenses

The Skin. The body's first barrier against disease is the skin, which normally prevents most pathogens from reaching its interior.

Linings Within the Body. The lining of the small intestine provides defense against organisms that enter the body through the digestive system, and the **mucous lining** of the nasal and respiratory passages traps a large proportion of organisms inhaled into the body.

Body Secretions. Part of the effectiveness of the skin barrier lies in its secretion of sweat and oils, which kill or repel disease-producing organisms. In addition, every entrance to the body (mouth, ears, nose, eyes, and so on) is protected by some sort of secretion. Tears, nasal secretions, and saliva all contain enzymes that can destroy bacteria. Furthermore, if an organism is swallowed, it must withstand the hydrochloric acid of the stomach and then the bile of the small intestine in order to survive.

Antibodies. **Antibodies** are proteins made by white blood cells that either neutralize the **toxins** (poisonous by-products) produced by germs or actually destroy the germs themselves.

Antibodies are produced in response to the presence of foreign molecules (usually proteins) but do not occur in the body otherwise. Foreign molecules that cause the production of antibodies are called **antigens.** A baby is born with antibodies acquired from the mother that provide protection against a number of diseases during the first months of life.

Once they are produced, certain antibodies provide a long-term (even a lifetime) immunity against disease. This is the reason most people get such "childhood" diseases as chicken pox or measles only once.

Interferon. Another disease-fighting chemical agent of the body effective specifically against viral diseases is called **interferon.** Though interferon does not neutralize a virus the way an antibody neutralizes an antigen, it appears to prevent the virus from reproducing itself within the cell.

White Blood Cells. In addition to mechanical and chemical barriers against invading pathogens, the body has specialized cells that fight infections. These *white blood cells* move toward the site of infection, engulf the germs, and destroy them. The number of white blood cells increases in the presence of bacterial infection. In the disease-fighting process a number of the cells will be killed. These destroyed white blood cells form part of the pus often seen at the site of infection.

Natural and Acquired Immunity

Some people inherit a **natural immunity** to certain diseases, such as tuberculosis. For this reason, the disease organism cannot thrive in their body tissues, even with repeated exposure.

If a person does not inherit immunity, he or she may acquire it. There are two ways of **acquiring immunity** to disease: actively and passively.

Active Acquired Immunity. Immunity in which the body produces its own antibodies is called **active immunity.** It may be acquired by the individual as the body manufactures antibodies and interferon in response to attack by disease organisms. These chemicals may remain in the body and destroy specific disease organisms if and when they again enter the body.

Active immunity may also be acquired through inoculation, which forces the body to produce antibodies against a specific disease such as smallpox, diphtheria, or poliomyelitis. The injected substance may be a **vaccine,** a preparation of killed or weakened bacteria or viruses, or a **toxoid,** a preparation of weakened toxins.

Passive Acquired Immunity. When a person already has a disease or has been exposed to a contagious disease in its incubation period, it is too late for inoculation with a vaccine or toxoid. The person's body may not be able to produce a sufficient quantity of antibodies to fight off the disease alone. However, the individual may still acquire immunity if he or she is injected with antibodies that have been produced in another person or animal. This type of immunity is known as **passive immunity.**

Passive immunity is acquired through the injection of a clear blood fluid

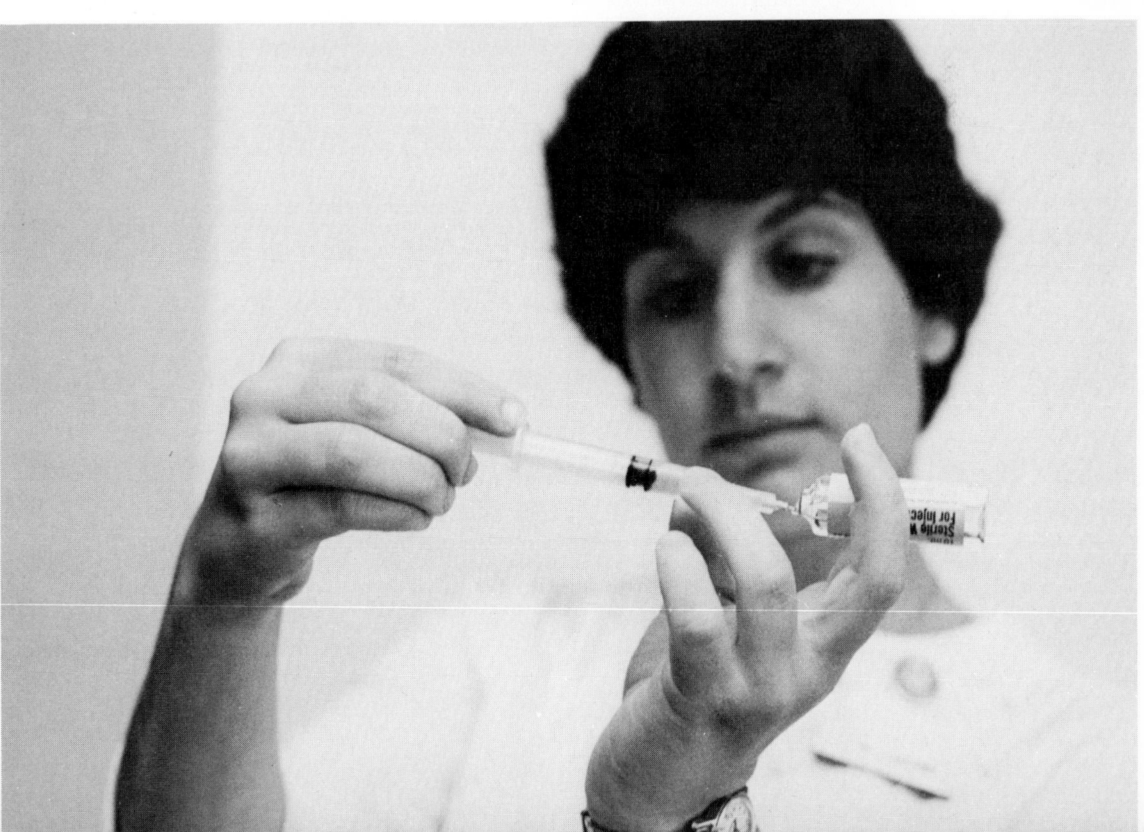

TABLE 15-1
Immunization Schedule for Children

Age	Diphtheria Pertussis Tetanus	Polio	Measles	Rubella	Mumps
2 mo	*	*			
4 mo	*	*			
6 mo	*	*(optional)			
15 mo			*	*	*
18 mo	*	*			
4–6 yr	*	*			

Notes: Measles, rubella, and mumps vaccines can be given in a combined form, at about 15 months of age, with a single injection. Children should receive a sixth tetanus-diphtheria injection (booster) at age 14–16 years.

MEASLES. Measles is an acute, highly contagious viral disease transmitted directly by coughing or sneezing, or indirectly by contact with articles contaminated with the nasal or respiratory secretions of an infected person. A vaccine confers immunity for about four years. Anyone who has once had measles is immune from further infection. A newborn baby whose mother has had measles is immune for about six months after birth.

POLIOMYELTIS. Poliomyelitis is caused by a virus that enters the body through either the mouth or the nose, reaches the bloodstream through the stomach or lungs, and then attacks the spinal cord. The development of the Salk and Sabin vaccines in the 1950s has brought this once-threatening disease almost completely under control. Those cases that still occur result most often from the failure of parents to immunize their children. Recent surveys indicate that more than 10 percent of school-age children have not been fully immunized.

RUBELLA (GERMAN MEASLES). Rubella is a mild, enervating viral disease transmitted from one person to another directly through the spray discharged into the air when an infected person coughs or sneezes, or indirectly through the contamination of food or water by the feces or urine of an infected person. Although death from rubella is rare, tragic complications may result when a woman in her first three months of pregnancy becomes infected. In perhaps 20 to 25 percent of such cases, the baby will be born defective in some way. The child may be mentally retarded or deaf, or have cataracts, a defective heart, or bone defects. For this reason, many countries recognize that an infection of German measles in a pregnant woman is sufficient cause for a therapeutic abortion. A vaccine confers immunity against the virus, but since it acts by producing a mild case of rubella, pregnant women should avoid it.

MUMPS. Mumps is a relatively mild viral disease that attacks the salivary glands. In about 15 to 25 percent of the cases involving males past puberty, however, the virus attacks the testes and renders the male sterile. In about 5 percent of females past puberty, it attacks the ovaries, producing sterility. Immunity can be provided by a vaccine.

DIPHTHERIA. Diphtheria is an acute infectious bacterial disease of the tonsils, throat, and nasal passages, leading to heart failure and death. Immunity for prolonged periods can be acquired by injections of a diphtheria toxoid.

PERTUSSIS (WHOOPING COUGH). Pertussis is an acute bacterial disease of the trachea, bronchi, and bronchioles. The development of vaccines against it has resulted in a marked decline in the number of cases and fatalities. All children should be inoculated against this disease.

TETANUS. The tetanus bacillus is ordinarily a harmless bacterium found in the intestines of animals and in soil. If, however, tetanus spores enter the body through a wound, they will germinate, and the living bacteria will release poisonous toxins. Death occurs in about 35 to 70 percent of all cases, depending on age, length of incubation period, and whether treatment is started before the appearance of symptoms. Treatment consists of inoculations of the tetanus antitoxin. Because tetanus spores are generally present in dust, soil, or animal feces, it is wise to be inoculated as a precaution when one's skin is broken by something unclean. However, it is better still to be immunized against tetanus prior to any injury. Immunity can be conferred for several years by a series of inoculations of tetanus toxoid.

Source: "Parents' Guide to Childhood Immunization" (October 1977), DHEW Publication No. (05) 77–50058.

called **antiserum** that contains antibodies that will protect the body against a specific disease. (It gives the same sort of passive immunity to a disease that is provided a newborn child by the antibodies of its mother.) Some antiserums are **antitoxins,** since they protect the body against the toxins released by the pathogens.

Immunization Schedule. Of the 14 million children from 1 to 4 years old in the United States (the years during which immunizations are recommended), many have not been immunized against one or more of the childhood diseases for which vaccines or toxoids are available. The figures range from 15 percent of our children who have not been immunized against **diphtheria, pertussis (whooping cough)**, and **tetanus** to 27 percent who are in danger of catching **mumps.** Figures for **poliomyelitis, measles,** and **rubella (German measles)** fall between those extremes. Some of these diseases can cripple a child and can even cause death. The U.S. Public Health Service and the overwhelming majority of medical experts believe that the benefits of complete immunization far outweigh the risks of side effects such as temporary fever, a sore arm, a rash, or even more serious reactions (see box: Vaccines and Their Side Effects). The Public Health Service strongly recommends that all healthy children be immunized against all of the vaccine-preventable childhood diseases. Table 15-1 shows the immunization schedule suggested by the U.S. Public Health Service for a child, starting at the age of 2 months.

PROBLEMS AND CONTROVERSIES: Vaccines and Their Side Effects

No vaccine is 100 percent safe, but the chances of becoming ill or suffering severe side effects from those in current use are so small that public health authorities decided long ago that they were little enough price to pay for the hundreds of thousands of cases of serious disease that vaccines prevented. For example, out of the 14 million children vaccinated each year against mumps, measles, rubella, and polio, about 10 experience moderately severe side effects, and 3 may contract polio from the polio vaccine.

Whooping cough vaccine, however, has in recent years caused about 43 cases of permanent brain damage (or 1 out of 300,000) in the United States annually. Because the majority of babies are vaccinated against whooping cough, the disease is rare in the United States. Most instances of it occur in teenagers who didn't get vaccinated as infants, and for them the disease is seldom serious. It is much more serious in infants, in whom it can lead to pneumonia and prove fatal.

It is understandable that parents, reading of cases of brain damage from whooping cough vaccine, should fear to have their babies vaccinated. They realize that whooping cough is not a very common disease, and think they would rather risk their baby's coming down with it than being brain-damaged by the vaccine.

Forty states do not permit children to enter school without having been vaccinated against whooping cough, but the most dangerous years for the disease are the preschool years. Public health officials worry that if enough parents leave their children unprotected against the disease, its incidence will rise, with a corresponding rise in infant deaths. (Something like this in fact happened in England in the 1970s.) They fear that parental resistance to vaccination could make whooping cough a very serious childhood disease once again.

SEXUALLY TRANSMITTED DISEASES (STDs)

The **sexually transmitted diseases,** also called **venereal diseases,** have as their common bond their method of contraction: They are contagious infections transmitted directly from person to person almost always during intimate sexual activity. In terms of potential consequences, AIDS (acquired immune deficiency syndrome) is the most serious, resulting in almost certain death. Two treatable STDs, syphilis and gonorrhea, can have serious consequences if left untreated. In terms of the number of new cases each year, chlamydial infections lead gonorrhea, followed by genital warts, genital herpes, and syphilis.

In view of the effectiveness of treatment for most of these diseases, it is somewhat surprising that such numbers of new cases of STD appear each year. Most forms are cured with little or no difficulty. But the situation is complicated by the myths surrounding STD, by the lack of effective educational programs, and by fears of disclosure and stigma.

Myths About STDs

Superstition, legend, and folklore abound in respect to STDs. Some believe, for example, that a person can become infected with an STD merely by sitting on a toilet seat recently vacated by an infected individual. This is most unlikely. The organisms responsible for most of these diseases are very delicate and can live only in a warm, moist place—which a toilet seat is not. They quickly die when exposed to the air. For this reason, it is also improbable that sharing a drinking glass or shaking hands with an infected individual will transfer a veneral infection.

Another misconception is that one can acquire an STD by kissing an infected person. In fact, it would be extremely unusual for this to happen. A person with a syphilitic infection may, during the early stages of infection, develop a sore on the lip or inside the mouth. In rare instances, if the infected individual kisses a person who has an open cut on the lip, the infection *may* be transferred.

Some believe that it is possible to fight off an STD by sheer physical vitality. This is untrue. Nor is it possible to go into a drugstore and buy a medicine off the shelf that will enable one to get rid of an STD quickly and privately.

Nor is it true that once a person has contracted and been cured of an STD he or she is immune from further infection. The person who has been cured with an antibiotic can be reinfected as soon as the drug has left his or her body.

Many think that only people who are unclean contract STDs. This, too, is false.

The myth that has perhaps done the most to hinder control of STDs is that "nice people don't get VD." The fact is that one in five persons in the United States will acquire an STD at some time. People living in small towns and large urban areas, adolescents and adults, rich and poor—no group is immune.

The Incidence of STDs

It is estimated that as many as 20 million Americans suffer from genital herpes and that another half million people contract it each year (see Figure 15-1). Some 3 million Americans a year are thought to contract chlamydial infections, including pelvic inflammatory disease (PID) and nonspecific urethritis. (PID is sometimes caused by chlamydia and sometimes by gonorrhea.)

FIGURE 15-1

Estimated new cases of STDs in 1986.

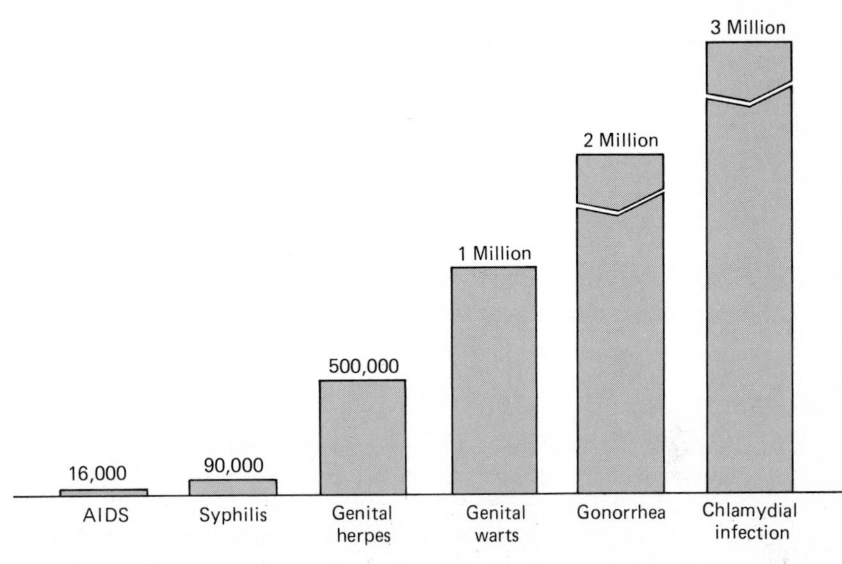

Since the introduction of penicillin in the treatment of syphillis there has been a steady decline in the percentage of the population that has the disease at any given time. This is a result of the effectiveness of penicillin and other antibiotics against the disease. Unfortunately, however, after a steady and dramatic decline in the rate of new cases of syphilis from the end of World War II until the mid-1950s, there has been a fairly constant increase so that the current annual rate of new cases is more than triple that of thirty years ago. The rate of new cases of gonorrhea also declined after World War II, though not so dramatically. But the resurgence of the disease since the mid-1950s has brought the rate of new infections to a point considerably above that of even the early postwar-years.

No figures can be exact because so many cases of STD go unreported. Though the law requires that the U.S. Public Health Service be informed of all cases of STD discovered by a physician or clinic, the number reported is grossly below the actual total. This is true for two reasons. First, many people who have contracted an STD do not know it, and therefore do not go to a physician or clinic. Second, physicians treating private patients do not always report these cases to their local public health authorities, in spite of the law. Many physicians prefer to spare the feelings of their patients by shielding them from public health investigators. The result is that others who have been in contact with the infected person may themselves be infected and continue to infect others. Current estimates are that more than two out of every three cases of venereal disease go unreported.

Who Is Likely to Become Infected?

The question likely to arouse the greatest interest for most teenagers and young adults is: What are the chances of my catching an STD?

The most important factor to consider is sexual habits. The greater the number of sexual contacts, the more likely a person is to contract an STD. Statistically, reported cases of both syphilis and gonorrhea are higher for men than for women, because men tend to have a greater number of different sexual partners than women. Another reason is that the symptoms of venereal disease are sometimes hidden in women, so they do not know they have become infected. STDs are especially widespread among teenagers and young adults. The highest rate of reported cases of syphilis is among 20- to 24-year-olds; for gonorrhea, the highest rate among males is in the same age group, but for females, the rate among 15- to 19-year-olds is slightly higher.

STDs are generally more prevalent in urban areas. This is not surprising since the larger number of people and the generally less restrictive sexual attitudes in urban areas make it likely that a greater number of sexual contacts will take place.

Why the Rate Remains High

There are several reasons for the continued high rates of STDs. For some people, there may be little dread of contracting an STD because therapy is usually effective and relatively easy. Another reason is that many people do not know the signs of infection. They may ignore the symptoms of gonorrhea or syphilis and unknowingly infect others. Also, many who suspect they have a disease are embarrassed to seek treatment.

Oral contraceptives have lessened considerably the risk of pregnancy, and thus have encouraged greater frequency of sexual contacts. Also, studies indicate that some of the new birth control methods tend to increase a women's chances of contracting gonorrhea. The Pill, for example, increases the moisture content of the vagina, providing an alkaline environment ideally suited for the growth of the gonorrhea bacterium. Older contraceptive methods did not have this effect. In fact, the acidic substances in contraceptive jellies are thought to offer some protection against the bacteria of STD. The condom, which more men used to wear during intercourse, blocks to some extent the transfer of disease organisms from one person to another.

The Control of STDs

STDs are so widespread that millions of dollars are allocated annually for their control. One approach has been to educate the public. In recent years government and private health agencies have been using pamphlets, posters, television, and radio to alert people to the dangers of STDs in a frank and informative manner. There are STD education classes in some schools. Many cities now have referral services where people can receive information about STDs over the telephone, anonymously.

An important method of controlling the spread of STDs is to pursue the chain of infection through which the disease is transmitted from person to person (see Figure 15-2). After a clinic or physician sends a report of syphilis to the local department of public health, an interviewer from the department will contact the infected individual and attempt to obtain the names of persons with whom he or she has had sexual intercourse recently. The investigator must then get in touch with whoever is named to recommend a checkup and, if necessary, treatment. He or she must also attempt to identify the recent sexual contacts of the new patients. One by one, the investigator must track

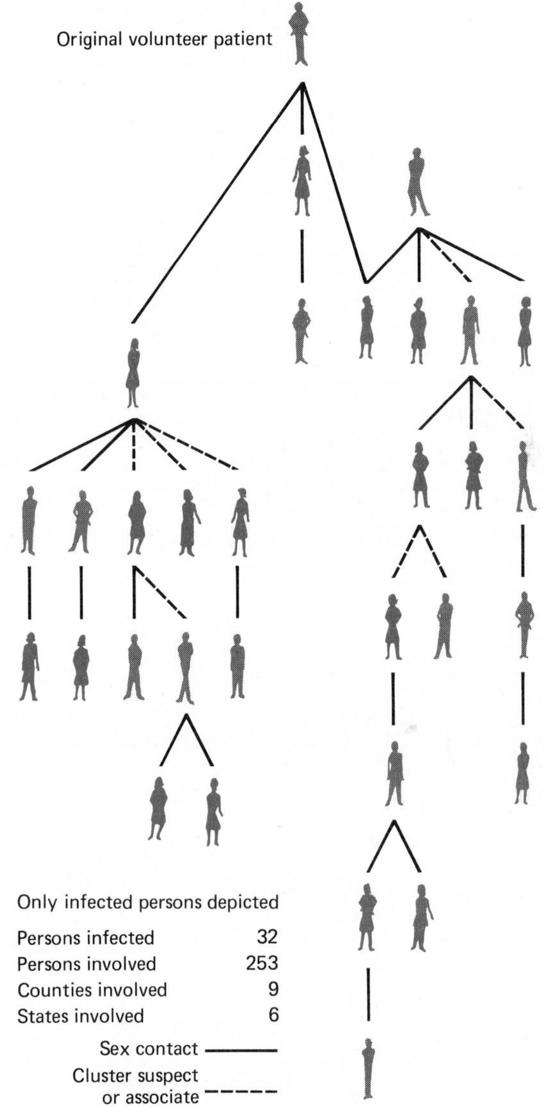

FIGURE 15-2

In the summer of 1972 one man initiated the spread of syphilis in a southern state. Before health officials could control the incidence of infection, 253 persons were exposed to the disease, and 32 were infected. By following the lines in the diagram, one can trace the development of the chain of infection.

Source: Adapted from *Today's VD Control Problem 1974*, p. 21. Courtesy of American Social Health Association.

down all those who might have been infected. A missing link in the chain means that the STD will spread to other people.

Because it has been learned that sexually transmitted diseases tend to concentrate within groups of people who know each other, a new interview technique called **cluster testing** has been developed. About 60 percent of all venereal infections are acquired from friends, so the interviewer attempts to find out the names of others in the same group of people who might have had the same general sexual experience as the infected individual. Following up the leads provided, the investigator is likely to discover that a high proportion of the people in that group also have an STD. In one case, interviews with 285 individuals belonging to the same general group of people in which one person was first found to be infected brought to light 153 other infections.

The problem of coping with the spread of STDs has been complicated by the reluctance of many people to seek treatment for fear their identities will be exposed. Of course, interviews with a public health investigator can be embarrassing, and a person may not want to "tattle" on friends; but the individual does have a responsibility to ensure that anybody he or she may have infected receives diagnosis and, if necessary, treatment. One recent trend should encourage teenagers and young adults to seek treatment: It is now possible for a minor to receive medical treatment for an STD without parental knowledge or consent in most states.

Syphilis

Syphilis is far less prevalent than gonorrhea, yet it has always been regarded as the more serious disease because its effects are more damaging to the body and far more insidious. The disease may attack almost any part of the body, but it does most damage to the heart and blood vessels and to the brain and nervous system. A person may not know he or she has syphilis until years after contracting the infection, and then the symptoms may be so diffuse that a physician might believe the disease is something entirely different. Syphilis has, for good reason, been called the "great imitator."

Syphilis is caused by an extremely small, corkscrew-shaped organism known as *Treponema pallidum*. *Treponema pallidum* is very sensitive to its environment. It requires warm, moist conditions and dies quickly if exposed to air, soap and water, alcohol, or excessive heat. Under the ideal conditions existing within the human body, however, the organism thrives and multiplies readily. It may even survive treatment and exist for the lifetime of the individual.

Because of its fragile nature, *Treponema pallidum* is almost always transferred from one person to another during the intimate bodily contact of sexual activity. It can then make its way through the delicate tissues that line the vagina and penis, through the anus or membranes of the mouth, as well as through other body areas. Whatever the route by which the organisms enter the body, once within, they reproduce rapidly, giving rise to a range of symptoms that appear at varying intervals after infection. These symptoms are manifested at the primary, secondary, and tertiary stages of the disease.

Primary Syphilis. The incubation period for syphilis is generally from two to three weeks, but it may be as long as eight weeks before the first signs of a chancre appear. The **chancre** is a hard, painless sore, varying in size from very small to an inch or two across, which will appear at the site of infection—the genitals usually, but sometimes the rectum, fingers, lips, nipples, or elsewhere. It is highly infectious, being filled with the spirochetes of syphilis. If it forms within the vagina or rectum, it can easily go unnoticed. Microscopic inspection of a smear of the chancre is the only way to diagnose syphilis at this time.

The chancre disappears after a few weeks, giving some people a false sense of security, but the infection continues to spread.

Secondary Syphilis. Some two to six weeks after the chancre disappears, secondary symptoms appear; these usually last no more than a few months. The symptoms are extremely varied, and may mislead an unsuspecting physician. Aching joints, headaches, a sore throat, and a painless rash are fairly common, but falling hair, whitish sores in the mouth and throat, and inflamed eyes with sensitivity to light can also occur. A blood test will detect syphilis at this stage.

Latent Syphilis. Following the symptoms of the second stage is a period of *latency,* which may last anywhere from a few months to twenty years or more, or even the entire lifetime of the individual. The disease will be infectious only during the first two years of latency, however. The individual may never become aware of having syphilis and may unknowingly transmit the disease to others during this infectious period. During latency the disease may be discov-

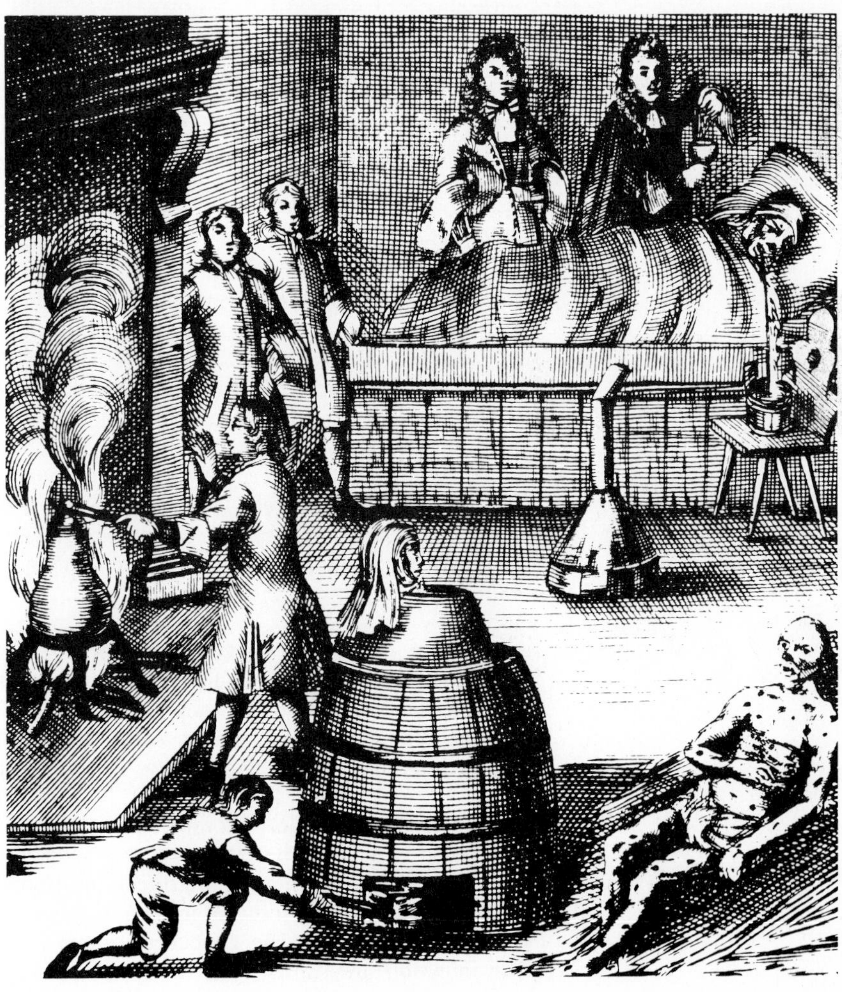

A seventeenth-century engraving showing syphilis sufferers undergoing various types of treatment, including mercury fumigation. A victim in the last stages of the disease is shown in the foreground.

ered as a result of a routine blood test—taken to obtain a marriage license, for example.

Tertiary or Late Syphilis. In about a third of the cases of untreated latent syphilis, tertiary symptoms will eventually occur. These are the most severe. Healthy tissues are killed and replaced by scar tissue, and the normal functioning of the body is upset. Symptoms of kidney disease, lung disease, stomach ulcer, or any of dozens of other disorders may appear.

Late syphilis frequently damages the aorta, the main artery leading from the heart. It can also affect the brain, eventually causing psychotic manifestations and hallucinations. In about 10 percent of cases late syphilis leads to death.

Congenital Syphilis. Syphilis in a pregnant woman often results in the transfer of the infection to her unborn child. If a fetus acquires syphilis during the early stages of pregnancy, a miscarriage or stillbirth may occur. Most of those fetuses that are born normally to women who have syphilis display the symptoms of **congenital syphilis,** or syphilis of the newborn child, by the fourth week of life.

If syphilis is discovered soon enough in the mother, treatment with penicillin will usually protect the child from any of the effects of the disease, and it will be born healthy and normal. In most states blood tests to detect syphilis are routinely given during pregnancy. Even if syphilis is undiscovered and the child is born with symptoms of it, treatment with penicillin will usually arrest the course of the disease immediately and prevent any further manifestations. But if the infection remains undiscovered and untreated, many of the disorders of the third stage may appear during childhood or adolescence.

Treatment of Syphilis. Penicillin is usually the preferred drug in the treatment of syphilis. In cases where a person is allergic or resistant to it, other antibiotics such as erythromycin and tetracycline are used. Following the penicillin injection, blood tests are taken at intervals for the next several months to make sure the blood reacts negatively. Generally, four to seven months are required before a negative reaction is registered. In third-stage syphilitic infections the blood test may never become negative, even though the penicillin has effectively halted the progress of the disease.

Gonorrhea

Gonorrhea is caused by the gonococcus organism *Neisseria gonorrhoeae*, a bacterium that is shaped rather like a kidney bean and is found in pairs in the body. To survive, the organisms require a moist, warm environment; if they are exposed to air or soap and water, they quickly die. They therefore are almost always transmitted from one person to another during sexual activity.

Gonorrhea in the Male. Compared to syphilis, with its deceptive and ambiguous symptoms, gonorrhea is usually easily diagnosed when it occurs in males. The pain and pus formation are direct and unmistakable symptoms. Following sexual contact with an infected individual, there is a two- to eight-day incubation period, during which the gonococci multiply in the body. Outward signs of the infection are usually evident by the second to fifth day. Ordinarily the

STDs and You

T or F

_______ 1. All STDs, if not treated, can lead to serious side effects.

_______ 2. Total fitness bestows total immunity to STDs.

_______ 3. The possibility of contracting an STD is proportionate to the number of sexual partners.

_______ 4. Though a person may suspect contraction of an STD, it is only a laboratory test that can verify it.

_______ 5. You can be vaccinated against STDs and in that way avoid the possibility of infection.

_______ 6. The outward signs of an STD may go hidden or unnoticed.

_______ 7. A person can have more than one STD at a time and can get a particular disease more than once.

_______ 8. A high intake of vitamin C has proven effective in preventing and curing gonorrhea.

_______ 9. It is more the exposure to a variety of partners than the frequency of sexual expression that renders a person vulnerable to contracting an STD.

_______ 10. There are several STDs that it is difficult, if not impossible, to cure.

_______ 11. The use of a condom can be an effective protection against the transfer of some STDs.

_______ 12. Unless a chancre is present, you can be sure that you have not been infected with syphilis.

_______ 13. A puslike urethral discharge is one of the early symptoms of gonorrhea.

_______ 14. The signs of gonorrhea are more readily noticed in the male than in the female.

_______ 15. Both steam baths and acupuncture have been used successfully in curing herpes.

Scoring: Statements 1, 3, 4, 6, 7, 9-11, 13, and 14 are true; 2, 5, 8, 12, and 15 are false. Anything less than a perfect score may bear serious consequences.

Source: Adapted in part from *Peer Education in Human Sexuality* (Planned Parenthood of Metropolitan Washington, 1108 16th Street NW, Washington, D.C. 20036).

organisms enter the body through the urethra. As the organisms multiply, the body's defenses react against this invasion. The walls of the urethra become inflamed, and pus forms as white blood cells rush into the infected area to engulf the gonococci. For the male, the first sign of infection is usually an intense burning sensation in the penis upon the attempt to urinate. There is a thin, watery discharge from the penis that becomes progressively more profuse and yellow in color.

Although the outward signs of gonorrhea soon disappear, the disease continues within the body. If left untreated, the infection may stop progressing (bacteria may stop multiplying) anywhere from six weeks to a year afterward, although this is not always the case. By that time, however, the infection will have already spread through the male's reproductive system, infecting the prostate gland and the testes. If the infection has reached the tubes that conduct sperm from the testes to the penis, the tubes may become blocked by the formation of scar tissue and the male will thus become sterile.

Gonorrhea in the Female. Unlike the dramatic pain that occurs in the male, the symptoms of gonorrhea in the female often go unrecognized. According to some estimates, nine out of ten women who contract gonorrhea do not know they have it. Sometimes there are no symptoms at all. More usually, there is a discharge from the vagina, perhaps accompanied by a mild burning pain. As in males, these symptoms lessen in time. And since so many women are often afflicted with mild, harmless infections of the vagina that produce similar discharges, they are likely to ignore evidence of a gonorrheal infection.

The infection usually remains localized in the vagina. But if it should spread beyond the cervix into the uterus, fever will develop, accompanied by abdominal pains. The symptoms are similar to those of appendicitis, and both the female and her physician are likely to suspect this is the cause. If gonorrhea is untreated, the infection may spread to the fallopian tubes and cause pelvic inflammatory disease (PID), discussed later in the chapter. PID can lead to sterility.

As in males, the disease may infect other organs, and a crippling form of arthritis is a common result. Heart disease is also a possibility.

If a woman with an undiagnosed case of gonorrhea gives birth to a baby, the infant's eyes may become infected with the gonococcus organisms as it passes through the cervix and vagina during birth. Within twenty-four hours an inflammation of the eyes occurs, which may permanently blind the infant. As a preventive measure, the law requires that the eyes of a newborn infant be treated immediately upon birth with a silver nitrate solution or antibiotic ointments.

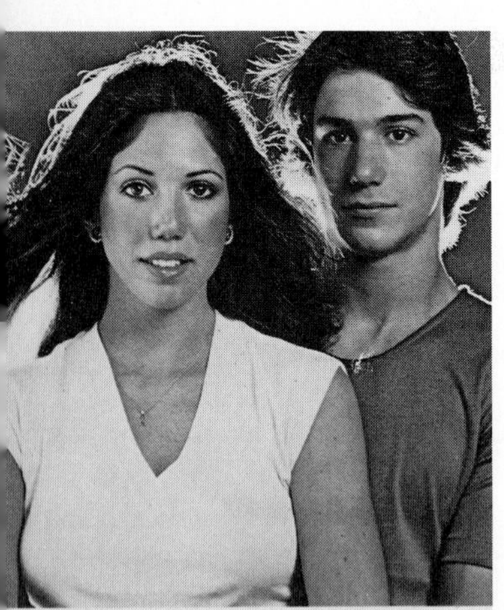

Adults, as well as infants, may lose their eyesight because of gonorrhea. If adults should rub their eyes while their hands harbor the gonococcus organisms, the bacteria may infect the eyes, producing a painful inflammation that can result in blindness.

Diagnosis and Treatment. The diagnosis of penile gonorrhea is simple enough; under a microscope the gonococci in the discharge can be seen clearly. Diagnosis in the female is more difficult, since the gonococcal discharge from the vagina is so similar to the discharge produced by other organisms. A smear of the substance is usually placed on a special culture medium and incubated for several days. If gonococci are present, they will multiply in the medium.

It is possible to acquire gonorrhea orally or rectally, in which case a smear test is the only sure method of detection. Sometimes there will be a sore throat or irritated rectum to indicate the presence of the gonococcus organism.

Antibiotics can cure gonorrhea rapidly and eliminate complications when they are used in early stages of the infection. Penicillin was formerly the best antibiotic; however, since the mid-1950s, penicillin-resistant strains of gonococci have developed, and some persons are sensitive or allergic to penicillin. Today a physician may use penicillin or another antibiotic such as Declomycin, erythromycin, tetracycline, or spectinomycin.

Genital Herpes

Most educated adults have long been aware of the danger of STDs such as syphilis and gonorrhea, but they have taken some comfort in knowing that early treatment can cure these infections. Since the late 1970s, however, an STD called **genital herpes** has caused widespread alarm among Americans who are sexually active. It is, so far, incurable.

Genital herpes is caused by a virus, herpes simplex type 2, which enters the body during sexual contact with an infected individual. It had been thought that the virus was spread only by those experiencing active symptoms of the disease. Recent research reported by the National Institutes of Health has shown, however, that "over time and throughout the population symptomless people apparently account for much of the spread of the disease." Once infected, a person is a carrier of the disease for life. Symptoms, if any, appear in from two to twenty days after exposure. Many people experience no symptoms; some may exhibit minor symptoms like those of jock itch; but others may develop one or more sores on the sex organs, the buttocks, or the thighs. These sores are usually painful blisters filled with fluid; they may be accompanied by fever, a mild burning sensation, swollen glands, and, in women, a vaginal discharge. Symptoms last from four to five days and then begin to heal; the healing is usually complete by the end of ten to twenty days.

The disease is not cured, however, and remains dormant. Some people never suffer a recurrence; others may be affected rarely; and still others may experience outbreaks at frequent and regular intervals. It is not yet understood what triggers a reactivation of the virus, but it is generally believed that poor health, low resistance, and even emotional trauma are contributing factors. Whatever the cause, the disease is at its most contagious when symptoms are present, and anyone experiencing symptoms should avoid sexual contact.

No direct relationship between the herpes virus and cancer has yet been established, but it is known that women with genital herpes are more prone to cervical cancer. Pregnant women who have herpes should inform their physicians, for if an infant comes into contact with herpes lesions while passing through the birth canal, there is a chance it will become infected.

STDs: Where to Go for Help

AIDS National Hotline
(800) 342-AIDS

American Social Health Association
260 Sheridan Avenue
Palo Alto, Calif. 94306
(415) 327-6465

VD National Hotline
(800) 227-9822
In California: (800) 982-5883

Source: *The Columbia University College of Physicians and Surgeons Complete Home Medical Guide* (New York: Crown Publishers, 1985), p. 803.

Herpes infections are usually diagnosed visually. There are laboratory tests, but they are unreliable and expensive. There is no screening test for people who have no lesions.

The pain, itching, and burning of herpes attacks can be relieved by acyclovir ointment. The same drug in capsule form can prevent recurrences as long as it is taken. As many as 40 million Americans are carriers of genital herpes, and an estimated 500,000 new cases of the disease are expected each year.

Nonspecific Urethritis (NSU)

The most common sexually transmitted disease is **nonspecific urethritis** (NSU), also known as *nongonococcal urethritis* (*NGU*). As the name suggests, the cause or causes of the disease are vague. According to the Centers for Disease Control, some 3 million Americans are infected with NSU each year.

In men the symptoms are frequently similar to those of gonorrhea—a thick white discharge and a burning sensation when urinating. Others might experience a clear discharge from the penis that is sometimes continuous, or sometimes present only in the morning before urinating. Usually there is mild to moderate pain when urinating.

In women the symptoms are often insignificant and hard to diagnose. Pain, itching, or burning around the vagina may be a sign of NSU.

NSU is probably not one disease, but several, all of which have similar symptoms. Chlamydia, a group of microscopic organisms that have characteristics of both bacteria and viruses, are thought to account for 50 percent of all NSU. Another cause might be bacteria; still another might be chemical irritation, such as, in men, when the meatus and urethra are irritated by certain soaps, deodorant sprays, or dyes from clothing. NSU is not, in the strictest sense, a sexually transmitted disease, nor even necessarily an infection, since it does not always require intercourse with an infected person to develop. It can, in fact, occur in two people who have never had intercourse with anyone else. Sometimes it seems linked to a change in sexual habits.

Any urethral or vaginal discharge should be tested for both gonorrhea and chlamydia. Chlamydial NSU has become easier to diagnose than it used to be: a new test became available in 1985. It should not be left untreated, for chlamydia can cause pelvic inflammatory disease in women, with serious effects. Because it is often spread by sexual intercourse, those who are diagnosed as having NSU should make sure that their sexual partners are tested for it too. NSU is treated with tetracycline or erythromycin.

Pelvic Inflammatory Disease (PID)

Untreated chlamydial or gonorrheal infections can spread to the cervix, uterus, fallopian tubes, ovaries, and other pelvic tissues, causing salpingitis, or *pelvic inflammatory disease* (*PID*). This disease can also develop from unknown causes. PID strikes over 1 million women a year, most under the age of 25. The symptoms of PID include severe pain in the lower abdomen, painful intercourse, irregular menstrual periods, and a profuse, odorous discharge. The disease can cause scar tissue to form in the fallopian tubes and thus result in infertility. It can also cause ectopic pregnancy, a condition in which the fertilized egg becomes implanted in the fallopian tube instead of moving down to the wall of the uterus. Severe PID infections can lead to blood poisoning, peritonitis

Pubic Lice ("Crabs")

Though not a disease, pubic lice ("crabs") are usually transmitted from person to person by close physical contact. It is also possible to become infested through bedding or towels that have been used by a carrier.

The crab louse is difficult to see with the naked eye. After feeding, when it is engorged with its host's blood, it is more visible as a rust-colored speck, hardly larger than a pinhead. The primary symptom signaling the presence of crab lice is an intense itchiness; this usually occurs in the pubic area, but crabs are also found on the scalp, armpits, and even eyelashes.

Several over-the-counter preparations are available and effective. Crabs can usually be eliminated within twenty-four hours.

(an inflammation of the membrane that surrounds the abdominal organs), and inflammation of the joints. Complicated cases may require surgery.

PID is treated with antibiotics—usually tetracycline, erythromycin, and penicillin—and bed rest. The sexual partners of infected women should be examined as well. Some may have nonsymptomatic chlamydia or gonorrhea.

Genital Warts

Genital warts are small pink or dark red swellings that grow rapidly and appear in cauliflowerlike clusters in the genital area. They are twice as common as genital herpes, afflicting over a million persons a year. Caused by the papilloma virus and transmitted through sexual intercourse, they usually appear between one and six months after initial contact. In men they are usually found on the head and shaft of the penis or inside the urethral opening. They may also occur in the anal area. In women they appear on the vulva, the walls of the vagina, the cervix, the anus, and the perineum (the area between the anus and genitals). They are also found in the larynx, trachea, and lungs of newborns who contract them from their mothers during delivery.

The treatment for genital warts, which must be given to both partners, varies with the severity of the condition. In simple cases, the warts are "painted" on alternate days with a chemical until they disappear. In more severe cases, warts may be removed by "freezing" with liquid nitrogen, by laser therapy, or by surgery. Care must be taken to remove all of them; otherwise they will reappear.

Genital warts are not as harmless as they might seem. They have been associated with cancers of the cervix, vagina, vulva, penis, and anus. Women who have had genital warts should have regular Pap tests. Since genital warts are extremely contagious, affected people should abstain from sexual relations until the warts have disappeared. Condoms are a recommended form of protection against genital warts.

Acquired Immune Deficiency Syndrome (AIDS)

An epidemic of a deadly new viral disease has erupted in the past few years. Intravenous drug users and men who engage in homosexual practices have been the most frequent victims in the United States, but the heterosexual population is increasingly coming under the threat of the disease as well. The disease is known as **Acquired Immune Deficiency Syndrome,** or **AIDS.** It is thought to have originated in Africa and is now found in some thirty countries of the world. Through 1986, nearly 30,000 cases had been reported in the United States, and between 1 and 1.5 million people had been infected by an AIDS virus. The Public Health Service estimated that by the end of 1991 there would be a cumulative total of 270,000 cases and 179,000 deaths.

Scientists have implicated a number of viruses in AIDS, many believing that it is caused primarily by a virus called the human T-cell lymphotropic virus, type 3, or HTLV-III, which suppresses the immune system. While HTLV-III infects many types of body cells, including brain cells, it is especially lethal to a kind of white blood cell—the T-helper cell—that enables the body to fight off disease-causing microorganisms. When the T-helper cells are destroyed, the body is left open to an array of diseases called *opportunistic infections*. They are opportunistic in the sense that they take advantage of the body's reduced ability to defend itself. People with AIDS can develop Kaposi's sarcoma, a rare cancer of the skin and mucous membranes, or *Pneumocystis carinii* pneumonia, an opportunistic protozoal infection.

Transmission of the AIDS Virus. The AIDS virus appears to be transmitted in two ways: through sexual contact and by inoculation. In both situations it appears critical that a virus-contaminated substance, such as semen or blood, gains access to the blood system of the victim for an infection to occur.

In the United States, sexually transmitted AIDS occurs primarily between males and most frequently among those who practice anal intercourse. Infected semen reaches the bloodstream of the victim through existing anal fissures or through fissures created in the act of intercourse. (Anal tissue is easily ruptured.) Presumably such semen could also reach the bloodstream through oral fissures during the act of fellatio. It is also possible for a male to transmit AIDS to a female during vaginal intercourse, and this appears to account for the high incidence of the disease among women in some foreign nations. How a female transmits the disease to a male during vaginal intercourse is not quite understood at this time.

A significant percentage of AIDS occurs among intravenous drug users and recipients of blood transfusions, particularly hemophiliacs. Recently introduced procedures for screening blood are expected to eliminate this last source of infection. And intravenous drug users have been warned of the risk they take in sharing a needle with others.

The Course and Symptoms of AIDS. Not everyone who is exposed to AIDS develops the disease. The best estimates are that 20 to 30 percent of those who are exposed will develop a fatal case of the disease. Another 20 percent will develop some symptoms. One thing that frightens those who think they may have been exposed is the long incubation period—an average of 4 years, at best estimate, but perhaps much longer. Those who are infected with the AIDS virus are thought to remain infected for the rest of their lives and therefore should consider themselves potentially infectious to others.

The occurrence of a particular cluster of symptoms can be indicative of the AIDS-related complex, or ARC. It should be remembered, however, that these symptoms also indicate diseases or conditions other than AIDS. People with ARC usually experience two or more of the following symptoms:

- Swollen lymph glands in two or more places in addition to the groin
- Recurrent fevers and drenching night sweats
- A heavy, dry, persistent cough that cannot be explained by smoking or minor illness
- Unexplained weight loss of more than ten pounds in less than two months
- Unexplained bleeding from any body opening; easy bruisability
- Profound fatigue that cannot be accounted for by physical activity or emotional stress
- Recurrent watery diarrhea
- Candidiasis, or thrush, a fungal infection that produces a thick white coating on the tongue or in the throat
- Neurological signs such as memory loss, disequilibrium, blurring of vision, loss of hearing

In most people with ARC these conditions clear up after a while, but between 9 and 30 percent of those who have ARC go on to develop AIDS.

It is also possible for AIDS to appear quite suddenly in people who have had no symptoms whatever. Awareness of the disease may occur when an individual demonstrates signs of ordinarily rare diseases such as Kaposi's sarcoma or *Pneumocystis* pneumonia.

Treatment. No successful treatment for AIDS has yet been discovered. AIDS specialists have tried to reduce the effects of the disease by treating the opportunistic infections with antibiotics. But while some of the infections are temporarily cured, it is only a matter of time before new infections appear because of the weakened immune system. Doctors have also used interferon and interleukin-2 (see box on page 394) in an effort to reinforce the immune system. The greatest success up through 1986 had involved the use of an antiviral drug, azidothymidine, which slows the progress of the disease in patients who are suffering from *Pneumocystis* pneumonia.

Blood-screening Tests. Tests employed in blood donor programs to screen out AIDS-infected individuals have been greatly misunderstood. The widely used ELISA test reveals whether a person has been exposed to the virus and formed antibodies to it; but this test produces a significant number of false positives. That is not a problem in blood donor programs, which as a precautionary measure discard any blood that tests positive, but it is not always understood by those who are tested. A positive result on the ELISA test may mean that (1) the test results were inaccurate and must be confirmed by a more elaborate and expensive test; (2) the person has been infected with the virus but has successfully fought it off and is now free of it, or immune to it, or both; (3) the person has both the live virus and antibodies to it but does not have the disease and may never develop it; (4) the person is infected with the virus and will develop AIDS. Thus the results of the current blood-screening test are highly uncertain, and because of this there has been considerable debate over how they should be interpreted and whether employers, government agencies, and health insurance companies should have access to the results (see box: Fears About AIDS).

Fears About AIDS

Fears about AIDS—especially uncertainties about how it is spread—have generated a near-hysteria in the nation. Principals and parents' groups have gone so far as to oppose the admittance to school of a child whose brother had AIDS. Adults with AIDS have lost their jobs or their homes when employers or landlords have learned that they have the disease. Many AIDS patients have been treated like pariahs by ambulance attendants and hospital personnel and have been unnecessarily subjected to strict quarantine procedures. The Justice Department has ruled that the civil rights laws will not protect AIDS victims from being fired if their employers fear that they will spread the disease.

The truth is that AIDS is not a very contagious disease. To cause infection, the AIDS virus must find its way into the bloodstream, usually through intimate sexual contact or the sharing of IV drug needles. The virus does not live long outside the body, and it does not penetrate the skin. It is therefore not spread by routine social contact—or even close casual contact such as being coughed on, sneezed on, or kissed lightly, as one large study of people with AIDS living at home revealed. Nor can a person become infected from the water in a public swimming pool, from handling something an infected person has touched, from food handlers, or even from sharing tableware and drinking glasses. Even those who have had the closest casual contact with AIDS patients remain free of infection. No doctor, nurse, or aide who has cared for an AIDS patient has ever come down with the disease.

Source: Adapted from Jane E. Brody, "Separating the Myths and Fears from the Facts on How AIDS Is and Isn't Transmitted," *New York Times*, February 12, 1986.

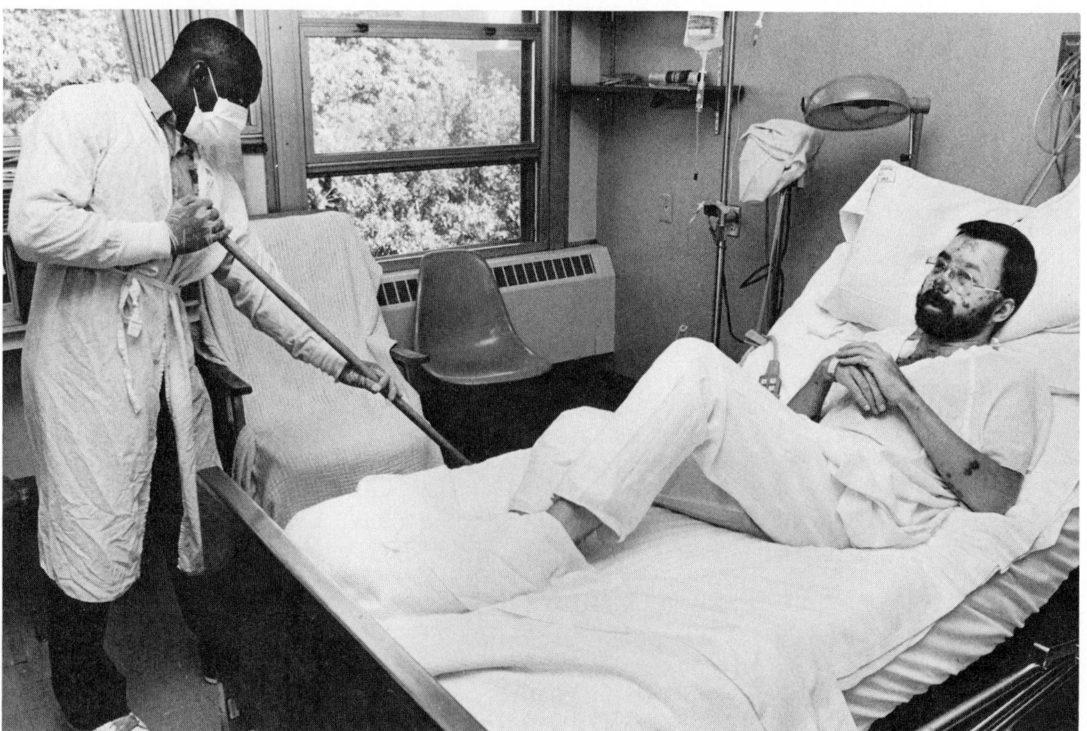

A hospital worker wears gloves and a mask while cleaning the room of an AIDS patient who has Kaposi's sarcoma. Such precautions are unnecessary.

Prevention Guidelines. With no viable vaccine in the immediate future, the only safe measure against AIDS is prevention. But what kind of prevention? For high-risk groups such as homosexual and bisexual men, simply reducing the number of sexual contacts is no answer when the exposure rate is so high. As the number of heterosexual carriers increases (AIDS is very widespread among prostitutes), heterosexuals are beginning to face high risks of infection from new sexual partners. The only safety appears to lie in abstention or in fidelity to a single partner who is free of infection. Since such self-discipline may not be a realistic expectation, the following guidelines will help to make sex safer:

- Do not have sexual relations with a prostitute of either sex.
- Avoid any direct anal, vaginal, or oral exposure to semen.
- Always use a condom; there is evidence that condoms can block the transmission of viruses. Diaphragms used together with spermicidal foams and gels are also thought to reduce the risk of infection.
- Avoid deep kissing; although saliva is not recognized as a source of infection, there may be some risk.

Other Sexually Transmitted Diseases

The following three sexually transmitted diseases are comparatively rare in the United States. Treatment for all three is with antibiotics.

Chancroid is caused by a bacillus, and generally produces an ulcer on the genitals and painful swollen glands after three to five days' incubation. Either sex can carry the infection without symptoms.

Lymphogranuloma venereum is caused by a small bacterium and can be contracted from infected bedding and clothing as well as from sexual intercourse. After five to twenty-one days' incubation, it produces a small genital blister or ulcer.

Granuloma inguinale is caused by a bacillus and is contracted sexually. After one to three weeks' incubation, it produces bright red painless genital sores.

Still another sexually transmitted disease is *trichomoniasis*, in which a purulent vaginal discharge may occur, causing itching and an unpleasant odor. It is caused by a protozoan, *Trichomonas vaginalis*. The disease responds readily to the drug metronidazole; because the organisms may also be in the male, sexual partners should be treated simultaneously.

OTHER COMMON COMMUNICABLE DISEASES

The following communicable diseases are of particular interest to young men and women living in restricted community situations such as campuses and dormitories. They range from such nuisances as the common cold to much more severe illnesses such as the lethal botulism.

The Common Cold

The **common cold** is a viral infection of the upper respiratory tract. The viruses responsible for the infection are transmitted directly through the spray discharged into the air when an infected person sneezes or coughs, or indirectly through articles soiled by the respiratory discharges of an infected person. The most frequent route of exposure has been discovered to be the hands. We shake hands with or otherwise touch a person who has a cold, and then transfer the germs to our own bodies by rubbing our eyes or nose.

Symptoms include a stuffy, achy feeling in the head, watering eyes, runny nose, chills, fever, and a general feeling of exhaustion. Most people have anywhere from one to six colds each year, usually in the fall, winter, and spring. Colds usually last from two to seven days.

There is no method of artificially immunizing oneself against colds, and for some reason the body is incapable of developing a permanent immunity against future infection. Part of the problem lies in the fact that there are so many different strains of cold virus—certainly as many as sixty. Researchers, however, are attempting to make more specific identifications of cold viruses so that it may be possible to develop a vaccine or some other means of immunization. At present treatment for a cold is rest, light diet, and the intake of plenty of fluids. The claim that massive doses of vitamin C can prevent colds has yet to be proven. Interferon sprays have been tested experimentally with promising results—they reduced the incidence of colds by 40 percent in test families who began to use them when one family member developed a cold—but they are not available on the market.

Influenza

Influenza is an acute viral infection of the respiratory tract. The viruses responsible for the disease (there are three major strains) are spread directly from person to person through coughing, or indirectly through the handling of articles that have been soiled by an infected person. There is an incubation period of from one to three days. The symptoms then appear abruptly and include fever, chills, headache, a sore throat, and exhaustion. A severe bronchial cough is characteristic of the disease. Serious complications such as bacterial pneumonia often occur after an attack of influenza. During the influenza epidemic of 1957–1958, for example, there were over 50,000 excess deaths—that is, unexpected deaths due to complications. In the 1972–1973 epidemic about 10,000 excess deaths occurred. Elderly people and those afflicted with heart and respiratory ailments are especially susceptible to complications. About 1,300 deaths from this disease occurred in the United States in 1984.

An influenza vaccine is available that confers immunity for about one year. Booster shots must be taken each year thereafter in order for the vaccine to remain effective. Also, a new vaccine must be created each time a new strain of influenza appears.

Pneumonia

Pneumonia, an acute infection of the lung, can be caused by bacteria, viruses, rickettsias, or fungi. It is a contagious disease, transmitted either directly, by inhaling the spray discharged into the air by an infected individual who coughs or sneezes, or indirectly, by handling the handkerchiefs or clothing soiled with the nasal or throat discharges of an infected person. Whatever the organism or mode of transmission, the symptoms are the same: the sudden appearance of chills, then fever and chest pains, a hoarse cough, and difficulty in breathing.

Pneumonia occurs most frequently in undernourished or weak individuals, such as the very young and the very old, and the lower-income inhabitants of large industrial cities. In infants the first symptoms are likely to be convulsions and vomiting. In the aged pneumonia is frequently a direct cause of death.

The mortality rate for persons suffering from pneumonia was at one time as high as 20 to 40 percent, but the use of antibiotics has reduced this enormously. Still, about 58,000 deaths from pneumonia occurred in the United States in 1984.

Tuberculosis

Tuberculosis is a chronic (long-lasting) disease caused by the tubercle bacillus. Though any part of the body may be infected (such as the bones, joints, or kidneys), the most common site is the lungs. The disease is usually transmitted directly from one person to another by the spray discharged into the air when an infected person coughs or spits. Most cases occur among young adults who live in poor and overcrowded conditions, and are discovered when a chest X ray is taken or a relapse of a long-dormant infection occurs.

Though the incidence of the disease is still high—between 25 and 30 million Americans are infected at present, and there are about 30,000 new cases each year—the mortality rate has declined dramatically, to about 1,300 deaths in 1984.

In the diagnosis of infectious mononucleosis, blood is tested for the presence of atypical white cells.

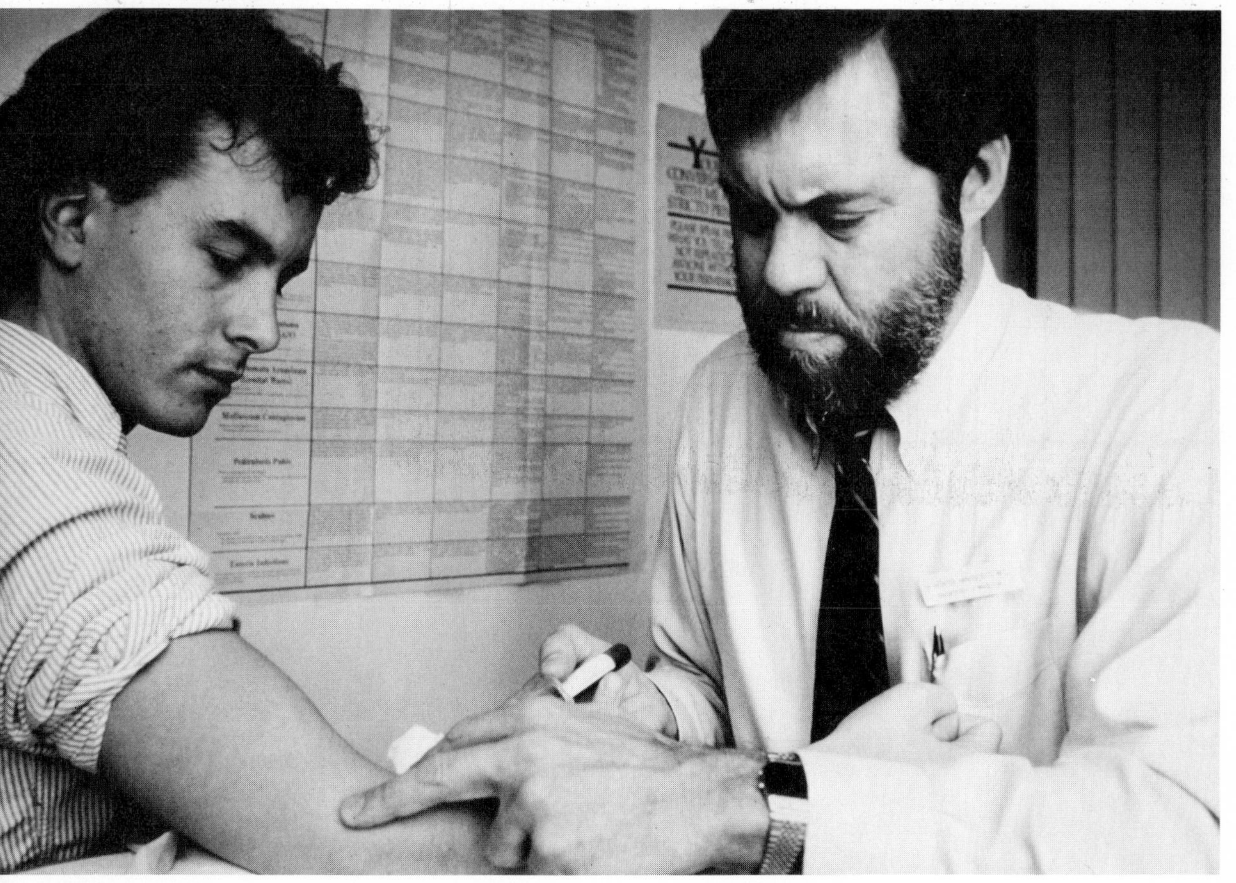

Infectious Mononucleosis

Infectious mononucleosis is an acute viral disease that often affects the lymph glands or the throat. How the disease is transmitted is uncertain, but it is likely that direct contact with an infected person, through touching or kissing, will transfer the infection.

About two to six weeks after invasion by the virus, the disease manifests itself in a fever, sore throat, swelling of the lymph glands (especially those in the back of the neck), fatigue, and an increase in mononuclear (single-nuclei) white blood cells.

Mononucleosis generally lasts from one to several weeks. It is seldom fatal, but it does bring on **jaundice** (yellowish pigmentation of the skin) in about 4 percent of those infected. It probably occurs most frequently in childhood as a minor infection, although it is diagnosed more often after adolescence when the infection is usually more severe. Although there is no evidence of permanent immunity, those who have been infected do seem to develop a resistance to the disease.

Hepatitis

There are three types of **hepatitis:** A, B, and non-A non-B. All are caused by a virus.

Infectious hepatitis (hepatitis A) is transmitted through respiratory discharges of the infected person or by fecal contamination of the food or water supply. There is an incubation period of about thirty days before the appearance of symptoms.

Serum hepatitis (hepatitis B) until recently was believed to be transmitted primarily by contaminated blood and used hypodermic needles, because it appeared in hospital patients requiring multiple transfusions and in drug addicts who shared needles. It now seems likely that the mode of transmission is broader than originally thought: Hepatitis B is fairly common in tropical countries, and is found in family clusters and in groups of sexually active persons. The incubation period ranges from 50 to 180 days.

The symptoms for both the A and B types of hepatitis vary widely. Initially, the infected person might feel tired, suffer loss of appetite, be nauseated, and suffer painful joints, a cough, sore throat, and low-grade fever. Often the first symptoms are mistaken for flu. Typically jaundice follows, beginning with the yellowing of the whites of the eyes and the skin, and lasts from six to eight weeks.

Less is known about **hepatitis non-A non-B.** Its incubation period is similar to that of hepatitis B, and it is also spread by contact with contaminated blood.

There is an enormous variance among hepatitis cases: Many are quite mild and never even develop jaundice; a very small percentage will progress to permanent liver damage (cirrhosis). In rare instances the disease can be fatal.

There is no specific treatment for hepatitis. Bed rest, avoidance of alcohol, and a high-calorie diet are usually prescribed. A serum, gamma globulin, when given to someone who has been exposed to the disease may prevent infection or lessen the severity of hepatitis A. A vaccine has been developed that provides immunity against hepatitis B. For all types of hepatitis, infection confers lasting immunity.

Food Poisoning Eating foods that have been contaminated by pathogenic bacteria or their toxins can cause food poisoning. There are four common forms of food poisoning: salmonella, *Clostridium perfringens*, staphylococcus, and *Clostridium botulinum*. In the common forms of food poisoning, the stomach and intestines become infected, causing the characteristic symptoms of abdominal pain, nausea, vomiting, and diarrhea. Treatment consists of bed rest and a liquid diet. Most people recover quickly.

Raw or partially cooked meats, eggs, and fish and food that is cooked in closed containers and later only partially reheated can easily become contaminated by pathogenic bacteria. Many foods can also be contaminated by an open infection on the person handling them.

A serious and often fatal food poisoning is **botulism**, which is caused by toxins that sometimes contaminate improperly canned foods. To avoid botulism, inspect food containers before you open them. Do not use any can that is bulging, broken, bent, or leaking. Avoid food that is unusual in color or odor. Do not taste a suspect food; even a small amount of botulism toxin can be fatal. Most cases of botulism result from eating home-canned foods.

SUMMARY

1. *Communicable diseases* are diseases caused by infectious microorganisms or by toxins, their poisonous by-products. Some of these diseases are contagious—that is, transferred directly from one person to another. Others, called *infectious diseases*, are transmitted by intermediaries, *vectors* or *vehicles* that carry the disease from one host body to another.

2. Natural body defenses against these diseases include the *skin*, internal body linings such as *mucous membranes*, body secretions, hydrochloric acid, antibodies, interferon, and white blood cells. A person may also have *natural*, or *inherited*, *immunity* to certain diseases.

3. Immunity to some diseases can be *acquired*. The *antibodies* and *interferon* manufactured by the body in response to certain diseases or to inoculations of vaccines and toxoids may give an individual *active immunity*. *Passive immunity* may be acquired with the injection of *antiserums* or *antitoxins*.

4. Among the most highly contagious and rapidly spread diseases are those which are *sexually transmitted*. This is all the more surprising because, in most cases, these diseases are easily diagnosed and their treatment is effective. The primary reason for the continued spread of such diseases is that, in spite of the recent sexual revolution, there remains a lingering haze of myth and misinformation around them. Many people are not familiar with the warning symptoms of sexually transmitted diseases, and others are too embarrassed to seek information or treatment.

5. The four major sexually transmitted, or *venereal*, diseases are syphilis, gonorrhea, herpes, and nonspecific urethritis (NSU).

6. *Syphilis* has three infectious stages: primary, secondary, and tertiary. Untreated tertiary syphilis can lead to a wide variety of disorders, and even death.

7. *Gonorrhea* is believed to occur ten times as frequently as syphilis. It is easily diagnosed in males but often goes unrecognized in females. Untreated gonorrhea can produce sterility, arthritis, heart disease, and other disorders.

8. *Genital herpes*, a viral infection whose symptoms disappear after about ten to twenty days, has spread alarmingly and so far is incurable.

9. *NSU* is the most common of all STDs. Its symptoms resemble those of gonorrhea, and it responds to treatment with antibiotics.

10. Untreated chlamydial and gonorrheal infections in women can lead to *pelvic inflammatory disease* (*PID*), a serious condition that can cause infertility, ectopic pregnancy, and blood poisoning; PID is treated with antibiotics. More common than herpes, *genital warts* are extremely contagious and have been associated with various cancers; they are treated by the application of a chemical solution or by surgery.

11. *Acquired immune deficiency syndrome*, or *AIDS*, is a new viral disease that cripples the body's immune system, leaving it open to opportunistic infections. It has spread rapidly among male homosexuals and IV drug users and is beginning to threaten the heterosexual population as well. It is always fatal, and there is no known treatment. It is transmitted almost entirely by infected semen during sexual intercourse or by contaminated blood and blood products.

12. Some comparatively rare STDs such as chancroid, *Lymphogranuloma venereum*, and *Granuloma inguinale* are cured by antibiotics. *Trichomoniasis*, an STD that causes a vaginal discharge, can also be easily cured.

13. Other common communicable diseases include the viral respiratory diseases such as the *common cold*, *influenza*, *pneumonia*, and *tuberculosis*. *Infectious mononucleosis* is another viral disease that affects the lymph glands and produces jaundice. Hepatitis is a serious viral disease, of which there are three types: A, or *infectious hepatitis*; B, or *serum hepatitis*; and *non-A non-B*. The first is transmitted by contaminated food and water, the second primarily, but not exclusively, by contaminated blood and hypodermic needles, and the third by contaminated blood. Contaminated food is responsible for various kinds of food poisoning such as *salmonella* and fatal *botulism*.

CONSUMER CONCERNS

1. A basic public health measure against communicable diseases is the immunization program. Since participants derive the benefits directly, why do so many parents fail to have their children immunized?
2. Do you feel that the continued prevalence of STDs is due more to indifference or to a lack of information? What role do guilt, fear, and stigma play?
3. Patients implore physicians to prescribe antibiotics, and physicians respond, even when there is no medical justification. What problems can this create?
4. Are you aware of the drugs to which you may be allergic? Do you ask questions about the side effects of drugs prescribed for you? How serious a problem is this?
5. The fear of AIDS has produced hysteria among many groups. What are some reasonable precautions that everyone should take?

16

Consumer Health

Problems of Medical Care
Selecting a Physician
Hospital Facilities
Nursing Homes
Financing Medical Services
Pharmaceuticals
Health, Science, and Decisions
Water Fluoridation
A Consumer Guide

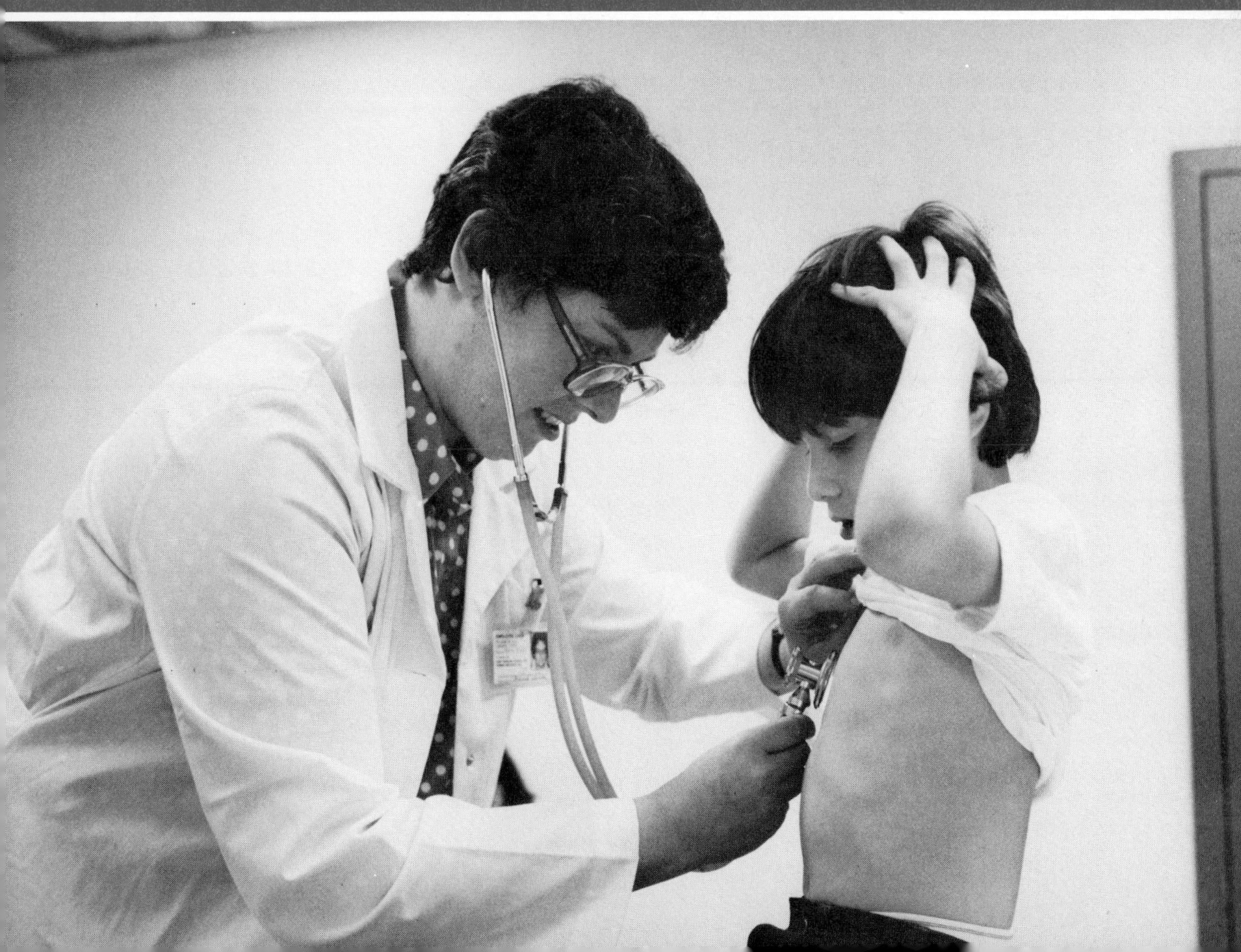

Consumers should approach the purchase of health services as they would any other commodity. Most consumers, however, do not really comprehend what is involved in the area of medical services. Moreover, they are apt to address their health problems only at a moment of crisis, when they are unable to think rationally about choosing physicians, hospitals, drugs, or insurance policies. Furthermore, adequate health services are a luxury a great many people in this country cannot afford.

Americans spent $387 billion for health care in 1984 (see Figure 16-1). The average cost for each of us was $1,580, paid by government agencies, insurance companies, and out of private pocketbooks. Federal, state, and local contributions paid nearly 40 percent of the bill; but millions of Americans had their savings wiped out in meeting rising medical costs.

Medical costs have risen steeply just at a time when the federal government has sharply reduced the number of health-care services. Consumer protection has also suffered, and consumer activists have experienced setbacks because of cuts in the funding of federal agencies established to protect consumer rights.

In this chapter we shall first examine how sound consumer practices can be applied to the purchase of health services. We shall discuss specific problems such as the distinctions among forms of health insurance; how to select a physician, hospital, or nursing home; and the controversial aspects of some current health practices and therapies. Although we cannot discuss all the forms of

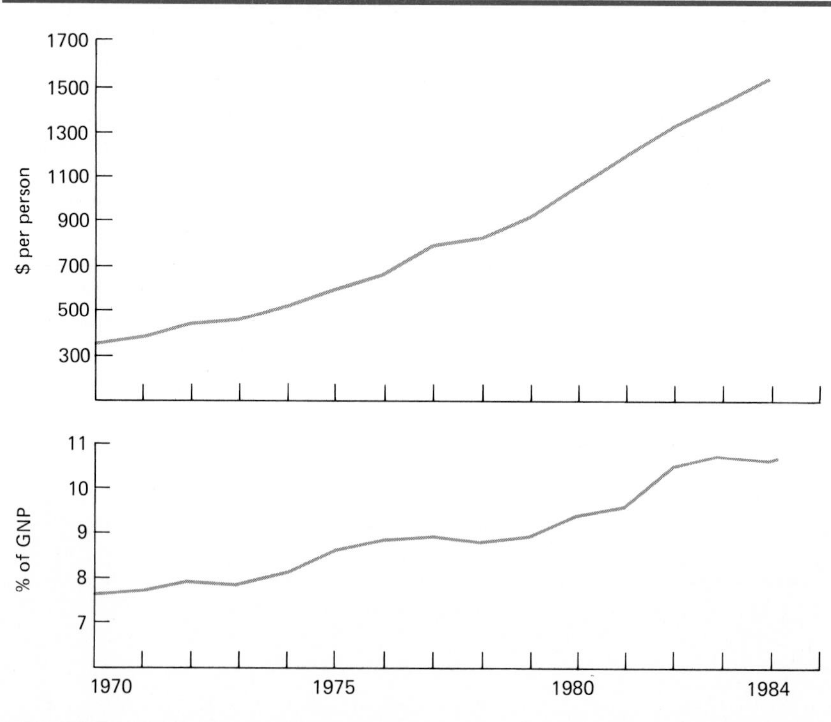

FIGURE 16-1

National health expenditures in the United States: Dollars per person and by percent of Gross National Product

Source: Health Care Financing Administration, 1986.

health quackery, we shall examine the increasing gullibility of many Americans who seek health cures. Health experts despair over the proliferation of charlatans in every area of cure and prevention. Purveyors of ineffective cures would not be in business—and opening new businesses every day—if they did not enjoy a ready market of uninformed consumers. The causes of this trend are hard to identify in a modern, technologically advanced, literate society such as ours. Some analysts believe that the daily reporting of conflicting findings in the media has confused the public and lowered its confidence in scientific documentation and recommendations from medical authorities.

Government regulation of unproven health remedies may be more important now than ever before. We shall examine the role of government in health care and then discuss the ways in which we can become knowledgeable consumer advocates.

PROBLEMS OF MEDICAL CARE

The most significant measures of the quality of medical care in a country are the **life expectancy** and **infant mortality rates.** Though the figures for life expectancy continue to rise in the United States, they are not as high as those of many other nations. We also continue to have higher infant mortality rates than many other developed countries (see Table 16-1). In addition, our maternal death rates are high. One explanation for this is that an estimated 33.7 million Americans who live at or below the poverty level cannot afford existing medical care. The difference in death rates between blacks and whites in the United States illustrates this clearly. Although there are more poor whites than poor blacks, a larger proportion of the black population is poor: 31 percent of black households as compared to 9 percent of white families. The mortality rate for black infants is almost twice that for white infants, and the maternal death rate among black women is more than three times that among white women.

The adverse nutritional and environmental conditions found among the poor affect their health at every level. The incidence of disability is almost three times higher among the poor, and chronic illnesses are seen four times as often.

Rapidly rising medical costs and the unequal distribution of doctors in this country have aggravated the problem of health care for rich and poor, though not equally for the two groups. Advances in medical knowledge have contributed to rising costs. As individual lives have been prolonged, the number of elderly persons requiring medical services has increased and will continue to do so as people in the baby-boom age group, now approaching their 40s, grow older and need more medical attention.

The disparity in medical care for the poor and nonpoor and the inadequate distribution of health services raises one final point: The United States ranks below many other developed countries in quality of health care. In countries like Sweden and Norway, which have national health programs, high-quality, state-subsidized medical services are made available to both rich and poor in urban and rural areas. This contrasts sharply with the situation in our own country, where adequate medical care is beyond the reach of many families. And when any segment of the population is chronically ill, other groups suffer as well.

TABLE 16-1
Infant Mortality Rates in Selected Countries

Country	Mortality Rate*
Japan	6
Iceland	7
Sweden	7
Switzerland	8
France	9
Canada	9
Spain	10
United States	11
USSR	32
Mexico	53
Algeria	109

* Deaths under 1 year per 1,000 live births.
Source: Population Reference Bureau, *1985 World Population Data Sheet* (Washington, D.C., 1985).

Unequal Distribution of Physicians

From a shortage of physicians nationally as late as 1970, we have gone to what may already be a surplus of doctors in many parts of the country. The cities and suburbs have always been well served; now more and more small communities can boast internists, family practitioners, and an increasing number of specialists. The most serious and complicated procedures still need to be performed in large medical centers, often connected with medical schools. But looked at as a whole, the supply of physicians is adequate in the United States and a surplus is rapidly appearing.

Still, if overall there are 220 active physicians for every 100,000 Americans, they are not distributed equally throughout the population. Physicians tend to cluster in urban areas, particularly where they have access to large hospitals and medical schools. Thus South Dakota and Wyoming, two of the least urban states, also have the fewest physicians per person, while Massachusetts and New York, two of the most urban states, have the greatest number per person.

Within the areas of greatest concentration of doctors, their distribution is still inequitable. When a census of physicians in private practice was made in the 1970s, New York's densely populated Central Harlem area was found to be served by a number of private doctors only one-fifth the national average. Harlem's mostly poor and mostly black residents were being served primarily in hospital emergency rooms. It is not surprising that most physicians prefer to locate their practices in more affluent areas, but their doing so greatly reduces the quality of our health care.

Specialization

There are twenty-five recognized medical specialties. Of the 502,000 active physicians in the United States in 1982, about 440,000 (88 percent) practiced specialties and only 62,000 (12 percent) were general practitioners (see Figure 16-2).

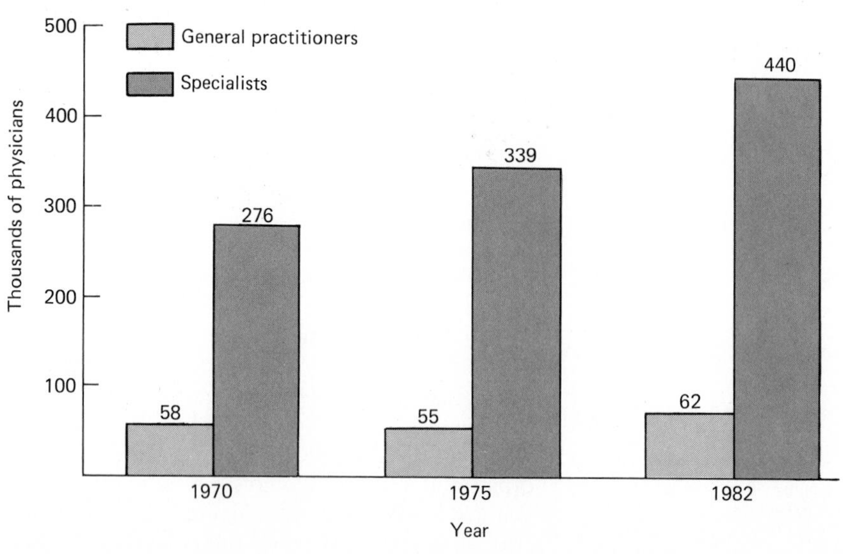

FIGURE 16-2

Trends in type of medical practice

Source: Statistical Abstract of the United States, 1986.

Why do physicians specialize? An important factor is the relatively recent explosion of medical knowledge. Today physicians are faced with an overwhelming mass of medical information. Forty years ago a physician could keep up with most of the new medical discoveries and methods of treatment, but the enormous number of medical research reports published annually now makes this impossible. Since physicians cannot keep abreast of all developments, they concentrate on what most interests them. Today even general practitioners are apt to have specialized medical interests and skills. Another great impetus to specialization is financial advantage. The average annual income for general practitioners is only about two-thirds that of obstetrician-gynecologists.

Specialization is absolutely essential if we are to obtain the best medical care. But it presents an important medical-care problem because there is often no one to look at the patient as a total person. It is conceivable that a patient will be sent to one specialist for a skin ailment, to another for a digestive complaint, to a third for a broken bone, and so on. The traditional family doctor who personally knew the patient and the patient's family and home life has for many people been replaced by a mosaic of specialists, who sometimes seem more concerned about their own square inch of patient than they are about the patient's total well-being.

Thus in this age of specialization people are faced with a double problem. First, they are forced to consult a number of physicians for a variety of complaints. This fragmentation of medical attention may provide heightened skill and knowledge, but it also creates a sense of personal detachment between physician and patient. Second, because individuals must arrange a separate examination for each type of ailment, their medical expenses are compounded. Instead of seeing one physician for all their ills and paying an inclusive fee, they visit several specialists, thereby multiplying the cost.

This problem is being coped with in at least two ways. First, there is an annually increasing number of graduates in a new medical specialty, **family practice.** Like the old-fashioned general practitioner, the specialist in family practice deals with the full range of medical problems that the family experiences, from delivering babies to setting broken bones. But unlike the general practitioner, the family practitioner has to complete a three-year residency, be certified in this specialty by passing a rigorous examination, and be recertified every six years.

Second, an increasing number of Americans are choosing to join health maintenance organizations (discussed later in this chapter). HMOs emphasize preventive care. Most HMO groups provide members with total health care through their organization of participating physicians. This closed structure theoretically enables physicians to know patients better than they are likely to under the "fee-for-service" system.

SELECTING A PHYSICIAN

Selecting a personal or family physician is not an easy task. It requires coolheadedness and sound judgment; therefore it should be undertaken when you are healthy and unstressed, not when you are in the midst of a medical emergency. There are many things to consider, beginning with the type of physician that will best serve your needs, where to find such a physician, what credentials and affiliations to look for, fees and payment schedules, and a number of important personal factors.

Primary-Care Physicians*

First, you must determine the type of primary-care physician you need. A **primary-care physician** is aware of your entire medical history and the specific details of your life: your family relationships, occupation, living conditions, and emotional stresses. He or she is the doctor you consult first when you have a medical problem, and the one who will refer you to a specialist or hospitalize you if necessary.

The two major kinds of primary-care physicians are family practitioners and internists. In addition, many women make their obstetrician-gynecologist their main medical-care provider, while many families choose a pediatrician to oversee the health of their children. However, **family practitioners** treat people of all ages and are able to take care of most routine medical problems. To be fully qualified, a family practitioner must have three years of internship and residency and receive special training in obstetrics, gynecology, internal medicine, dermatology, and pediatrics. **Internists,** on the other hand, focus on the general care of adults, particularly diseases of the heart, lungs, liver, stomach and intestines, urinary tract, and endocrine glands. They also receive special training in chronic diseases such as arthritis and diabetes.

* This section is based in part on suggestions contained in The Columbia University College of Physicians and Surgeons *Complete Home Medical Guide* (New York: Crown, 1985).

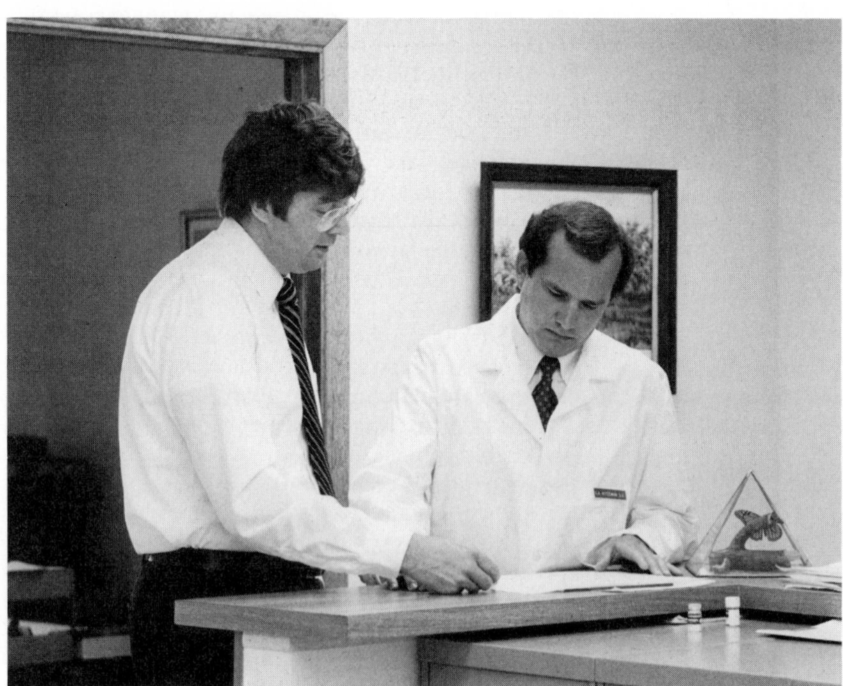

In looking for a primary-care physician, a good source is the staff of a teaching hospital. Such doctors usually maintain a private practice as well.

Sources of Names. Probably the best place to look first for the name of a qualified primary-care physician is a good hospital, especially a teaching hospital, or a medical school. Most doctors who teach also maintain private practices. The next best source is the *AMA Directory* or the *Directory of Medical Specialists*; both can be found in a public library. Friends and relatives are not always reliable sources of information; while they can describe a doctor's office manner or personality, they are not really competent to judge how well a doctor has handled a difficult medical problem.

Qualifications. Once you have the names of one or two doctors, you should look into their background. The medical school a physician has attended should be fully accredited; this is particularly important if it is one located outside the United States, Canada, or Western Europe. Also important is a physician's place of internship and residency, particularly if the medical school attended is not familiar. Most qualified physicians are members of a local medical society; and if specialists, they should be board-certified. A board-certified family practitioner, for example, is required to keep up-to-date on the latest medical knowledge and must be periodically recertified. Hospital affiliation is another important consideration. Hospital affiliation permits a doctor to have patients admitted and treated through the hospital's facilities; and if it is an accredited hospital or a teaching hospital, such affiliation is a reliable indicator of a physician's quality and competence.

Some Practical Matters. A number of practical considerations will also determine what physician you choose. One of the most important is fees and payment schedules. You should not hesitate to ask about a doctor's range of fees for services, including office visits, complete physical exams, and the occasional necessary house call. You should also inquire whether a physician demands cash payment for each visit, accepts Medicare and Medicaid patients, and is agreeable to deferred methods of payment. You should also ask if the doctor is willing to answer questions over the phone once in a while. If the doctor is not part of a group practice, find out who covers when he or she is out of town.

Some Personal Matters. Because you will be disclosing intimate details of your personal life to a physician, it is essential that he or she be someone you can talk to freely; for this reason, many people prefer a doctor of their own sex. And since this person will be your primary-care provider and medical-history keeper for many years to come, you may want to choose someone young enough to outlive you.

The Physical Examination. The way a doctor conducts a physical exam reveals a lot about his or her competence and methods. A thorough physical exam involves a medical history followed by a complete visual inspection of the unclothed body head to toe. It should take no less than thirty minutes and most often requires an hour. In addition to questioning you about your physical health, your doctor should ask about your family situation, finances, employment, emotional problems, and smoking, eating, drinking, and exercise habits. He or she should avoid jargon and explain medical matters in language you can understand.

Many people are intimidated by physicians and lack the courage to assert themselves in a doctor's office. As a patient, you have a right to question any proposed medical procedure and to be told its risks and benefits; you also have a right to be told the results of all tests, what they mean, and how accurate the results are. If you disagree with a diagnosis, you should say so; you should also demand more information when you feel a doctor is giving you only partial or evasive answers.

Unwarranted Surgery

Concurrent with a decrease in general practitioners in this country is the enormous increase in the number of surgeons. With this greater number of surgeons goes an exceptionally high number of operations, many of them unwarranted. Compared to Great Britain, for example, the United States has, proportionally, double the number of surgeons—and double the annual rate of operations. Most unwarranted operations are tonsillectomies and hysterectomies (the latter with a fatality rate of 200 per 100,000 operations). In a survey of several thousand hysterectomies performed in New England, Dr. Osler Peterson of the Harvard Medical School discovered that a normal uterus had been removed in about 50 percent of the cases.

To help prevent unnecessary surgery, insurance carriers have begun paying for second opinions when a physician recommends nonemergency, elective surgery. Medicare also pays for second opinions. It is now becoming acceptable to seek a third opinion, should the first two be in disagreement. According to one study conducted by Blue Cross/Blue Shield of Greater New York, this

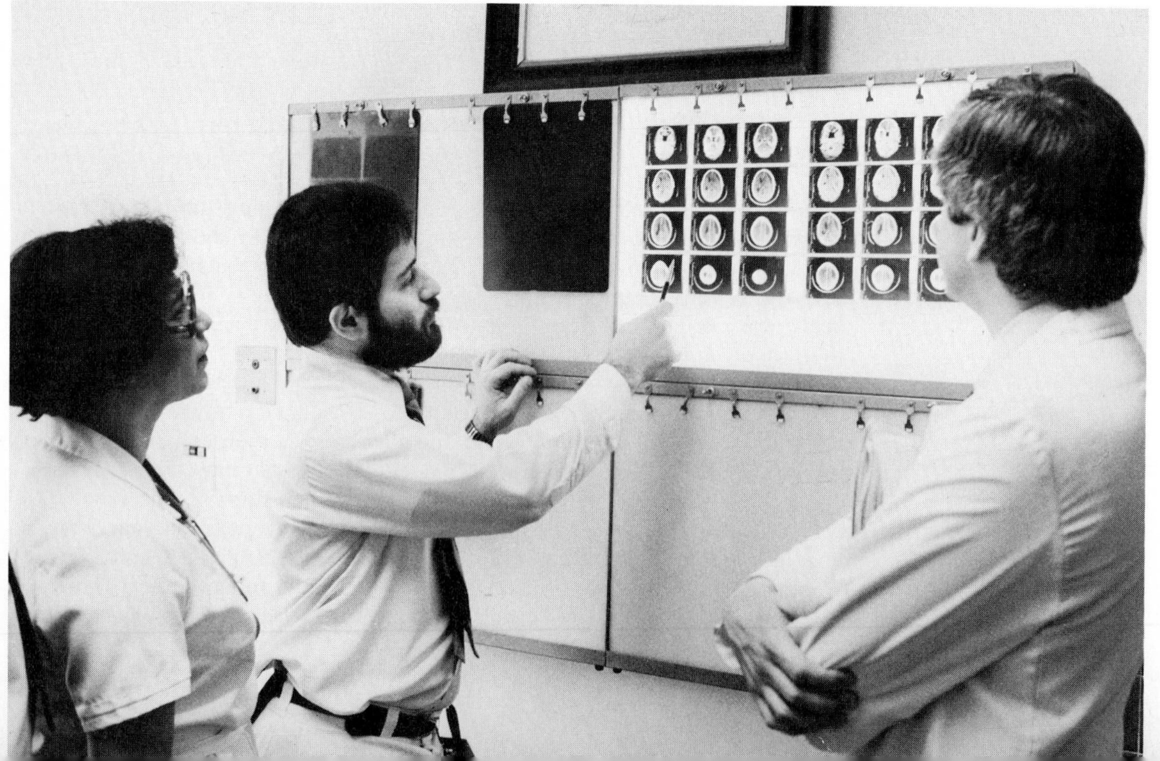

Advances in medical technology—such as the CAT scans being examined here—have made possible improvements in medical diagnosis but have also raised the cost of health care.

PROBLEMS AND CONTROVERSIES: *Malpractice Insurance—Is Everybody at Fault?*

As the image of the kindly family physician dedicated to human service has given way to that of the uncaring and avaricious specialist, the number of malpractice suits against physicians has tripled over the last ten years, and the average award to a plaintiff in such a suit has become astronomical. As a result, malpractice insurance premiums have skyrocketed, the costs of health care have risen sharply, and many medical specialists have simply discontinued practice.

Physicians' groups blame overly sympathetic juries and the legal profession for the size of the awards (the average is now over $1 million). Plaintiffs are being compensated not only for out-of-pocket costs such as medical expenses and time lost from work, but also for "pain and suffering." And they are often given enormous settlements not only when the physician was neglectful or incompetent, but also when the physician performed a medical procedure correctly but the patient suffered a "bad result." Physicians say they are unfairly being held accountable for consequences that are not predictable and that many patients today feel entitled to rich compensation if it can be had.

Physicians also blame personal injury lawyers for many of their malpractice problems. The fact that some lawyers openly advertise their availability in such cases encourages many to pursue legal recourse. Contingent fees—the practice whereby a lawyer represents a plaintiff in return for a share of any damages won—are also seen as a potent force in the trend toward multimillion-dollar suits.

Lawyers say that if they did not work on a contingency basis, poor people who have been injured by incompetent doctors would never receive justice because they could not afford to advance a retainer's fee for legal counsel. Lawyers also claim that there are not that many really large settlements, and that those few are justified. More than two-thirds of the multimillion-dollar awards, they say, have been for serious injuries such as permanent paralysis or death.

To protect themselves from malpractice suits, doctors are ordering many more diagnostic tests for patients. Such "defensive medicine" is adding $15 billion to $40 billion a year to health-care costs in the United States. To protect themselves from the heavy financial drain of multimillion-dollar awards, insurance companies claim that they have had to raise their premiums by 400 to 600 percent. The average physician in many states is now paying about $16,000 a year in malpractice premiums, and such specialists as obstetricians, orthopedists, and neurosurgeons are paying between $40,000 and $100,000 a year. Obstetricians have been the most frequently sued doctors, and as a result 3,000 of them have abandoned their specialty.

Several remedies for the problem of large medical malpractice awards are under consideration. Some states are recommending putting a limit on the amount of damages a plaintiff can collect in any suit—for example, Missouri has already limited "pain and suffering" awards to $300,000. To discourage lawyers from seeking huge damages for clients, several states want to impose a sliding scale that would diminish the percentage of a lawyer's share of damages as the amount of the award increases. Other states are establishing pretrial review boards of medical specialists to decide beforehand whether a malpractice case has sufficient merit to go to court.

Sources: "Sorry, Your Policy Is Canceled," *Time*, March 24, 1986, pp. 16–26; "An Epidemic of Malpractice Suits," *Newsweek*, January 28, 1985, p. 62; Nicholas D. Kristoff, "Insurance Woes Spur Many States to Amend Law on Liability Suits," *New York Times*, March 31, 1986, pp. A1, A13.

practice has called into question the advisability of as many as one in every four operations currently performed.

Many hospitals in this country, it is true, do have review groups or "tissue committees" to oversee the type of surgery being performed. Thus if it appears that a particular surgeon has been removing an unusual number of healthy organs, he or she may be censured by colleagues. However, this type of review doesn't help the patient because it occurs after surgery has already taken place.

Medical Incompetence

While most American physicians are well trained, the group has its share of incompetents. A 1986 report of the U.S. Health and Human Services Department estimated that anywhere from 5 to 15 percent of U.S. physicians ought not to be practicing or require some form of disciplinary action.

Medical incompetence leads to poor care; in addition, it can result in unnecessary expenditure. The Public Citizen's Health Research Group, directed by Ralph Nader, estimated that $21.5 billion is spent annually on needless surgery, X rays, and drugs. Some 30,000 hospital deaths annually are attributed to adverse reactions to drugs.

Under the present system, incompetent doctors are supposed to be disciplined by a variety of agencies such as state medical boards, private medical societies, hospital medical staffs, and peer review agencies. The problem is that those who know the most about professional incompetence—doctors, hospitals, and medical societies—are reluctant to come forward with the information.

Although the number of malpractice suits and complaints to medical boards has risen to an all-time high, many state medical boards spend most of their time investigating the credentials of foreign-trained physicians who are applying for state licenses. They do not have the personnel to investigate the vast backlog of complaints against practicing doctors.

The American Medical Association, long considered a conservative force and resistant to outside policies, has itself called for a nationwide peer review system for monitoring the performance of doctors in hospitals. As things stand now, incompetent doctors who are discharged from one hospital are free to begin practicing at another. In its 1985 report the AMA called for increasing the investigative and disciplinary powers of state licensing boards, and entering the results of investigations into a national computer registry; thus doctors who lose their license in one state would be unable to practice in others.

The 1986 Health and Human Services Department report recommended a number of changes in the laws and regulations affecting hospitals and physicians. For example: Hospitals that do not report incompetent physicians to state medical boards should be prevented from receiving Medicare payments; physicians who have been disciplined by state boards should also be denied Medicare payments; and finally, state boards should be required to report incompetent doctors to the federal government.

One of the surest ways to ensure high-quality medical service is to make physicians undergo periodic reexaminations. At present several states no longer license physicians for life, but instead renew licenses only upon proof of further education through course work and attendance at scientific meetings.

HOSPITAL FACILITIES

Hospitals can be divided into two broad groups: general and specialty. General medical and surgical hospitals provide for the diagnosis and treatment of a wide range of conditions. Eighty-seven percent of these hospitals are classifed as short-term institutions. Institutions that admit individuals with specific conditions or diseases are specialty hospitals. In contrast to general hospitals, most specialty hospitals are classified as long-term-care hospitals. The majority of these institutions treat psychiatric conditions, tuberculosis, or chronic diseases.

Types of Hospitals

The financing of a hospital determines whether it is classified as voluntary, government, or private. (Figure 16-3 shows the percentage of each type in the total number of hospitals in the United States.) **Voluntary hospitals** are public, nonprofit general-care hospitals run by religious or charitable organizations or by individuals. They admit more than two-thirds of all hospital patients and treat many emergency cases and welfare patients under local government contracts. **Government,** or **public, hospitals** are maintained by federal, state, and local governments. They care for military and Public Health Service personnel, American Indians, and merchant seamen. They handle narcotics addiction and long-term illnesses such as tuberculosis or leprosy, provide psychiatric care, and treat other special medical problems. In addition, local government hospitals provide general and emergency medical care and treat welfare patients. **Private,** or **proprietary, hospitals** are operated by individuals or corporations as a profit-making business. They treat patients with short-term illnesses and usually do not accept those unable to pay. Proprietary hospitals are often smaller than voluntary hospitals and are not as well equipped or staffed; only about one-third are accredited.

How to Evaluate a Hospital

Three major points should be considered in evaluating a hospital: accreditation, affiliation with a medical school, and size. To be accredited by the Joint Commission on Accreditation, the major hospital-monitoring body in the United States, a hospital must meet minimum standards for staff training and performance, equipment, surgical methods, food-service facilities, pharmaceutical facilities, and medical recordkeeping. Any hospital that is affiliated with a medical school—a *teaching hospital*—almost always provides high-quality medical care. Experienced physicians act as teachers and the staff is highly qualified. Some unaffiliated hospitals that have training programs for physicians and interns also provide quality care. As for size, small hospitals can offer only a few services and have

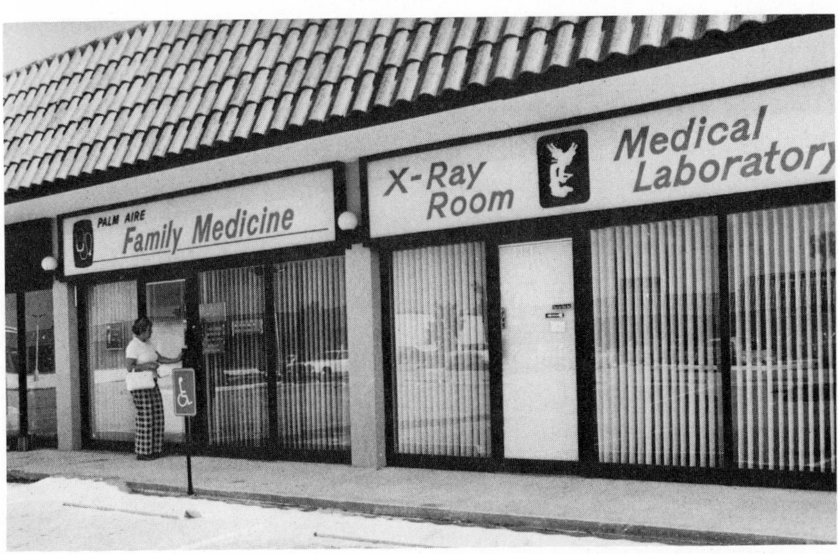

A community health center in Florida.

A Patient's Bill of Rights

1. *The patient has the right to considerate and respectful care.*
2. *The patient has the right to obtain from his physician complete current information concerning his diagnosis, treatment, and prognosis in terms the patient can be reasonably expected to understand. When it is not medically advisable to give such information to the patient, the information should be made available to an appropriate person in his behalf. He has the right to know, by name, the physician responsible for coordinating his care.*
3. *The patient has the right to receive from his physician information necessary to give informed consent prior to the start of any procedure and treatment. Except in emergencies, such information for informed consent should include but not necessarily be limited to the specific procedure and/or treatment, the medically significant risks involved, and the probable duration of incapacitation. Where medically significant alternatives for care or treatment exist, or when the patient requests information concerning medical alternatives, the patient has the right to such information. The patient also has the right to know the name of the person responsible for the procedures and/or treatment.*
4. *The patient has the right to refuse treatment to the extent permitted by law and to be informed of the medical consequences of his action.*
5. *The patient has the right to every consideration of his privacy concerning his own medical-care program. Case discussion, consultation, examination, and treatment are confidential and should be conducted discreetly. Those not directly involved in his care must have the permission of the patient to be present.*
6. *The patient has the right to expect that all communications and records pertaining to his care should be treated as confidential.*
7. *The patient has the right to expect that within its capacity a hospital must make reasonable response to the request of a patient for services. The hospital must provide evaluation, service, and/or referral as indicated by the urgency of the case. When medically permissible, a patient may be transferred to another facility only after he has received complete information and explanation concerning the needs for and alternatives to such a transfer. The institution to which the patient is to be transferred must first have accepted the patient for transfer.*
8. *The patient has the right to obtain information as to any relationship of his hospital to other health care and educational institutions insofar as his care is concerned. The patient has the right to obtain information as to the existence of any professional relationships among individuals, by name, who are treating him.*
9. *The patient has the right to be advised if the hospital proposes to engage in or perform human experimentation affecting his care or treatment. The patient has the right to refuse to participate in such research projects.*
10. *The patient has the right to expect reasonable continuity of care. He has the right to know in advance what appointment times and physicians are available and where. The patient has the right to expect that the hospital will provide a mechanism whereby he is informed by his physician or a delegate of the physician of the patient's continuing health care requirements following discharge.*
11. *The patient has the right to examine and receive an explanation of his bill regardless of source of payment.*
12. *The patient has the right to know what hospital rules and regulations apply to his conduct as a patient.*

Source: *A Patient's Bill of Rights*, published by the American Hospital Association, copyright © 1972. Reprinted with permission.

few specialists on their staffs. A large hospital, with a minimum of 200 beds, usually offers the best medical services.

Centers for Minor Surgery and Emergencies

Two new medical facilities have been devised for patients who do not require hospitalization. **Ambulatory surgical centers,** or **surgicenters,** perform minor, low-risk procedures such as tissue biopsies, cosmetic surgery, hernia repairs, abortions, and D&Cs (dilation and curettage). Local anesthesia is used, and patients go home the same day. In communities that are far away from hospitals, small private **freestanding emergency centers,** or **urgicenters,** provide many of the same services as hospital emergency departments but at far less cost. Most are open twenty-four hours a day, seven days a week, and treat simple bone fractures, sprains, bruises, wounds that need stitches, and respiratory infections. About half are operated by nonprofit hospitals; the rest by physicians' chains and other for-profit organizations. Before using either of these facilities, however, one should check the qualifications of their physicians, determine whether they are affiliated with a good hospital in case a transfer is necessary, and learn whether they have established, thorough follow-up procedures.

The Patient

In 1972 the American Hospital Association compiled a set of guidelines indicating what a patient should expect from a hospital. These constitute *A Patient's Bill of Rights* and include the patient's right to receive respectful care; to be given complete information regarding diagnosis, treatment, and prognosis; to receive information necessary for consent prior to any procedure; to refuse treatment; to enjoy privacy regarding care and records; to be granted requests for services within reason; to be advised of any experimental procedure; to expect continuity of care; to receive explanation of the bill; and to know which hospital regulations are applicable to the patient.

These guidelines are timely, because the average hospital patient feels anxious and insignificant in the impersonal atmosphere of a hospital. What is worse, diagnosis and treatment are often performed without the patient's knowing the details of the illness or the type of medication to be received. Many physicians feel this kind of information is beyond the patient's understanding and will only cause anxiety. The result of such "protection" is that the physically ill patient feels emotionally upset as well.

An individual who moves frequently from one community to another may have come into contact with dozens of doctors and numerous hospitals. Each of these physicians and institutions has a record of visits or stays; but no comprehensive, continuous record of care exists. Thus costly diagnostic procedures may have to be repeated. There is also the chance that improper or conflicting medications may be prescribed.

Many doctors believe that having a systematized record of all medical care for each individual is the answer. Such a record would be a complete personal reference source for the patient, to be shared with physicians and hospitals. Continuity of treatment could be assured, and patient access to medical records could be improved.

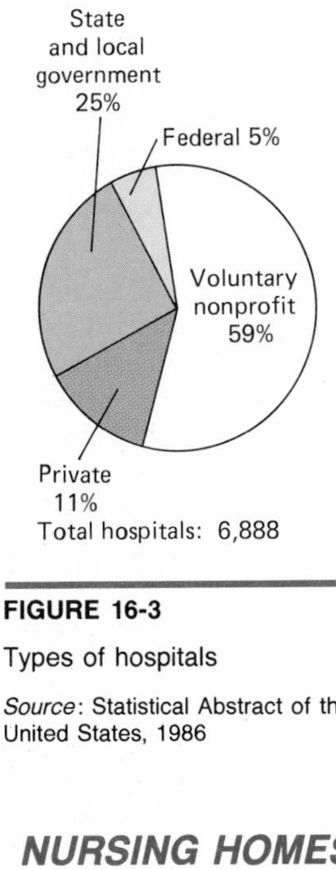

FIGURE 16-3

Types of hospitals

Source: Statistical Abstract of the United States, 1986

NURSING HOMES

Nursing homes, while not designed exclusively for the care of the elderly, draw the great majority of their patients from the ranks of the aged (see Chapter 10). And since the U.S. population is an aging one, the need for this type of health service will certainly increase in the near future. The past two decades

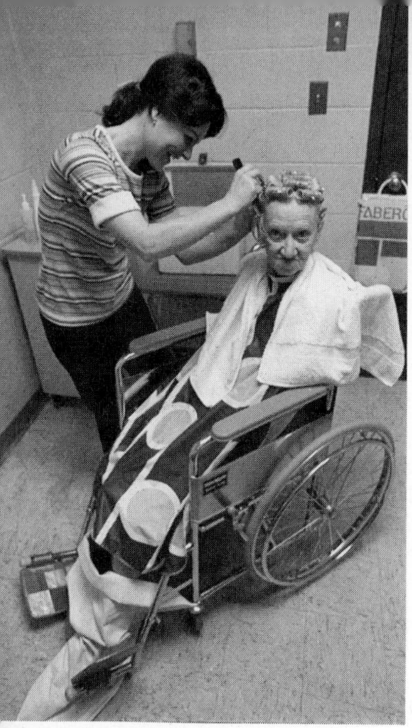

In a good nursing home a resident receives loving attention.

have already witnessed an explosive growth in this particular type of facility, partly because of the availability of Medicare and Medicaid funds. This sudden access of funds caught people in government and the health-care field unprepared, and subsequently a number of substandard operations were permitted to flourish. The hazards and abuses to patients in such establishments have been well documented. As early as 1974 a New York investigation turned up shocking instances of patient abuse, neglect, and fraud. And each year since, there have been revelations of proprietors taking advantage of helpless old people.

When selecting a nursing home, the consumer should make use of all existing sources of counsel—the local health department, social agencies, the medical profession, nursing associations, and friends who have undergone a similar experience. Personal visits should be made to prospective nursing homes, and checklists should be kept on critical factors such as: the quality of administration; the physical layout of the facility and its degree of practicality and cleanliness; the facility's manner of operation, as defined in terms of programs, attentiveness to patients, and visiting hours; services such as medical attention, availability of nurses, and, importantly, financial arrangements.

Because of the growing high cost of nursing-home care—and the growing number of people who will need it as the baby-boom generation reaches retirement age—the government is looking for solutions. Long-term nursing-home care is the most rapidly rising cost for Medicaid. Either costs must be lowered or alternatives must be found. The principal alternative under investigation is home care; communities and families would take over functions now left to institutions.

FINANCING MEDICAL SERVICES

Most people, even those with above-average incomes, worry more about how they are going to pay for medical services than about choosing a physician or hospital. The cost of medical care amounted to 10.6 percent of GNP in 1984, or $1,580 per American. Without insurance, many people could not afford the medical care they need, and a major illness or operation could spell financial disaster for all but the very wealthy.

In 1940 only 9 percent of Americans had even the simplest form of health insurance; today 85 percent of Americans are insured. However, this still leaves some 35 million of us uninsured, and the rest of us liable in varying degrees for medical costs that could be devastating.

Choosing a Nursing Home

The American Health Care Association provides a 135-point checklist for choosing a nursing home. The brochure, available from the association at 1200 15th Street NW, Washington, D.C. 20005, suggests, among other things, that you check a prospective home at an unguarded moment: Stop by on a Saturday evening and ask to taste the supper.

Source: *The (Bergen County, N.J.) Record*, March 15, 1985.

Important Insurance Terms

- *Deductible*: A deductible is the amount you must spend within a stated period of time before you become eligible for benefits from an insurance company. The higher the deductible, the less the benefit of the policy.
- *Exclusion*: Many policies do not cover psychotherapy, cosmetic surgery, and other services. Check your policy to see what is and is not covered.
- *Limitation*: There is often a limitation on the amount an insurance company will pay for certain services such as office visits and some kinds of surgery. Insurance companies also limit the number of consultations during a hospitalization and the total number of hospital days that are covered.

Medical services are usually financed by one of four methods: (1) private health insurance; (2) public tax-supported insurance such as Medicare and Medicaid; (3) prepaid comprehensive programs such as those offered by health maintenance organizations; and (4) national health insurance, as found in most major industrial countries other than in the United States.

Private Health Insurance

Insurance companies sell private health insurance plans to groups and to individuals. While group plans offer a wide range of benefits and are less expensive than individual plans, the benefits cannot be tailored to a person's special needs. There are a number of other shortcomings in both group and individual plans. First, besides being expensive, they often have a high deductible (see box: Important Insurance Terms) and put a ceiling on the amount of money they will pay. Second, they often exclude high-risk individuals. And third, group coverage may cease when a person becomes unemployed or changes jobs.

Most private health insurance is provided by group plans, usually through places of employment. The premium may be paid entirely by the employer or it may be divided between employer and employee. The benefits may be paid to the patient after he or she submits a bill from a doctor or hospital, or directly to the doctor or hospital.

Six types of policies are offered by insurance companies:

- Hospital insurance
- Medical-surgical insurance
- Major medical insurance
- Disability insurance
- Medicare supplementary insurance
- Dental insurance

Hospital Insurance. Hospital insurance plans such as Blue Cross cover part of the expenses for room and board, nursing services, drugs, anesthetics, and the use of an operating room and laboratory for a specified number of days. They do not reimburse for private-duty nurses or for physicians' fees; and they do not cover additional hospitalization, should an illness run over the maximum number of days allowed.

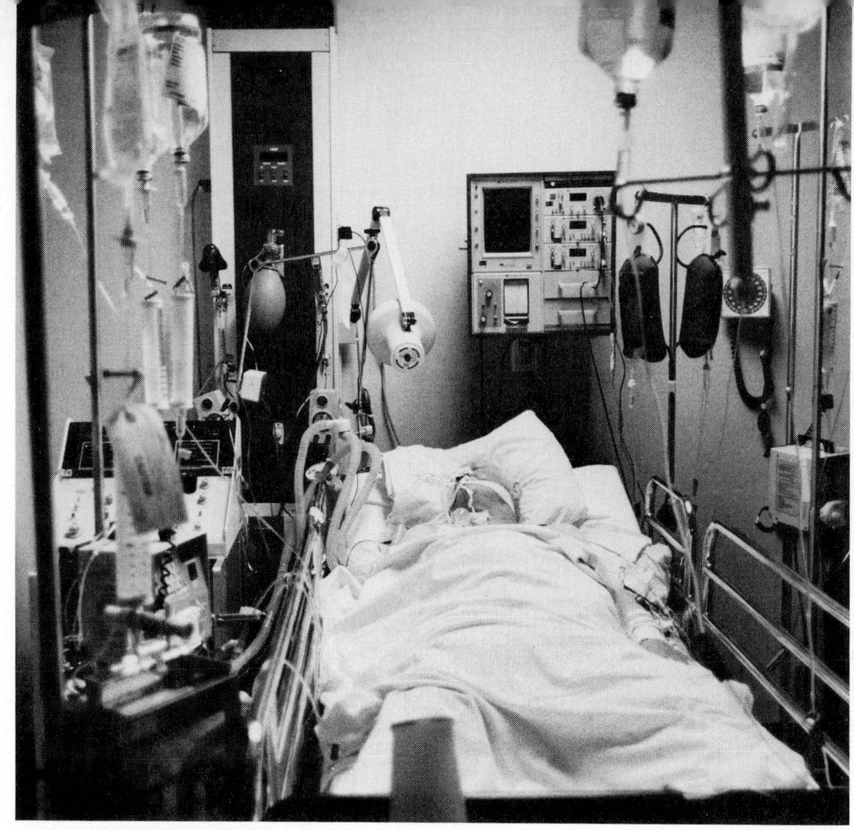

Medical-Surgical Insurance. Medical-surgical insurance plans such as Blue Shield cover physicians' medical and surgical services in a hospital, anesthesia and maternity services, care for accidential injuries, second-opinion consultations, and often physicians' services in a skilled nursing facility or home-care program. Such plans usually pay fixed fees for covered services; however, these fees may not cover costs. Medical-surgical plans do not cover house calls and office visits, diagnostic services, or dental services.

Major Medical Insurance. Major medical plans pay for most medical expenses not covered by hospitalization or surgery plans. They take effect after a deductible amount has been reached and typically pay 75 to 80 percent of uncovered expenses, usually to a maximum of $250,000. Major medical insurance protects the insured against catastrophic medical bills caused by severe illness or injury, and often makes the difference between solvency and destitution.

Disability Insurance. Disability insurance replaces part of the income lost due to sickness or disability. Short-term policies often require a two-to-three-week waiting period and then pay a set amount for a specified number of weeks, often thirty. Long-term policies may have a six-month waiting period and then pay a set amount per week for a specified number of years or until the policyholder reaches 65.

Medicare Supplementary Insurance. Many older people covered by Medicare (see the discussion below) buy private insurance to pay for medical costs that Medicare does not cover, including its annual deductibles, expenses that are incurred when Medicare coverage runs out, and the difference between Medicare coverage and the doctor's actual charges.

Dental Insurance. Dental insurance plans are usually group plans and provide limited coverage for regular dental care—that is, they pay a percentage of covered services beyond the deductible. Most dental insurance plans do not cover cosmetic dentistry.

How to Buy Private Health Insurance. A medical insurance company should be reliable and financially stable. In addition, it should have a high loss ratio—that is, the higher the percentage of premiums it pays back in benefits, the better the company. Check *Best's Insurance Reports* in your local library for loss ratios, and ask a stockbroker about the insurance company's financial standing.

After reviewing any coverage that you carry with your employer, decide what kind of additional coverage you need. Then check the brochure the insurance company publishes on the provisions of its policies. How long is the waiting period—the amount of time that must elapse before a policy goes into effect? Check also for the exclusion of coverage of "pre-existing conditions," benefit-reduction clauses, and provisions for emergency care. You should also notice the age limitations that are imposed and the cancellation and renewal privileges that apply.

The Scope of Voluntary Health Insurance. Most medical insurance plans cover hospital costs; individuals usually still pay for most preventive medicine and doctor's fees. Besides not providing total coverage, most insurance plans have a rate schedule that lists the maximum they will pay for a service; this maximum often becomes the minimum charged by hospitals and physicians, which thus raises health-care costs. Moreover, physicians often recommend unnecessary hospitalization because many policies go into effect only when a patient is hospitalized. And of course, the poorest people cannot afford to pay insurance premiums, or even the deductible, and thus remain unprotected. The American College of Healthcare Executives concluded on the basis of a 1986 survey that "access to care is today's most critical health-care issue." One million uninsured American families, it is estimated, had a family member who could not obtain needed medical care in 1985 because of inability to pay.

Tax-Supported Insurance and Assistance

In 1965 Congress set up two programs, Medicare and Medicaid, to provide medical care to the elderly, the disabled, and the needy. **Medicare** is an *insurance* program that pays most of the hospital and medical expenses for the disabled and for persons over 65. **Medicaid** is an *assistance* program that provides medical treatment for those unable to pay. The costs of Medicare are met by Social Security taxes; Medicaid is financed by federal and state funds.

Medicare. Under its Part A, Medicare provides hospital insurance for certain disabled people and for eligible persons over 65. Those who turned 65 before 1968 are covered automatically; those who became 65 thereafter have to be eligible for Social Security or railroad retirement benefits in order to qualify.

Medicare Part A carries a deductible and requires a copayment by the insured after sixty days' hospitalization for any "spell of illness." Before 1983 reimbursements to hospitals under Medicare were based on the hospitals' charges for the services they provided. In 1983 the method of payment was changed to a flat rate per patient that varies according to illness.

Upon being admitted to a hospital, a Medicare patient is categorized in one or more of 468 **diagnosis-related groups (DRGs).** The government pays a fixed sum of money based on the average cost of treating that illness or condition, no matter how long the patient is hospitalized. If the patient can be treated at a lower cost than that mandated by the DRG, the hospital keeps the difference. Hospitals thus are under pressure to employ the most economical treatments and to discharge patients quickly. Since 1984 the average length of a Medicare patient's hospital stay has decreased from 9.5 days to 7.5 days.

The DRG system of payment has aroused considerable controversy. While some applaud its reduction of hospitalization costs, others claim that thousands of patients are being discharged "sicker and quicker"—that is, they are being forced out of hospitals before they have fully recovered from their illnesses.

Medicare's Part B is available to almost everyone over 65, whether or not he or she is eligible for Social Security, upon payment of a monthly premium. After an annual deductible has been met, Part B covers 80 percent of approved charges for doctors' services, outpatient physical therapy and speech pathology services, home health care, and some other services and supplies. Payments to doctors under Part B are limited by a complex formula and may be less than the actual current charges by physicians for covered services.

Medicaid. Financed by federal and state governments, Medicaid assistance is available to needy people of all ages. Although benefits vary from state to state, Medicaid pays for hospital care and services, nursing-home care, visiting nurses, and doctors' fees. In many states it also covers clinic visits, diagnostic tests, prosthetic devices, drugs, eyeglasses, and dental care. For needy older people who are eligible for Medicare, Medicaid may pay the deductible charge that Medicare does not pay, as well as other costs not covered by Medicare.

Health Maintenance Organizations

Prepaid medical-care plans are another form of health financing. They are referred to as **health maintenance organizations,** or **HMOs.** About 21 million Americans are currently estimated to belong to 310 HMOs in the United States; two of the best known are the Kaiser-Permanente plan in some Western and Midwestern states and the Health Insurance Plan in New York State.

Under a federal law passed in 1973, employers of more than twenty-five persons must provide HMO coverage—if it is available—as an alternative to traditional health insurance. Most HMO subscribers join through such an employer-sponsored group plan. For a fixed annual sum paid in installments, HMOs provide comprehensive medical care to enrolled persons. The annual sum charged is based on the HMO's estimates of the cost of treating an average patient for a year. Most HMOs are of the type known as *closed-panel* plans, consisting of a group of salaried physicians who work in a single facility. (When costs can be controlled, these physicians share in the profits of the operation above and beyond their salaries.) Services provided include physician consultation, routine examinations, emergency care, diagnostic tests, and outpatient and inpatient hospitalization. (Psychiatric treatment, cosmetic surgery, dental care, and treatment for alcoholism and drug addiction are often excluded.) HMOs stress preventive medical care and therefore cover the costs of Pap smears, vaccinations, and screening for bowel and breast cancer. Thus with HMOs, unlike other health plans, a patient need not be ill to be eligible for medical attention.

Independent Practice Associations (IPAs). Another kind of HMO, called an **independent practice association (IPA)** or *open-panel* plan, provides medical services to HMO patients through a group of physicians who work in their own offices. Under a contract agreement with the IPA, each physician is paid in advance a preset amount for each HMO patient seen; and the physician agrees to be responsible for the cost of treating the patient. Since these physicians work in their own offices, they also see fee-for-service patients.

In terms of patient care, the various types of HMOs have resulted in less hospitalization, fewer diagnostic tests with less duplication, and better focused medical attention. As a result, HMOs are, on the average, 15 percent cheaper than other forms of fee-for-service health insurance. With their full coverage and prevention orientation, HMOs have proven their value against the standard crisis-oriented system of health insurance.

Preferred Provider Organizations

A criticism of HMOs is that they may provide inadequate care for their more seriously ill subscribers in an effort to keep costs down and provide greater profits for their member physicians. An alternative to the HMO that answers this criticism is the **preferred provider organization.** Under a PPO an insurer contracts with a group of physicians and health-care institutions to pay a set fee for a detailed list of medical services. Subscribers to the PPO are given a list of the "preferred providers" who have agreed to the fee schedule, and choose among them when they need medical care. The PPO thus pays a separate fee to participating doctors for each service that they render, but costs are held down. PPOs are a recent innovation in health-care financing, and are gaining in popularity.

National Health Insurance

It must not be forgotten that some 15 percent of Americans have no health insurance coverage whatever. Ironically, this group includes the people who need coverage the most because of their high rate of illness and disability. People in this segment of the population have no private insurance because they are unemployed; they are not eligible for Medicare because they are younger than 65; and they often are not eligible for Medicaid either, because of eligibility requirements that vary from state to state.

People who have no health coverage, as well as those who are covered by current programs but are unable to pay additional required sums, are faced with a financial situation that often denies them access to medical service or that affects the quality of the service they do receive. Many foreign countries have overcome these economic barriers by adopting systems of national health insurance. Germany was the first to do so, a century ago in the Bismarck era.

Since then, some form of national health plan has been instituted in nearly every country in Europe, both Eastern and Western, and in other nations, including Canada, Australia, New Zealand, and Japan. National health insurance plans continue to be proposed from time to time in the U.S. Congress. Although opposition by the medical profession is often blamed for the lack of national health insurance in this country, recent surveys have shown that more and more physicians are in favor of some form of national health insurance, and most view it as inevitable. The inequities of our current system appear to make national health insurance not only necessary, but unavoidable.

PHARMACEUTICALS

The consumer health movement has made it increasingly evident in recent years that consumers require guidance and protection when dealing with the vast numbers of pharmaceutical products now available to them. Drug firms, because of the enormous funds at their disposal, are especially able to affect consumer buying habits in ways that are not always in the best interest of the individual.

The profits made by drug firms, as a percentage of their net worth, are the largest of any industry in the United States. Industry spokesmen justify these profits by pointing out that much of their funds is spent on research. Critics

Herbal Remedies: "Natural" Cures or Dangerous Drugs?

Distrusting doctors and modern medicine in general, some people turn to herbal remedies as an alternative to antibiotics or from other health beliefs. Some who want to avoid caffeine look to herbal teas as a safe alternative to tea and coffee. Both are misguided, however, for many herbs are very dangerous substances. In fact, the plant kingdom contains a tinderbox of powerful cathartics, allergens, carcinogens, and poisons that can bring on severe illness or mental disturbance.

Pharmacologists remind us that herbs have been employed medicinally for thousands of years in both the Old World and the New. Until the beginning of this century, they were dispensed in pharmacies where an element of control was established. With the exception of a few herbal remedies, however, such as digitalis, the remainder have been displaced by modern antibiotic therapy. The present vogue of herbal usage should cause concern. Purchased freely at health-food stores and supported by popular literature full of half-truths and dubious claims, these herbs are as yet untested by the FDA, so their capacities are mostly still unproven.

While many herbal preparations like peppermint or rose-hip tea are harmless, many others previously considered safe have proven to be dangerous. Sassafras bark, for example, has been found to contain a potent carcinogen. Others, like calamus and tonk bean, have been shown to be poisonous even in small doses. A popular herbal weight-reducing formula was revealed to contain mandrake and pokeroot, both highly toxic substances. Nutmeg and jimsonweed, when made into tea, can be powerful hallucinogens with a number of unpleasant side effects. Even "harmless" camomile tea can bring on a strong allergic reaction in people who are sensitive to ragweed. Pharmacologists, pointing out that even mild herbal teas can counter the effects of prescription drugs, suggest that anyone who is taking prescription medication avoid drinking herbal teas. To avoid treating yourself for even minor illnesses with herbal home remedies is sound advice.

Source: Tim Larkin, "Herbs Are Often More Toxic Than Magical," *The FDA Consumer* (October 1983), HHS Publication No. (FDA) 84–1112; Jane E. Brody, "Herbal Teas: Source of Potent Drugs," in *The New York Times Guide to Personal Health* (New York: Avon, 1983), pp. 268–271.

note, however, that drug firms spend far more money advertising their products than they do researching them.

The two large categories of drugs sold by pharmaceutical houses may be distinguished by the way they are distributed to the consumer. The first, **over-the-counter drugs,** are those that can be sold without a doctor's prescription; the second, **prescription drugs,** are those that can be bought only with a physician's prescription.

Over-the-Counter Drugs

A variety of pharmaceutical products can be sold without a prescription because the drugs they contain are not known to be harmful in the amounts usually taken. These are over-the-counter (OTC) drugs. They include aspirin, antacid prescriptions for upset stomach, cold "remedies," bromides that have a mild relaxing effect (sold as sleeping aids), cough medicines, lotions for sunburn or sore muscles, dandruff removers, and the like. Over-the-counter drugs are the property of the firms who own the trade names under which they are sold; different manufacturers may charge widely varying prices for virtually the same product.

Enormous amounts of money are spent by manufacturers to advertise their products by brand names. They believe—with justification—that consumers will spend more to buy a familiar product and will not be too concerned with what the product contains. Some OTC drugs do not have any of the curative effects suggested in advertisements. Patented acne and psoriasis remedies, baldness cures, and the like do nothing except offer gullible consumers a new way to spend their money. Other OTC drugs can temporarily alleviate symptoms, but their effectiveness as therapies is questionable. Aspirin, for example, remains the most effective drug one can take for reducing fever and relieving the discomfort of a headache; but aspirin does absolutely nothing about the basic cause of the headache, nor can it help cure a cold, in spite of what television commercials may imply.

Self-medication. For the short-term treatment of minor ailments, most of us rely on over-the-counter drugs. But even such a useful product as aspirin can be misused.

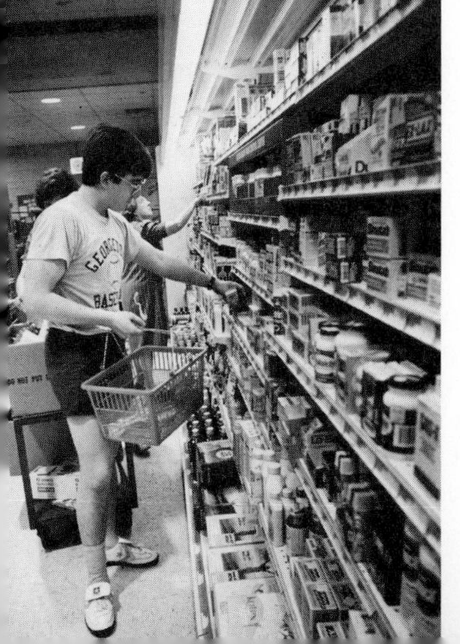

Some OTC drugs seem to be effective for the same reason that quack devices sometimes are—because the individual taking them believes they will work. The so-called **placebo effect** is well documented: Controlled studies have shown that some individuals who are given a neutral substance (the placebo) will experience a relief of bothersome symptoms.

Although most over-the-counter drugs are relatively harmless in themselves, their overuse or misuse can have serious consequences. Excessive intake of aspirin, for example, can cause gastrointestinal bleeding. Children with flu or chicken pox who are given aspirin run an increased risk of contracting Reye's syndrome, a deadly viral infection; and so labels on aspirin containers now warn against use of the drug in those cases. Laxative overuse may adversely affect the entire digestive tract. Professional diagnosis and treatment of serious disorders is often tragically delayed when people prescribe their own drugs. These persons are sometimes lulled into believing that relief from discomfort or pain through the use of OTC medications is equivalent to a cure for their illness. Furthermore, people who do not correctly diagnose their symptoms may unwittingly take a drug that seriously aggravates a physical disorder. For example, taking a mild laxative is usually harmless; but if the user's symptoms are caused by appendicitis, this self-treatment becomes hazardous. Despite all these dangers, however, self-diagnosis and self-medication continue as a form of self-inflicted quackery.

Home Tests: Is Self-Monitoring a Sound Health Practice?

People have been taking their temperature, measuring their pulse rate, and weighing themselves for a long time. Monitoring one's body processes is therefore not a particularly new idea. Now, however, home test kits are enabling people to perform many procedures that used to require a trip to the doctor's office. With the help of home test kits, for example, diabetics are able to monitor their blood sugar before it reaches a dangerous level, infertile women can determine the best time for conception, and others can test their stool to see if they are in the early, most treatable stages of colorectal cancer.

Sensing a lucrative market in such devices, commercial interests have launched a major effort to popularize the self-measurement of blood pressure, blood cholesterol, sexually transmitted diseases, menopause, and urinary tract infections. Other tests, such as ones for herpes and strep throat, are in the process of being developed. Kit manufacturers are looking forward to a $500-million-a-year market by 1990.

Doctors have mixed feelings about the worth of these tests. Because new genetic engineering techniques have made some tests much more accurate and reliable, conditions such as colorectal cancer, pregnancy, and diabetes can be monitored much more closely. But no home test, even the best, is a substitute for the careful analysis a physician can perform. Furthermore, doctors warn that a negative result on some tests can lull a person into a false sense of security. The V.D. Alert test, for example, is considered to be dangerous: While it may reliably indicate that a person does not have gonorrhea, it says nothing about whether the person has syphilis or some other STD that can be passed on to others.

Source: Based in part on "Medicine-Chest Labs," *Newsweek*, May 27, 1985, p. 85.

Prescription Drugs

Each year in the United States retail sales of prescription drugs approach $10 billion. Because prescription drugs can be purchased only through a doctor's prescription, drug companies invest much of their income in massive selling campaigns aimed at physicians. The drug industry spends several thousand dollars per doctor each year for medical journal advertising, highly paid salesmen, literature mailings, and free samples.

Does this kind of selling work? In several surveys physicians were asked where they had first heard of new drugs. From 50 to 75 percent answered they had learned about them from manufacturers' advertisements or salespersons. From 50 to 60 percent said they were persuaded by these sources to prescribe the drugs for their patients.

Most of the prescription drugs sold by competing firms are identical—penicillin, for example, is penicillin, no matter who makes it. But the approximately 3,000 prescription drugs available today are marketed under some 22,000 brand names. This multiplicity results in a grossly inflated and competitive drug industry—and increased expense to the consumer.

Generic Names. The **generic name** of a drug is the name used to identify the drug by its chemical content. It is generally a simplification of the drug's more complex chemical name. The **brand name** of a drug, on the other hand, is the name arbitrarily given a drug by its manufacturer as a means of associating the drug with the producer and making its name easy to pronounce and remember. Hardly anyone, for example, has heard of the generic name *meprobamate*, while doctors and patients alike are familiar with specific brands of this widely prescribed "tranquilizing" drug: Miltown and Equanil.

Generic drugs are screened by the Food and Drug Administration for safety and effectiveness in the same way that brand-name drugs are; when they are used in place of brand-name drugs, consumer savings can be substantial. Physicians are legally required to note on prescription blanks whether substitution

Drugs for the Home Medicine Cabinet

Every household, large or small, should have a basic supply of medicines on hand for emergencies and for the care of routine aches, pains, and other short-term, self-limiting ailments. The contents of the home medicine chest will vary with the nature of the household. People with children will want to have baby aspirin, antidiarrhetics, and emetics immediately available. The elderly, on the other hand, may need linaments or mild laxatives, while adolescents may want skin cleansers.

As a general rule, antibiotics should not be kept longer than a year, and other medicines should be discarded if they start to crumble, change color, harden, melt, or separate. Any medication that has lost its label should also be thrown out.

Here is a list of drugs and supplies that a family of adults should have on hand, with a few items for children.

analgesic	Aspirin or acetaminophen to reduce fever and pain; only aspirin, however, can reduce inflammation. Stronger preparations with codeine need a prescription.
emetics	Syrup of ipecac to induce vomiting in case of accidental poisoning (read the instructions carefully).
antacid	Preparations such as Maalox or Mylantin that contain aluminum hydroxide or magnesium hydroxide for indigestion and heartburn.
laxative	A mild laxative such as Milk of Magnesia for constipation.
antiseptics	A bottle of 70 percent rubbing alcohol.
antibiotic cream	Any ointment or cream such as Mycitracin or Polysporin containing bacitracin or polymyxin.
anti-inflammatory/ anesthetic ointment	A hydrocortisone cream like Cortaid to reduce inflammation and temporarily soothe pain.
antipruritic lotion or spray	Calamine lotion for poison ivy or insect bites and other skin irritations.
lubricant	Petroleum jelly.
antidiarrhetic	Preparations with pectin or bismuth salicylate such as Pepto-Bismol or Kaopectate.
cough syrup	A nonsuppressant type is best.
decongestant/ antihistamine	For colds and allergic symptoms.
bandages	Band-Aids, gauze, tape, etc.

All of the above preparations are for the short-term treatment of minor ailments. If symptoms persist longer than a week, call your physician; his or her number should be on an emergency phone list near every telephone in the house or taped inside the medicine cabinet door.

Source: Annabel Hecht, "Does Your Medicine Chest Need First Aid?" *The FDA Consumer* (April 1982), HHS Publication No. (FDA) 82–3123; Hamilton Southworth, M.D., "The Home Medicine Chest," in *The Columbia University College of Physicians and Surgeons Complete Home Medical Guide* (New York: Crown Publishers, 1985), pp. 768–771.

may be made for brand-name drugs. If these substitutions are allowed, generic equivalents may be supplied and the resultant savings passed on to the consumer.

Pharmaceuticals and Side Effects. There is no such thing as a totally harmless drug, for all drugs may adversely affect certain people. Some authorities estimate that about 1.5 million Americans are admitted to hospitals every year because of the adverse side effects of drugs prescribed for them—enough to make harmful reactions a major health hazard in themselves. With prescription drugs, in particular, these side effects must always be weighed against the drug's benefits. Unfortunately, the sheer number of new drugs being developed makes it almost impossible for physicians to keep abreast of the side effects of the drugs they may prescribe. Many doctors have only a superficial knowledge of these drugs; and this knowledge itself is derived from drug industry sources rather than from more comprehensive and impartial scientific and medical journals and reports.

The overuse of antibiotics has come in for recent criticism. Because many doctors have prescribed antibiotics when they were not really necessary, strains of bacteria resistant to these drugs have multiplied and new antibiotics must constantly be developed to cure ills that existing ones no longer affect.

Federal Rules and Regulations. For years public officials and private citizens had expressed their concerns about various aspects of the pharmaceutical industry. In order to protect the public, Congress passed the Kefauver-Harris Drug Amendment Act in 1962, containing the following provisions:

1. All manufacturers must comply with strict standards of quality control.
2. Automatic certification for a new drug, when the FDA failed to examine it in a specified period of time, was abolished. FDA approval of a drug must be obtained.
3. Drugs must be proved not only safe but effective. A drug must live up to the claims made for it. (Before this, the only concern was whether a drug was harmful, not whether it was efficacious.)
4. The generic name of the drug must be included on all labels and promotional materials in letters at least half as large as the trade name.
5. All advertising must contain a summary of side effects, contraindications (conditions that make use of the drug inadvisable), and effectiveness.
6. Drugs may not be tested on humans without first being tested on animals and meeting certain safety specifications.
7. Manufacturers must report promptly to the FDA any adverse effects of drugs discovered after the drug is marketed.

HEALTH, SCIENCE, AND DECISIONS

It is often difficult for us as laypeople to distinguish among the variety of existing health practices, products, and practitioners because we may not have access to adequate information or because the information we receive may be contradictory. Nevertheless, for our own protection it behooves us to be as informed as possible about present health choices. The health practice that

The Scientific Method

Modern medicine is a science based on an accumulated body of proven knowledge. Medical researchers and scientists, employing accepted techniques of objective research, have established the validity of this body of knowledge to the satisfaction of medical authorities. From this proven basis, new theories emerge and are subjected to the same degree of scientific scrutiny. Mere claims or countless testimonials do not qualify a new concept for acceptance within this body of knowledge without conclusive testing and proof according to established research techniques. By rigidly adhering to the scientific method, the medical profession can help to protect the world community from the hazards of unfounded therapies and the exploitation of unscrupulous therapists.

we adopt for its supposed benefits is often the very one that places our health in the greatest jeopardy.

But where should we turn for counsel? The tragedy of our health delivery system is that counseling and preventive health measures are not an integral part of it at present. We are left to our own devices.

The charlatan, the huckster, and the exploiter of health delivery thrive in this atmosphere. They appear to be everywhere. And these persons, speaking with the utmost assurance of the product or service they promote, can be very convincing. Furthermore, we tend to accept as proven the claims made by products and services that are widely advertised—despite their lack of adequate validation—just because they are so familiar to us. Therefore we are forced to make decisions that affect our health with little authentic guidance and a great deal of misinformation. Among our options are some services that exist despite the opposition of medical authorities, some whose role remains to be defined, and at least one health measure that continues to be attacked by critics despite its complete endorsement by medical authorities.

Some of the terms with which we should be familiar are the following: faith healing, gadgetry, acupuncture, holistic medicine, chiropractic, and water fluoridation.

Faith Healing

Faith healing is practiced by individuals who profess the ability to produce cures through a spiritual force. Although faith healing has been repudiated by recognized religious leaders, the "faith healer" continues to operate in the United States with great financial success. One well-known faith healer was "the lady of love with the healing hands," Mrs. Susie Jessel, who enjoyed an average income of $500 a night for her curative services. "Susie," as her patients called her, made no guarantees. She stated to her audiences: "I dedicate my hands to the Lord. . . . The Lord gave me the gift; and He did not give it in vain. If He chooses at times to make it so they don't heal, we must remember that we cannot be a winner all the time." Faith healers draw large crowds—and incomes—for their "services."

It is difficult to assess the healing powers of these persons because of the absence of accurate medical diagnoses. In addition, there is the difficulty of conducting any type of followup on those who "recovered." Physicians are

Pain

At any given time, about 10 million Americans are in chronic pain. Because of it, 550 million days are lost from work each year and $60 billion is drained from the national economy.

Acute pain is short, sharp, and sudden; it is brought on by injuries, infections, or other organic conditions that resolve themselves, usually within hours, days, or weeks. Chronic pain is long lasting and persistent and disrupts our daily physical and mental functioning. It can be caused by long-term conditions such as arthritis or cancer; it can also be brought on by severe emotional stress.

Because pain is a subjective experience, it is impossible to measure. Some people cannot tolerate the slightest discomfort; others can ignore it. Our perception of pain is very much influenced by the mind—by attitudes, moods, and expectations. A toothache hurts more at night when we have nothing else to think about than during the day when our minds are occupied with other things. In repeated tests one-third to one-half of those given a placebo they believe to be a painkiller report that their pain has lessened or vanished.

Most Americans regard pain as catastrophic—certainly not to be endured. So when we are in pain, we demand *fast relief*—words that are featured, not surprisingly, in the advertisements for most over-the-counter painkillers. We do not question the method as long as it produces results.

Traditional medical methods for treating pain include anesthesia (both general and local), analgesics (both prescription drugs like morphine and codeine and over-the-counter drugs like aspirin and acetaminophen), electrical stimulation of nerves that block pain, and, as a last resort, surgery to cut the nerves that are transmitting the pain. Hypnosis, biofeedback, and behavior modification have been used successfully in the treatment of low back pain and migraine headache. Practitioners of less orthodox methods such as acupuncture and Hatha Yoga have achieved quick, dramatic results in relieving some forms of chronic pain. And most people who resort to chiropractors do so because of pain.

Most reputable pain clinics are affiliated with a major hospital or medical center. Dozens of small pain centers, on the other hand, have sprung up around the country offering cures based on various unproven techniques. The best advice about relief from pain is the same as that for any medical decision: Check the credentials of any practitioner carefully before you spend your money. Pain is the quack's delight.

Source: Jane E. Brody, "Pain: Almost No One Escapes It," in *The New York Times Guide to Personal Health* (New York: Avon, 1983), pp. 486–492; "Headache for a Pain Remedy," *Newsweek*, July 9, 1984, p. 53.

rarely, if ever, permitted to examine a patient after "therapy." Therefore the nature of the patient's illness as well as the "recovery" are open to question.

Gadgetry

The income from worthless health machines and devices contributes considerably to the annual multibillion-dollar swindle of the health-minded consumer. All kinds of strange devices have been invented by the quacks.

Some create mystical lighting effects; some employ "therapeutic" vibrations. Other gadgets promise self-hypnosis through the use of a "brain-wave synchronizer," and there is even a device that "directly heats the blood." Coin-operated blood pressure machines are some of the most dangerous gadgets on the market. Even though they are similar to the familiar sphygmomanometers found in doctors' offices, they often provide incorrect blood pressure readings, which may give consumers a false impression about their health. Gadgets promising quick weight loss, increased bust size, dramatic leg reshaping, and the overnight disappearance of wrinkles also guarantee disappointment and may cause serious medical problems.

Acupuncture has been used successfully as an anesthetic and for the relief of chronic pain, but claims for it as a cure for disease have no scientific basis.

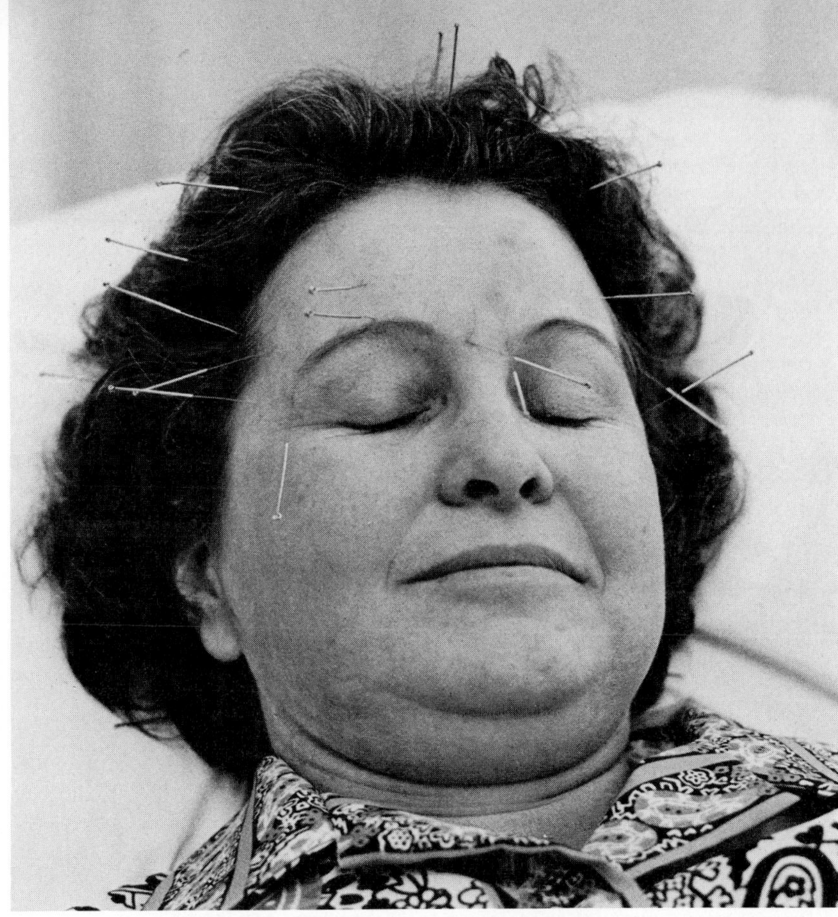

Acupuncture

Acupuncture is the practice of inserting needles into the body at particular points in order to anesthetize parts of the body or to treat disease. The points of insertion are called loci, and there are from 500 to 800 loci that the acupuncturist can use. Although acupuncture (from the Latin *acus*, "needle," and *pungere*, "to pierce") has been practiced in China for about 5,000 years, it has only recently attracted considerable interest in the West.

Electrical equipment is frequently used in conjunction with the acupuncture charts to determine the position of the loci. It has been found that these points have twenty times less electrical resistance than other sites on the body. Electrical instruments are also sometimes used to stimulate the needles once they are inserted.

While Chinese acupuncturists have claimed successful treatment of such illnesses as blindness and polio, these claims are difficult or impossible to substantiate. The effectiveness of acupuncture as an anesthetic technique, however, has been documented by respected U.S. doctors and surgeons. Many kinds of operations have been performed with acupuncture as the sole anesthetic.

At present the Food and Drug Administration considers acupuncture a technique in the experimental stage. (Even in China an anesthesiologist always stands by while an operation is being performed in case acupuncture fails.) Many patients use acupuncturists for relief of chronic back and arthritic pain, but the safety and reliability of the technique have not been firmly established. Acupuncture definitely should not, for example, be considered a cure for such

Protect Yourself Against Quackery

This year, we Americans will spend billions of dollars on products that do nothing for us—or may even harm us. And we'll do it for the same reason people have done it since ancient times . . . we want to believe in miracles. We want to find simple solutions and shortcuts to better health.

It's hard to resist. All of us, at one time or another, have seen or heard about a product—a new and exotic pill, device, or potion—that can easily solve our most vexing problem. With this product, we're told, we can eat all we want and still lose weight. We can grow taller or build a bigger bustline. Or we can overcome baldness, age, arthritis, even cancer.

It sounds too good to be true—and it is. But we're tempted to try the product in spite of all we know about modern medical science—or perhaps because of it. After all, many treatments we take for granted today were once considered miracles. How can we tell the difference?

• • •

Apply the "it-sounds-too-good-to-be-true" test to ads for health products by watching for these common characteristics of quackery:

- A quick and painless cure.
- A "special," "secret," "ancient," or "foreign" formula, available only through the mail and only from one supplier.
- Testimonials or case histories from satisfied users as the only proof that the product works.
- A single product effective for a wide variety of ailments.
- A scientific "breakthrough" or "miracle cure" that has been held back or overlooked by the medical community.

Before buying a suspect product or treatment, find out more about it. Check with one or more of the following:

- Your doctor, pharmacist, or other health professional
- The Better Business Bureau
- Your local consumer office
- Your state's attorney general
- The Federal Trade Commission, Washington, D.C. 20580
- Your nearest office of the Food and Drug Administration
- Your postmaster or the Postal Inspection Service.

Source: Excerpted from U.S. Department of Health and Human Services, Public Health Service, Food and Drug Administration HFI-40, HHS Publication No. 85–4200.

diseases as cancer, sickle-cell anemia, or cerebral palsy. As an anesthetic, however, acupuncture could become invaluable, since there are numerous operations in which conventional general anesthesia poses serious threats to the patient's well-being and others in which it is desirable to have the patient conscious. Extensive research is now being conducted on the effects of acupuncture, and it is likely that a medical consensus will soon develop. In the meantime, since only 14 states license acupuncturists, extreme caution should be exercised to avoid the fraudulent practitioner.

Holistic Medicine

The contemporary holistic health movement revives an old belief in the totality of the individual. In contrast to therapy-oriented medicine, it encourages positive approaches toward health and promotes courses of action designed to preserve health and achieve maximum levels of wellness.

Unfortunately the direction of this creditable movement has become diffused, leading government officials to state that "at present nobody knows how many practitioners call themselves 'holistic,' exactly what services they provide, how many people use them, their costs, or their outcomes on health."

The major drawbacks to holism, and a significant concern for the individual, are the movement's all-embracing nature and its lack of discernment. Demanding no evidence of the proven merit of a method, holism appears ready to accept any approach as long as it claims to promote well-being. This lack of judgment concerns those who otherwise accept the value of such positive approaches to health.

Chiropractic

Chiropractic is currently a licensed occupation in all fifty states. It was originally based on the theory that manual adjustment of the spinal vertebrae eliminates disease. Today this approach has been expanded to include methods involving the use of heat, light, water, exercise, and electricity.

The medical profession has continually disputed the authenticity of chiropractic as a healing art because there is no evidence in medical literature to support the chiropractic theory. Claims of some chiropractors to be able to treat cancer, diabetes, and heart disease are viewed as dangerous. Additionally, standards of admission to schools of chiropractic and the quality of chiropractic training have been questioned. In 1979, however, the American Medical Association, while repeating that there is no scientific evidence that disease can be treated by spinal manipulation, stated that this in itself does not mean that "everything a chiropractor may do is without therapeutic value, nor does it mean that all chiropractors should be equated with cultists." Since that time chiropractors have been admitted to practice in a few accredited hospitals in the United States.

WATER FLUORIDATION

Quacks and cultists usually come to our attention because they advocate therapies or practices unsupported by scientific evidence. The exact opposite is true, however, regarding the fluoridation of water. The dental benefits of natural or artificial fluoridation have been attested to by more than seventy-five dental, medical, nursing, scientific, and educational organizations, and the Public Health Service has set a goal of fluoridated water for at least 95 percent of the population by 1990. That goal will not be met, however, because antifluoridation cultists and their allies continue to oppose the extension of these benefits and would like to put a stop to all water fluoridation programs.

To underscore this resistance, fluoridation opponents have attempted to mislead the public into believing that the drinking of fluoridated water poses a health hazard. But to date, not one of the prospective dangers cited by these opponents has materialized, and sixty-one percent of the U.S. population is currently enjoying the benefits of fluoridation.

As reported in a recent study of nearly 1 million people conducted by the Center for Disease Control in Atlanta, water fluoridation has been responsible for a 65 percent reduction of tooth decay among children. And adults who have consumed fluoridated water throughout their lives have less tooth decay, fewer extractions, and fewer dentures. Also reported, and confirming all prior studies, is the absence of any ill effects upon the health of those who drink water fluoridated at the one-part-per-million level, the concentration typically used in the artificial fluoridation of water.

Fluoridation of water has two advantages over the direct application of fluorides to the teeth: It is more effective and it is cheaper to the consumer. But everyone should also use a fluoride toothpaste as a further protection against decay.

A CONSUMER GUIDE

We should become better informed about the products and services we purchase to solve our health problems. We should be wiser, more aware, and more judicious in our choices and demands; more aggressive and outspoken about our rights as consumers; more alert to the protection we have under the law; and more involved in the lawmaking process itself.

Obtaining Information

The United States government traditionally has not only encouraged the consumer movement, but has also assisted it with information and advice (see box: The Regulatory Agencies). According to a recent report, there are 362 consumer offices in the United States, Guam, Puerto Rico, and the Virgin Islands.

Consumer agencies have been created at all government levels to provide information, receive complaints, and generally assist consumers. Local offices are often listed in the phone book under the heading of Office of Consumer Affairs or Consumer Protection Division (or Department or Unit); sometimes they can be reached through the office of the state's attorney general. The United States Office of Consumer Affairs publishes the *Consumer's Resource Handbook*, available free from the Consumer Information Center, Pueblo, Colorado 81009, which contains a mine of information on the names and addressses of city, county, and state consumer agencies and the consumer complaints addresses of hundreds of corporations.

The agencies listed under Federal Sources of Consumer Aid and Information in this chapter are all excellent sources of information and assistance for personal consumer needs. The Consumer Information Center in Pueblo, Colorado, is a particularly bountiful source. Its *Consumer Information Catalog* lists pamphlets available on nutrition, health care, pharmaceuticals, child care, safety, and other topics related to health. Most of the pamphlets are free or available for a nominal charge.

The two best-known nongovernment sources of consumer information are *Consumers Research* and *Consumer Reports*. *Consumers Research*, established in 1927, evaluates products of use to consumers and rates them as "recommended," "intermediate," or "not recommended." Prices are given but do not affect the ratings.

Consumer Reports is the publication of the Consumers Union, established in 1936. The Consumers Union also tests and rates consumer products, taking price into consideration in giving ratings such as "best buy," "recommended," or "not recommended."

The growing interest in consumer affairs has also prompted colleges and universities to offer courses on the subject.

The Regulatory Agencies

PCBs, asbestos, toxic waste sites, and acid rain. Laetrile, toxic shock syndrome, and factory recalls. These are all words that have become familiar to us in the past decade by virtue of the research of some governmental agency. In each case an agency has revealed a factor that poses a danger to the safety or health of the public. These agencies, called regulatory, are empowered to issue restrictions or bans for the protection of the public.

The list of words above gives a notion of the regulatory agencies' very broad scope of concern in our lives. Their most extensive concern is the environment. Monitoring the environment is a tremendous task. It involves measuring the level of pollutants in the air we breathe, in the water we drink, and in the soil in which our food crops are grown. Monitoring, furthermore, is only a part of regulation. The authority to issue rules and to implement the law is just as significant. And in the long run, the degree to which the law is enforced is the critical factor.

The regulatory agencies responsible for monitoring, testing, and enforcing at the national level have included the Environmental Protection Agency, the Occupational Safety and Health Administration, the Consumer Product Safety Commission, the Federal Trade Commission, and the Food and Drug Administration. Other agencies serve these functions at the national level as well, but to a lesser extent.

What has been happening to these agencies? Ironically, at a time when life is becoming more complex and the need for regulation is becoming more essential, their influence and the protection they are empowered to provide have been sharply reduced. This has occurred in various ways. In some cases, administrative policies have directed these agencies not to take the initiative in enforcing regulations. In other situations, legislative action has weakened an agency by reducing its sphere of influence. The most common method of disabling a regulatory agency has been to slash its budget, thereby decreasing its staff and limiting its scope of operations.

The undermining of these organizations in this fashion has adversely affected the health of our nation, as the following examples show:

- The number of food poisoning cases has almost doubled in the last few years. Critics of government and industry say that the Agriculture Department has lowered its inspection standards in order to help the food industry boost its productivity. As a consequence, more contaminated meat and poultry are being sold to consumers than ever before.

- Although 16 children died and 118,000 were injured in 1985 as a result of playing with defective toys, the current head of the Consumer Product Safety Commission has stated that consumers, not toy manufacturers, should bear the burden of responsibility for toy safety. That is, it is parents' duty to see that their children do not play with dangerous toys, not the manufacturers' obligation to stop making them.

- Thirty-eight infants died in 1984 as a result of being given an illegally marketed vitamin E supplement. When informed that the drug was being sold without its approval, the FDA nevertheless delayed action for four months. The agency explained later that it had mistakenly believed the supplement to be similar to another with a long history of safe use. However, it had not yet completed a safety review of the entire class of drugs to which the supplement belonged. Critics charge that the FDA, wishing to inconvenience the drug industry as little as possible, has deliberately failed to monitor the marketing of many new drugs.

- In 1985 the federal government refused to fund a program of one of its own agencies, the National Institute of Occupational Health and Safety, to inform workers of the extent of their exposure to carcinogenic substances on the job. Among the reasons the agency gave was that if workers were made aware, they might sue their employers.

Federal Sources of Consumer Aid and Information

1. *U.S. Consumer Product Safety Commission (CPSC)*
   Office of Information and Public Affairs
   Washington, D.C. 20207
   Toll-free hotline: (800) 638-2772
   Maryland only: (800) 492-8104

CPSC's primary goal is to reduce injuries associated with consumer products in or around the home, schools, and recreational areas. The commission assists consumers to evaluate the comparative safety of consumer products, develops uniform safety standards for consumer products, and promotes research on product-related deaths, illnesses, and injuries.

2. *Food and Drug Administration (FDA)*
   Department of Health and Human Services
   5600 Fishers Lane
   Rockville, Maryland 20852
   (301) 443-3380

The FDA enforces laws to ensure the purity and safety of foods, drugs, and cosmetics, the safety of therapeutic devices, and the truthful, informative labeling of such products. Many products, such as food additives and prescription drugs, are subject to premarketing approval by the FDA. The agency also enforces radiation safety standards for products such as color television sets, sunlamps, microwave ovens, and medical devices.

3. *National Highway Traffic Safety Administration (NHTSA)*
   Department of Transportation
   400 Seventh Street S.W.
   Washington, D.C. 20590
   (202) 426-1828

The NHTSA enforces safety standards for motor vehicles and some of their parts. The agency enforces manufacturer compliance with federal standards, provides fuel economy standards for passenger cars and light trucks, and assists states with motor vehicle safety programs.

4. *Federal Trade Commission (FTC)*
   Pennsylvania Avenue at Sixth Street N.W.
   Washington, D.C. 20580
   (202) 523-3598

The FTC enforces antitrust laws and consumer protection statutes, including those prohibiting false advertising, fraud in credit (lending), and the circulation of inaccurate or obsolete credit reports.

5. *Public Health Service (PHS)*
   5600 Fishers Lane
   Rockville, Maryland 20852
   (301) 443-2404

The PHS is concerned with various areas of health research, regulation of health-related products, delivery of health care, and improvements in mental health.

6. *Department of Education*
   400 Maryland Avenue S.W.
   Washington, D.C. 20202
   (202) 245-3192

The Department of Education guides national education policies and administers most federal assistance to education.

7. *Agriculture Department*
   14th Street and Independence Ave. S.W.
   Washington, D.C. 20250
   Animal and Plant Health Inspection Service (202) 447-2511
   Agricultural Marketing Service (202) 447-8998
   Food and Nutrition Service (703) 756-3276

The Agriculture Department inspects and grades meats, poultry, fruits, and vegetables. It also provides nutrition information through labeling requirements, administers the food stamp program, and carries out studies on human nutrition.

8. *Treasury Department*
   Bureau of Alcohol, Tobacco, and Firearms
   1200 Pennsylvania Avenue N.W.
   Washington, D.C. 20226
   (202) 566-7777

This agency has jurisdiction over alcohol, tobacco, firearms, and explosives.

9. *Environmental Protection Agency* (*EPA*)
   401 M Street S.W.
   Washington, D.C. 20460
   (202) 382-2090

The EPA sets standards for air and water quality. It also regulates the disposal of hazardous wastes and the manufacture and use of pesticides.

10. *Nuclear Regulatory Commission* (*NRC*)
    1717 H Street N.W.
    Washington, D.C. 20555
    (301) 492-7000

This agency regulates the commercial nuclear energy industry, inspecting and licensing all nuclear energy facilities.

11. *Occupational Safety and Health Administration* (*OSHA*)
    200 Constitution Avenue N.W.
    Washington, D.C. 20210
    (202) 523-8017

OSHA has responsibility for safety and health in the workplace.

12. *Office of Consumer Advisor*
    Department of Agriculture
    14th Street and Independence Avenue S.W.
    Washington, D.C. 20250
    (202) 382-9681

This office coordinates USDA actions on problems and issues of importance to consumers.

13. *General Services Administration* (*GSA*)
    Consumer Information Center Program
    Eighteen and F Streets N.W.
    Washington, D.C. 20405
    (202) 566-1794

Registering a Complaint: Taking a Course of Action

In spite of carefully researching a product, examining the credentials of a therapist, or scrutinizing the fine print of a service contract, we may still feel that we have been denied full service or have been a victim of fraud or exposed to personal hazard. What can we do about it?

The first course of action is to complain directly to the person or organization involved. All documents, such as orders, contracts, or receipts, supporting our claim should be assembled, with duplicates prepared if it is necessary to submit them so that we may retain the originals. If this direct approach fails, the next step is to approach a business or trade group that is able to exert pressure: A government office of consumer affairs can be of great assistance; the state attorney general's office is another possibility.

The offices of almost all state attorneys general are equipped to handle consumer complaints and are willing either to assist consumers directly or refer them to the appropriate agency for help. In most cases, the state unfair or deceptive trade practice statutes are also enforced by the office of the state attorney general. The National Association of Attorneys General at 3901 Barrett Drive, Raleigh, North Carolina, 27609, distributes a special report, *Placement of State Consumer Protection Programs*, which deals with schemes and frauds that move from state to state.

If these approaches bring no satisfaction, legal help may be necessary. Small claims court is a legal, yet informal, way to pursue complaints. Generally for a fee of less than $15, a claim can be filed and a case presented without the aid of an attorney. If a claim is large and complicated, there may be no alternative but to hire a lawyer. This is, of course, an expensive course of action.

The Consumer Movement

The federal government has recognized the right of consumers to be involved in the decision-making processes that affect health delivery systems. It has mandated the inclusion of consumers on the health councils of every government tier from county to federal, in an effort to help eliminate waste and improve the delivery of primary care.

State legislatures and Congress are under constantly increasing pressure from vested interests that attempt to influence the passage or defeat of bills. Similar pressure is being exerted on public agencies. Individuals and organizations wishing to influence the creation of laws or government policy have an opportunity to do so at public hearings. Legislative bodies and governmental agencies conduct hearings in order to provide interested parties the chance to express their viewpoints. The federal government has even provided financial assistance to citizens to enable them to appear at hearings. *A Guide to Consumer Action*, an instruction manual on the techniques of organizing and exerting influence, is available from the Consumer Information Center Program in Pueblo, Colorado (HSS publication [OE] 77–15800).

The techniques of educating, as well as exercising, influence through the use of lobbyists is very much a part of the political system. It is estimated that lobbyists spend $1 billion a year to influence Washington opinion, plus another $1 billion to sway public opinion. It is not surprising that lobbyists have been referred to as "the fourth branch of government."

In contrast to the well-financed business interests, the interests of consumers have been represented by only a few groups, such as the Consumer Federation of America, Congress Watch, The National Consumers League, Common Cause, and Consumers Union. The $3 million per year that is spent by these groups for lobbying is only about .3 percent of the amount that is spent by business in grass-roots lobbying alone.

Out of this inequity arose the call for the establishment of a Federal Consumer Protection Agency. Although some thirty-five federal agencies have officials handling consumer matters, many consumer leaders felt that such representation possessed more form than substance. The purpose of the proposed agency was to provide consumer representation before regulatory bodies, gather information, and act as a clearing house for complaints. After five years of debate and despite widespread public support, the bill to establish this agency was defeated.

But as consumer champion Ralph Nader states, "You can't put a cap on consumer interest. Every time someone goes into a store or a clinic or into a deal and gets rooked—that's the stuff of which the consumer movement is made. And health is the fundamental consumer issue."

SUMMARY

1. The *infant mortality* and maternal death rates of the United States are higher than those of many other industralized countries, and our *life expectancy* rate continues to lag as well. Affecting these figures are America's 33.7 million poor, who are unable to afford proper health care. Another factor involved is the unequal distribution of physicians throughout the nation.

2. Selecting a personal or family physician is not an easy task. Many factors should be considered before arriving at a decision, including credentials and hospital affiliations, fees, and personal factors. Unwarranted surgery and medical incompetence are fairly serious problems.

3. Hospitals are classified as *voluntary* (nonprofit), *government,* and *private* or *proprietary.* Most are *general,* short-term institutions. *Specialty* hospitals offer long-term care. *Ambulatory surgical centers* do minor procedures on an outpatient basis; *freestanding emergency centers* provide many of the same services as hospital emergency centers, at far less cost, in communities without hospitals. *Nursing homes* are primarily for the care of the aged.

4. Soaring health care costs have been partly offset by private and public (Medicare and Medicaid) insurance plans. *Health maintenance organizations* (HMOs) are prepaid medical-care plans that provide preventive care as well as diagnostic and emergency care and hospitalization.

5. Massive advertising campaigns by drug manufacturers induce the public into unnecessary purchases of and unwarranted reliance upon *over-the-counter drugs*. In a similar fashion, physicians often recommend *prescription drugs* for their patients based solely upon the information provided them by the sales representatives of the pharmaceutical companies.

6. The *generic name* of a drug identifies its chemical structure. The *brand name* is given to the drug by its manufacturer. By requesting a prescription from your physician for a generically equivalent drug rather than a brand name drug, you can often purchase a similarly effective drug at less cost.

7. The great variety of medical abuses and the harmful side effects of drugs make it necessary to regulate the drug industry and medical profession. Federal regulatory agencies include the Food and Drug Administration (FDA) and the Federal Trade Commission (FTC). State and local agencies, citizens' groups, and individual action can also do much to curb quackery.

8. There is a great deal of exploitation in the health field today, ranging from ineffectual *faith healing* to possibly harmful *gadgetry*. In between are techniques such as *acupuncture* and *chiropractic* whose purpose and effectiveness are not precisely established.

9. The consumer movement, assisted by the federal government, is continually growing in the United States. Consumer agencies have been created at the municipal, state, and federal levels to provide information, receive complaints, and assist consumers in general. As consumer champion Ralph Nader has said, "Health is the fundamental consumer issue."

CONSUMER CONCERNS

1. When purchasing a prescription drug, are you in the habit of inquiring about its side effects or asking for a customer insert describing them? Do you feel that adequate attention is given to this matter?
2. There are standards by which to gauge the preparation and competency of medical doctors. These include college and medical school degrees, recognition by colleagues, and hospital affiliation. By what standards would you measure the competency of practitioners who are not medical doctors?
3. A correct diagnosis is the basis for successful therapy. What qualifications do you seek in a practitioner that give you confidence in his or her ability to make a correct diagnosis?
4. Do you feel that regulatory agencies that protect your health, such as the FDA, FTC, CPSC, and OSHA, exercise too much authority, or do you believe that situations still exist that warrant more stringent control?
5. What factors prompt people to risk their well-being through unproven remedies and unsound health practices?

17

Environmental Health

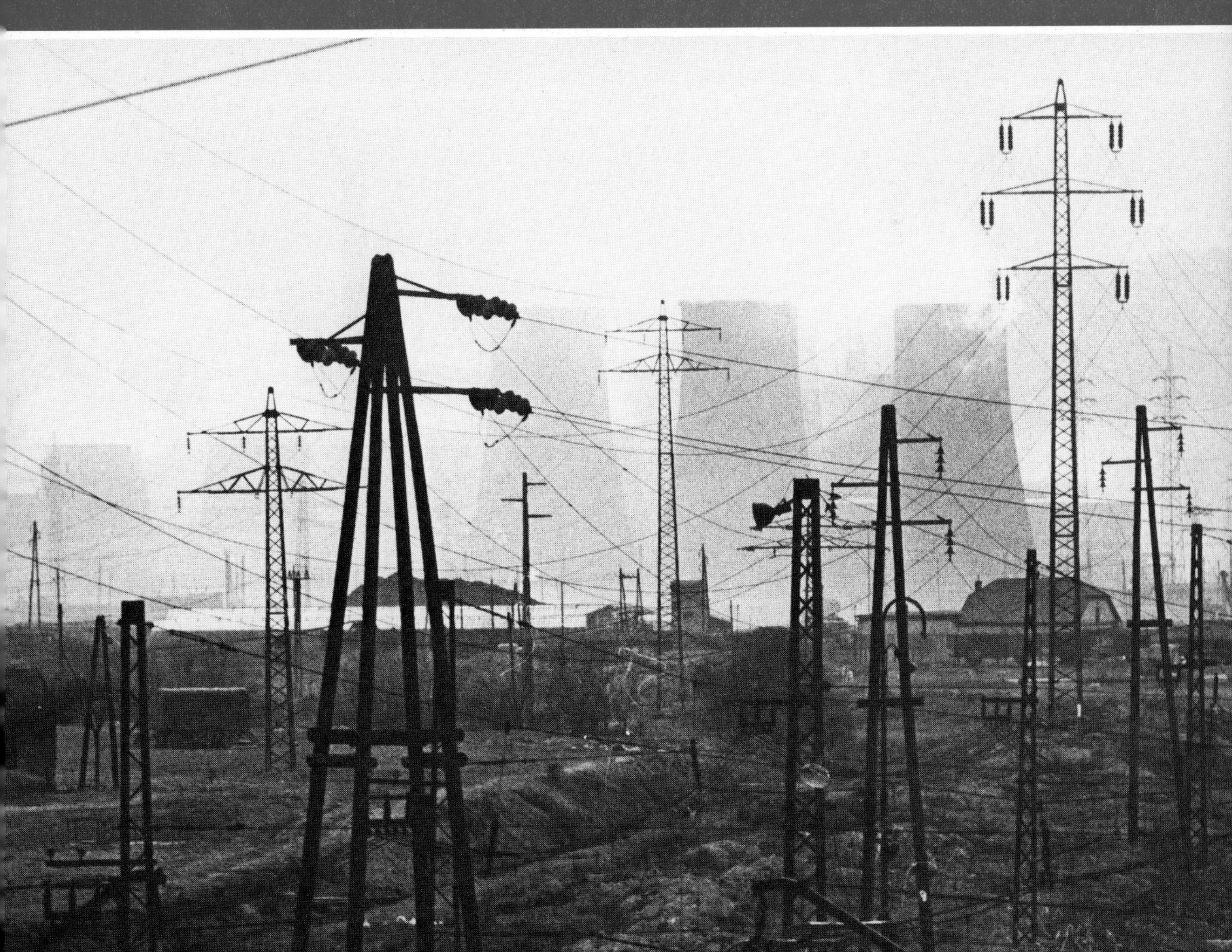

The earth, for all its size and abundance of growth and resources, has its own natural limitations. Although most of the earth's surface is covered by water, over 97 percent of it is salt water, which is unfit for drinking or agriculture. Furthermore, most of the potential fresh water from natural sources remains locked up in glaciers. At present, after the requirements of agriculture and industry have been met, only a relatively small amount of water is left over for drinking.

The air we breathe is an essential resource that is becoming globally polluted. No longer is pollution restricted to urban or industrial areas; space satellites show a brownish haze in every part of the earth's atmosphere. Industrialization has rapidly depleted our mineral resources, and there are now shortages of many substances considered vital to our way of life.

The final, and perhaps most critical, challenge is the struggle for existence in the greater part of the world that has an ever-increasing population. It is anticipated that by the year 2000, the earth's population will exceed 6 billion people.

Given these facts, we can only conclude that the earth's capacity to support life is decreasing, while the amount of life the earth is required to support is increasing. Unless significant changes are made in these conditions, prospects for the quality of life in the future appear grim.

These are people working to conserve our natural resources, to preserve species of plants and animals, and to protect the purity of our air and water. These people are called conservationists or environmentalists, and they have become politically active in an effort to influence the passage of legislation designed to curb practices that harm the environment. There also exist various government bureaus, such as the Environmental Protection Agency (EPA) in Washington, D.C., whose responsibility it is to monitor and control our impact on the environment.

Until recently, the passage of protective legislation was not difficult. The enforcement of this legislation, however, was constantly delayed and compromised. Of course, any bargaining with polluters to postpone the meeting of target dates or to reduce the levels of compliance occurs at the expense of the public's health. In light of the mounting evidence linking environmental pollution to cancer and other diseases, the EPA, for example, began to assume the role of a public health agency, instead of a mere antipollution enforcement bureau. Both roles have been threatened, however, by budget cuts in recent years, despite poll results showing strong opposition to weakening environmental regulations.

In this chapter we shall consider first the various forms of pollution, the health hazards they represent, and the efforts being made to control them. Then we shall survey the overall state of our environment and discuss some important steps that need to be taken to preserve it. Finally, we shall look at world population trends, their effects on our supplies of natural resources, and some solutions to the population problem.

THE SCIENCE OF ECOLOGY

Ecology is the branch of biology that deals with the relation between living organisms and their environment. The actual environment we interact with is much smaller than might be supposed. It consists of a thin layer of soil, water, and air near the earth's surface called the **biosphere.**

The Biosphere

The biosphere is composed of **biotic communities,** which consist of plants and animals in organized relationships, each exchanging life-sustaining raw materials with the other. The biotic communities are the living segment of larger units called **ecosystems,** which encompass air, water, soil, and all earthly and atmospheric substances. In an ecosystem interaction is based on *cycles of exchange*. Plants convert substances such as carbon dioxide and energy from the sun into food, animals consume the plants, bacteria decompose the waste products of plants and animals, and plants utilize this waste to perpetuate the cycle. In such a system nothing is superfluous; every element is an essential part of the whole. Because all ecosystems are interrelated, no one part of nature can be altered without affecting other parts.

AIR POLLUTION

Of the resources needed to sustain life in the biosphere, air is the most vital. Deprived of air, we cannot survive for more than a few minutes. Each day the average person breathes 35 pounds of air, most of which comes from the lowest 7 feet of the 15,000-foot-high oxygen-rich atmosphere. Considering these facts, it is hard to understand why societies carelessly spew into the air more than 200 million tons of pollutants each year. **Air pollution** is the contamination of the atmosphere by waste products at levels that are unhealthy to human beings and their environment. Air pollution first came to public attention in 1930, when a heavy fog blanketed the Meuse Valley in Belgium. Despite the weather, factories and industrial plants continued to pour out smoke; five days

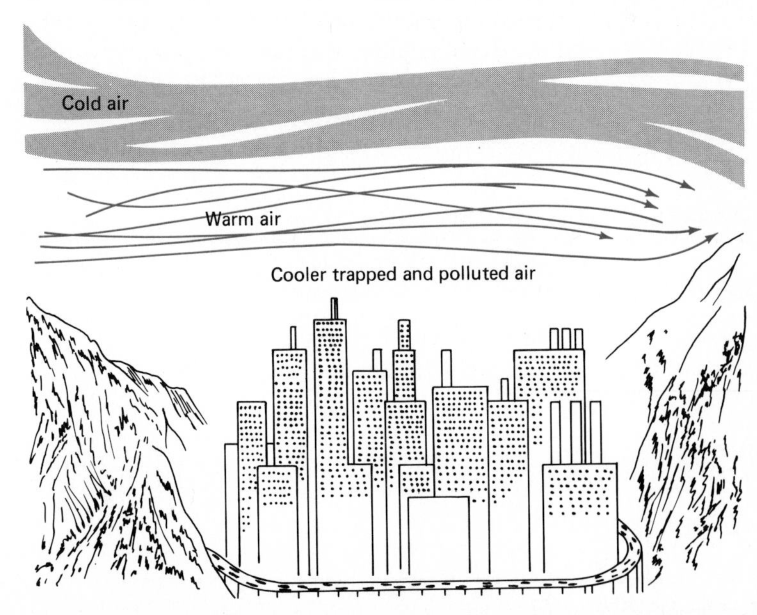

FIGURE 17-1

A temperature inversion occurs when a warm air mass moves over cooler air below. The cooler air becomes trapped with whatever pollutants it contains. The warm air layer is, in turn, prevented from rising by a layer of cold air pressing down from above.

later the heavily poisoned air had taken more than 60 lives and caused the illness of 6,000 inhabitants.

The condition that brought on this destruction was a combination of smog and a temperature inversion. **Smog** is a mixture of smoke and fog, but its meaning has been generalized to include many varieties of chemical and industrial pollution. A **temperature inversion** occurs when a warm air mass moves over cooler air near the ground below. Warmed air and smog rising from the ground stop at the level of the still warmer air and are trapped. Thus pollutants are not dissipated in the atmosphere; if pollution continues, the level of pollutants will rise (see Figure 17-1). Situations similar to the Belgian smog have occurred repeatedly in all parts of the world since 1930. Presently, smog, as measured by the general decrease in visibility, is being reported all across the nation, in metropolitan, rural, and even remote areas. National Park officials reported in 1985 that visibility in even the most remote parks was being affected by pollution 90 percent of the time.

The Sources of Air Pollution

Air pollution can be attributed to three major sources. In order of quantity, these are (1) motor vehicles; (2) factories and power plants; and (3) refuse disposal (see Table 17-1).

Motor Vehicles. By far the greatest source of air pollution is motor vehicles, which expel about 100 million tons of pollutants into our air each year. Because a car's engine cannot utilize all the fuel it receives, a portion of this fuel escapes into the air in the form of poisons. Pollution from burned gasoline emitted from exhaust pipes accounts for more than half of all atmospheric wastes.

Factories and Power Plants. Industrial installations such as iron and steel mills, chemical plants, oil refineries, smelters, phosphate plants, pulp and paper mills, and many others are major polluters of the air. They generate air pollutants such as sulfur and nitrogen gases, which are produced by burning heavy fuel oil and coal for low-cost industrial power and heat. If fuel consumption increases over the coming decades, this source of emission may produce even higher

TABLE 17-1

Major Sources of Air Pollution (in millions of tons per year)

Category	Carbon Monoxide	Sulfur Oxides	Hydrocarbons	Nitrogen Oxides	Particulates
Transportation	47.7	0.9	7.2	8.8	1.3
Fuel combustion (stationary)	7.0	16.8	2.1	9.7	2.0
Industrial processes	4.6	3.1	7.5	0.6	2.3
Solid-waste disposal	12.0	—	0.6	0.1	0.4
Miscellaneous	6.3	—	2.5	0.2	0.9
Total	67.6	20.8	19.9	19.4	6.9

Source: Statistical Abstract, 1986.

levels of harmful materials. However, if existing technology is employed to control these emissions, their unhealthful consequences can be minimized.

Refuse Disposal. Each year pollutants, chiefly in the form of carbon monoxide, are produced by refuse disposal. Belching incinerators, smoldering city dumps and municipal facilities, and private trash burning all contribute pollutants, foul odors, and smoke to the air.

The Harmful Effects of Air Pollution

Direct and indirect effects of air pollution take a toll on the private and public sectors of the economy as well as on human health and longevity. Individuals exposed to a pollution crisis—a temperature inversion, for example—suffer immediate harm; but air pollution also affects crops, forests, fish, and livestock many miles away from industry. And private and public property may be irreparably damaged by air pollutants.

Human Health. The main effect of air pollution on human health is the increasing incidence of respiratory disease. Because of air pollution, the incidence of pulmonary emphysema is increasing; and chronic bronchitis, bronchial asthma, pneumonia, and the common cold have become more widespread, particularly in urban areas. Although the main cause of lung cancer is cigarette smoking, air pollution compounds the problem. Pollution may also contribute to heart disease by impairing the body's ability to take in oxygen; it can cause irritation of eyes and throat, coughing, difficulty in breathing, headaches, dizziness, chest pains, nausea, and vomiting; and it may affect the unborn fetus and even cause genetic damage.

With every pollution crisis, hospital admissions rise, absenteeism from school and work increases, and the death rate becomes abnormally high. Those who suffer the greatest harm are infants and young children, the very old, and people with heart or lung ailments. No one entirely escapes some health impairment during an acute pollution crisis. Even long-term exposure to low-level pollution can contribute to the development of certain respiratory and heart diseases, or make them worse. It is also important to note that many of the health effects of pollution are a result of exposure to pollution over only the past thirty years. Unless the enormous quantities of pollutants that exist today are eliminated, the incidence of disease will be much higher in the future.

Vegetation, Crops, and Livestock. Pollutants carried in the wind from industrial areas and cities can affect farm crops many miles away. Pollution damages vegetation by retarding growth, discoloring leaves, interfering with pollination, and destroying plant tissue. Indirectly, too, pollution can lead to plant destruction by killing beneficial predatory insects, thus leaving plants vulnerable to harmful insects.

Pollution also reduces crop yields. Many crops have suffered from air pollution: spinach, grapes, beans, lettuce, cotton, beets, grains, and others. Thousands of acres of citrus groves have been ruined, and the annual crop damage has been estimated to be in the hundreds of millions of dollars.

Farm animals, like crops, have been seriously affected. The contaminants that settle on grazing grasses and plants have harmed cattle, sheep, and other farm animals that rely on them for food.

Private and Public Property. Air pollution takes a costly toll each year because it causes the deterioration of virtually every kind of property. The costs of laundering fabrics soiled by contaminants and of washing cars are on the increase. The expense of repainting soot-blackened, discolored, or peeling house exteriors is also rising. More subtle but equally costly damage occurs when pollutants cause fabrics and leather to wear out or rot, auto finishes to pit and stain, rubber tires to crack, windshield-wiper blades to disintegrate, and metals to corrode.

Public property fares little better. Priceless sculptures, monuments, and stone buildings suffer irreparable damage from air contaminants that eat away marble and limestone and destroy glass, brick, and other construction materials. Metals such as copper, aluminum, zinc, brass, iron, and steel corrode many times faster in polluted areas; such corrosion damages bridges and transportation systems. Repair costs are ultimately passed on to the public in the form of increased taxes.

Air Contaminants

Many different substances contaminate the earth's atmosphere, and they have distinct effects on the environment and upon our health. Only a partial listing is given below. Technological advances constantly produce new air pollutants.

Sulfur Oxides. First in terms of danger to human health is a compound called *sulfur dioxide* (SO_2), a colorless gas that has a pungent, irritating odor. Its major source is the combustion of fuel in homes and factories. SO_2, which is a major element of smog, is a strong irritant to the human lungs, respiratory tract, and cardiovascular system, and a primary cause of damage to plant life. Combining with water and other materials in the air, sulfur dioxide forms sulfuric acid, which destroys stone surfaces, rots fabrics, and corrodes steel. It is also a major element in acid rain, discussed below.

Particulates. A second pollutant, which may be equally dangerous, is **particulates**—minute particles, solid or liquid, that are dispersed in the atmosphere. Produced mainly from combustion, particulates include tiny pieces of ash, oil and grease, and metal and carbon materials; they are visible in the air as fly ash, smoke, haze, and dust.

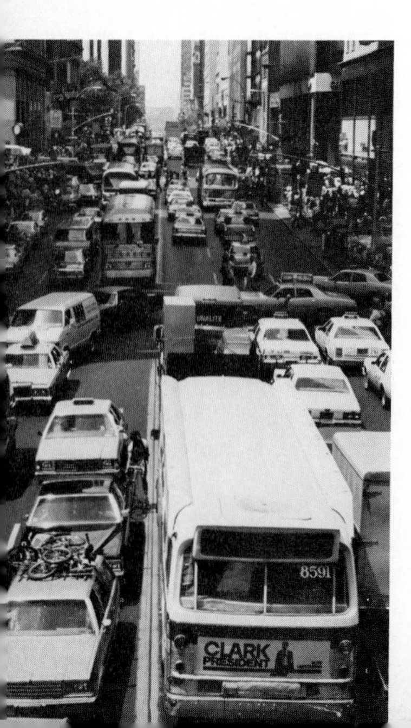

Often found in smog conditions, particulates greatly increase the damage sulfur oxides do to the respiratory tract by providing a vehicle to carry the oxides deep into the lungs. In similar fashion, particulates combine with SO_2 to increase the destruction of building and stone materials by pitting, soiling, and disfiguring them. Particulates damage vegetation by forming hard crusts on leaves and killing plant tissue. High levels of particulates in the air are chiefly responsible for the visibility problems during smog conditions.

Carbon Monoxide. Produced through imperfect gasoline combustion in motor vehicles, *carbon monoxide* (CO) is the most extensive pollutant of our air. CO is a colorless, odorless, and highly poisonous gas that can affect the level of oxygen in the bloodstream and produce death by asphyxiation. For this reason it is extremely dangerous in heavy traffic, tunnels, and garages, where concentrations can build up. In small quantities CO causes dizziness, headache, and tiredness. People with heart conditions, asthma, anemia, and other diseases involving the respiratory and cardiovascular systems are particularly susceptible to its toxic effects.

Smoking is the most impairing source of CO. According to the National Center for Health Statistics, smokers as a group have four times the level of CO in their blood as people who have never smoked.

Nitrogen Oxides. Two of the various nitrogen oxide compounds present a serious threat to air quality: *nitrogen dioxide* (NO_2) and, to some extent, *nitric oxide* (NO). Nitrogen dioxide is a foul-smelling brown gas produced when engine heat breaks up nitrogen molecules and combines them with oxygen. Attributed mostly to motor vehicle emissions and chemical manufacturing processes, NO_2 can irritate the nose and eyes, cause plant damage, shut out sunlight, and reduce visibility. Combined with other pollutants in smog, it can endanger health and crops.

Hydrocarbons. Although produced from many sources, *hydrocarbons* are found mainly in automobile exhaust. Suspected of being cancer-producing agents, hydrocarbons are most dangerous when they combine with other pollutants to create smog.

Ozone. Nitrogen dioxide and hydrocarbons combine in sunlight to produce *ozone*, a gas with a chlorinelike smell that is highly active chemically and extremely poisonous. A principal component and the most toxic element of smog, ozone irritates the nose and throat, causes eyes to burn, produces lung disease after long exposure, deteriorates clothing, causes tires and often rubber products to crack, and destroys crops. (The ozone layer in the atmosphere, however, serves to protect us from the sun's harmful ultraviolet rays. It has been so threatened by a number of chemicals, such as fluorocarbons, used as propellants in aerosol cans, that the government has imposed a ban on their use.)

Asbestos. *Asbestos* is a mineral that was once widely employed in manufacturing and construction. It was also used in automobile brake linings, talcum powder, and building materials. From these sources, asbestos fibers and dust still escape into the air, where they become particulate matter. When inhaled over a long period of time, asbestos causes serious respiratory disorders, including lung cancer. Fortunately, asbestos is now less widely used since its dangers have become known, and the Environmental Protection Agency initiated a program in 1986 to phase out its use altogether.

Vinyl Chloride. *Vinyl chloride* is a gas used as a propellant in aerosol products. It is also used in some manufacturing processes. Prolonged exposure to vinyl chloride has been linked to cancer, particularly cancer of the liver. For this reason, federal law requires that workers exposed to significant levels of vinyl chloride be offered periodic health examinations at the expense of their employers.

Acid Rain. *Acid rain* is a recent environmental concern that combines several pollutants. Nitrogen and sulfur oxides from auto emissions and coal-burning industries circulate in the upper air and combine with water vapor to form nitric and sulfuric acid. These acids are carried far from their highway and industrial sources and fall as rain and snow on rivers, lakes, and forests across the United States and Canada. Acid rain is believed by many experts to have a devastating effect on marine and plant life.

Ironically, the high smokestacks designed by pollution-control experts to better disperse factory pollutants in the wind may contribute to acid rain. The Canadian government has complained that U.S. industrial pollution has created intolerable levels of acidity in thousands of Canadian lakes and streams. Acid rain over the Adirondacks has been linked to the absence of fish in hundreds of mountain lakes and to the blight of red spruce trees near their shores. More recently, mountain lakes in the western United States hitherto thought free of pollution have shown high levels of acidity.

The problem will be very expensive to solve. The national government continues to favor more study, pointing to the multibillion-dollar cost of refitting coal-burning utility and industrial plants in the Midwest, which are thought to be responsible for much of the acid rain in the Northeast. As a start toward a solution, the U.S. and Canadian governments in 1986 agreed to a $5 billion program for developing new technologies to burn coal more cleanly.

Controlling Air Pollution

Controlling air pollution is complex and expensive. Repeated polls show, however, that U.S. citizens see pollution as a serious problem and are willing to pay to have it solved. Still, industry too often continues to resist meeting federal standards. And the administration's introduction of cost-benefit concepts, whereby the dollar cost of an antipollution measure is weighed against its dollar benefit, has helped to blunt the implementation of effective controls. (Though

Clean Power from High-Sulfur Coal

Coal-burning steam turbines now generate over 50 percent of the electric power in the United States. Unfortunately, much of the coal used is of the high-sulfur variety, which when burned produces sulfur dioxide and nitrogen oxides, the major pollutants found in acid rain. Now, however, a nonpolluting technology for generating electricity from high-sulfur coal is being developed in California. In the new method pulverized high-sulfur coal, mixed with water and oxygen, is converted into a gas from which the sulfur is extracted before it is burned as a fuel to produce electricity. The developers of the process describe it as the leading long-term solution to the acid-rain problem.

Because the new technology produces clean energy from the country's most abundant fuel, and because the plants can be built quickly and cheaply, power companies all over the United States have invested in the project. The first five-year test is due to end in 1989; at that time these companies will decide whether they will adopt the system.

Source: Walter Sullivan, "Power Plant Shows Promise in Cleaner Burning of Coal," *New York Times,* April 1, 1986, p. C5.

cost-benefit ratios may be regarded as commonsense business calculations, they assume a different dimension when the benefit is no longer dollars, but lives.)

Control of Automotive Pollution. Under the Clean Air Act of 1970, the Environmental Protection Agency was established and given the power to set and enforce standards for air quality that would protect public health. One of the EPA's concerns was automotive pollution.

New, lowered pollution levels for automobiles were set quickly, but the automotive industry succeeded in having deadlines for meeting them postponed, so it was not until the late 1970s that new cars were complying with EPA regulations. Since that time there has been a marked decrease in the amount of carbon monoxide, in particular, that new automobiles emit. In fact, the amount of CO emitted by new cars today is only 10 percent of what it was in 1970.

That is progress indeed. But two factors have kept CO levels from decreasing as much as they might have. First is the simple fact that there are more cars on our roads today than when the Clean Air Act was passed. Though each car produces less pollution, the total amount released into the air remains high. Second is that antipollution devices (primarily the catalytic converter) installed in new cars have to be maintained or pollution levels will increase as the cars get older. Four out of five states have passed mandatory vehicle inspection laws to ensure that automobiles continue to comply with EPA standards, but the rules do not apply to older cars. These cars do not have catalytic converters and may still use leaded gasoline. Furthermore, an EPA study in 1985 showed that emission-control devices in nearly one in four newer cars had been tampered with and that one in six cars designed to be driven with lead-free gasoline had leaded gas in their tanks. These statistics reveal very clearly that without universal, ongoing programs of automobile inspection to monitor the effectiveness of emission-control devices, all other efforts will be severely compromised.

Perhaps the ultimate step to reduce air pollution would be to reduce our dependence on the automobile. To this end, several different mass transportation systems are now being studied. Some cities have also raised tolls and car-use taxes and have passed parking restrictions in an attempt to reduce car use. Many concerned citizens are fighting air pollution by reporting pollution law violations, supporting the concept of improved mass transportation, and forming energy-saving car pools or reducing their use of automobiles. Many states now provide parking facilities ("park-ride") to enable commuters to make better use of public transportation and to encourage car pooling.

Control of Factory and Power Plant Pollution. The Environmental Protection Agency is also empowered to deal with industrial air pollution. The EPA sets emission standards for industry; that is, it limits the amount of pollutants that each factory or plant is permitted to discharge. If a polluter cannot meet the emission standards immediately, the state government imposes a compliance schedule that spells out when the changes will be made.

In compliance with these laws, industries have begun to find ways of cutting down on pollution. Refineries have developed a technique to capture sulfur dioxide and convert it into sulfur or sulfuric acid. The steel industry has begun replacing open-hearth furnaces with oxygen furnaces that reduce emission of iron oxide. Electrostatic precipitators installed by the electric power industry are catching a major portion of the fly ash emitted; and the substitution of low-sulfur fuel oil, higher smokestacks, and charcoal filtration are aiding in the control of sulfur dioxide emission and odor. A low-pollution method of producing electricity from high-sulfur coal, first put into commercial use in 1986, shows promise for reducing a major cause of acid rain (see box: Clean Power from High-Sulfur Coal). As with auto pollution, however, control of industrial pollution has been hampered by the resistance of industry and the reluctance of government to implement the law.

Control of Refuse Disposal. In order to cut down on air pollution, many localities have banned the outdoor burning of refuse, and in many places compactors have replaced incinerators in apartment houses. But the problem of what to do with refuse has not been satisfactorily solved.

Two types of solution have been proposed: (1) *resource recovery*, which means making some productive use of the refuse, such as burning trash as a source of energy in power plants and recycling metal, paper, and glass; and (2) *source reduction*, which means cutting down on refuse by banning throwaway bottles and cans, eliminating overpackaging, and improving the durability of products.

Some progress has been made in both areas. There are already plants that use wastes for fuel, and pilot projects to convert solid refuse to fuel oil or gas by subjecting it to intense heat are under way. At the same time, concerned citizens are beginning to demand that manufacturers cut down on their excess

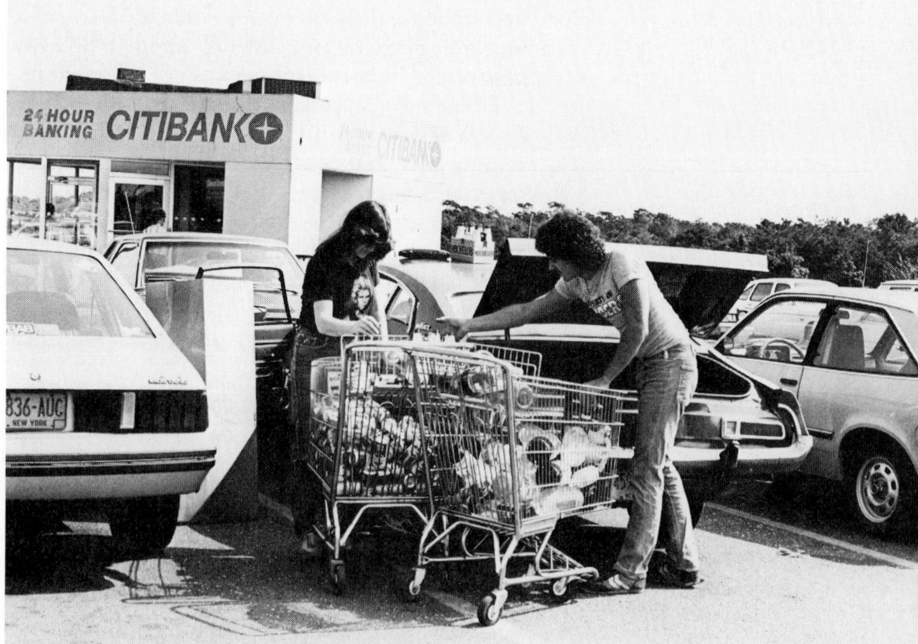

Bottle bills passed in some states have stimulated the return of beverage containers for the refund of deposits. The welcome result has been less litter on our highways and beaches.

packaging. Bottle bills requiring a deposit to be paid on beverage containers have been enacted in many states, with a resulting reduction in trash on roadsides and in state parks.

Recent Problems of the Clean Air Act. The battle between the federal government and environmentalists has centered on the Clean Air Act of 1970, which gave the EPA enough muscle to force the states to comply with federal standards. The administration has been accused of inadequate enforcement of the Clean Air Act in the belief that full compliance would hinder the country's economic growth. Environmentalists, on the other hand, have argued that economic growth can be spurred just as effectively by the new antipollution industry and the employment it provides, as well as by the lower medical costs in a population that breathes cleaner air.

Environmentalists continue to fight any legislation that proposes to reduce the power of the Clean Air Act or lower its standards. Since 1970 improvements have resulted from the steady increase in standards: Particulate matter in the atmosphere has been halved, and sulfur dioxides and carbon monoxide have both been reduced by a fourth.

Environmentalists look to future global problems as well as to the immediate health of American citizens. A problem looming in the future and recognized by the American Association for the Advancement of Science—one of the most prestigious scientific organizations in the world—is the **greenhouse effect.** According to the greenhouse theory, air pollution is forming a layer of carbon dioxide in the atmosphere that retains heat, much as a greenhouse does. The prediction is that global air temperatures will rise in the twenty-first century and cause the polar ice caps to melt, thus raising the sea level to a dangerous degree and causing both droughts and coastal flooding. Only if all the industrialized countries in the world agree to very strict air pollution controls, some geophysicists argue, can this course of events be avoided.

Between these two poles of opinion, and with time running out, the Clean Air Act has become the center of heated controversy. Our quality of life depends on both economic security and environmental health—two goals that seem to be at cross-purposes. The critical question for the future is whether the goals will be continually compromised, or whether the United States will find the means to gear economic progress to environmental progress, thus making both goals possible.

WATER POLLUTION

Like air, water is a vital resource for human existence. Without water, a human being cannot survive for more than five days. And yet people have dumped wastes of every description into nature's waterways. Today virtually every pond, stream, river, lake, and sea inlet in this country has been affected by such indiscriminate pollution. Ironically, as water pollution increases, so does our need for consumable fresh water. But this resource is strictly limited. Only 3 percent of the world's water supply consists of fresh water, and of this amount 98 percent is frozen in the polar ice caps.

Sources of Water Pollution

Water pollution occurs when wastes accumulate in a body of water to the point that the water's natural purification processes cannot break them down into harmless and inoffensive forms. There are four major water polluters: (1) industry, (2) municipalities, (3) agriculture, and (4) navigational craft.

Industry. By far the greatest polluters of water are factories and industrial plants. Industry needs water for cooling, for power, as an ingredient in products, and for transporting raw materials and finished products. Very large quantities of water are used in making everyday products. For example, 100,000 gallons of water are used in the manufacture of one automobile. Industry is now using hundreds of billions of gallons of water each day, and its requirements are increasing.

As industry's need for pure water grows, so does the amount of industrial waste being spewed into the waterways. Industrial sources, it is estimated, produce 60 percent of the pollution in the national water supply. Such major industries as paper manufacturing, petroleum refining, steel, and organic chemicals account for three times as much waste as is discharged by all Americans living in communities with sewers. Construction of facilities to process industrial wastes is lagging. To make the situation worse, plants and facilities tend to cluster together in the same area, so that local lakes and streams become heavily polluted. EPA tests of underground drinking-water supplies of nearly a thousand cities have shown contamination in 29 percent of the samples. Other EPA studies identified more than 80,000 U.S. sites with contaminated surface-water pools, 90 percent of which were thought to be potential threats to groundwater supplies.

The development of new products brings with it an endless array of new pollutants. Nearly 1,000 new chemicals are developed each year in the United States alone; and, according to one congressional study, more than a ton of hazardous chemical waste for every man, woman, and child in the United States is dumped into the nation's environment each year. Among the materials discharged into U.S. waters are some extremely toxic substances, including radioactive wastes. In many cases, the techniques for processing such waste materials have not been developed as quickly as the waste itself.

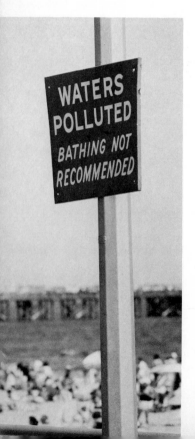

Many of these chemicals, once released, tend to remain in the environment and in human tissue. They are absorbed into the human body through the food chain, through drinking water, and through the air. Of particular concern have been *PCBs*, or *polychlorinated biphenyls*, used in transformers, capacitors, and other electrical equipment. PCBs have been found to cause tumors, reproductive disorders, and other problems in test animals and are regarded as a threat to human health. Though federal regulations banned the production of PCBs in 1976 and required that their existing uses be phased out, 99 percent of all Americans are thought to have some detectable PCBs in their body tissues and the chemicals are still in evidence in the food chain. As late as 1986 commercial catches of striped bass were banned off Long Island in New York because the fish were found to contain dangerous levels of PCBs.

Accidental pollution, too, is very hard to prevent and control. Oil leaks from land and offshore drilling, storage equipment and pipelines, and accidental spills can cause widespread damage. Mine drainage, accounting for millions of tons of toxic waste each year, largely from abandoned mines, is another industrial source that is difficult to manage.

Municipalities. Considering today's generally high living standards, it is shocking that almost three in ten people in the United States live in areas that have no waste-treatment facilities. And many of the facilities that exist are poorly maintained, inefficient, or overloaded. Many cities still dump raw sewage into the freshwater supply.

Primary sewage treatment, the most basic form of waste processing, is at present used in systems serving some 34 million people. This method decays sewage by speeding up natural bacterial processes, using mechanical, biological, or chemical means. The process removes sediment, and chlorination reduces disease-causing bacteria; only 40 percent of the organic matter is removed, however.

Secondary sewage treatment goes a step further. Serving about 124 million people in the United States, this measure destroys organic matter more completely and more quickly by introducing extra bacteria to decompose it. An additional 40 to 50 percent of the organic material is removed by this process. If chlorination is included, the method is 80 to 90 percent efficient.

Tertiary sewage treatment, used mainly in large metropolitan centers or major industrialized areas, involves chemical treatment to remove sediments and phosphates, filtration to remove turbidity, absorption to remove stubborn organic matter, and a procedure called *electrodialysis* to remove dissolved salts. Only about 5 million people are served by this form of treatment.

Sewage disposal is a major problem in this country. The federal government, realizing its dimensions, has spent $50 billion over the past decade to fund construction of new sewage-treatment plants nationwide. And there have been heartening results, with fish returning to waters formerly too polluted to support animal life. Still, the volume of waste is expected to increase over 400 percent in the next fifty years, leaving even the newest plants inadequate to the task. Pollution from the many communities that lack sewers and rely on septic tank disposal has also grown, and there is evidence of groundwater pollution.

Even as they process contaminants, most municipal waste-treatment facilities add to water pollution. The end products of primary and secondary sewage treatment are mainly nitrates and phosphates, which kill fish and other aquatic life.

A final source of pollution in municipalities is the sediment, silt, and sand that build up in rivers and streams as a result of *nonpoint pollution*: runoff from city streets and construction sites. Nonpoint pollution from cities and farms (see below) has gone largely uncontrolled and is thought to be responsible for half the total pollution of our waterways nationwide.

Agriculture. To make farmlands and livestock more productive, farmers are using modern methods of irrigation and fertilization; to control insects, rodents, and unwanted vegetation, they are using pesticides and herbicides. All these techniques contribute to water pollution.

Irrigation of croplands sometimes causes a condition known as **irrigation return flow.** Water draining through the soil dissolves salts and minerals; with repeated use of the same water supply, harmful concentrations are built up. The water becomes unfit for further use until these pollutants have been diluted.

Synthetic fertilizers, pesticides, and herbicides can also have wide-ranging

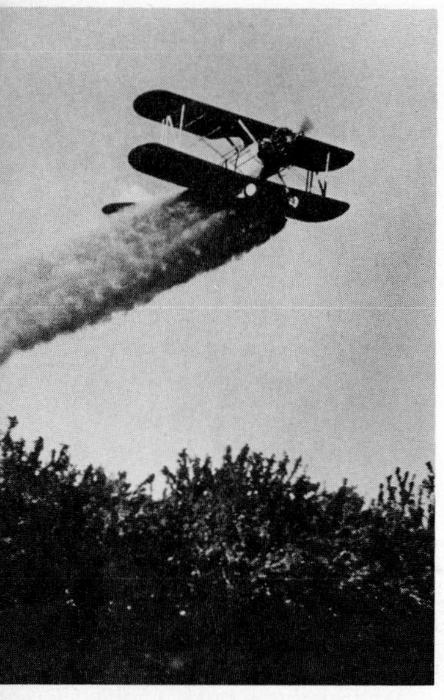

Pesticides dusted onto crops are carried by runoff from rain into our streams, where they have damaged marine life.

side effects. These chemicals are carried by the rain into streams. Here they do great damage to fish and other wildlife, plants, and aquatic insects. They may also be transmitted up the food chain and eventually affect human beings through biological magnification, a process described below.

Sedimentation and cropland and pasture area erosion also create pollution. Such conditions are reflected in the dirty brown appearance of a stream following a rainstorm. Poor agricultural techniques have been estimated to increase normal land erosion rates from four to nine times.

The increase in the number of livestock being bred and fed also affects water purity. Large herds of animals bunched in small feeding areas produce a great deal of animal waste—partly because of the highly enriched food they are fed. Washed into our rivers and streams by rains, animal wastes can kill fish and promote excessive plant growth. They also introduce undesirable tastes and odors, clog water-treatment facilities, and allow harmful bacteria to enter the water supply.

Navigational Craft. Another important cause of water pollution is the wide variety of navigational craft that use our waterways. There are some 13 million recreational craft, and few of them are equipped with disposal systems to process galley and toilet wastes. Exhaust materials discharged from motorboats also contaminate water surfaces. Larger ships pollute the environment with bilge and ballast water, garbage, sanitary wastes, and littering. Few commercial ships navigating U.S. waterways have systems for collecting and treating shipboard pollutants. The sewage they release into the water presents a hazard to shellfish and to recreational areas.

Harmful Effects of Water Pollution

Water pollution has far-reaching effects on human well-being, wildlife, recreational areas, and the economy.

Human Health. Typhoid fever, dysentery, cholera, and intestinal disturbances are just a few of the diseases that may be transmitted by polluted water. Insects that frequent polluted streams, and animals that drink from and swim in them, may carry bacteria and viruses into human food and habitats. Viruses from human waste can cause diseases such as infectious hepatitis. Other human ailments may be caused by the cumulative toxic effects of chemical and metal particles that enter the body through drinking water. Sodium ions are suspected of being related to heart disease, and chlorides may aggravate high blood pressure. The presence of cancer-producing agents in polluted water is also considered a possibility. Asbestos fibers have been found in the water of several municipalities; these can cause cancer when ingested by mouth. Radium, a known cancer-causing agent, has been found in drinking supplies. There is also a possibility that genetic damage or birth defects are caused by water pollutants.

Wildlife. Water pollution attacks fish, birds, and animals, causing them to sicken and die. It can alter the balance of the ecosystem, fertilizing algae and other plant life until they choke the waterways. It can kill off some species and thus permit others to proliferate. And it can destroy plankton, which provide food for other creatures.

Water pollution directly affects fish; it can slow their reproduction, change their growth rate, blanket their breeding areas and food supplies, or simply poison them. Massive fish kills and the reduction of fish species have already resulted from water pollution. Continuing up the food chain, waterfowl, wild animals, and human beings may eat contaminated fish and be poisoned by the toxic substances in them.

Recreation. As urbanization increases, more and more people seek the change of pace offered by water recreation and outdoor activities—swimming, water skiing, sailing, fishing, and boating. But pollution threatens to make beaches unusable through contamination by disease-causing organisms or by unattractive, bad-smelling substances such as visible sewage.

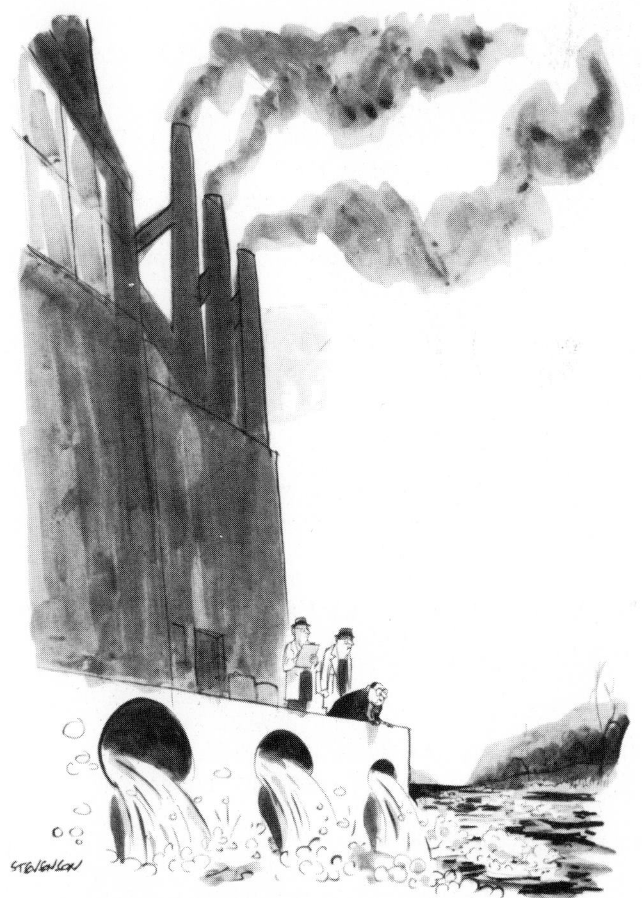

"*So* that's *where it goes*! *Well, I'd like to thank you fellows for bringing this to my attention*."

Pollutants that kill fish also threaten fishing, a pastime enjoyed by millions of anglers, serious and casual. Boating, too, has suffered from the effects of water pollution. Vile-smelling waters, as well as contaminants that deteriorate the hulls and coatings of watercraft, diminish the carefree enjoyment of yet another recreational activity.

Economic Considerations. Pure water is essential for many economic reasons. Commercial fisheries are threatened when fish species are reduced or destroyed. Communities that derive income from recreational facilities are harmed by the closing of beaches; waterfront property is devaluated; manufacturers and sellers of equipment for boating, fishing, camping, and swimming suffer from lowered sales; the communities that want industrial plants to locate in their towns cannot offer essential water resources. Damage to farmlands, crops, and livestock by polluted irrigation waters is also an important economic factor. The cost of controlling water pollution is high, but the cost of continuing it is higher still.

Water Contaminants

Many different toxic substances pollute our waterways, and their sources are frequently difficult to control. Some of the most critical ones are discussed here.

Nitrogen and Phosphorus Compounds. Two major pollutants that can bring death to lakes and slow-moving waterways are **phosphates** and **nitrates.** Present in detergents, fertilizers, municipal sewage, human wastes, and industrial discharges, these compounds of nitrogen and phosphorus, even in small quantities, can result in huge fish kills, foul-smelling beaches, and bad-tasting drinking water. Lakes and slow-moving rivers suffer the greatest damage, for they cannot disperse the materials.

Phosphates and nitrates serve as fertilizers or nutrients in the water, stimulating the growth of algae and aquatic weeds. This gradual increase in plant nutrients is called **eutrophication.** As eutrophication continues, water plants proliferate and soon clog the shorelines and advance into the lake's center. The dying plants eventually begin to pile up on the lake's bottom, making it shallower and smaller. As these plants decay, the supply of oxygen in the water is gradually removed until it cannot support life. Soon the only living organisms are of the lowest, most primary forms.

The gradual death of Lake Erie is one example of the process of eutrophication. Used as a dumping ground for several hundred million pounds of detergents, chemicals, and sewage from industries and municipalities, this Great Lake gradually choked to death on its own overfertilized plant life. And not only was the lake virtually dead, but the rivers flowing into it also became despoiled by industrial pollution. In recent years, however, progress has been made in restoring Lake Erie to life. The reappearance of fish in the lake is a clear sign of what can happen when efforts are made to reduce pollution.

Insecticides, Pesticides, and Herbicides. Several hundred synthetic chemicals are used to exterminate insects, weeds, rodents, and other unwanted organisms. Some examples are arsenic, chlordane, heptachlor, dieldrin, aldrin, endrin, and malathion. Many of these chemicals are sprayed directly into the water to kill weeds, insect larvae, and unwanted fish species. Others are sprayed on crops or vegetation and carried by rainwater or groundwater into rivers and streams. Through a process called **biological magnification,** concentrations of long-lasting toxins *increase* as they move up the food chain. A study of radioactivity in the Columbia River showed that concentrations in the water were not harmful. However, river organisms such as plankton showed levels 2,000 times greater than the water; fish that ate the plankton, 15,000 times greater; and ducks, 40,000 times greater. Concentrations of insecticides and other poisons also increase as they ascend the food chain

Such chemicals can sicken humans and animals, destroy or damage crops, poison well water, and kill huge numbers of fish, fish-eating waterfowl, and wildlife. Residues of these poisons can linger and actually build up in the water or combine with other chemical pollutants to render even harmless substances toxic.

The killing of water life, intended or accidental, has repercussions for the whole aquatic environment. The effect of poisons is not always selective, and numerous innocent species of aquatic life may be the unintentional recipients of these destructive agents. The accidental destruction of food sources may also wipe out organisms that are dependent on them.

Another problem causing great concern is the infiltration of insecticides into public water supplies. Present water-treatment facilities are not adequate to remove all the complex chemicals introduced into the water. Though only small quantities of these agents may exist in public drinking water now, some of them can be stored within the body until dangerous levels build up.

Mine Acids. *Iron sulfide* is found in coal beds. In combination with air and water it produces an acid that can cause much ecological damage. Recognizable as a bright yellow deposit on rocks or a reddish sediment in streams, **mine acid** can be highly toxic to fish, cutting down their growth rate and reproductive

A strip mine in North Dakota.

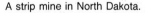

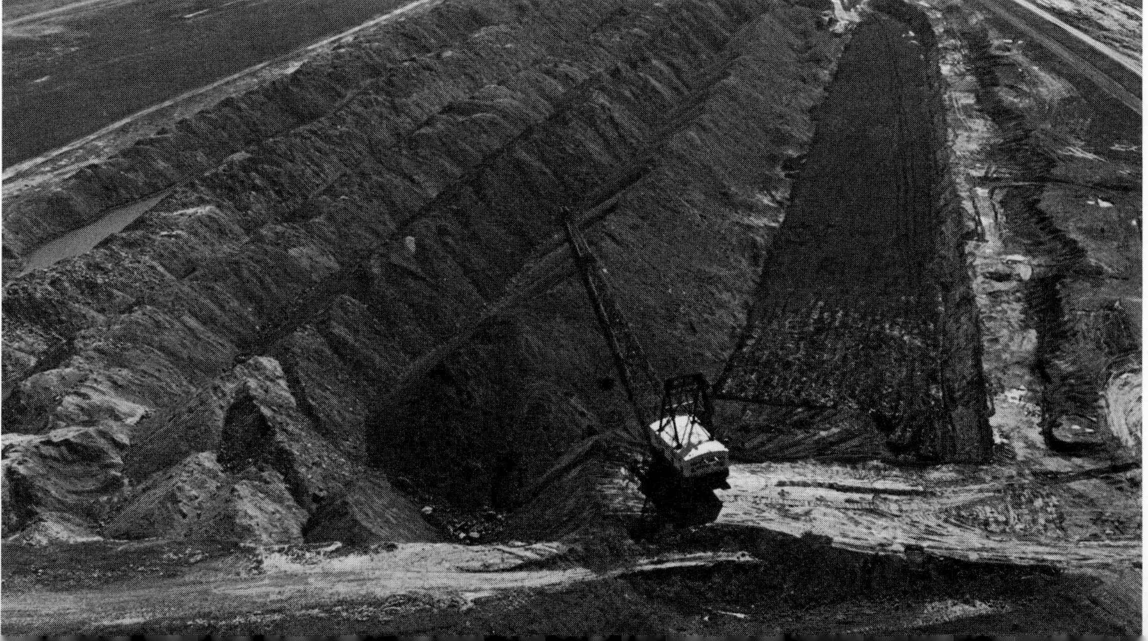

capacity; it can corrode bridges, boats, and piers, and reduce the aesthetic and recreational uses of water. Mine acid is one of the major causes of fish kills in this country, and over 4 million tons of this sulfuric acid equivalent are produced each year. Each day a single mine may discharge as much as 10 million gallons of water contaminated by mine acid.

Sediment and Silt. The pollution of water by suspended solids in various forms is a serious problem. From farms and woodlands, city streets, construction sites, and other erodable areas, large volumes of **sediment** (materials that settle to the bottom of water) and **silt** (fine particles suspended in water) are washed into rivers and streams, giving them a murky brown color. These materials destroy fish habitats by covering over their nests and food supplies. They clog waterways and reduce the water capacity of reservoirs, and they prevent sunlight from penetrating the water. Sediments can also damage crops, spoil water recreation, and clog water used for power equipment.

Oil Spills. Oil spills are the accidental loss or seepage of oil from pipelines, transport vessels, drilling operations, or other operations that discharge oil into the sea or onto the land. A large number of spills have resulted from the collision or grounding of transport vessels. And as these vessels continue to be built on a larger scale, the amount of oil that they are capable of spilling

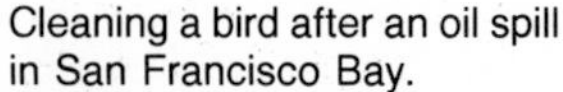

Cleaning a bird after an oil spill in San Francisco Bay.

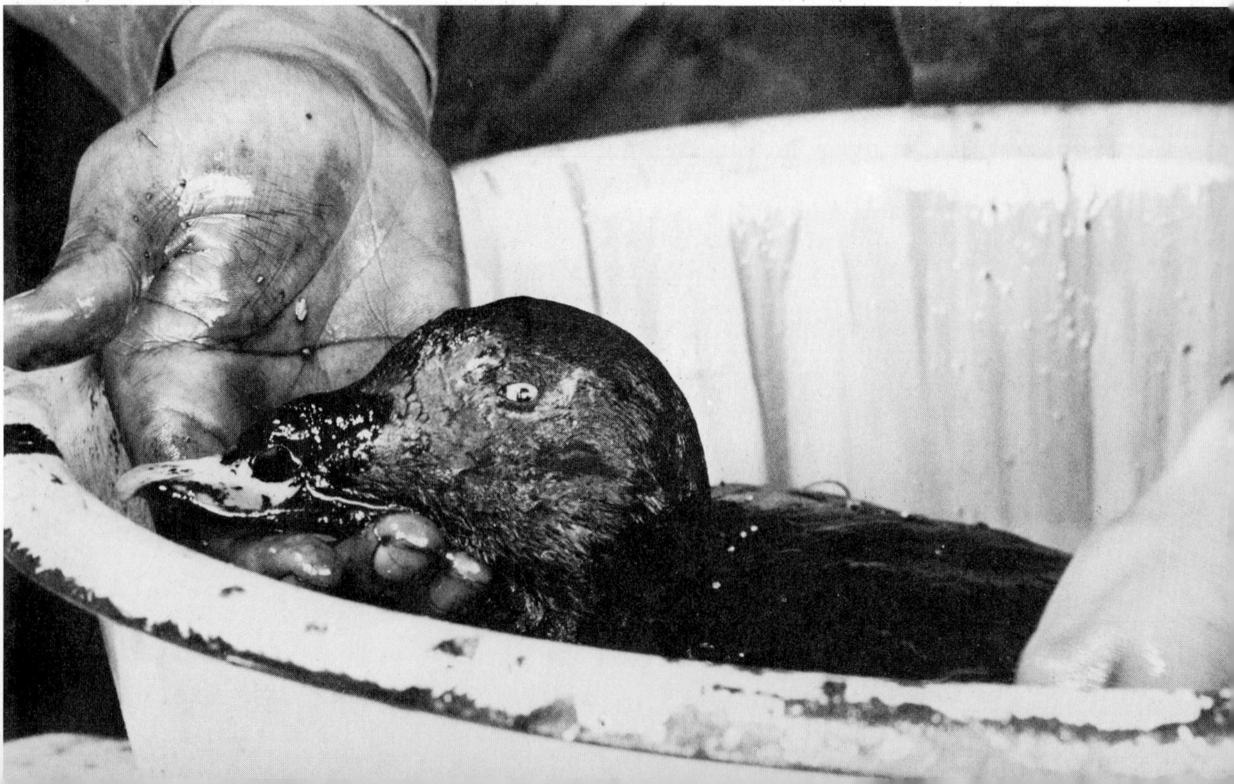

increases as well. The *Amoco Cadiz*, a supertanker, was torn apart off the coast of France in 1978, spilling its entire cargo of over 200,000 tons of oil into the water and thereby creating the largest accident of its kind to date.

Despite all precautions, offshore drilling accidents increase with the proliferation of these operations. The largest spill in history occurred in 1979, when an oil rig in the Gulf of Mexico blew out and, before it was capped, released about 100 million gallons of oil into the surrounding waters.

The damage done to the environment following any major oil spill is far-reaching and tragic. Thousands of birds become coated with the material and drown or starve because they cannot fly. The bodies and gills of fish become covered with oil and large numbers die. Beaches are defaced and made unusable. Waterfront property is damaged. Fire hazards are created, and freshwater supplies are endangered. Although attempts are made to cleanse the water and rescue the wildlife, much of the damage cannot be reversed.

Heated Water. **Thermal water pollution,** produced when large quantities of water are used to cool electric generators, can have an adverse effect on aquatic life. Power-generating facilities may discharge very hot water—up to 115°F—raising the temperature of rivers as much as 30°F for several miles downstream.

Temperature changes of even a few degrees can affect the ecological balance of a river and kill fish. When the temperature of river water has been raised to 95°F, its ability to contain oxygen diminishes. As a result, the river is no longer able to assimilate wastes efficiently, plant growth increases, and the water becomes foul-tasting. As the demand for electric power continues to increase, thermal pollution becomes a more serious problem.

Organic Sewage. When organic wastes—that is, animal or vegetable waste—are released into waterways (mainly from sewage or from animal feed lots), they are generally decomposed by bacteria that depend on oxygen. But an overabundance of such pollutants may lower the oxygen content of the water. Such oxygen depletion kills off bacteria and thus lessens the water's natural ability to cleanse itself. Fish and other aquatic organisms die; plant life diminishes, thus continuing the oxygen depletion; toxic microorganisms proliferate; filtration systems become clogged; and waterways become heavily polluted.

The disposal of *sludge*, or human waste, remains a problem. For many coastal cities, the ocean has been a convenient dumping area, but federal law has attempted to halt this practice because of its overfertilizing and polluting effect upon the ocean floor. Controversy surrounds the implementation of these laws, mostly because of the cost to municipalities.

Controlling Water Pollution

The Federal Water Pollution Control Act Amendments of 1972 established a system to limit water pollution. Under this law, it is illegal to discharge any pollutant into the nation's waters without a permit. The permit sets limits on the nature and quantity of pollutants that may be discharged. Violations are punishable by fines or prison sentences. The ultimate goal of the 1972 law was to eliminate entirely the discharge of industrial pollutants into our waterways. It is a task that has yet to be accomplished.

Technology and research are needed to develop better, cheaper, and more desirable methods for dealing with water pollution problems. Some specific controls are already known. Hot-water pollution, for instance, can be reduced by using cooling towers or ponds, by selecting more appropriate sites for plant construction, and by improving plant efficiency. Mine-acid pollution can be regulated by renovating mine areas, regrading and replanting, sealing off mines, using chemical or biological controls to reduce acid formation, or adding neutralizers. The presence of sand and sediments in our waterways can be reduced through erosion prevention techniques that include crop rotation, stream bank stabilization structures, and the sloping and contouring of river banks. Salts and minerals from irrigation can be cut down by lining canals and using desalination equipment. And sewage from watercraft can be eliminated by trapping it in holding tanks and disposing of it onshore. Of course, the citizen's role is most important. Funds for federal, state, and local regulatory agencies are allocated in response to public pressure. Citizens can also function as monitors to ensure that pollution guidelines are being met.

NOISE POLLUTION

Modern living has intensified an old problem: *noise pollution*. In the street, in our homes, and on the job, the noise of daily living can be frustrating and harmful to our well-being. Every ten years, according to recent estimates, the intensity of noise in our environment doubles. At this rate, we are fast approaching the point at which more noise will be intolerable to the human auditory system. Noise pollution is emerging as a serious problem and one that demands prompt attention.

The intensity of sound is measured in **decibels** (db). One decibel is the smallest difference in sound intensity detectable by the human ear; every ten-decibel increase is perceived as a doubling of loudness. Common sounds range from a whisper (20 db) to live rock music (115 db) to the roar of a jet plane on takeoff (140 db or more); normal conversational tones fall at a middle range of about 60 decibels. Sounds below 80 decibels are generally considered safe. Unfortunately, many of the sounds we hear every day are much louder (see Figure 17-2).

Sources of Noise Pollution

Noise is a by-product of human activity, and some noise is virtually unavoidable. But the excessive noise most of us hear comes from certain common sources. The noise of automobiles, trucks, trains, motorcycles, buses, and airplanes is a fairly common nuisance. Many people, especially those who live or work in cities, become used to the roar of traffic. The sound of motors, engines, and equipment being used in construction and demolition can be very hazardous. Our own homes fail to provide a haven from noise. Stereos, television sets, air conditioners, and vacuum cleaners are among household noisemakers; and the kitchen is likely to be the noisiest room in the house. Even a small device like a food blender may operate above safe noise levels. Adding to the din, noises from neighbors may intrude into nearby homes and adjoining apartments. The machinery of many industries is extremely noisy, and many people must

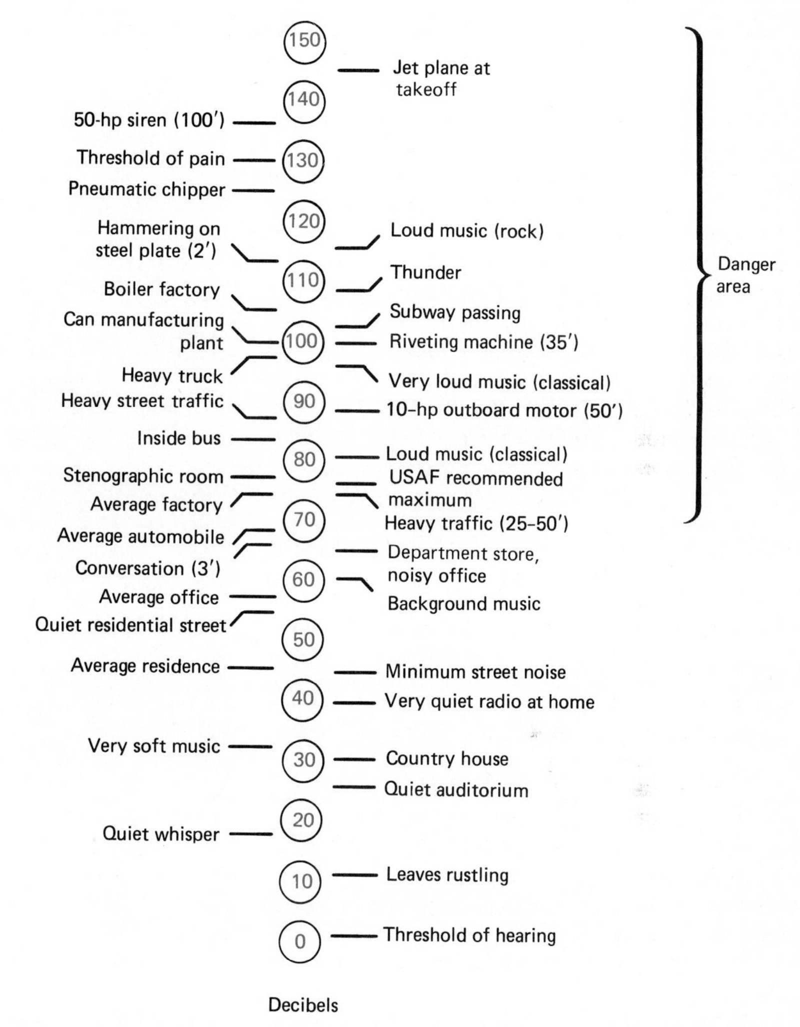

FIGURE 17-2

Decibel values of common sounds.

Source: Richard H. Wagner, *Environment and Man*, 2nd ed. (New York: W. W. Norton, 1974). Used by permission. Copyright © 1971, 1974 by W. W. Norton & Company, Inc.

work long hours in environments that have dangerous noise levels. For this reason, partial deafness is an occupational hazard in some kinds of work. This is understandable when one looks at the noise ratings of some common industrial equipment.

Harmful Effects of Noise Pollution

A full understanding of noise pollution has yet to be achieved, but researchers are focusing more attention on this environmental problem as it increases and becomes more annoying and harmful.

Human Health. Sound pollution may affect human health in more diverse ways than any other kind of pollution. More than 16 million Americans now

Noise Pollution

In trying to track a suspected Soviet submarine [in 1982], the Swedish Navy had difficulty finding sailors who could hear well enough to operate the listening devices. The hearing of vast numbers of young people, a navy captain said, apparently has been permanently damaged by years of listening to loud rock music.

Whether or not music is the culprit in Sweden, similar hearing losses have been noted among American high school and college students who are rock music aficionados or who frequent discotheques; and hearing loss resulting from abusive noise has become a matter of pressing concern in this country.

For example, Dr. David Lipscomb, head of the noise laboratory at the University of Tennessee, recently found that more than 60 percent of 1,410 college freshmen had significant hearing loss in the high-frequency range, a deficit he believes is increasing at an alarming rate. Just one year earlier he had found high-frequency hearing loss in 33 percent of the freshmen tested. He described the students as "two or three decades ahead of themselves in hearing deterioration."

While noisy work environments have long been the focus of research and regulatory efforts, in recent years avocational *noise has been attracting more attention. The explosive rise of noisy equipment in and out of American homes—ranging from snowmobiles, rock bands, and chain saws to hair dryers, food processors, and stereo headphones—has made nearly every American potentially vulnerable to noise damage.*

Source: Jane E. Brody, "Noise Poses a Growing Threat, Affecting Hearing and Behavior," *The New York Times,* November 16, 1982, pp. C1, C5. © 1982 by The New York Times Company. Reprinted by permission.

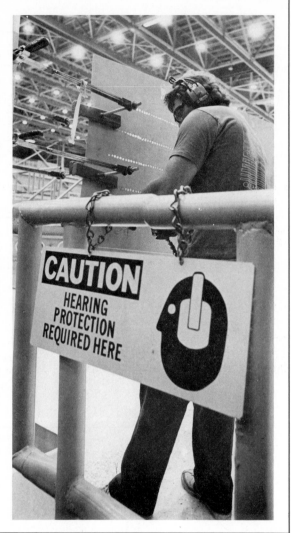

suffer some degree of hearing loss caused by excessive noise. Immediate symptoms include discomfort, pain, and ringing in the ear. Permanent hearing damage may result from exposure to excessive noise for a long period of time.

Besides deafness, noise causes other physical reactions. Researchers have noted a rise in blood cholesterol and blood pressure, dilation of pupils, constriction of blood vessels, and unnatural brain-wave rhythms. Side effects of noise pollution include loss of sleep and of relaxation.

Psychological symptoms may also appear. Irritability, fatigue, unsociability, and nervous exhaustion often result from exposure to noise. Under such conditions, changes in the nervous system cause accelerated heart rate, constricted blood vessels, and skin pallor.

Other Effects. Studies now under way suggest that noise has some potentially dangerous effects on wildlife, buildings, property values, and the economy. Current research is also aimed at exploring the relationship between noise stress and prenatal development. One of the most important lines of research links noise pollution with learning impairment among schoolchildren. A 1982 study in New York City found that the reading scores of students improved after subway noise near the classroom was reduced.

Controlling Noise Pollution

Unlike some other environmental pollutants, noise pollution can be eliminated through existing technology. Many sound-dampening devices and techniques are available, including sound- and vibration-absorbing materials for motors and engines, soundproofing materials for building construction, and baffles and exhaust silencers for power generators.

Perhaps the most effective means for getting these products into use is to enact local noise-control ordinances. One problem is how to enforce them: Identification and proof of violation are difficult to obtain. Police and other personnel need to be instructed in the use of detection equipment and noise meters. (Police and fire departments and ambulance companies should also be made aware of the noxious effects sirens have on city residents.) Another problem is the reluctance of municipalities to provide the extra funds needed for noise-controlled equipment. This may change, as the high noise level of cities has been one factor in the recent migration of some Americans from urban to rural areas.

Federal regulatory agencies can make a difference. In 1980 the EPA reported that more complaints were made by citizens about motorcycle noise than any other traffic noise. The EPA thereupon passed regulations limiting the noise level of motorcycles to 80 decibels by 1986, an average reduction of 5 decibels, a not inconsiderable amount when one remembers that 10 decibels equals a doubling of perceived noise.

The establishment of the federal Office of Noise Abatement and Control was another important step toward solving the noise pollution problem. Its program includes analysis of the causes and effects as well as the ecological implications of noise, compilation of existing local laws and regulations, and identification of criteria for acceptable noise levels. New legislation has also been proposed that would expand this agency's power to set standards for products, to carry on needed research, to enforce the labeling of products for noise, and to punish violators with fines.

GOVERNMENT AGENCIES AND POLLUTION CONTROL

The vital issue of controlling environmental pollution has divided those concerned into two opposing camps, each operating under a different set of values and priorities. The real issue is not what causes pollution, nor even the effects of pollution; these factors have been studied thoroughly and elicit little general disagreement. The real issue is compliance, and the degree of willingness or determination to actually do something about pollution.

If government regulations were stringently enforced, polluters would be obliged to discontinue or adjust operations that adversely affect the quality of air, soil, or water. But continual fencing between polluters and regulatory agencies has delayed the enforcement of these laws. The polluter's response is generally an argument based upon economic grounds: The cost of adjustment and modifications would be enormous and would have to be passed along to the consumer, and adherence to the new regulations would require lowering production and laying off employees. Industry often claims that the cost of environment safeguards is altogether prohibitive and unjustified; and its solution to the problem is to adopt a strategy of minimal response.

Those on the opposite side of this issue emphasize the consequences of pollution. Pollution causes substantial damage to buildings and equipment. It also affects plant and animal life, our air and water—indeed, everything around us. Of primary concern, however, is the effect pollution has on human health and the enormous costs of treating pollution-induced illnesses.

In terms of jobs, environmentalists claim that strict adherence to EPA standards would create many new jobs within the economy. Industry, however, questions the basic willingness of the American public to pay the costs of compliance with environmental regulations. But public response to polls has revealed a wide margin of support for environmental protection. Even many corporate executives—who are generally unsympathetic to environmental concerns—have advocated tougher environmental policies.

Membership and contributions have significantly increased for many environmentally concerned organizations, such as the Sierra Club, the National Wildlife

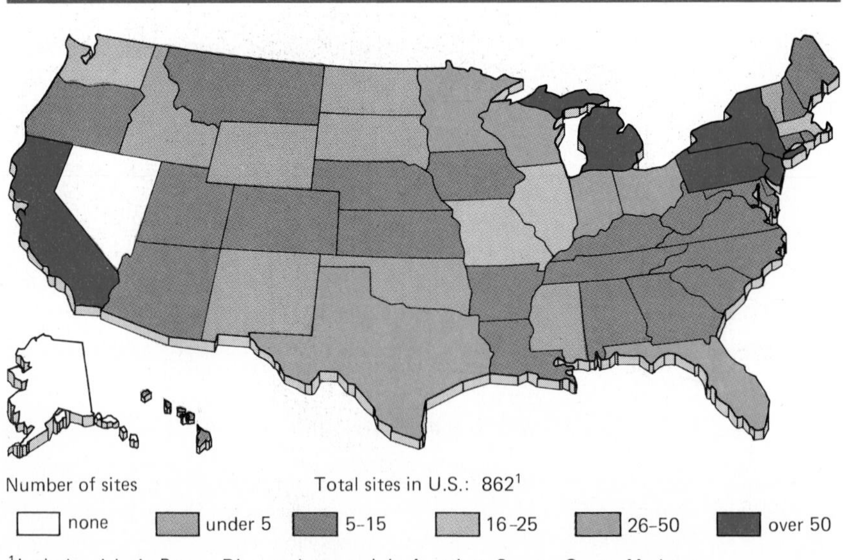

FIGURE 17-3

Hazardous waste sites on the superfund priority list: number by state.

Source: U.S. Environmental Protection Agency, September 1985.

Federation, and the National Audubon Society, each of which vigilantly observes and reports on environment-related activities in Washington.

Government agencies are the instrument by which pollution-control legislation and regulation could be implemented. But this has been the very Achilles' heel of the environmental movement. Although a great deal of valuable environmental legislation has been passed, the agencies responsible for the enforcement of these provisions have been, in the main, reluctant to insist upon compliance. In 1980, for example, Congress established a "Superfund" of $1.6 billion to clean up the worst toxic waste sites in the United States, but six years later only 6 of the 862 designated sites had been cleaned up (see Figure 17-3).

A great hindrance to progress has been the influence of lobbyists, who have been repeatedly successful in blunting the impact of environmental legislation. The relatively few proconservation lobbyists in Washington have been unable to match the power and influence of the lobbyists representing the various industrial interest groups that constitute the opposition. Therefore the pressure upon legislators and administrators has been distinctly one-sided.

A legality that no one has yet been able to circumvent is the obligation to submit an environmental impact statement before any project involving the use of federal funds may begin. This is also true in the various states that have adopted this concept at their own governmental level.

THE STATE OF THE ENVIRONMENT

The National Environmental Policy Act of 1970 and the Environmental Protection Agency have become the vehicles for the expression of the American public's concern. Despite intense lobbying and obstruction by the opposition, environmentalists have found their constituency and have made themselves heard at public hearings and through letters, petitions, phone calls, organizing campaigns, and citizens' lawsuits.

While American industry argued at first that pollution abatement and control were too difficult and expensive to achieve, it has gradually been forced to acknowledge the necessity of environmental reform and to change many of its traditional methods of operation. Conditions have improved; but seen in the cold light of actuality, governmental agencies are too often ineffectual, and industry continues its delaying tactics by tying up reforms in the courts.

The scope of environmental concern has broadened in the past decade. In fact, public consciousness has been raised to the point that numerous reforms have been implemented since 1969; but at the same time, it is becoming increasingly evident that we still have a long way to go. What follows is an inventory of environmental quality in the United States as measured by the National Wildlife Federation's Environmental Quality Index.

Wildlife Resources

The effects of pollution on our wildlife constitute perhaps the most sensitive index of environmental damage. Even though our wildlife is being protected increasingly by the courts, and species recently on the verge of extinction have been allowed to proliferate once more, the list of endangered species in the United States has grown to 225.

Conservationists cite widespread habitat loss as the greatest challenge of the future in this area. Strip-mined lands must be reclaimed and cut-over national forests must be correctly replanted. Pollution and the drainage of wetlands are also major causes of habitat loss, as is residential and industrial development. Even though important new laws and conservation programs are in effect, loss continues to increase.

Air Quality

Nearly 7,000 stations throughout the United States monitor air pollution, and over 90 percent of all major factories in the country are currently complying with pollution laws. The result of this progress has been a general improvement in air quality.

But 90 million Americans are exposed each year to unsafe levels of ozone created by automotive and industrial emissions. And though the levels of sulfur dioxide in the air are decreasing each year, the full danger of the substance is just now being realized.

The Soil

Despite recent federal expenditures of more than $20 billion to control soil erosion, the average acre of U.S. cropland loses nearly seven tons of topsoil each year to wind and water erosion. The result is poorer soil, lower crop yields, and the need for more chemical fertilization. Further soil loss can be attributed to the growth and expansion of suburbs, highway systems, shopping centers, industrial parks, and parking lots. As former farmlands are lost to these and other uses, new and more fragile areas are being farmed that are more susceptible to erosion.

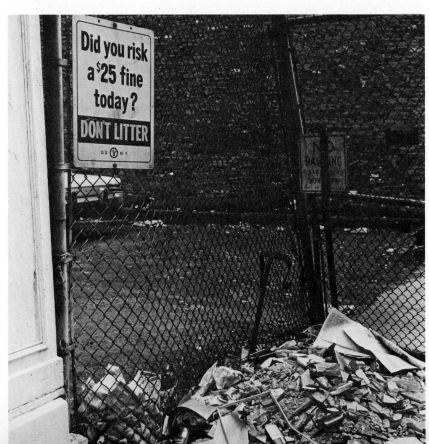

U.S. farmers export some $35 billion in grain and other products annually. Not only does the health of the U.S. economy depend on these exports, but an increased world population relies on them for food. (There are 1.25 billion more people on the earth today than there were only fifteen years ago.) If farmlands are not protected and soil erosion is not somehow managed, this source of food for the world's nonfarm countries will be endangered.

Forests The United States is still growing more wood than it cuts, and as public and commercial forests are harvested, new trees are planted. Environmentalists see several areas of concern, however:

- Many commercial forests have been heavily harvested, and there is a resulting pressure on the federal government to license the cutting of more and more trees on federal lands each year.
- Thousands of acres of privately owned forests are being converted to cropland and suburbs each year.
- As mature forests of trees of mixed species and age are cut down, they are being replaced with seedlings of only one or two species—all, of course, of the same age. The result is a decrease in the habitat available for wildlife and a forest more susceptible to devastation by a single pest or disease.
- There is evidence that acid rain is killing trees in the Northeast. Acid rain has been linked to widespread forest kills in central Europe, and experts worry that the same problem may occur in the United States.

Living Space Several recent measures have helped protect our living space in important ways. Many coastal areas are now under federal protection. Highway construction in some scenic areas has been suspended. Many antilitter laws have been passed. Environmentalists have used the Endangered Species Act and the requirement for environmental impact statements to delay or halt some potentially disastrous housing developments and highway projects.

But where people have moved from urban areas to rural communities, they have taken their pollution with them. Formerly rural areas of New Hampshire are experiencing increased air pollution. Many small communities nationwide are finding their sewage-disposal plants and freshwater supplies inadequate for expanding populations. As manufacturing moves south, so do the sources of industrial pollution. In short, the population shift means that problems already partially solved in some parts of the country are being created all over again in others.

Water Quality Much progress has been made in cleaning up the lakes, streams, and rivers of the United States over just the past decade. Most of the nation's waterways are now "fishable and swimmable" as a result of new sewage and industrial-treatment plants mandated by the federal government.

Two continuing problems have already been discussed: 1) the lack of regulation of nonpoint water pollution—runoff from farms, construction sites, and city streets; and 2) the effects of acid rain, particularly in the Northeast. Another concern is the rapid depletion of subsurface water supplies in great areas of

The EPA and Groundwater Pollution

Presently, more than half of all Americans rely on underground supplies for drinking water. In rural areas, the figure may be as high as 90 percent. But years of carelessness and ignorance are threatening those precious reservoirs.

"Society was pretty casual in the way it handled chemicals in the post-World War II era," observes Victor J. Kimm, head of the EPA's drinking water program. "And we have a fair amount of groundwater that is contaminated. Now we must find the problems and deal with them.

In May of 1985 the U.S. Geological Survey reported that almost one in five of the 124,000 wells it tested were unnaturally high in levels of nitrates, largely because of uncontrolled agricultural drainage. One in 16 exceeded the federal safety standard for the toxic substances, which are suspected of causing cancer in adults and a potentially fatal blood disorder in infants. "The question is," remarked Geological Survey official David W. Moody, "if you have nitrates, what else do you have?"

A month later, EPA researchers reported that 63 percent of rural Americans may be drinking water tainted by pesticides or other contaminants. A single pesticide, DBCP, has so contaminated California's lush Central Valley that state officials have closed more than 1,400 wells there since 1979—the year the pesticide was banned.

In other areas, leaking toxic waste dumps pose an equally dangerous dilemma. In one study, congressional researchers reported in 1985 that nearly half the 1,246 hazardous waste dumps surveyed showed signs of groundwater contamination. Unfortunately, the subcommittee report added, EPA monitoring of the sites is "inaccurate, incomplete, and unreliable."

A drinking water source tainted with pesticides or other chemicals is not necessarily unfit to use—at least according to the EPA's few safety guidelines for water pollutants. For many contaminants, however, the agency does not yet know what constitutes a "safe" level of consumption for humans. Thus far, more than 200 foreign substances have been detected in the country's groundwater supplies, but the EPA has set standards for only 22 of them.

The first controls aimed specifically at toxic water pollutants went into effect in 1985, requiring electroplating companies, such as automakers and jewelry manufacturers, to reduce levels of certain contaminants in their wastewater. The controls were the first in a series of regulations that, according to mandates of the Clean Water Act, will be enforced primarily by the states. They will eventually require industry to reduce toxic pollution in this country by 96 percent.

Source: "Environmental Quality Index," *National Wildlife*, February-March 1986, p. 32. Reprinted by permission.

the country. The underground aquifer that supplies the Great Plains is dropping at the rate of a foot a year and could run dry in forty years if conservation measures are not adopted. Finally, all over the country underground water supplies are being found to be contaminated by toxic chemicals that have seeped down from pesticides, municipal landfills, and illegal waste dumps. The extent of this problem is not known, but it is one of increasing concern (See box: The EPA and Groundwater Pollution).

THE POPULATION PROBLEM

A high rate of population growth is a comparatively recent cause for worry. In fact, during most periods in human history the concern was that birth rates were too low and population growth too small. Until the last few decades a variety of diseases caused a high infant mortality rate and a shorter life span. Famine and warfare also reduced the human population. Now, among other factors, the increase in medical knowledge and facilities, the expansion of health programs, the reduction of mortality rates, and the temporary stabilization of major political systems have resulted in a burgeoning of the world population. For the first time it has become necessary to make conscious decisions about limiting human reproduction.

Explosive Population Growth

According to recent estimates, world population is now 4.8 billion and growing at the rate of 200,000 a day. Even if population growth is somehow curtailed, the world population is expected to reach 6.1 billion by the year 2000 and 7.8 billion by 2020.

The total world population in 1850 was approximately 1 billion people. It is estimated that it must have taken over eighteen centuries for the human population to grow from 250 million in the year 1 A.D. to the 1 billion point. But at present-day rates of population increase, almost 1 billion people are added to the human family each decade.

World Population Trend

Although the earth's population continues to increase at a dangerous rate, the speed of this growth has for the first time begun to slow down. In most developing countries the birth rate has been in decline since 1950; but because of improvements in medical services, the death rate has been declining even more rapidly. Since 1960, however, global birth rates have declined faster than death rates, resulting in a net drop in the population growth rate.

The decline in the growth rate has been virtually universal, with the sole exception of the continent of Africa, which continues to register a slight increase. Especially notable declines have taken place in Sri Lanka, the Philippines, Thailand, and Korea. Significant decreases have also occurred in Colombia, South Africa, the People's Republic of China, and Turkey.

The drop in the birth rate of countries that have heretofore been seen as seedbeds for an imminent population explosion, such as China, India, Indonesia, and Egypt, is attributed to expanded birth control programs.

This recent trend provides the first encouragement that a world population crisis is avoidable and that a balance between the birth and death rate could come to pass by the second decade of the next century.

U.S. Population Patterns

The **fertility rate** of American women—that is, the number of live infants born to women of childbearing age—had been declining during the Depression of the 1930s. After World War II, however, America experienced a "baby boom." The fertility rate rose steadily through the 1950s, and by 1957 American families averaged nearly four children. After 1957 the fertility rate again declined. By 1973 American families averaged fewer than two children. **Zero population growth (ZPG)**—the birth rate level at which births will eventually equal deaths (2.1 children per family)—had been reached and surpassed. However, because the baby-boom generation is now at the child-producing age and because people are living longer, our population continues to grow.

The United States is an urban society: 75 percent of us live in the cities and suburbs. And the suburbs continue to absorb almost three-fourths of the country's population growth. Middle- and upper-income people have settled in suburbia in increasing numbers. Today most inner-city residents belong to low-income groups.

But changes in geographical distribution are becoming apparent. People are moving from the old population centers in the Northeast to the Pacific Coast, the Southwest, and the South. Topography, availability of resources, accessibility, and climate, as well as economic opportunities—all influence the development of population centers in any given area. Since 1970 northeastern and central parts of the country have experienced the slowest population gains, and the South and West the most rapid. However, in spite of these recent trends, the northern and central areas continue to be major population centers.

The Future. If we maintain our zero population growth, the population of the United States will level off at over 300 million by the middle of the twenty-first century. This would have a significant impact on America's future. For one thing, the pressure on our social and economic institutions would be reduced. In the area of education, for example, the two-child family norm would produce a 50 percent lower elementary-school enrollment in the year 2000. And the nation's economy would have to produce 20 percent less to maintain a population based on the two-child family norm in the year 2000 than it would to maintain the three-child family norm at the same standard of living (see Figure 17-4). Furthermore, less crowded conditions would result in an aesthetically more pleasing life style, with easier access to wilderness areas and recreational facilities. We would have more resources to devote to raising the standard of living of low-income Americans, confronting social problems, and providing services for the population. Finally, environmental pollution might be reduced to a manageable level.

On the negative side is a serious social problem that the Office of Management and Budget is now addressing: how to provide services for the enormous popula-

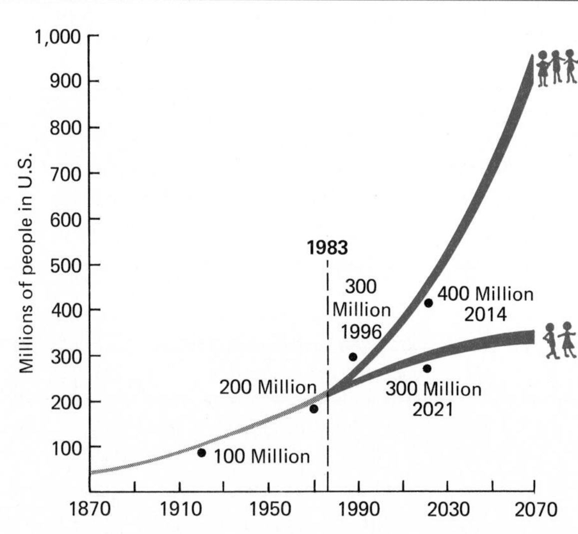

FIGURE 17-4

Will the United States add an extra 100 million to its population? Effect of a three-child family versus a two-child family.

Source: Commission on Population Growth and the American Future, *Population Growth and America's Future*.

tion of the elderly that will occur as soon as the baby-boom generation reaches retirement age. As long as members of that generation are in the work force, they will provide income for the smaller age groups that retire ahead of them. However, when *they* retire and require extensive social services, such as housing and medical care, the work force supporting them will be a much smaller population. Only massive social planning on the part of government today will prevent a crisis in the future. The baby-boom group will become an impressive and forceful voting block of "gray power" in the years to come.

NATURAL RESOURCES AND POPULATION

Resource exhaustion poses serious problems worldwide. Water supplies are rapidly dwindling, and mineral and energy reserves are being used up at an alarming rate. Recent famines in Africa and Latin America portend serious global food shortages in the future. In many cases, these problems have been caused or aggravated by overpopulation and too-rapid industrialization, and part of the solution lies in reducing consumption. In other cases, such as the food shortages, part of the solution lies in making better use of existing resources.

Food Supplies

Hunger and malnutrition are widespread throughout the developing world. Almost half a billion people are living close to starvation, and more than a billion are malnourished. And yet none of this need happen; there could be plenty of food to go around. Nutritionists and land-use experts at the United Nations and the World Bank agree that the problem is due not so much to overpopulation or lack of food supplies as to poverty and the misallocation of existing resources. They point out that the world's agriculture can now easily produce two pounds of grain a day—more than 3,000 calories—for every human being on earth.

The world food shortage has also been adversely affected by the agricultural policies and eating habits of the industrialized countries. In order to maintain food prices at a high level, for example, the U.S. farm supply program pays farmers not to grow as much as they could. This has hindred our ability to help some starving countries. Production is not the only problem, however. Even when food supplies are available for foreign aid, inefficient storage and distribution cause spoilage, waste, and loss of foodstuffs. In addition, as one of the world's leading meat-eating countries, we consume annually about 175 pounds of meat per capita, which is equivalent to 1,400 pounds of grain. A country like India, on the other hand, consumes about 350 pounds of grain per capita.

Water

As the American population grows, more water is drawn from our rivers and streams and from underground aquifers. By far the greatest amount is used for irrigation, but other uses, including industrial, are increasing as well. The regions of the country that are experiencing the biggest population boom—California and the Southwest—are also the regions with the least water. Worldwide, the problem of dwindling freshwater supplies is aggravated in many developing countries by the use of inefficient agricultural techniques.

Energy Sources

Energy and mineral resources are being depleted all over the world, but the problems are different in different countries. In some developing nations forests are being cut down for new croplands and firewood much faster than they can ever be replaced. In other nations nonreplaceable fossil fuels are being depleted at an ever greater rate. The United States alone is responsible for about a third of the *world's* annual consumption of mineral and energy resources, an amount vastly disproportionate to its population. Some of this energy, to be sure, is used to grow food that is exported to feed the world's hungry, but much of it is used to support the world's highest standard of living. As the developing countries industrialize and as their population continues to grow, their own energy needs will increase as well. The only ways in which this problem can be solved are through decreased consumption of our nonrenewable energy resources, the development of renewable resources, or a slowing of the growth of the world's population.

The United States, like the rest of the world, did not make a major effort to solve "the energy problem" until the Organization of Petroleum Exporting Countries began to raise oil prices in the 1970s. The Department of Energy, established in 1977, included in its program a declaration that, in view of the limited availability of domestic oil and the high price of foreign oil, "for the next decade the United States will rely mainly on strict conservation and the two 'bridging fuels,' coal and conventionally produced nuclear energy."

The promotion of coal over oil and gas meant that two conditions had to be met in order to maintain existing environmental standards. The first was that land would be restored to a useful condition once strip mining had taken place. The second was that increased coal burning should not violate air quality

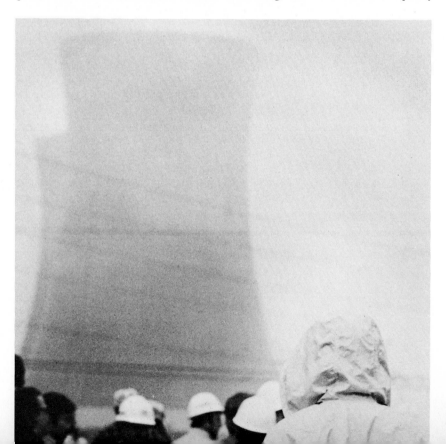

The nuclear plant at Three Mile Island in Pennsylvania soon after the accident of 1979.

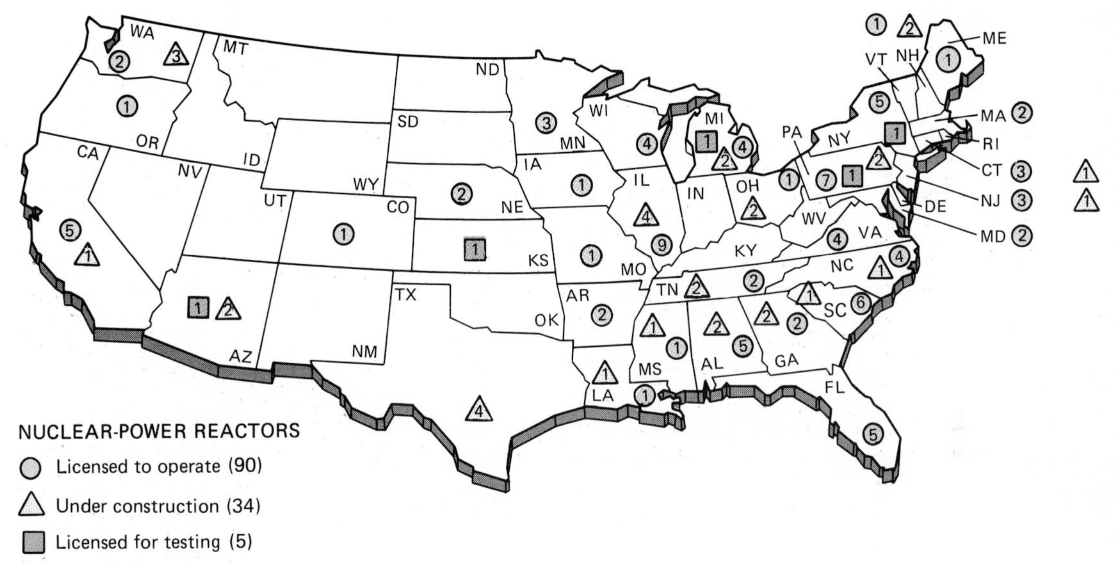

FIGURE 17-5

Commercial nuclear power reactors in the United States.

Source: U.S. Department of Energy, 1985.

standards, and that coal-using concerns should install the most modern antipollution equipment, including the costly "scrubbers" that sharply reduce smokestack emissions.

The promotion of nuclear power was shortly dealt a severe blow by a nuclear accident at a plant at Three Mile Island, Pennsylavania, in 1979. The accident raised many questions concerning the wisdom and safety of the nuclear program, as well as grave doubts about the general credibility of its advocates. Suddenly, after the incident, alarming facts were revealed regarding the number of nuclear plant accidents that had previously occurred across the nation; and also regarding the effectuality of a control system that could permit a seemingly minor malfunction to escalate so rapidly into a near-disaster. As a result of these grim facts—and because of rapidly rising costs of nuclear plant construction—plans for new plants were dropped and many plants already under construction were canceled (see Figure 17-5). A further nuclear accident at Chernobyl in the Ukraine in 1986 made people realize once more that nuclear technology is far from foolproof.

Dr. Alice Stewart, a British radiation epidemiologist, has registered her grave concern about the dangers of long-term exposure to low-level radiation. She has drawn particular attention to the statistics concerning the cancer deaths of workers who had been exposed for long periods of time to radiation that was within permissible federal limits. Dr. Stewart expressed fear that nuclear energy's advocates might be too busy promoting its benefits to reflect upon its attendant hazards.

Studies concluded a generation after experimental atomic tests in southwestern Utah revealed that an unusually high number of youngsters in that area who were exposed to nuclear fallout had died of leukemia. Similarly, military personnel who observed these tests at close range had experienced high cancer rates. At the same time, other investigators discovered a high incidence of cancer among workers who overhauled nuclear submarines at the Portsmouth Naval Shipyard in Maine.

Another unresolved issue is the matter of nuclear waste disposal. Should the production of nuclear energy merely continue at its present level, by the year 2000 there will be 190,000 metric tons of nuclear wastes. And by that same time, fifteen obsolete nuclear facilities will have to be dismantled—all of them highly radioactive. Nuclear wastes emit dangerous radiation for tens of thousands of years. To date, no one has been able to devise an absolutely safe lodging place for radioactive material. (See boxes: Disposing of Nuclear Wastes, and Low-Level Radioactive Waste.)

The cost of dismantling an obsolete nuclear reactor is roughly equal to the

PROBLEMS AND CONTROVERSIES: *Disposing of Nuclear Wastes*

The disposal of nuclear wastes is one of the most troublesome problems that faces the United States today. Ten thousand tons of highly radioactive spent fuel rods are currently being stored at nuclear power plants all across the country, and some plants have already run out of space. At the present rate, they will have 40,000 tons on their hands by the year 2000.

Originally, the problem was not meant to arise at all: The rods were to have been decontaminated and used again. But the nuclear power industry does not have a sufficient number of plants in operation to make such a process economically feasible, and so the search goes on for large permanent storage sites.

Because spent fuel rods remain dangerously radioactive for at least 10,000 years, they must be kept in geologically stable, leakproof repositories. The places of choice are rock or salt domes 2,000 to 4,000 feet underground. The plan was to truck the wastes to the sites in steel and concrete containers, deposit them in the deep holes, and then monitor them for the next fifty years before permanently sealing them.

Foreseeing the problem in 1982, Congress ordered the Department of Energy to locate nine suitable sites, to narrow that list to three, and from those to pick one site for the first nuclear waste shipments, which must begin by 1998. In 1986 the DOE removed from consideration all but three sites: one at Hanford, Washington; one at Yucca Mountain, Nevada; and one in Deaf Smith County, in the Texas panhandle.

However, environmentalists and officials in each of these states claim that serious technical and environmental problems must be resolved first, and they have mounted a fierce campaign against disposing of nuclear waste at any of the three sites. They say that the Hanford site is unsafe because it is located in volcanic rock that is susceptible to fracture by earthquakes; there is also a possibility that the wastes could contaminate the groundwater and pollute the nearby Columbia River. The Yucca Mountain site is shaken frequently by vibrations from nuclear test explosions that take place just a few miles away. The burial of wastes at the Deaf Smith County site poses a hazard to the aquifer that furnishes drinking and irrigation water to a vast area in the Midwest.

While everyone agrees that underground burial is probably the best method of disposing of nuclear wastes, everyone wants them buried somewhere else. The problem is not likely to be resolved easily or soon.

Sources: "U.S. Suspends Plan for Nuclear Dump in East or Midwest," *The New York Times*, May 29, 1986, p. A1; "Too Hot to Handle?" *Newsweek*, December 31, 1984, pp. 35–36, condensed from *Newsweek*, copyright 1984.

Low-Level Radioactive Waste

Some 14 million cubic feet of low-level radioactive waste (LLRW) is generated each year in the United States, about a fourth of it from hospitals and medical research facilities. Radioactive materials are routinely used in the diagnosis of disease and are vital in the development of new drugs. Where will all of the contaminated test tubes and protective gloves be stored?

As Drs. James Adelstein and Kenneth McKusick point out, "The United States currently has only three sites for storage of LLRW. . . . The states where they are located—Washington, Nevada, and South Carolina—have objected to being the nation's sole repositories for LLRW." But six years of battle have not produced alternative solutions. Unless the problem is solved in the fairly near future, "the effects will be felt on all aspects of medical care. At least four years are required to prepare an adequate disposal site. If negotiations continue at their present sluggish rate, we may well find that our national commitment to better health care at a reasonable cost is sabotaged. . . . Medically important radioactive materials may not be produced because of the storage problem. And those that are produced may become prohibitively expensive."

Source: James Adelstein and Kenneth McKusick, " 'Not in My Back Yard': Low-Level Radioactive Waste and Health," *Harvard Medical School Health Letter*, April 1986, pp. 4–6. Excerpted by permission.

cost of constructing a new one. Economic considerations have often been cited to justify continued support for the nuclear energy program. But how economical is nuclear power when we tally all of the costs, apparent and hidden, that are involved? Consider the following: the costs of constructing and dismantling nuclear reactors; the cost of safely storing a dangerous substance whose radioactive life is virtually endless; and the health costs to those who suffer from the consequences of exposure to radioactivity—a health hazard of unknown dimensions.

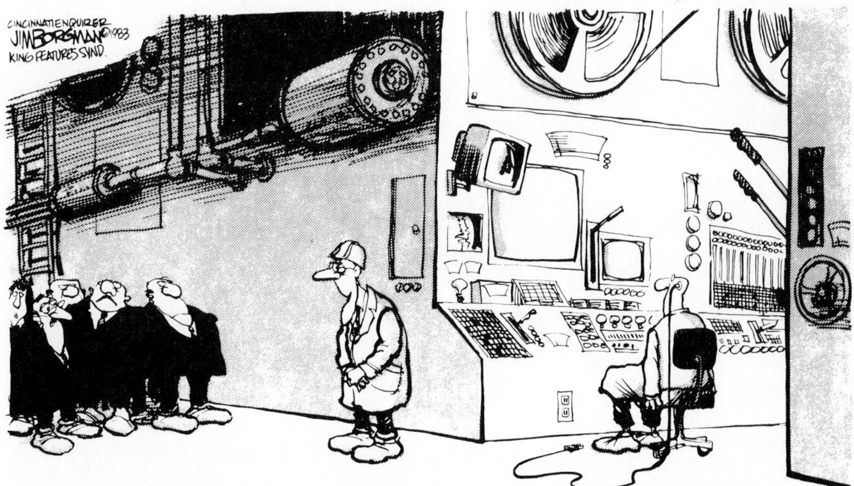

"So you see, your fears are unwarranted! The technology in a nuclear power plant is absolutely foolproof!"

The doubts that have recently arisen about the costs and safety hazards of the nuclear program may encourage the pursuit of renewable energy. Already the United States gets more than 9 percent of its energy from renewable resources. Many new programs are being actively developed, according to reports of the National Wildlife Federation*:

- *Solar power* is already well established. Economically costly, it is expected to become cheaper in the 1990s.
- *Geothermal heat*—released from beneath the earth's crust through hot springs and geysers—already is being harnessed by twenty countries to produce the annual energy equivalent of nearly 100 million barrels of oil.
- *Wind power*—in the form of centralized wind farms operated by and for utilities—produced some 250 million kilowatt hours of electricity in the United States in the first half of 1985 alone.
- *Hydropower* already produces a fourth of the world's electricity, and the output is expected to double by the end of the century. Small-scale hydroelec-

* *National Wildlife*: "Environmental Quality Index," February-March 1986, p. 33; "We're Living for Today . . . and Buying Trouble for Tomorrow," March–April 1984, p. 38.

The solar panels on the roof of this house in New York State power a heat pump.

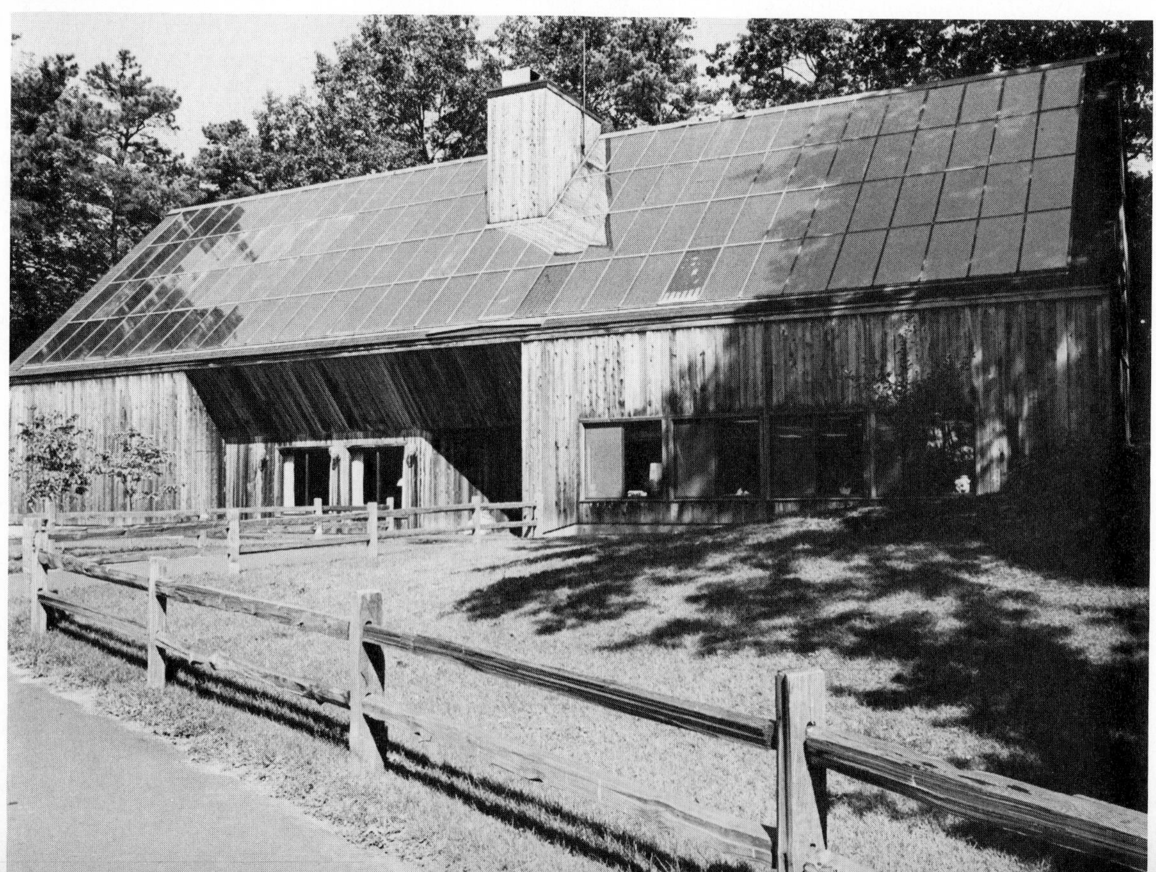

tric plants are being built in many countries at a greater pace than in the past: China has 90,000 such projects.

- *Wood waste* is a basic source of fuel in some parts of the Third World, but it is underutilized in industrialized countries. Sweden and Finland plan a massive shift to wood as an energy source in the 1990s.
- *Sugar cane*, a renewable resource, can be used to produce ethanol to replace gasoline as an automotive fuel. Brazil runs a fourth of its cars on ethanol produced in this manner.

Even ocean waves are the subject of several projects. One of these uses the ocean's surface movement in order to capture the energy contained in passing waves. Another approach attempts to tap the energy produced by the ebb and flow of the tides. And in yet another water experiment, scientists are attempting to exploit the energy potential of the current in the Gulf Stream.

SOLUTIONS TO THE POPULATION PROBLEM

An ever-increasing world population poses many problems, not least of which is the question of our capacity to create a food supply adequate to nourish the numbers of people it is anticipated will occupy the earth in future years. Thomas Malthus summed up the problem in 1798 in his *Essay on the Principles of Population*. He noted that population grows geometrically (2, 4, 8, 16, 32) whereas the food supply increases, field by field, arithmetically (1, 2, 3, 4, 5). Therefore the tendency is for population to exceed its food supply. That this does not happen, he stated, is a result of the contravening effect of disasters such as famine, disease, and war, which hold the population in check. But since Malthus's day medical science has intervened, and the controlling effect of plagues and pestilence no longer occurs. The result has been a universal decline in the death rate of such magnitude that not even the successful birth control programs initiated in many countries can halt the population growth that is occurring. The present hope is that agricultural techniques will increase our capability to feed all the world's inhabitants through a "green revolution."

Agricultural Technology

The prospects for feeding the world's growing population do not have to be so grim, as we have already seen. The past few decades have also produced several possibilities for developing new sources of food to feed humankind. The most promising of these are the new varieties of rice, grain, sorghum, corn, and wheat that produce yields twice as high as those of traditional varieties. Their development is called the **green revolution.** However, these grains require huge quantities of fertilizer; their widespread use therefore depends on stable and affordable oil prices. Many food firms are at work producing livestock product substitutes made from grains and vegetables. Margarine is an example of such a substitute. Current efforts are also directed toward producing milk and meat substitutes that will be nutritionally equivalent to the real products.

Many experts believe that the oceans are another valuable potential source of food for human consumption. In addition to supplying fish products, the oceans might be "farmed" for plant life that is rich in protein.

Birth Control

While some experts believe that better land-use policies and technological advances can increase food production, many others are not so optimistic and insist on the necessity of population control. Dr. Norman E. Borlaug, an American scientists and winner of the Nobel Prize for his work on developing new and better human food sources, made the following statement upon accepting his award. "The green revolution . . . has won a temporary success in man's war against hunger and deprivation; it has given man a breathing space. If fully implemented, the revolution can provide sufficient food for sustenance during the next three decades. But the frightening power of human reproduction must also be curbed; otherwise, the success of the green revolution will be ephemeral only."

One possible vehicle for the dissemination of birth control information to the public is health organizations. Women might be reached at hospitals after they have had their first or second baby, or undergone an abortion, and be offered birth control services. Public health programs might regularly disseminate birth control information as part of their regular health education programs, stressing the need to curtail population and the individual's responsibility for doing so. It is only through a massive, worldwide effort that the population

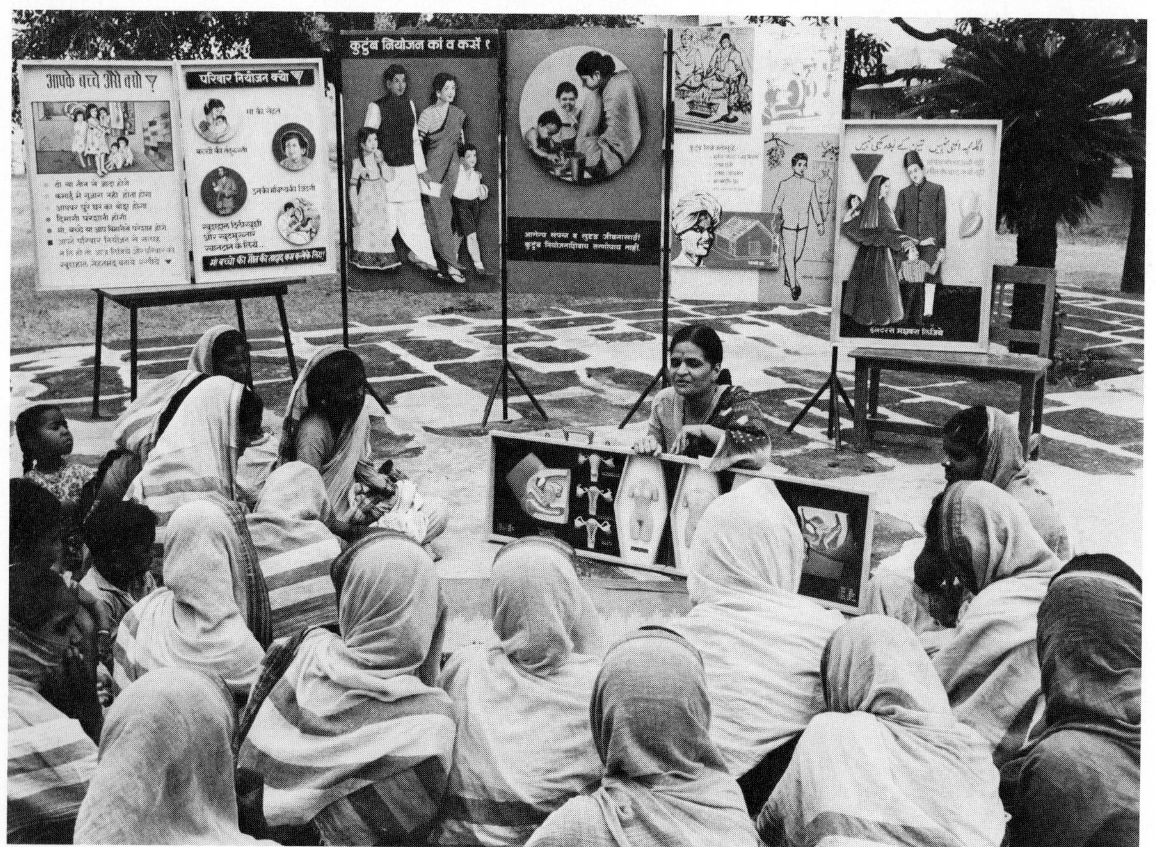

Instruction in family planning in India, a country that has been in the lead in developing birth-control programs.

problem can be solved. Such programs have been successful in many developing countries, particularly in Asia.

Changing Attitudes

The problems of overpopulation and pollution cannot be solved without a change in our cultural attitudes. Until now we have been extravagant in our use of natural resources and materials. We have wasted food, consumed enormous amounts of energy, and contaminated our air, our water, and our soil without considering how these resources can be replenished. Now we must try to disengage ourselves from our commitment to a constant economic growth rate that creates ever-increasing pollution. Such a change in attitude cannot be imposed by government but must originate in the thoughts and actions of individual citizens. Such widespread change in attitudes can be promoted only by individuals who are willing to practice responsible consumption of goods, actively work for the passage of environmental legislation, monitor and report violations of pollution laws, and support political candidates with a strong interest in the environment.

SUMMARY

1. We think of the earth as abundant in resources, but it has its own natural limitations. And if we do not begin to conserve and replenish our resources on a larger scale, and stop polluting the *biosphere*, we shall not be able to support increasing populations. Our present methods of industrial waste disposal and our pursuit of certain alternatives to fossil fuels are threatening the *ecology* of the planet. Many industrial wastes have long-lasting effects and, through *biological magnification*, increase their harmful effects as they travel up the food chain.

2. *Air pollution* is the contamination of the atmosphere by waste products at levels unhealthy to humans and their environment. Sources of air pollution include *motor vehicles*, *factories and power plants*, and *refuse disposal*. Air pollution undermines human health, destroys vegetation, crops, and livestock, and damages public and private property. Steps toward controlling air pollution include federal legislation monitored by the Environmental Protection Agency (EPA), which has relaxed some of its regulations because of economic policies and pressure from industry.

3. *Water pollution* occurs when so many wastes in a body of water accumulate that natural purification processes cannot break them down into harmless forms. Sources of water pollution include industry, municipalities, agriculture, and navigational craft. Water pollution damages human health, destroys wildlife, and ruins recreational areas. Water pollution control is monitored by the EPA.

4. Noise pollution ruins the lives of countless millions of people. Noise intensity is measured in *decibels*. Many everyday sounds are louder than the 80-decibel level that is considered safe. Sources of noise pollution include transportation, construction machinery, household appliances, and industry. Noise pollution can cause serious hearing losses and a variety of other health problems. It can be controlled with the use of existing technology.

5. The many pollution-control regulations are not enforced properly. Polluters are often slow to comply with federal regulations. The influence of powerful lobbies has frequently blunted the impact of environmental legislation and encouraged underfunding of regulatory agencies, despite the numbers of Americans who favor pollution control.

6. The nature and extent of our environmental abuses are just now coming to light, but it is already clear that much remains to be done in the fight against environmental pollution. In the very near future the

United States must greatly increase its conservation efforts and obtain a far greater degree of compliance from major industrial polluters. Some means must be found to bring the goals of economic growth and pollution control into harmony. Currently, progress toward one goal is viewed as harmful to the other.

7. The United States has reached *zero population growth*—the birth rate level at which births will eventually equal deaths. At this rate population will level off at 300 million by the middle of the next century.

8. Population growth in developing countries has come about largely because of improved medical care, which has resulted in lower death rates and a rise in life expectancy. The greatest increase in population is now in developing areas. A fast-growing population faces the problem of allocating existing resources more wisely. Contamination of air, deterioration of soil, lack of abundant water, and depletion of mineral and energy reserves are also major concerns.

9. Factors that would ease the problem include growing more staple crops, developing new sources of food and energy, and promoting birth control. Most important of all, people must change their attitudes and become dedicated to conserving and replenishing natural resources. For the first time in recorded history, the world's population growth rate has declined, even in the overpopulated countries. This decline is attributed to birth control programs, and it offers the hope that a world population crisis may after all be avoided.

CONSUMER CONCERNS

1. Viewed in retrospect, the environmental movement has achieved recognition in a rather brief period of time. Do you feel that the movement has lost momentum of late, or, conversely, are its goals better understood and its purposes more accepted? In other words, could there be a return to the conditions and attitudes that existed prior to the environmental movement?
2. Environmental organizations often evaluate state and federal elected officials on the basis of their voting record on selected environmental issues. Are you aware of these ratings and do you consider this an important standard by which to judge a candidate for office?
3. Implementation of environmental legislation has been threatened by the introduction of the concept of cost-benefit ratios. That is to say, if the cost of complying with environmental regulations were judged to be high in comparison with the health benefits or lives saved, it might justify noncompliance or partial compliance. To what extent do you agree with this logic?
4. The nuclear industry was born against the wishes of a good portion of the public. Its advocates promised a reasonable and reliable source of energy. Now that things are turning out differently, the public is being obliged to bear the expense of repairs and the cost of purchasing the power the nuclear plants cannot produce. Should this be the financial responsibility of the public?

Appendix: First Aid

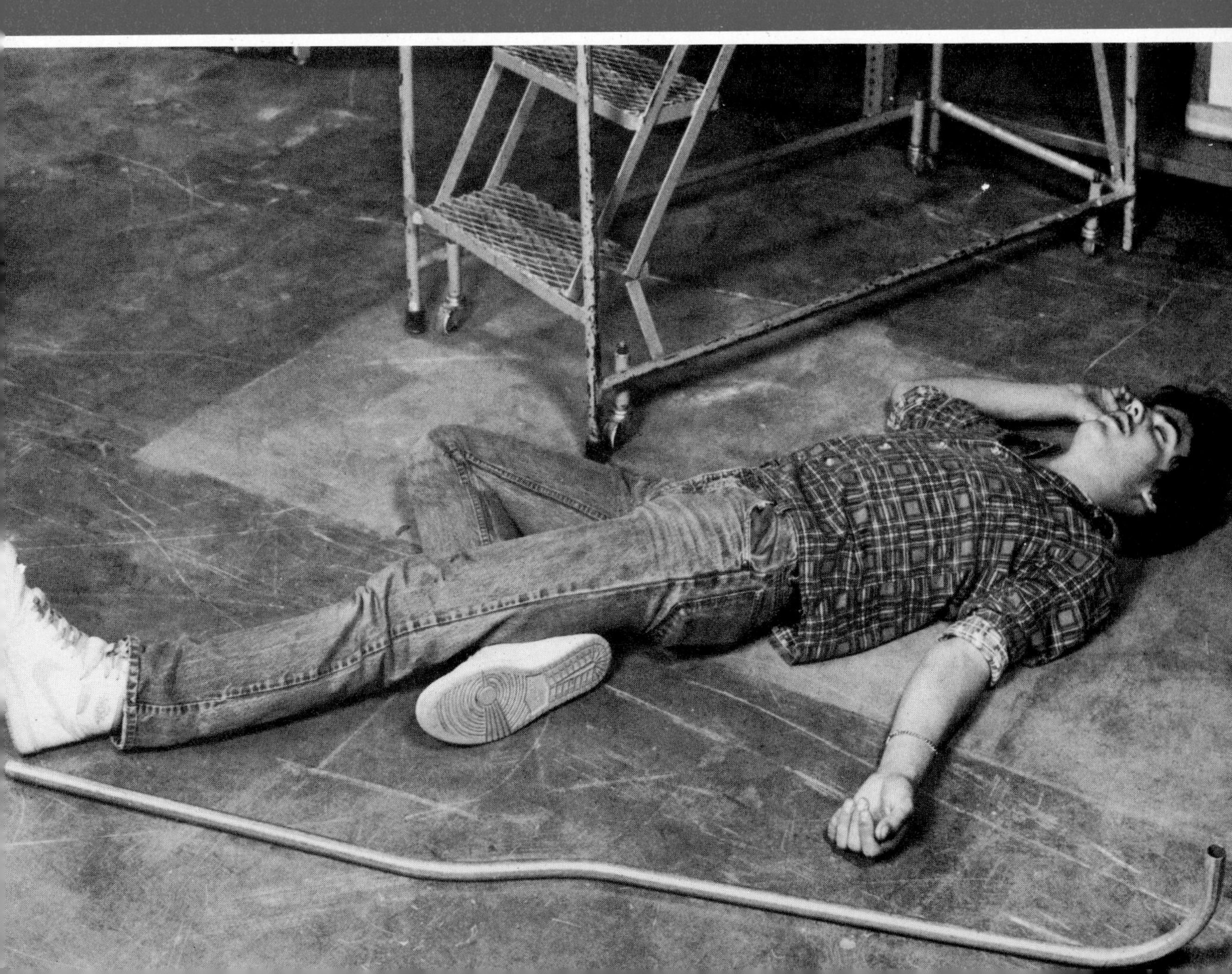

The purpose of first aid is to save life, prevent worsening of injuries, protect the victim until medical help is reached, and reduce pain. Sophisticated first-aid techniques should not be attempted unless one is trained in their use. An inexperienced rescuer will probably harm the accident victim if he attempts anything more than the elementary lifesaving techniques described here. First-aid training can and should be obtained through the American Red Cross or other reputable agencies.

The victim of an accident must first be checked to make sure the vital function of breathing is not impaired. Any signs of bleeding must be noted and attended to. The victim should also be examined for fractures, burns, or other injuries. If the accident involves the ingestion of poison, appropriate countermeasures must be taken. The victim should be made to rest quietly and comfortably, and those in attendance must remain alert for signs of shock. The victim should be kept warm by being completely wrapped (underneath as well as on top) in a blanket or other cover. In more serious cases, medical aid should be summoned to the accident site, rather than an attempt made to move the victim to a hospital or doctor's office.

A person giving first aid should check a victim for evidence of a chronic condition that might explain the situation or might be an important consideration in treatment. Many individuals with conditions such as diabetes, heart impairment, epilepsy, and so on belong to an organization called Medic-Alert. They wear an identifying tag, such as a bracelet or neck pendant, that contains critical information about their medical problem and a phone number where their medical history can be obtained.

ARTIFICIAL RESPIRATION

A person who ceases to breathe will become unconscious and may die within a very few minutes. To reestablish breathing, artificial respiration must be given immediately. The mouth-to-mouth technique is the most efficient. Fears of contracting AIDS through administering artificial respiration to a stranger do not appear to be well-founded; the Centers for Disease Control have not reported a single case of AIDS attributable to exposure to infected saliva.

1. Place the victim on his or her back.
2. Open the victim's mouth and pull the tongue forward.
3. Clear the mouth of any obstructions.
4. Pinch the nostrils together.
5. Place your mouth over the victim's to form a tight seal and breathe into it quickly until the victim's chest rises.
6. Remove your mouth and listen for air leaving the victim's chest. If no air leaves, try again.

Note: Some material in this appendix is drawn from *First Aid* (U.S. Department of Labor, Mine Safety and Health Administration, National Mine Health and Safety Academy), Safety Manual No. 3, reprinted 1985. Other material is based on recommendations contained in the American Red Cross's *Standard First Aid and Personal Safety*, 2nd ed. (Garden City: Doubleday, 1979).

7. If there is still no air exchange, turn the victim on his side and slap his back between the shoulder blades. Again check the mouth for obstructions and start over. Continue this process until an air exchange is felt.
8. Now breathe into the victim's mouth (with the nostrils held shut) until the chest rises, at a rate of 12 times a minute, removing your mouth each time to let air escape. (For infants, breathe shallowly into both the mouth and the open nostrils at a rate of 20 times a minute.)
9. Continue until the victim is breathing normally or until help arrives.

SHOCK

An accident victim may go into shock rapidly as a result of trauma to the nervous system. Shock may directly accompany other injuries or may appear as a delayed symptom hours later. It has been estimated that more people die from shock following accidents than from the actual physical injuries received.

Shock symptoms do not always follow a set pattern. Common signs include paleness, rapid but weak pulse, clammy skin, shallow breathing, and cold perspiration on the face and hands. Treatment procedures are simple, but if untreated the victim can lapse into unconsciousness. The preferred method is:

1. Make sure the victim's airway is open.
2. Take measures to control any bleeding (see "Bleeding," below).
3. Keep the victim lying down.
4. Elevate the feet.
5. Place blankets both over and under the victim.
6. Do *not* give the victim anything by mouth, especially stimulants or alcoholic beverages.
7. Reassure the victim that help is on the way.
8. If possible prevent the victim from seeing the extent of his or her injuries.

UNCONSCIOUSNESS

Unconsciousness can be divided according to three categories, depending on the general color of the victim: red (caused by sunstroke or head injury), blue (caused by suffocation), and white (caused by injuries, fainting, burns, poisoning, shock, or heart failure). All categories are extremely dangerous and medical assistance should be sought immediately.

For red unconsciousness, the treatment is:

1. Elevate the victim's head and shoulders.
2. Apply cold compresses to the victim's head.

For blue and white unconsciousness, the treatment is the same as for shock, items 1 through 5, above. For white unconsciousness, the **CPR (cardiopulmonary resuscitation)** technique is recommended. This combination of mouth-to-mouth resuscitation and heart massage reproduces the function of the heart and lungs until the victim's own cardiopulmonary system functions once more. In this manner, a person may be revived without having incurred brain damage.

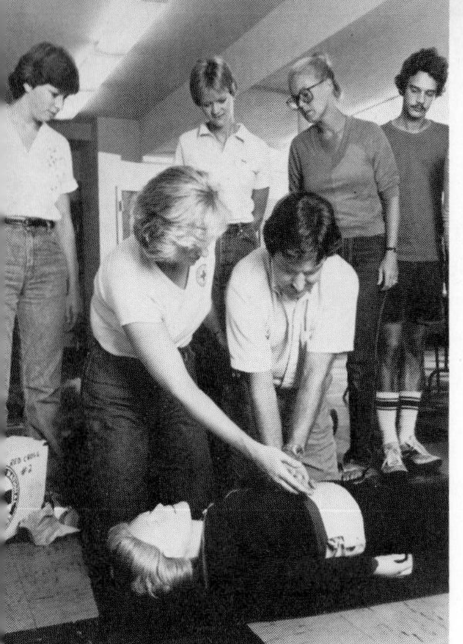

By blowing air into the victim's lungs, oxygen is put back into the blood; the additional manual compression of the heart forces blood into the arteries, and the release of this same pressure causes the veins to fill the heart with blood.

Only 20 to 30 percent of those who have been given CPR revive. But that percentage represents persons who would otherwise have died from a sudden arrest of pulmonary function. Nurses who are taught CPR are told that the technique should be stopped only: 1) if the patient revives; 2) if a doctor says to stop; 3) when the rescuer becomes too exhausted to continue; 4) if the patient has not responded after an hour.

There is a special CPR technique used for small children; and the standard technique should never be practiced on real persons (a life-sized dummy is used), because it is possible to damage the stomach, spleen, and liver, as well as to crack the ribs or chestbone.

CHOKING

For the purpose of our discussion, choking may be defined as a stoppage of normal breathing due to an obstruction of the windpipe, or esophagus. A large number of deaths occur each year as a result of this form of choking, and it is only recently that something has been done about it.

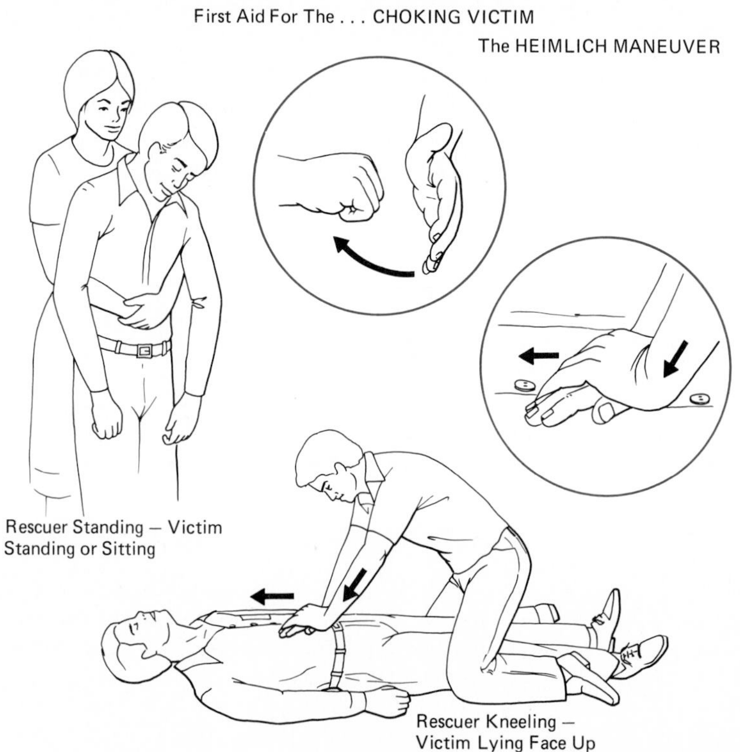

FIGURE A-1

The Heimlich Maneuver.

The Heimlich Maneuver, developed in 1973 by a Cincinnati throat surgeon, is an emergency first-aid technique that causes a sudden burst of air through the esophagus to expel an obstruction (see Figure A-1). Pressure is exerted upon the victim's breastplate, just below the rib cage; quick thrusts of pressure are applied until the obstructing matter is expelled from the windpipe.

BLEEDING

Because a victim may bleed to death very quickly, first aid should be applied immediately to stop any rapid loss of blood. Bleeding from capillaries or a vein can usually be stopped by direct pressure on the covered wound, and this is the preferred technique. (If capillaries have been cut, blood will ooze from the wound. If a vein has been cut, the blood flow will be continuous and dark red.)

The direct pressure method is to:

1. Cover the wound with the cleanest cloth available.
2. If the wound is on an arm or leg, elevate the limb above the level of the victim's heart, unless there is evidence of a broken bone.
3. Place the palm of the hand over the dressing and apply continuous pressure.
4. If blood soaks through the dressing, apply another on top of the blood-soaked one and continue to apply pressure with your hand. Do not remove the first dressing, because it helps to allow the blood to clot.

If an artery has been cut, bright red blood will spurt from the wound, and direct pressure alone may not stop the bleeding. In this case, pressure must be applied by the hand or finger at a point on the artery between the heart and the wound. Pressure on the supplying artery should not substitute for direct pressure on the wound but should supplement it, and then for as short a time

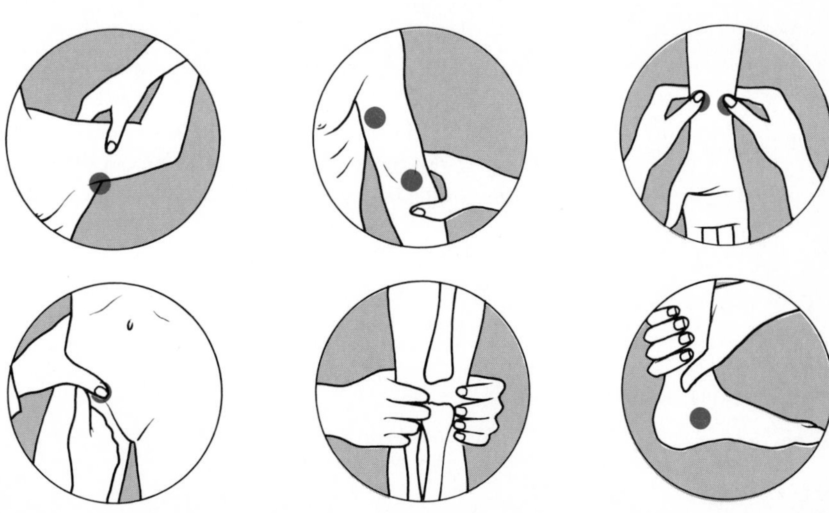

FIGURE A-2

Arterial pressure points for controlling bleeding in the limbs and extremities.

Source: *First Aid* (U.S. Department of Labor, Mine Safety and Health Administration, Safety Manual No. 3).

as possible, because it stops circulation within the affected limb. Arterial pressure points for the arms and legs are shown in Figure A-2.

A third method of stopping the flow of blood, application of a tourniquet, is often used incorrectly and dangerously. A tourniquet will cut off the blood supply to an extremity, causing it to become gangrenous and die. The rule is that tourniquets should be used only when an extremity has already been partially or completely severed or when arterial bleeding refuses to respond to the pressure-point method. The American Red Cross states that "The decision to apply a tourniquet is in reality a decision to risk sacrifice of a limb in order to save life." A tourniquet is formed by tightly tying a cloth or piece of tubing close above the wound.

POISONING

When it is apparent that the victim has swallowed a poisonous substance, the first action is to determine the nature of the poison. Advice can then be sought as to the correct antidote.

If the victim is unconscious:

1. Maintain an open airway.
2. Administer artificial respiration if necessary.
3. Call an emergency squad as soon as possible.
4. Do not force fluids down the victim's throat or induce vomiting.
5. Save the poison container, if you can find it, and save a sample of any vomited material to give to the emergency squad.

If the victim is conscious:

1. Dilute the poison by giving the victim several glasses of water or milk, but discontinue this procedure if the victim becomes nauseated.
2. If possible, get the label or the container of the suspected poison to read to the emergency-care provider.
3. Call the nearest poison control center or the local emergency service number (911 or 0). Describe the poison and the circumstances of the poisoning—how long ago, what the symptoms are, etc.
4. Have available the three most frequently helpful first-aid medications for poisonings, to use on the advice of the poison control center: a) syrup of ipecac, to induce vomiting; b) activated charcoal, to deactivate the poison; c) Epsom salts, as a laxative.
5. Follow the advice of the poison control center.
6. If the patient vomits, save a sample of the vomited material for analysis at the hospital or emergency center; this is particularly necessary if it is not certain what poison was swallowed.

If you cannot get to a phone, you must decide on your own whether to induce vomiting in the victim. The rule is:

7. If the victim has swallowed a petroleum product such as gasoline or a highly corrosive substance such as lye, *do not* induce vomiting; if the patient has swallowed something else, *do* induce vomiting.

BURNS

The pain accompanying burns and scalds received in an accident is caused by injury to the nerve endings of the affected area. For all severe burns:

1. Separate any burned areas that might come in contact with each other when bandaging (fingers or toes from each other, ears from head).
2. *Do not* break blisters: this can lead to infection.
3. *Do not* use petroleum jellies or ointments—they must be removed before medical treatment is possible.
4. Get medical attention as soon as possible.

For burns caused by contact with chemicals:

1. Remove any clothing that may be impregnated with the chemical.
2. Flood the affected area with cool water for at least 5 minutes.

For burns caused by heat:

1. First-degree, or minor, burns (symptom: reddened skin): Immerse the affected area quickly in cold water or apply ice until the pain stops.
2. Second-degree burns (symptoms: reddened skin, blisters): Immerse the burned area in cool water until the pain goes away; blot the area dry; apply a sterile dressing. Watch for symptoms of shock.
3. Third-degree burns (symptoms: charred skin, damaged tissue): a) Remove loose clothing but not clothing that adheres to the burn; b) cover the burned area briefly with cool, moist dressings to bring the temperature down; c) elevate burned limbs; d) treat the victim for shock; e) summon an emergency service to take the victim to a hospital.

HYPOTHERMIA

Hypothermia is a lowering of temperature of the entire body as a result of exposure to extreme cold, whereas frostbite is the effect of cold upon a limited portion of the body such as the face, fingers, or toes. The symptoms of hypothermia may include shivering, numbness, drowsiness, mumbling, incoherence, muscular weakness, slowed respiration, and slowed, irregular, and ultimately arrested heartbeat, the last resulting in death. First aid procedures are:

1. Get the victim to a warm place as quickly as possible.
2. Give artificial respiration if necessary.
3. Remove wet clothing.

4. Warm the victim's body by placing him or her a) in a warm tub of water, b) between prewarmed blankets, c) between two warm people, or d) next to one warm person.
5. If the victim is conscious, administer a warm, nonalcoholic drink.
6. Get medical help as quickly as possible.

Glossary

abortion The termination of a pregnancy before the fetus can live outside the uterus; often, but not necessarily, refers to an artificially induced termination.

acquired immunity Resistance to an infectious disease that is acquired during a person's lifetime, as opposed to being inherited.

active acquired immunity Acquired immunity in which the body produces its own antibodies, either in response to attack by disease organisms or as a result of inoculation.

acupuncture A traditional Chinese method of anesthesia and treatment of disease based on the insertion of needles into the body at particular points.

addiction A condition in which individuals are physically dependent upon a particular substance and suffer withdrawal symptoms when it is denied to them.

additives Substances intentionally or incidentally introduced into food to improve, alter, or preserve it.

adrenal glands A pair of glands located above each kidney that, among other things, influence the development of primary and secondary sex characteristics.

aerobic "With oxygen"; applied to physical activities that place a demand upon the cardiovascular and respiratory systems.

aerobic capacity The maximum ability to take in oxygen.

afterbirth The umbilical cord, placenta, and remnants of the chorion and amnion that are expelled from the uterus shortly after the delivery of a baby.

ageism Discrimination, prejudice, and stereotyping directed against older people.

air pollution The contamination of the atmosphere by waste products at levels that are unhealthy to human beings.

alcohol A colorless, pungent liquid produced by the process of fermentation; also a highly addictive psychoactive drug.

alcoholic A person who cannot control his or her consumption of alcohol. *See also* prealcoholic symptomatic phase; prodromal phase; crucial phase; chronic phase.

Alcoholics Anonymous (AA) An informal society of alcoholics that meets in local groups for mutual support in overcoming their problem with alcohol through abstinence.

alpha-fetoprotein testing (AFP) An examination of amniotic fluid and maternal blood for the diagnosis of neural-tube defects such as anencephaly and spina bifida.

ambulatory surgical center Medical facility for minor, low-risk, surgical procedures, usually performed with local anesthesia; may be independent or hospital-related.

amniocentesis The process of withdrawing a small sample of amniotic fluid to check for congenital defects in the fetus.

amnion A thin membranous sac filled with fluid in which the embryo is suspended.

amniotic fluid A light, straw-colored fluid contained within the amnion that insulates the embryo, protects it against physical shock, and allows it to change position.

amphetamines Synthetic stimulants of the central nervous system used to overcome fatigue and to suppress appetite; also called "pep pills."

analgesic A painkiller.

anaphylactic shock A hypersensitive reaction to an intravenously administered drug, characterized by heart arrest, collapse of the circulatory system, and sometimes death.

androgens Male sex hormones that are responsible for the maturation of the reproductive system and the development of secondary sex characteristics.

anemia A deficiency of red blood cells or hemoglobin.

angina pectoris Pains over the heart, and often over the left side of the chest and along the left arm, caused by insufficient oxygenation of the heart muscles.

anorexia nervosa A life-threatening condition in which a person loses too much weight by refusing to eat. *See also* bulimia.

antibodies Proteins made by white blood cells that destroy germs or neutralize their toxins.

antigens Foreign molecules, usually proteins, that do not normally exist in the body, and whose entrance into the body causes the production of antibodies.

antiserum Blood serum containing antibodies against a specific antigen.

antitoxin Blood serum containing antibodies that neutralize toxins.

anxiety A feeling of apprehension and insecurity arising from perceived threats to one's safety or well-being.

aorta The principal artery in the body; carries blood from the heart for distribution throughout the body.
apoplexy *See* stroke.
appetite depressants Drugs such as amphetamines and tranquilizers that are supposed to reduce a person's desire for food.
arterial system The system of blood vessels that carries blood from the heart to the lungs and all other parts of the body.
arterioles The smallest arteries, ending in capillaries.
arteriosclerosis An uncommon hardening and thickening of artery walls; also called hardening of the arteries. *See also* atherosclerosis.
artificial insemination The process of impregnating a woman by injecting concentrated amounts of sperm close to the cervix.
assertiveness training A behavior therapy method in which a therapist rewards assertive responses from the patient and gives no approval for passive behavior.
atherosclerosis A type of arteriosclerosis in which fatty plaques build up within the arteries, eventually restricting blood flow.
aversion therapy A form of drug therapy in which alcoholics are simultaneously administered a nausea-inducing drug and an alcoholic beverage to condition them to associate illness with alcohol.

bacteria Single-celled microorganisms found virtually everywhere; some are pathogenic.
barbiturates Synthetic drugs used in the treatment of emotional disorders; sedatives.
Bartholin's glands Two glands located within the labia minora that secrete a lubricating fluid during sexual excitement.
basal metabolic rate (BMR) The amount of energy used to support basic body functions.
basic food groups The four major classifications of food: milk, meat, vegetables and fruits, and grains.
beer An alcoholic beverage created from the natural fermentation of grains.
behaviorism A theory of human behavior that holds that psychological problems are the result of learning wrong responses to situations, as opposed to unconscious desires or any internal mental state.
benign A term frequently used to describe tumors that are nonmalignant.
beriberi A painful nerve disease caused by a deficiency of vitamin B_1.
biological magnification A process in which concentrations of long-lasting toxins increase as they move up the food chain.
biosphere A thin layer of soil, water, and air at or near the earth's surface that comprises the zone of life.
biotic communities Communities of organized plant and animal relationships for the exchange of life-sustaining raw materials.
birth canal The dilated cervix and vagina through which a baby passes during childbirth.
bisexuality A behavior pattern that includes both homosexual and heterosexual expression.
blackout The inability to recall events that occurred during a period of time. Alcoholics experience blackouts.
blood alcohol level The amount of alcohol in the bloodstream.
blood pressure The pressure of the blood against the walls of the arteries.
body image The physical and emotional picture we have of ourselves and how we appear to others.
bone cancer Either of two types of sarcoma affecting the bones; symptoms may include pain in the bones, fever, and gradually developing tumors.
botulism An often fatal form of food poisoning caused by eating food that has been contaminated by botulism bacteria or their toxins.
brand name The name arbitrarily given by a manufacturer to a product such as a drug.
breast cancer A carcinoma characterized by the development of a lump or growth in the breast.
breech presentation The fetal position at childbirth in which the feet or buttocks precede the rest of the body.
brewing The process of producing beers and ales in which malt is added to grain to convert starch to sugar and thus cause fermentation.
bronchi Two large tubes through which air travels to and from the lungs and where most cases of lung cancer originate.
bulimia An eating disorder that usually affects young women; sufferers go on prolonged eating binges and then purge themselves in order not to gain weight. *See also* anorexia nervosa.

calorie The unit by which the energy content of food is measured.
cancer A disease of the cells, characterized by a change in basic cell behavior and appearance, and by the unrestricted growth and spread of malignant cells.
capillaries Fine hairlike blood vessels that connect the arterioles and venules and through whose walls substances enter and leave the blood.
carbohydrates Chemical compounds of carbon, hydrogen, and oxygen that are the body's principal source of energy.
carbonation The presence of carbon dioxide in a beverage.
carcinogens Cancer-causing agents.
carcinoma Cancer that affects the epithelial cells.

carcinoma in situ Cancer of the epithelial tissue that has not yet penetrated to deeper tissue.
cardiopulmonary resuscitation (CPR) An emergency procedure that is started immediately after a person experiences a heart attack; uses a combination of mouth-to-mouth breathing and closed-chest heart massage.
cardiovascular disease Any of a variety of diseases of the heart and blood vessels.
carrier A person who carries a gene for a certain trait without manifesting it; the trait, however, can be passed on to the person's offspring. Also, a person or animal that is immune to a disease, shows no symptoms of it, but transmits it to others.
cavernous tissue Tissue such as that composing the penis, which contains hollow spaces that fill with blood during erection; also known as erectile tissue.
cephalic presentation The fetal position at childbirth in which the head precedes the rest of the body.
cerebral hemorrhage The rupture of an artery in the brain.
cervical cancer A carcinoma affecting the cervix which, if left untreated, can spread into the uterus and upper part of the vagina.
cervical cap A contraceptive device similar to the diaphragm that fits over the cervix and is held in place by suction.
cervix The small necklike portion of the uterus that opens into the vagina.
cesarian delivery Delivery of a child at birth through a surgical incision in the mother's abdomen.
chancre A hard sore that appears at the site of the entrance of syphilis organisms during the primary stage of syphilis.
chemotherapy The treatment of cancer by means of drugs.
child abuse Unrestrained punishment, either physical or psychological, inflicted upon a child.
chiropractic A form of therapy based on manipulation (subluxation) of the spine; has not been scientifically validated.
cholesterol A fatty substance manufactured by the body and also present in certain animal foods and products.
chorion The thick membrane that surrounds the amnion.
chorionic villi Fingerlike projections from the chorion into the endometrium through which nutrients, antibodies, and other substances in the mother's blood are diffused and absorbed by the embryonic system, and through which wastes from the embryo are absorbed by the maternal system.
chromosomes Threadlike bodies in the nuclei of cells that carry genetic information; in humans, all cells but the sex cells contain twenty-three pairs of chromosomes.
chronic bronchitis A respiratory disease frequently caused by cigarette smoking; symptoms include lung congestion, phlegm, and difficulty in breathing.
chronic conditions Illnesses of significant duration.
chronic phase The fourth stage of alcoholism, characterized by addiction, mental and physical deterioration, severe emotional problems and personality changes, loss of motor coordination, and fear of withdrawal symptoms.
cilia Small hairlike projections that protrude from certain cells, such as those lining the fallopian tubes and the surface of the lungs.
circulatory system The system of blood circulation, which is comprised of the blood, blood vessels, and heart.
circumcision The surgical removal of the foreskin or prepuce.
cirrhosis of the liver A fatty degeneration and hardening of the liver.
climacteric A period of declining sexual function in the male.
clitoris A small cylindrical mass of erectile tissue buried in the flesh near the joining of the labia minora in the female.
cluster testing An interviewing technique used to trace the chain of STD infection by contacting a cluster of the infected individual's contacts.
cocaine A stimulant and local anesthetic extracted from the leaves of the coca plant (not related to the cacao plant).
codeine An opium derivative, usually extracted from morphine, that has milder but similar effects to both drugs and is used as a cough suppressant.
coitus Sexual union, or the mating act; copulation; intercourse.
coitus interruptus A contraceptive method in which the penis is withdrawn from the vagina prior to ejaculation; also called withdrawal.
colon cancer A carcinoma affecting the colon and rectum whose symptoms include a change in bowel habits, bleeding at the anus or blood in the stool, and loss of appetite accompanied by nausea and vomiting.
colostrum The first fluid secreted by the mammary glands after childbirth.
common cold A viral disease of the upper respiratory tract whose symptoms include runny nose, chills, fever, watery eyes, and fatigue.
communicable disease A disease caused by microorganisms that can be transmitted directly from person to person, or indirectly through the agency of a plant, animal, or the environment.
community psychology An approach to the prevention and treatment of mental illness that provides means for the early detection of emotional problems and makes available a variety of treatment facilities.

compensation Making up for one's feelings of inferiority in one area by striving to succeed in other areas.
complete protein food Food that contains essential amino acids in the amounts and proportions required by the human body.
compulsive habit Any practice or behavioral pattern over which individuals have little control.
condom A sheath of very thin rubber or animal tissue that fits over the penis and traps the semen expelled during ejaculation.
congeners Chemical agents that are usually produced during the aging process of alcoholic beverages and that are responsible for many of the symptoms of hangover.
congenital heart disease Any heart disease that is present at birth.
congenital syphilis Syphilis passed from a mother to her unborn fetus.
constitutional obesity Obesity that begins in infancy; is most likely due to prenatal or genetic factors.
Consumer Product Safety Commission A federal agency created in 1973 to remove hazardous consumer items from the marketplace.
contagious disease A communicable disease that is transmitted from one person to another either by direct contact or by contact with an infected object.
contraceptives Devices or drugs used to prevent pregnancy.
coping Making the adjustments necessary to bring physical or mental functioning back into balance.
copulation Sexual union, or the mating act; coitus; intercourse.
coronary arteries Two arteries that branch off from the aorta where it emerges from the heart and that supply the heart muscle with blood.
coronary occlusion Blockage of a coronary artery by plaque or a blood clot.
coronary thrombosis The blocking of a coronary artery by a blood clot.
corpus luteum A yellowish mass of endocrine tissue that produces estrogen and progesterone and that is formed from the ruptured Graafian follicle after ovulation.
cortex The outer layer of the ovum, adrenal gland, etc.
Cowper's glands A pair of glands located alongside the urethra that secrete a lubricant during sexual excitement, facilitating the passage of sperm.
crash diet A diet designed to produce rapid weight loss; crash diets are nutritionally unsound and have no lasting benefit.
cross-tolerance A form of drug resistance that occurs when tolerance produced by one drug generalizes to all other chemically similar drugs.
crucial phase The third stage of alcoholism characterized by total addiction to alcohol, loss of control over the urge to drink, drinking sprees, and mental and physical deterioration.
cunnilingus Using the mouth and tongue to stimulate a woman's genitals.
cystic fibrosis An inherited disease that damages the lungs and digestive system; most prevalent among whites.

daydreaming Engaging in fantasy while awake.
decibel (db) The unit of measure of sound.
defense mechanism Constructive, self-protective strategies people use to cope with unacceptable desires, reactions, and emotions.
deinstitutionalization The policy of bringing people considered eligible from situations of confinement and isolation into the open community.
delirium tremens (D.T.'s) A disorder afflicting alcoholics that is characterized by hallucinations and uncontrollable shaking.
densitometry A method of measuring body fat using the principle of water displacement.
deoxyribonucleic acid (DNA) The basic chemical of the gene that enables it to carry the information of heredity.
dependence The physical psychological commitment to a drug, obligating an individual to its continued use.
depressants Drugs that act to decrease body cell activity and induce drowsiness and sleep.
depression A feeling of sadness, hopelessness, worthlessness, apathy; symptoms may include insomnia and loss of appetite. *See also* neurotic depression; psychotic depression; postpartum depression.
desirable weight A recommended weight range based upon height, build, sex, and age that is considered to be most healthful.
detoxification The sudden and total discontinuation of an abusable substance upon which an individual is dependent. *See also* withdrawal symptoms.
developmental obesity Obesity as a result of childhood eating patterns and emotional disturbances.
diabetes mellitus A disease in which the body's ability to use sugar and carbohydrates is impaired because of inadequate secretion of insulin.
diagnosis-related group (DRG) One of 468 categories of ailments for which Medicare pays a fixed sum of money to hospitals based on average cost of treatment.
diaphragm A cuplike contraceptive device that fits over the cervix and prevents sperm from entering the uterus.
diastole The period in the heartbeat cycle during which the heart muscle relaxes.
diastolic blood pressure A measurement of arterial blood pressure at the moment when the heart is in the relaxed stage.

dietary fiber The parts of grains, vegetables, and fruits that cannot be broken down by the digestive system.
dilation and curettage An early abortion procedure in which the cervix is dilated and the embryo scraped from the inner lining of the uterus.
diphtheria An acute contagious disease of the tonsils, throat, and nasal passages caused by a bacillus bacterium and characterized by fever, sore throat, swollen tonsils or lymph glands, and a sore and swollen neck.
distillation A process of boiling a mash made from potatoes or grains to create a vapor that, after condensation, results in ethyl alcohol.
distilled spirit An alcoholic beverage such as rye, scotch, or gin, which has been produced through distillation.
distress The negative, or harmful, response to stress.
diuretics Drugs that cause an increased excretion of urine.
DNA *See* deoxyribonucleic acid.
Down's syndrome (mongolism) A nonhereditary genetic defect that causes severe mental retardation in children; the risk of having a child with Down's syndrome increases with the mother's age.
drug abuse The taking of any drug for a purpose other than that for which it is intended, and in any way that could damage the user's health or ability to function.
drugs Natural or synthetic chemicals that alter the biological functions of the body in some way, usually to prevent or cure disease and to relieve pain and discomfort.
drug-sensitive cancers Cancers with many cells in the dividing state, which are more responsive to drug treatment than slower-growing cancers.
dyspareunia Painful coitus, more common among women than among men.

ecology The branch of biology that deals with the relation between living organisms and their environment.
ecosystem A system of interacting relationships among plant and animal life, air, water, soil, and all earthly and atmospheric substances.
egg The female reproductive cell, also known as the ovum.
ejaculation The ejection of semen from the penis by means of a series of muscle contractions.
ejaculatory ducts Ducts through which sperm and fluids from the seminal vesicles flow to the prostate gland.
electrocardiogram (EKG) A record of electric impulses produced by contractions of the heart.
electroencephalogram (EEG) A record of brain waves.
embolus A blood clot or other particle circulating in the blood.
embryonic period The period of prenatal development lasting from the second to the eighth week after conception.
emphysema Obstruction of the small bronchial tubes brought about by smoking; symptoms include impaired exhalation, coughing, and bloating of the chest cavity.
empty-calorie foods Foods with high caloric value but little or no nutritive value; for example, soft drinks, candy, alcoholic beverages.
endocarditis An inflammation of the inner lining of the heart and heart valves.
endocardium A thin layer of cells lining all the internal surfaces of the heart.
endometrial cancer A carcinoma that affects the lining of the uterus.
endometrium The layer of cells along the inner lining of the uterus that is shed in menstruation if conception has not occurred.
endurance The capacity to conduct prolonged activity; stamina; the principal measure of physical fitness.
enzymes Complex organic compounds that bring about or accelerate a chemical change.
epidemic The widespread occurrence of an infectious disease among a population.
epididymis An extremely fine tube coiled on the upper side of the testis where sperm are collected before they move toward the penis.
episiotomy An incision in the tissue between the vagina and rectum performed to avoid vaginal tearing during the birth process.
epithelial cells Skin cells and cells lining many body organs.
erectile tissue *See* cavernous tissue.
erection The rigid condition of the penis resulting from the engorgement of cavernous tissue with blood during sexual arousal.
erogenous zones Areas sensitive to sexual stimulation.
essential amino acids Nine amino acids that are not manufactured by the body but must be obtained from protein foods.
estrogens Female sex hormones produced primarily by the ovary; estrogens prepare the uterus for receiving the fertilized egg and contribute to the maturation of the reproductive system and the development of secondary sex characteristics.
eustress The positive, or constructive, response to stress.
eutrophication The destruction of a body of water by the fertilizing action of nitrogen and phosphorus compounds on plant life, and the subsequent exhaustion of the oxygen supply as the dying plants decompose.
Ewing's tumor A type of bone cancer whose symptoms are pain in the bone, fever, and gradually developing tumors.
excitement phase As identified by Masters and Johnson, the first phase in the sexual response cycle.
extended family The traditional family structure of

agrarian societies that includes parents, numerous children, grandparents, uncles, aunts, and cousins.
extinction In behavioral theory, the process of not rewarding a certain behavior in order to make it disappear.

fad diet Any reducing program that limits an individual to certain foods and promises a rapid weight loss.
faith healing Healing endeavors performed by individuals who claim spiritual powers.
fallopian tubes The tubes through which the ova pass after ovulation and which lead into the uterus.
family practice A medical specialty that corresponds roughly to general practice, but requires a three-year residency, certification, and frequent recertification.
family practitioner A new type of medical specialist who deals with the full range of medical problems experienced by families.
fantasy Mental images that fulfill a psychological need.
fasting Depriving the body of all food or of almost all food for a period of time to promote rapid weight loss; prolonged fasting may cause serious medical problems.
fatigue A feeling of tiredness caused by physical activity; occurs when the concentration of lactic acid and carbon dioxide reaches a certain level in the blood.
fats A major category of energy-producing nutrients, found in meats, dairy products, and plant oils.
fellatio Using the mouth and tongue to stimulate a man's genitals.
female orgasmic dysfunction According to Masters and Johnson, the inability of a woman to go beyond the plateau phase in sexual response.
fermentation The growth of yeast in a sugar-and-water solution to produce alcohol.
fertility rate A measure of the fertility of a population based on the number of live infants born to women of childbearing age.
fetal stage The period from the ninth week of prenatal development to the moment of birth.
fetoscopy The direct examination of the fetus and placenta by means of a small device inserted through the woman's abdomen.
fetus The unborn child in any stage between the ninth week of development and birth.
fibrotic lesion A harmful change in tissue occurring in tertiary syphilis, characterized by the development of hard fibrous tissues in place of healthy tissue.
fight-or-flight reaction The natural response to any stressor; the body actively prepares to fight the threat or to escape it; involves a complex series of chemical reactions.
foreplay Petting that precedes intercourse.
foreskin *See* prepuce.
for-profit hospitals Hospitals that are owned by individuals or corporations and are designed to make a profit.
fortified wine A wine to which alcohol has been added to increase its alcohol content.
freestanding emergency center Private facility that performs many of the same services as a hospital emergency center but at less cost.
fructose A simple sugar resulting from the breakdown of carbohydrates by the digestive system. It occurs naturally in fruit juices and honey.
functional impotence An occasional inability to achieve or maintain an erection owing to factors such as fatigue.
fundus The top portion of the uterus.
fungi A class of parasitic plants lacking chlorophyll, such as molds, rusts, and mushrooms, and including several organisms that cause disease in humans.

galactose A simple sugar resulting from the breakdown of carbohydrates by the digestive system.
General Adaptation Syndrome (G.A.S.) Selye's term for the nonspecific response the body makes to any form of stress; has three stages: alarm reaction, resistance, and exhaustion.
general effect An effect achieved when a drug is absorbed by the blood and circulated throughout the body; systemic effect.
generalized cancer A cancer that either begins as a widespread condition or becomes widespread very soon after its onset.
generic name The name used to identify a drug by its chemical content.
genes The basic DNA-containing units of heredity found in the chromosomes.
genetic code The hereditary information transmitted in the genes.
genital herpes A highly contagious incurable viral disease that may cause painful sores around and on the sex organs; other symptoms include fever, swollen glands, and vaginal discharge.
German measles A mild viral disease characterized by a rash, low fever, headache, fatigue, sore eyes, and cold symptoms.
glans penis The head or tip of the penis.
glucose One of the end products of digestion, resulting from the breakdown of carbohydrates; it is the usual form in which carbohydrates are assimilated.
glycogen A compact form of glucose that is stored by the body as a reserve supply of energy.
gonads The sex glands; ovaries and testes.
gonorrhea One of the most prevalent of the sexually transmitted diseases; is caused by the organism *Neisseria gonorrhoeae*.

government hospitals Hospitals financed by federal, state, county, or city governments and equipped to care for patients with long-term illnesses; also called public hospitals.
Graafian follicle A large, fluid-filled structure that contains the maturing ovum.
greenhouse effect A theory that continuing air pollution will build up a layer of carbon dioxide in the atmosphere, which in turn will cause air temperature to rise and the polar ice caps to melt, thus raising the sea levels to a dangerous degree.
green revolution The development of new high-yield grains that are expected to revolutionize food production.
GRAS "Generally recognized as safe"; the FDA's term for food additives that no longer require regulation.

habituation *See* psychological dependence.
hallucinogens The name for various substances that alter consciousness and cause hallucinations. *See also* LSD; peyote; marijuana.
health maintenance organization (HMO) A plan that provides comprehensive medical care in one location for a fixed annual sum.
heart A muscular organ located in the chest cavity that is responsible for pumping blood throughout the circulatory system.
heart murmur An unusual rushing sound heard through a stethoscope when the heart valves do not function properly.
hepatitis A general name for three types of viral disease. *See* serum hepatitis; infectious hepatitis; hepatitis non-A non-B.
hepatitis non-A non-B A form of hepatitis whose incubation period is similar to that of serum hepatitis; also thought to be spread by contaminated blood.
heredity The process by which certain physical traits and intellectual, emotional, and psychological tendencies are biologically transmitted from patient to child.
heroin An addictive, euphoria-inducing opiate that has no medically accepted application.
high A state of euphoria (n.); under the influence of drugs (adj.).
high-calorie diet A diet that requires about 3,000 to 3,500 calories a day.
high-density lipoproteins (HDL) A blood factor that transports cholesterol to the liver, from whence it leaves the system; now believed to provide protection against heart disease.
homeostasis Adjustments the body makes to keep itself working in a balanced way.
homosexual A person who prefers to have sexual relations with members of the same sex.
hospices A method of caring for the terminally ill that emphasizes relief from pain and involvement with family and friends.
host The organism within or upon which a parasite lives.
hymen A thin membrane at the opening of the vagina.
hypersensitivity Increased reactivity to a drug arising from an unknown allergy; may lead to symptoms ranging from nausea and diarrhea to anaphylactic shock.
hypertension High blood pressure; rarely produces warning signals but leads to stroke, heart disease, and kidney failure.
hypnotics Strong barbiturates that induce euphoria, drowsiness, and sleep.

idealization The positive interpretation of something or someone in accordance with one's desires rather than with reality.
identification Incorporating within oneself the values, beliefs, and attitudes of others.
implantation The spread of poorly adhering cancerous cells that slough off of tumorous growths within body cavities and lodge in nearby organs; also the process by which the zygote buries itself in the endometrium.
impotence The inability to achieve or maintain an erection. *See also* functional impotence; primary impotence; secondary impotence.
independent practice association (IPA) A plan that provides medical services to health maintenance organization members through a group of physicians who work in their own offices and are paid on a fee-for-service basis.
infant mortality rate The death rate of infants, born alive, within the first year of life.
infectious disease A communicable disease that is transmitted through the agency of an animal or insect vector or such vehicles as food or water.
infectious hepatitis (hepatitis A) An infectious viral disease characterized by fever, exhaustion, loss of appetite, and jaundice.
infectious mononucleosis An acute viral disease that affects mostly children and young adults; suspected of being caused by herpes-like virus. Symptoms are fever, fatigue, headaches, and chills.
infertility Inability to have children.
influenza A viral infection of the respiratory tract characterized by fever, chills, headache, sore throat, cough, and exhaustion.
insulin A hormone secreted by the pancreas that is essential for the metabolism of carbohydrates.
interferon A protein produced by the cells that blocks the ability of a virus to reproduce within an infected cell.
intercourse Sexual union, or the mating act; coitus; copulation.

internist A physician who focuses on the general care of adults, particularly diseases of the heart, lungs, liver, stomach and intestines, urinary tract, and endocrine glands.
intoxication A condition of diminished control over physical and mental powers resulting from the action of alcohol on the brain.
intramuscular injection An injection into a muscle.
intrauterine device (IUD) A birth control device such as a coil of plastic or metal that is inserted into the uterus.
intravenous injection An injection into a vein.
invasion The escape of cancer cells from their site of origin and their entry into tissue elsewhere.
in vitro fertilization Process in which egg cells are removed from the woman's ovary and put into a glass dish, where they are fertilized by the man's sperm; after undergoing a few cell divisions, the embryos are inserted into the woman's uterus, where they may become implanted and continue to develop normally.
involuntary muscles Those muscles that cannot be consciously controlled.
iron-deficiency anemia A disease characterized by a shortage of red blood cells or hemoglobin; is caused by an iron deficiency or excessive loss of blood due to internal bleeding.
irrigation return flow The buildup of harmful concentrations of dissolved salts and minerals after repeated use of the same water for irrigation of croplands.

jaundice Yellowish discoloration of the skin and body fluids.

Korsakoff's syndrome "Wet brain"; an advanced state of mental deterioration shown by long-term alcoholics.

labia majora Two thick folds of flesh that lie on either side of the vaginal opening.
labia minora Two thin lips of flesh within the labia majora that cover the vaginal opening when pressed together.
labor The process of childbirth, involving contractions of the uterine muscles to force the infant through the birth canal.
lactation The production of milk within the mammary glands.
lacto-ovo vegetarians Vegetarians who accept milk and eggs in their diet.
lean body mass (LBM) A measure of excess fat arrived at by subtracting the fraction of free-fat tissue and its water and then calculating the percentage of excess body fat.
lesbian A female homosexual.
lesion An abnormal change in body tissue.
leukemia Cancer of the blood-forming organs characterized by aberrations in the production of white blood cells; symptoms include anemia, bleeding from mucous membranes, and weakness.
leukocytes *See* white blood cells.
life expectancy The anticipated number of years of life of a person or group of people, based on statistical probability.
low-carbohydrate diet A diet that calls for a drastically reduced number of carbohydrates and an unlimited intake of high-protein foods.
LSD (d-lysergic acid diethylamide-25) A semisynthetic hallucinogen that may produce insightful experiences and exhilaration; may also intensify psychotic reactions or cause panic reactions.
lung cancer A cancer of the lungs characterized by persistent and nagging cough, shortness of breath, chest pains, coughing up of blood, and eventual loss of strength and body weight.
lymphoma Cancer of the infection-fighting organs; symptoms include enlargement of the lymph nodes, sore throat and difficulty in swallowing, and pain in the back, legs, or abdomen.

macrobiotic diet A diet based upon the consumption of large amounts of carbohydrates, particularly grains, at the expense of other nutrients.
maintenance dose A dosage of a drug such as methadone that must be ingested every day to prevent withdrawal symptoms.
major tranquilizers A potent class of drugs that are effective in treating the symptoms of schizophrenia and other psychoses.
malignant Cancerous.
malt A grain, usually barley, that has been steeped in water to germinate and is used in the brewing of beer.
mammary gland A milk-secreting gland in the breast.
mammography A cancer-detection procedure involving the use of X rays to discover abnormal growths in the breast.
mania An episode of excitement that may be marked by a flow of words and ideas, hyperactivity, and elation.
marijuana The leaves, stems, and flowering tops of the female Indian hemp plant, *Cannabis sativa*; produces mild hallucinogenic effects and euphoria when smoked or ingested.
masturbation Self-manipulation of the genitals to induce orgasm.
measles A highly contagious viral disease characterized by fever, inflamed eyes, cold symptoms, bronchitis, and blotchy rash.
Medicaid A federal-state health assistance program that provides medical treatment for the needy of all ages.
Medicare A federally administered public health insurance program that offers partial payment for

hospitalization and medical expenses for persons aged 65 or older.
medulla The thin inner layer of tissue of an ovum.
megavitamins Vitamins in abnormally large doses.
melanoma A tumor of the pigment-carrying skin cells.
menarche First menstrual flow.
menopause Cessation of menstruation and the production of mature ova; usually occurs between the ages of 46 and 51.
menses Menstruation.
menstrual extraction A procedure in which the contents of the uterus are removed by a suction device.
menstruation The expulsion of blood, mucus, and cells of the endometrium over a period of four to seven days at the end of the menstrual cycle; also called the menses.
mescaline A hallucinogenic drug derived from the peyote cactus that produces changes in sensory perception.
metabolism All the chemical processes that are involved in converting food into energy and protoplasm for the repair and growth of cells.
metastases New colonies or secondary growths of cancer that have spread from the site of origin.
metastasis The spread of cancerous cells from the site of origin through the bloodstream or lymph system to other parts of the body, where they establish new colonies.
methadone A synthetic opiate used to counteract heroin addiction; resembles morphine in most of its effects.
midwife Individual who is specifically trained to deliver babies.
migraine headache A severe, throbbing pain in the head caused by constriction of the arteries; often accompanied by distorted vision, nausea, and vomiting.
mine acid A chemical equivalent of sulfuric acid, produced by the action of air and water on the iron sulfide found in coal beds; is highly toxic to fish and can corrode bridges and ship hulls.
minerals Inorganic compounds that constitute a major category of body-building nutrients.
minor tranquilizers Antianxiety drugs such as Librium and Valium that depress the central nervous system and help relieve tension; they are highly addictive and frequently abused.
miscarriage A spontaneous or involuntary termination of pregnancy.
modified nuclear family Families consisting of childless couples or single parents and their children.
mons veneris A mound of fatty tissue above the female's pubic bones that is covered with pubic hair and protects the genital area.
morning sickness A slight feeling of nausea experienced by women in the early stages of pregnancy.
morphine An opium derivative used as a painkiller; is highly addictive.
mucous lining A lining of mucus—in the respiratory system and elsewhere—that traps foreign organisms that enter the body.
multiple myeloma A type of bone cancer that develops in the bone marrow.
mumps A mild viral disease characterized by fever and swelling of the salivary glands and occasionally of the testes, ovaries, or pancreas.
myocardial infarction A small area of dead heart muscle caused by a coronary thrombosis or coronary occlusion.

narcotics Drugs that affect the central nervous system to dull the senses, relieve pain, and induce sleep.
National Traffic and Motor Vehicle Safety Act The 1966 law that resulted in a variety of automobile safety reforms.
natural foods Foods that contain no synthetic or artificial ingredients and that have undergone a minimum of processing.
natural immunity The inherited ability to resist specific infectious diseases.
navel The involuted piece of skin that remains after an infant's umbilical cord is removed.
neurosis A psychological disorder characterized by inappropriate emotions and behavior.
neurotic depression Depression marked by long-lasting, extreme hopelessness; is usually brought on by a relatively minor event.
niacin One of the B vitamins; a deficiency causes pellagra.
nicotine An addictive drug found in tobacco smoke.
night blindness An inability to see in dim light that is caused by a deficiency of vitamin A.
nitrates Nitrogen compounds present in detergents, fertilizers, human wastes, and industrial discharges.
nocturnal emission A spontaneous discharge of semen that occurs during sleep; also called a "wet dream."
nonmarital cohabitation Living with a person of the opposite sex outside of marriage.
nonspecific urethritis (NSU) A common sexually transmitted disease that causes a watery discharge and, in males, pain on urination.
nuclear family The immediate family consisting of parents and their children. *See also* modified nuclear family; extended family.
nutrients Chemical substances in foods that nourish the body.
nutrition The entire process by which the body takes in and makes use of foods.

obesity Excessive fatness; a body weight 20 percent or more above the desirable weight range.
obsession The constant, irrational, and uncontrollable fixation of thoughts or ideas on a particular idea or image.

Occupational Safety and Health Act The law passed in 1971 that promulgated mandatory safety and health standards in almost all industries.
oils Liquid fats.
one-emphasis diets Diets that are limited to one or a few specific foods.
open hysterotomy An abortion procedure used in advanced stages of pregnancy in which the fetus is removed through an incision in the abdomen.
opium A depressant, analgesic, and addictive narcotic extracted from a variety of poppy plant. *See also* codeine; morphine; heroin.
oral contraceptives Pills that contain progesterone or estrogen (or both) that prevent ovulation.
organically grown foods Foods that have been grown in soil enriched with natural fertilizers, have not been sprayed with pesticides, and have had no artificial substances added to them.
orgasm The sensation of pleasure and release experienced at the culmination of intercourse.
orgasmic phase Masters and Johnson's term for the third phase of the sexual response cycle.
ovaries Glands in the female that produce ova and sex hormones.
over-the-counter drugs Drugs that can be sold without a physician's prescription.
overweight A body weight 10 to 20 percent above the desirable weight range.
ovulation The release of the ovum from the Graafian follicle.
ovum The female reproductive cell, which is fertilized by a sperm; also called the egg.
oxidation Combination of a substance with oxygen; the process by which alcohol is metabolized within the body, primarily through the action of the liver.

pacing The modification of the intensity or rhythm of a physical exercise in order to prevent exhaustion and build endurance.
Pap smear A painless test for uterine cancer in which a sample of discharge from the cervix and vaginal area is examined for traces of cancerous cells.
parasite An organism that lives within or upon another organism.
particulates Minute solid or liquid particles produced by combustion.
passive acquired immunity Acquired immunity in which antibodies produced in another person or animal are injected to counteract a specific antigen.
passive smoking Exposure to tobacco smoke in the environment.
pathogen A disease-producing agent, particularly a microorganism.
PCP Phencyclidine; a tranquilizer banned on account of its side effects; also known as "angel dust."
penis The male copulative organ.
pep pills *See* amphetamines.
perineum The tissue between the external genitalia and anus.
pernicious anemia A severe anemia resulting from failure to absorb sufficient vitamin B and characterized by abnormally large red blood cells.
personality The totality of traits, attitudes, and ways of behaving that make each person unique; tends to remain stable throughout life.
pertussis *See* whooping cough.
petting Any form of sexual contact between individuals that does not involve intercourse.
peyote The button of the peyote cactus, which contains mescaline, a hallucinogenic drug.
phobia An irrational fear of objects or situations, usually as a result of an earlier traumatic experience.
phosphates Phosphorous compounds present in detergents, fertilizers, human wastes, and industrial discharges; often found in water pollutants.
physical dependence A need for a drug that can cause an addict physical discomfort or illness if the drug is withdrawn; addiction.
pinch test A test to determine the degree of body fat by pinching the back of the upper arm.
pituitary gland A small gland below the brain; among other functions, it controls the production of sex hormones and stimulates the production of sex cells.
placebo effect The relief of physical symptoms produced by a medication that the patient believes to be an effective drug, but that is actually a neutral substance.
placenta A vascular organ partially surrounding the embryo and uniting it with the uterus. Maternal nutrients and fetal waste products are exchanged by osmosis through the tissue of the placenta. *See also* chorionic villi.
placental aspiration A method of sampling fetal blood by means of a hollow needle inserted into the placenta.
plaque Fatty deposits on the interior walls of blood vessels. The main ingredient of plaque is cholesterol.
plasma A clear, yellowish, cell-free liquid that constitutes about 55 percent of the blood.
plateau phase Masters and Johnson's term for the second phase of the sexual response cycle.
platelets Irregularly shaped fragments of larger blood cells that play an important part in clotting.
pneumonia A contagious disease characterized by chills, fever, chest pains, hoarse cough, and difficulty in breathing.
Poison Prevention Packaging Act The 1970 law requiring that hazardous substances be sold in child-resistant containers.
poliomyelitis An infectious virus disease that attacks the

nervous system and causes symptoms ranging from stiffness to permanent paralysis and death.
postpartum depression The sensation of anticlimax experienced by some women for a few weeks after childbirth.
potentiator A drug that intensifies the effect of another drug.
prealcoholic symptomatic phase The first stage of alcoholism, marked by drinking for relief from tension, depression, or boredom, or to induce positive feelings such as courage, happiness, or relaxation.
preferred provider organization (PPO) A plan whereby an insurer contracts with a group of physicians and health-care institutions to pay a set fee for a list of medical services provided to subscribers.
premature ejaculation The inability to delay ejaculation long enough to satisfy a normally responsive partner in at least 50 percent of the occasions of sexual intercourse.
premenstrual syndrome A cluster of symptoms, including headaches, acne, and tenderness of the breasts, that many women experience before menstruation begins.
prepuce A fold of skin that covers the glans penis and secretes smegma; also known as the foreskin.
prescription A written order from a physician authorizing the purchase of a restricted drug and providing instructions for its use.
prescription drugs Drugs that can be bought only with a physician's prescription.
primary effect The desired effect for which a drug is introduced into the body; for example, to fight infection or kill pain.
primary follicle The primordial ovum with its covering of cells; one primary follicle develops into a Graafian follicle during each menstrual cycle.
primary impotence A condition in which a man has never been able to achieve or maintain an erection.
primordial ovum The immature ovum found within the cortex of the ovaries.
prodromal phase The second stage of alcoholism, marked by blackouts, increasing preoccupation with alcohol, secret drinking, rapid drinking, and guilt.
progesterone The female sex hormone that prepares the endometrial lining of the uterus for pregnancy; the lack of progesterone causes menstruation.
projection The attribution to another person of one's own emotions, traits, or impulses.
proof The arbitrary standard strength of an alocholic beverage as measured on a scale in which 100 proof signifies a spirit containing 50 percent alcohol by volume.
proprietary hospitals *See* for-profit hospitals.
prostatic cancer A carcinoma affecting the prostate gland; symptoms include pain during urination and blood in the urine.
prostate gland A small spongy gland surrounding the neck of the male urethra that secretes a thin, milky fluid; this fluid comprises the bulk of the semen, neutralizes the acidity of the vagina, and activates the sperm cells.
protein Complex compound of amino acids that is the basic structural unit of all living cells.
protozoa Single-celled animals that can reproduce sexually and asexually, such as the amoeba.
psilocybin A hallucinogen derived from certain mushrooms, including *Psilocybe mexicana.*
psychoactive substance A substance that affects the central nervous system and produces an altered state of mind and, often, feelings of euphoria.
psychological dependence An emotional need for a drug that can result in nervousness and psychological discomfort if the drug is withdrawn.
psychoses Serious mental disorders in which a person is disabled owing to a breakdown in thinking ability or mood or both.
psychosomatic disorder A physical disorder in which there is an intimate connection between physical symptoms and emotional states.
psychotic depression A crippling state of sadness in which a person loses appetite and sexual interest and experiences severe sleep disturbances.
puberty The age when mature reproductive life begins, usually at about the 12th year in the female and the 13th year in the male.
public hospitals. *See* government hospitals.
pulse rate The measure of the pulsations taken at pressure points in the wrist or neck; is similar to the heart rate.

radiation therapy The use of X rays, radioisotopes, cobalt, or laser beams to destroy cancerous tissue.
radioisotopes Radioactive chemical elements that release destructive gamma rays and alpha and beta particles; can be used for radiation treatment of cancer.
rationalization The process by which a person justifies an action or event by distorting the real reasons for its occurrence.
reaction formation The outward expression of attitudes that are diametrically opposed to an individual's true, but suppressed, feelings.
reactive obesity Obesity as a response to stress of emotional conflict.
rectal cancer *See* colon cancer.
red blood cells Disk-shaped, red, oxygen-carrying cells that contain hemoglobin; also called erythrocytes.
reducing clubs Clubs that advocate well-balanced, low-calorie diets and provide group support for weight reduction.
refractory period Masters and Johsnon's term for the postorgasmic period during which males are unable to achieve another orgasm.

regression The escape from an anxiety-producing situation by returning to an earlier form of behavior.
reinforcement The process by which a behavior is learned. Behavior that is rewarded and associated with pleasure is repeated; that which is associated with pain is not repeated.
remission The temporary disappearance of disease symptoms.
repression The pushing into forgetfulness of painful experiences and unacceptable desires.
resolution phase Masters and Johnson's term for the fourth phase in the sexual response cycle.
rheumatic heart disease Heart disease caused by rheumatic fever; produces endocarditis, which damages heart valves to the point where they cannot close properly.
Rh (rhesus) factor A substance in the red blood cells that causes the production of antibodies. *See also* sensitization.
Rh negative The absence of the Rh factor in the blood.
Rh positive The presence of the Rh factor in the blood.
rhythm method A contraceptive method involving abstention from intercourse immediately before and after ovulation.
riboflavin One of the B vitamins, also known as vitamin B_2 or vitamin G; helps the body make use of the energy in glucose.
ribonucleic acid (RNA) The chemical messenger that transmits the genetic code from the DNA in the nucleus of a cell to the cytoplasm surrounding it.
rickettsias Microorganisms intermediate in size between bacteria and viruses that can be transmitted to human beings by an insect vector.
rubella *See* German measles.

saline instillation (injection) A late-term abortion procedure involving the replacement of a pint of amniotic fluid by a saltwater solution.
sarcoma A cancer affecting the connective tissue of the body, such as the bones, muscles, and cartilage.
saturated fats Fats in which all chemical linkages between adjacent carbon atoms in the molecules are occupied by hydrogen atoms.
scrotum A thin-walled sac of skin and muscles located behind the penis that contains the testes.
scurvy A disease affecting the gums, skin, and mucous membranes caused by a deficiency of vitamin C.
secondary effect An effect of a drug that occurs in addition to the primary effect and that may or may not be harmful; a side effect.
secondary impotence Masters and Johnson's term for a condition that exists when a man is unable to achieve or maintain an erection in 25 percent of his sexual encounters.
sedatives Drugs that depress the central nervous system and cause relaxation without inducing sleep; barbiturates.
sediment Materials that settle to the bottom of water; sediments can clog water-powered equipment and damage crops.
semen The mixture of sperm and glandular fluids ejected from the penis during ejaculation. *See also* prostate gland.
seminal vesicles Two glands located below the bladder that secrete a clear fluid that forms part of the semen.
seminiferous tabules The extremely fine sperm-producing tubes contained within each compartment of the testes.
sensitization The development of antibodies in the blood of an Rh negative mother after the birth of a first child; these antibodies may attack the real blood cells of subsequent Rh positive fetuses.
serum hepatitis (hepatitis B) A viral disease characterized at first by fever, nausea, vomiting, and jaundice.
sex flush A flushing of the skin that appears on most women and some men during intercourse.
sex-linked characteristics Characteristics such as color blindness or hemophilia that are inherited because the genes for them are carried on the X chromosome.
sexual dysfunction The repeated inability to maintain an erection or to achieve orgasm.
sexually transmitted diseases (STDs) Any of a group of highly contagious diseases spread through sexual intercourse, such as syphilis, gonorrhea, nongonococcal urethritis, herpes, and AIDS.
sickle-cell anemia A hereditary blood disease that affects mainly the black population and usually causes death before the age of 20.
silt Fine particles suspended in water that can destroy fish habitats and clog waterways.
skeletal muscles *See* voluntary muscles.
skin cancer A carcinoma affecting the epidermis; begins with a sore or growth that may bleed, form a crust, and be slow to heal; the sore eventually grows inward to form a tumor.
skinfold measurement *See* pinch test.
smegma A lubricant secreted by the prepuce.
smog A combination of smoke and fog, or any of a number of chemical and industrial pollutants.
socialization The adaptation to cultural attitudes, expectations, and behavioral patterns exhibited by others in one's country, geographical area, and social and economic class.
solid tumor cancer Cancer characterized by the formation of a primary growth that generally spreads by metastasis.
sperm Spermatozoon.
spermatic cord A thick tube containing blood vessels, nerves, and ducts leading from the testes.
spermatozoon (pl. spermatozoa) The male reproductive cell, which fertilizes the female egg, or ovum; also known as the sperm.
spermicide A chemical substance, in the form of a tablet, jelly, foam, or cream, that kills sperm.

spore A hard-coated seedlike structure that contains a bacterium in a dormant or resting state.
spouse abuse Physical or psychological assault by one member of a marital couple upon the other.
starch A complex carbohydrate stored in vegetable roots.
sterilization The process of surgically rendering a person incapable of reproduction.
stimulants Drugs that excite body cells to increased activity and stimulate the central nervous system.
stomach cancer A carcinoma affecting the stomach whose symptoms include loss of appetite, chronic stomach discomfort, dark stools, anemia, and weight loss.
stress The nonspecific response of the body to any demand.
stressor Any factor that causes stress.
stroke A cardiovascular disease in which a part of the brain receives insufficient blood; also called apoplexy.
subcutaneous injection An injection under the skin.
sublimation The replacement of a socially unacceptable goal with a socially acceptable one.
surgicenter *See* ambulatory surgical center.
surrogate mother A woman who agrees to help an infertile couple by being artificially inseminated with the husband's sperm, bearing the child, and then turning it over to the contracting couple.
synergistic reaction An effect produced in the body when two substances interact powerfully and with unpredictable results.
syphilis A contagious sexually transmitted disease caused by the organism *Treponema pallidum*.
systematic desensitization A behavior therapy method for phobias in which patients are first taught relaxation techniques and then taught to approach the object or situation that causes fear.
systole The period in heartbeat during which the heart muscle contracts.
systolic blood pressure The blood pressure produced by the contracting ventricle during systole.

tar Particulate matter found in tobacco smoke, composed largely of carcinogens.
Tay-Sachs disease An inherited disorder that affects mainly Eastern European Jews; results in loss of coordination, blindness, and eventually death.
temperature inversion An atmospheric condition in which a cool air mass close to the ground is trapped by a warm air mass above, thus preventing pollutants from being dissipated in the atmosphere.
testes Testicles.
testicles Two egg-shaped glands contained in the scrotum that produce sperm and testosterone; also known as the testes.
testosterone The primary male sex hormone that influences maturation of the reproductive system, stimulates the development of secondary sex characteristics, and influences the male sex drive.
tetanus An acute, often fatal communicable disease resulting from bacterial contamination of a wound; is characterized by painful and persistent contraction of the muscles, especially of the neck and jaw.
thalassemia An inherited anemia in which the red blood cells lack sufficient hemoglobin; prevalent among Asians and people whose ancestors came from around the Mediterranean.
THC Tetrahydrocannabinol; the active ingredient in marijuana.
thermal water pollution The release of very hot water from industrial or power plants into the waterways, raising their temperatures and increasing the growth of aquatic plants.
thiamine One of the B complex vitamins, also known as vitamin B_1; essential to normal metabolism.
thin fat people People who succeed in losing weight but are continually preoccupied with food, dieting, and weight.
thrombosis A condition in which a thrombus, or blood clot, is formed within a blood vessel.
tolerance A condition that develops when the body becomes accustomed to a drug and no longer responds to the original dosage.
toning down A period after vigorous exercise during which the body can relax gradually and return to its normal condition.
topical administration Administration of a drug to the specific body area under treatment in order to achieve a localized effect.
toxemia A condition in which toxic waste products accumulate in the bloodstream.
toxicity The tendency of a drug used in long-term chemotherapy to damage healthy cells.
toxins The poisonous by-products manufactured by certain pathogenic bacteria.
toxoid A preparation of weakened toxins used for inoculations to stimualte the production of antitoxins.
training effect The increase in the body's capacity to adjust to meet the demands of physical activity.
tranquilizer A nonbarbiturate depressant that is used for sedation and to relieve anxiety.
transference A process in psychoanalysis in which the patient resolves emotional conflicts by shifting them temporarily onto the person of the analyst.
transverse presentation The fetal position at childbirth in which the shoulder or chest precedes the rest of the body.
tricyclic drugs A class of antidepressant drugs.
tubal ligation The surgical sterilization of a female in which the fallopian tubes are tied off or cauterized.
tuberculosis A chronic, contagious bacterial disease characterized by lesions in the lungs, swollen lymph glands,

persistent coughing, chronic low-grade fever, weight loss, hoarseness, and chest pain.

tumor A lump or mass of excess tissue resulting from uncontrolled cell division; may be benign or malignant.

Type A personality A behavioral type characterized as being prone to heart disease; individuals of this type are aggressive, competitive, restless, impatient, and mistrustful.

Type B personality A behavioral type characterized as relaxed and unhurried, and much less prone than a Type A to heart disease; Type B individuals are calm and accepting, and adjust well to change or unforeseen events.

ultrasound A method of examining the uterus, placenta, and fetus by means of high-frequency sound waves.

umbilical cord The cord connecting the fetus with the placenta; contains blood vessels that conduct nutrients to and wastes from the fetus.

unconscious A vast, submerged area of the mind containing the basic drives that motivate human behavior and also repressed thoughts and desires.

underweight A body weight that is more than 10 percent below a person's desirable weight range.

unsaturated fats Fats such as vegetable oils that are liquid at room temperature.

urethra The duct that carries off the urine from the bladder, and that, in the male, discharges semen.

urgicenter *See* freestanding emergency center.

uterine aspiration An early abortion procedure in which the embryo is pulled off the wall of the uterus by a suction device.

uterine cancer A carcinoma affecting the uterus whose symptoms include irregular bleeding and unusual discharge.

uterus The womb, or organ that carries the fetus during pregnancy.

vaccine A preparation of weakened or dead bacteria or viruses used for inoculations.

vagina A thick-walled tube connecting the uterus to the external genitalia or vulva.

vaginal insert A small white oval tablet that, when inserted into the vagina, acts as a spermicide.

vaginismus A powerful and often painful contraction of the vaginal muscles.

varicocele A swollen vein inside the scrotum that increases the temperature within the scrotum and sometimes causes infertility.

vascular system The body's network of blood vessels and capillaries.

vascular tissue Tissue of the circulatory system.

vas deferens (pl. vasa deferentia) A duct through which sperm pass from the epididymis to the seminal vesicles.

vasectomy The surgical sterilization of a male in which the vasa deferentia are tied off or severed.

vector The organism responsible for carrying a communicable disease from one host to another.

vegans Vegetarians who eat only fruits, vegetables, and grains.

vehicle A medium, such as food and water, through which an infectious disease can be spread.

venereal diseases *See* sexually transmitted diseases.

venules Minute veins connecting the capillaries to larger veins.

vestibule The area surrounding the vaginal and urethral openings.

virulent Endowed with a great capacity for producing illness.

virus The smallest known parasitic organism; survives by entering a living cell and taking control of its metabolic machinery.

vitamin An organic chemical compound essential in minute quantities for the nourishment and functioning of the body.

vitamin A A fat-soluble vitamin found particularly in milk products and fish-liver oils; prevents night blindness.

vitamin B complex A group of water-soluble vitamin compounds that includes niacin, riboflavin, and thiamine.

vitamin C A water-soluble vitamin found in fresh fruits and vegetables; prevents scurvy; also known as ascorbic acid.

vitamin D A fat-soluble vitamin found in fish-liver oils, milk, eggs, butter, and sunlight.

voluntary hospitals Public, nonprofit hospitals run by religious groups or other philanthropic organizations or individuals.

voluntary muscles Muscles such as the skeletal muscles that respond to an act of will.

vulva The external genitalia of the female; i.e., the labia majora, labia minora, Bartholin's glands, clitoris, and mons veneris.

warm-up A pre-exercise period in which the joints and muscles are limbered up in order to prevent sprains and to increase respiratory and circulatory rates.

water An essential substance whose presence enables the chemical machinery of the body to work.

water pollution The condition in which wastes have so accumulated in a body of water that natural purification processes cannot break them down into harmless forms.

wet dream *See* nocturnal emission.

white blood cells Blood cells that do not contain hemoglobin and whose primary function is to protect the body against foreign microorganisms; also called leukocytes.

whooping cough (pertussis) An acute bacterial infection of the trachea, bronchi, and bronchioles characterized by cold symptoms, a hard, dry cough, wheezing inhalation of breath, and sometimes vomiting.

wine An alcoholic beverage created from the natural fermentation of fruit juice, usually from grapes.
withdrawal *See* coitus interruptus.
withdrawal symptoms Physical discomfort and illness resulting from the denial of a substance to which a person is addicted.
zero population growth The state in which the birth rate equals the death rate; in the United States this will occur if the birth rate remains at 2.1 children per family or less.
zygote The fertilized ovum.
zygote stage The first two weeks in the development of the fertilized egg.

Select Bibliography

Chapter 1: Mental Health

"Abandoned." *Newsweek*, January 6, 1986, pp. 14–19.
Arieti, G., ed. *American Handbook of Psychiatry*. 2nd. ed. New York: Basic Books, 1974.
Braceland, F. J., and D. I. Farnsworth. "Depression in Adolescents and College Students." *Maryland State Medical Journal*, 18 (April 1969), 67–73.
A Consumer's Guide to Mental Health Services. DHHS publication no. (ADM) 80–214. Washington, D.C.: National Institute of Mental Health, 1980.
Craig, G. J. *Human Development*. 4th ed. Englewood Cliffs, N.J.: Prentice-Hall, Inc., 1986.
Darley, J. M., et al., *Psychology*, 3rd ed. Englewood Cliffs, N.J.: Prentice-Hall, Inc., 1986.
Eaton, W. W. *The Sociology of Mental Disorders*. 2nd ed. New York: Praeger, 1985.
Erikson, E. *Childhood and Society*. Rev. ed. New York: Norton, 1964.
Fromm, E. *Escape from Freedom*. New York: Avon, 1971.
Gelman, D., and M. Hager. "Psychotherapy in the '80s." *Newsweek*, November 30, 1981, pp. 70–73.
Janis, I., et al. *Personality: Dynamics, Development, and Assessment*. New York: Harcourt, 1969.
Lazarus, R., and A. Monat. *Personality*. 3rd ed. Englewood Cliffs, N.J.: Prentice-Hall, Inc., 1979.
"Lessons in Bringing Up Baby." *Time*, October 22, 1984, pp. 97–98.
Liebert, R. M., et al. *Developmental Psychology*. 4th ed. Englewood Cliffs, N.J.: Prentice-Hall, Inc., 1986.
Lindzey, G., et al., eds. *Theories of Personality: Primary Sources and Research*. 2nd ed. New York: Wiley, 1973.
"Mental State of the Union." *Newsweek*, October 15, 1984, p. 113.
Morris, C. G. *Psychology: An Introduction*. 5th ed. Englewood Cliffs, N.J.: Prentice-Hall, Inc., 1985.
Nelson, B. "Despite a Blur of Change, Clear Trends Are Emerging in Therapy." *The New York Times*, March 1, 1983, pp. C1f.
Penrod, S. *Social Psychology*. 2nd ed. Englewood Cliffs, N.J.: Prentice-Hall, Inc., 1986.
Plain Talk about Adolescence. Washington, D.C.: National Institute of Mental Health, 1981.
Plain Talk about Feelings of Guilt. Washington, D.C.: National Institute of Mental Health, 1977.
Plain Talk about Raising Children. Washington, D.C.: National Institute of Mental Health, 1981.
Rachman, S. *Phobias: Their Nature and Control*. Springfield, Ill.: Charles C Thomas, 1968.
"Raising Children Who Care." *Newsweek*, March 12, 1984, p. 76.
Rogers, D. *Adolescents and Youth*. 5th ed. Englewood Cliffs, N.J.: Prentice-Hall, Inc., 1985.
Rycroft, C. *Anxiety and Neurosis*. Garden City, N.Y.: Doubleday, 1970.
Sarason, I. G., and B. R. Sarason. *Abnormal Psychology*. 4th ed. Englewood Cliffs, N.J.: Prentice-Hall, Inc., 1984.
Sass, L. "The Borderline Personality." *The New York Times Magazine*, August 22, 1982, pp. 12ff.
Sears, D. O., et al. *Social Psychology*. 5th ed. Englewood Cliffs, N.J.: Prentice-Hall, Inc., 1985.
Szasz, T. *Ideology and Insanity*. Garden City, N.Y.: Doubleday, 1970.
——. *The Myth of Mental Illness*. New York: Harper, 1974.
Taube, C. A., and S. A. Barrett, eds. *Mental Health, United States 1985*. Rockville, MD. U.S. Department of Health and Human Services, 1985.
Ullmann, L., and L. Krasner. *A Psychological Approach to Abnormal Behavior*. 2nd ed. Englewood Cliffs, N.J.: Prentice-Hall, Inc., 1975.
Waldinger, R. *Handbook of Psychiatry for Legal and Health Care Professionals*. Washington, D.C.: American Psychiatric Association, 1985.
Worchel, S., and W. Shebilske. *Psychology: Principles and Application*. 2nd ed. Englewood Cliffs, N.J.: Prentice-Hall, Inc., 1986.

Chapter 2: Stress

Anderson, D. B., and L. J. McClean, eds. *Identifying Suicide Potential*. New York: Behavioral Publications, 1971.
Asimov, I. *The Human Brain*. New York: Signet, 1963.
Benson, H., and M. Z. Klipper. *The Relaxation Response*. New York: Morrow, 1975.
Brown, B. B. "New Mind, New Body." *Psychology Today*, August 1974, pp. 45–56f.
Cannon, W. B. *The Wisdom of the Body*. 2nd ed. New York: Norton.
Craig, L., and R. Senter. "Student Thoughts about Suicide." *Psychological Record*, 22 (1972), 355–58.
Frederick, A. B. "Tension Control in the Physical Education Classroom." *Journal of Health, Physical Education, and Recreation*, September 1967, pp. 42–44f.
Friedman, M., and R. Rosenman. *Type A Behavior and Your Heart*. Greenwich, Conn.: Fawcett, 1981.
Gellhorn, E. "Motion and Emotion: The Role of Proprioception in the Physiology and Pathology of the Emotions." *Psychological Review*, 71 (1964), 457–72.
Girdano, D. A., and G. S. Everly, Jr. *Controlling Stress and*

Tension: A Holistic Approach. 2nd ed. Englewood Cliffs, N.J.: Prentice-Hall, Inc., 1986.
Gottschalk, E. C., Jr. "Stress Is More Severe for Collegians Today." *The Wall Street Journal*, June 1, 1983, p. 1f.
Grollman, E. A., ed. *Suicide*. Boston: Beacon, 1971.
Holmes, T. H., and R. H. Rahe. "The Social Readjustment Rating Scale," *Journal of Psychosomatic Research*, 11 (1967), 213–18.
"How Long Will You Live?" *Time*, November 2, 1981, p. 106.
Jacobson, E. *Progressive Relaxation*. 3rd ed. Chicago: University of Chicago Press, 1974.
——. *You Must Relax*. 5th ed. New York: McGraw-Hill, 1978.
——. *The Human Mind*. Springfield, Ill.: Charles C Thomas, 1982.
Lazarus, R. "Little Hassles Can Be Hazardous to Your Health." *Psychology Today*, July 1981, pp. 59–62.
Luthe, W. "Autogenic Training." *American Journal of Psychotherapy*, 17 (1963), 174–95.
Melzack, R. "Promise of Biofeedback: Don't Hold the Party Yet." *Psychology Today*, July 1975, pp. 18–22ff.
Michaels, R. R., et al. "Evaluation of Transcendental Meditation as a Method of Reducing Stress." *Science*, 192 (1976), 1242–44.
Naranjo, C., and R. E. Ornstein. *On the Psychology of Meditation*. New York: Viking, 1971.
Seliger, S. "Stress Can Be Good for You." *New York*, August 2, 1982, pp. 20–24.
Selye, H. *Stress Without Distress*. Philadelphia: Lippincott, 1974.
——. *The Stress of Life*. 2nd ed. New York: McGraw-Hill, 1978.
Simeons, A. T. W. *Man's Presumptuous Brain*. New York: Dutton, 1962.
Wallis, C. "Stress: Can We Cope?" *Time*, June 6, 1983, pp. 48–54.
Wolpe, J. *The Practice of Behavior Therapy*. 3rd ed. Elmsford, N.Y.: Pergamon, 1982.

Chapter 3: Accidents and Safety

Carper, Jean. "Feud over Treatment of Food-choking Victims." *The Sunday Record* (Bergen County, N.J.) April 29, 1979.
"Choosing a Small Car: The Safety Question. "*Consumer Reports*, April 1974, p. 294.
"Green Light for Air Bags." *Time*, July 11, 1977.
"The Gun under Fire." *Time*, June 21, 1968, p. 13.
"Guns Against Society." *The New York Times*, January 2, 1975, p. 26.
Hicks, Nancy. "Fight over Gun Control." *The New York Times*, April 8, 1975, p. 16.
Insurance Institute for Highway Safety. *Key Issues in Highway Loss Reduction*. 1970 symposium. Washington, D.C., 1970.
Lindsay, Robert. "Traffic Toll Still Declines despite Increased Travel." *The New York Times*, January 2, 1975, p. 66.
Metropolitan Life Insurance Company. *Your Child's Safety*. New York: Metropolitan Life Insurance Company, 1970.
——. *Statistical Bulletin*. September 1974.
Nader, Ralph. *Unsafe at Any Speed*. Rev. ed. New York: Grossman, 1972.
National Safety Council. *Accident Facts*. Chicago: National Safety Council, 1986.
"A New Prohibition." *Newsweek on Campus*, April 1985, p. 7.
"One Less for the Road?" *Time*, May 20, 1985, pp. 76–78.
Schultz, Terri. "Someday You Are Going to Need an Ambulance." *Today's Health*, July 1974, p. 47.
Sourcebook of Criminal Justice Statistics, U.S. Department of Justice, July 3, 1978.
Thygerson, A. L. *Essentials of Safety, 3rd ed*. Englewood Cliffs, N.J.: Prentice-Hall, Inc., 1986.
——. *Safety: Principles, Instruction, and Readings*. 2nd ed. Englewood Cliffs, N.J.: Prentice-Hall, Inc., 1986.
U.S. Department of Health, Education, and Welfare, Office of Child Development. *Young Children and Accidents in the Home*. Washington, D.C.: Government Printing Office, 1974.
U.S. Department of Health, Education, and Welfare, Public Health Service. *Home Accident Prevention: A Guide for Health Workers*. PHS publication no. 261. Washington, D.C.: Public Health Service.
U.S. Department of Housing and Urban Development. *Fire Safety*. Washington, D.C.: Government Printing Office, 1974.
U.S. Department of Transportation. "The Hazards of 'Mixing' Tire Types." Fact sheet. Washington, D.C.: National Highway Traffic Safety Administration, January 1972.

Chapter 4: Physical Fitness

Burt, J. J. "Cardiovascular Health." *Journal of Health, Physical Education, and Recreation*, November-December 1968, pp. 36–37.
Cooper, K. H. *The New Aerobics*. New York: Bantam, 1970.
Cooper, M., and K. H. Cooper. *Aerobics for Women*, New York: Evans, 1973.
Falls, H. B., ed. *Exercise Physiology*. New York: Academic, 1968.
"Fitness, Corporate Style." *Newsweek*, November 5, 1984, pp. 96–97.
Glover, B., and J. Shepherd. *The Runners' Handbook*. New York: Penguin, 1978.
Greenberg, J. S., and D. Pargman. *Physical Fitness: A Wellness Approach*. Englewood Cliffs, N.J.: Prentice-Hall, Inc., 1986.
"Learning to Take Exercise to Heart." *The* [Bergen County, N.J.] *Record*, December 19, 1982, p. 31.
Morrow, L. "The Great Bicycle Wars." *Time*, November 24, 1980, p. 110.
Reed, J. D. "America Shapes Up." *Time*, November 2, 1981, pp. 94ff.
Royal Canadian Air Force Exercise Plans for Physical Fitness. Rev. U.S. ed. New York: Pocket Books, 1976.
Schweufeld, Y., et al. "Walking: A Method for Rapid Improvement of Physical Fitness." *JAMA*, 243:20 (May 23-30, 1980), 2062–63.
Special Issue on Physical Fitness. *Journal of the Florida Medical Association*, 67:4 (April 1980), 367–434.
Successful Jogging. National Jogging Association, 1910 K Street, N. W., Suite 202, Washington, D.C. 20006.
"A Third of All Runners Face Injury." *The* [Bergen County, N.J.] *Record*, December 19, 1982, p. 24.
Vaughan, T. *Science and Sport*. Boston: Little, Brown, 1970. "The Weaker Sex? Hah!" *Time*, June 26, 1978, p. 60.

"Woes of the Weekend Jock." *Time*, August 21, 1978, pp. 50–51.

Chapter 5: Nutrition

"America's Diet Wars." *U.S. News & World Report*, January 20, 1985, pp. 62–69.
Birch, G. G., et al., eds. *Health and Food*. New York: Elsevier, 1972.
Burros, M. " 'Natural' Food: Telling the Real from the Artificial." *The New York Times*, August 18, 1982.
The Confusing World of Health Foods. Washington, D.C.: U.S. Government Printing Office, 1981.
Conserving the Nutritive Values in Foods. Rev. ed. Home and Garden bulletin no. 90. Washington, D.C.: U.S. Government Printing Office, 1971.
Consumer's Guide to Food Labels. Washington, D.C.: U.S. Government Printing Office, 1981.
"Dietary Fiber." *Harvard Medical School Health Letter*, August 1986, pp. 1–4.
Family Fare: A Guide to Good Nutrition. Rev. ed. Home and Garden bulletin no. 1. Washington, D.C.: U.S. Government Printing Office, 1978.
Fenner, L. "Salt Shakes Up Some of Us." *FDA Consumer*, March 1980. Reprinted as HEW publication no. (FDA) 80-2129. Washington, D.C.: U.S. Government Printing Office, 1981.
Food. House and Garden bulletin no. 228. Washington, D.C.: U.S. Government Printing Office, 1979.
Food Additives. Washington, D.C.: U.S. Government Printing Office, 1981.
Jacobson, M. *Nutrition Scoreboard: Your Guide to Better Eating*. Washington, D.C.: Center for Science in the Public Interest, 1973.
Kart, C. S., and S. P. Metress. *Nutrition, the Aged, and Society*. Englewood Cliffs, N.J.: Prentice-Hall, Inc., 1984.
Kreutler, P. A. *Nutrition in Perspective*. Englewood Cliffs, N.J.: Prentice-Hall, Inc., 1980.
Lecos, C. "A Compendium on Fats," *FDA Consumer*, March 1983. {HHS Publication No. (FDA) 83-2171}
Lecos, C. W. "Sugar: How Sweet It Is—and Isn't." *FDA Consumer*, February 1980. Reprinted as HEW publication no. (FDA) 80-2127. Washington, D.C.: U.S. Government Printing Office, 1981.
Long, P. J., and B. Shannon. *Nutrition: An Inquiry into the Issues*. Englewood Cliffs, N.J.: Prentice-Hall, Inc., 1983.
Martin, E. A., and A. A. Coolidge. *Nutrition in Action*. 4th ed. New York: Holt, 1978.
Miller, R. W. "There's Something to Be Said for Never Saying 'Please Pass the Meat.' " *FDA Consumer*, February 1981. Reprinted as HHS publication no. (FDA) 81-2144. Washington, D.C.: U.S. Government Printing Office, 1981.
Nutrition and Family Planning. Washington, D.C.: U.S. Department of Health, Education, and Welfare, 1980.
Nutrition and Your Health: Dietary Guidelines for Americans. Home and Garden bulletin no. 232. Washington, D.C.: U.S. Government Printing Office, 1980.
Nutritivé Value of Foods. Washington, D.C.: U.S. Government Printing Office, 1981.
"Primer on Food Additives," *FDA Consumer*, May 1973. Reprinted as DHEW publication no. (FDA) 74-2002. Washington, D.C.: U.S. Government Printing Office, 1973.
Robinson, C. H., and M. R. Lawler. *Normal and Therapeutic Nutrition*, 6th ed. New York: Macmillan, 1982.
Roughage. Washington, D.C.: U.S. Government Printing Office, 1980.
Saccharin, Cyclamate, and Aspartame. Washington, D.C.: U.S. Government Printing Office, 1981.
Salt. Washington, D.C.: U.S. Government Printing Office, 1981.
Some Facts and Myths About Vitamins. Washington, D.C.: U.S. Government Printing Office, 1981.
Sugar. Washington, D.C.: U.S. Government Printing Office, 1981.
Vegetarian Diets. Washington, D.C.: U.S. Government Printing Office, 1981.
Wallis, C. "Salt: A New Villain?" *Time*, March 15, 1982, pp. 64–71.
"The Wide World of Mineral Supplements." *Newsweek*, January 27, 1986, p. 53.
Willis, J. "Please Pass That Woman Some More Calcium and Iron," *FDA Consumer*, September 1984. {HHS Publication No. (FDA) 85-2198}

Chapter 6: Weight Control

Adams, C. F., and M. Richardson. *Nutritivé Value of Foods*. Rev. ed. Home and Garden bulletin no. 72. Washington, D.C.: U.S. Government Printing Office, 1981.
"After the 'Last Chance' Diet." *Consumer Reports*, February 1978, pp. 92–95.
"America's Sweet Tooth." *Newsweek*, August 26, 1985, pp. 50–56.
"Base Anorexia Nervosa Dx on Positive Findings." *Clinical Psychiatry News*, 10:2 (February 1982).
Beller, A. S. *Fat and Thin: A Natural History of Obesity*. New York: Farrar, Straus and Giroux, 1977.
"Block Those Starch Blockers," *Time*, July 26, 1982, p. 41.
Bloom, W. L. "To Fast or Exercise." *American Journal of Clinical Nutrition*, 21 (December 1968), 1475–79.
Bray, G. A., ed. *Obesity in America: A Conference*. DHEW publication no. (NIH) 80-359. Washington, D.C.: U.S. Government Printing Office, 1980.
Bruch, H. "Anorexia Nervosa." *Nutrition Today*, September/October 1978, pp. 14–18.
——. *Eating Disorders: Obesity, Anorexia Nervosa, and the Person Within*. New York: Basic Books, 1979.
"Dieting: The Losing Game." *Time*, January 20, 1986, pp. 54–60.
Eating for Better Health. Washington, D.C.: U.S. Government Printing Office, 1981.
Exercise and Weight Control. Washington, D.C.: U.S. Government Printing Office, 1979.
"Fat Is an Energy Issue." *The New York Times*, November 14, 1978, p. C2.
Fenner, L. "Cellulite: Hard to Budge Pudge." *FDA Consumer*, May 1980. Reprinted as HHS publication no. (FDA) 80-1078. Washington, D.C.: U.S. Government Printing Office, 1980.

The Hassle-Free Guide to a Better Diet. Washington, D.C.: U.S. Government Printing Office, March, 1980.

Kanack, E. B., et al. "Relation of Body Weight to Development of Coronary Heart Disease: The Framingham Study." *Circulation*, 35 (1967), 734–44.

Kiell, N., ed. *The Psychology of Obesity*. Springfield, Ill.: Charles C Thomas, 1973.

Kreutler, P. A., et al. "The Overweight Condition." In R. B. Howard and N. H. Herbold, eds., *Nutrition in Clinical Care*. New York: McGraw-Hill, 1978.

Lowenberg, M. E., et al. *Food and People*. 3rd ed. New York: Wiley, 1979.

Mann, G. V. "The Influence of Obesity in Health." Parts I and II. *New England Journal of Medicine*, 291 (July 25, 1974), 178–85; 291 (August 1, 1974), 226–32.

Mayer, J. "Liquid Protein: The Last Word on the Last Chance Diet." *Today's Health*, 10 (January 1978), 40–41.

Mayo Clinic, Committee on Dietetics. *Mayo Clinic Diet Manual*. 5th ed. Philadelphia: Saunders, 1981.

Mirkin, G. "The Impossible Dream?," *The Runner*, October 1979, pp. 14f.

"Overweight and Obesity: The Associated Cardiovascular Risk." *Minnesota Medicine*, 52 (August 1969), 1265–70.

"Pass the Eclairs, Please." *Time*, March 14, 1983, p. 75.

Powers, P. S. *Obesity*. Baltimore: Williams and Wilkins, 1980.

Schachter, S. "Some Extraordinary Facts about Obese Humans and Rats." *American Psychologist*, 26 (1971), 129–44.

Stunkard, A. J. et al. "A Twin Study of Obesity," *JAMA*, July 4, 1986, pp. 51–54.

"Why Kids Get Fat." *Newsweek*, February 3, 1986, p. 61.

Chapter 7: Reproduction and Birth Control

"Another Barrier to Pregnancy." *Time*, January 26, 1981, p. 57.

Begley, S., and J. Carey. "How Human Life Begins." *Newsweek*, January 11, 1982, pp. 38–43.

Birth Defects: Tragedy and Hope. The National Foundation/ March of Dimes, 1977.

Brody, J. E. " 'Barrier' Methods of Birth Control." *The New York Times*, December 31, 1980.

Caffeine and Pregnancy. HHS publication no. (FDA) 81-1081. Rockville, Md.: Public Health Service, 1981.

Calderone, M. S., ed. *Manual of Family Planning and Contraceptive Practice*. 2nd ed. Baltimore: Williams and Wilkins, 1970.

Contraception: Comparing the Options. HEW publication no. (FDA) 78-3069. Rockville, Md.: Public Health Service, 1978.

"Contraceptive Efficacy among Married Women Aged 15–44 Years: United States." *Vital and Health Statistics*, Series 23, No. 5, May 1980. DHHS publication no. (PHS) 80-1981. Washington, D.C.: U.S. Government Printing Office, 1980.

"The Contraceptive Sponge." *Consumer Reports*, January 1985, p. 11.

"Doctors Debate Surgery's Place in the Maternity Ward." *The New York Times*, March 24, 1985, Section IV, p. 24.

"Female Fertility: A Sharp Dip after 30." *Newsweek*, March 1, 1982, p. 79.

Ferber, A., and W. L. Ferber. "Vasectomy." *Medical Aspects of Human Sexuality*, 2 (June 1968), 29–35.

Golden, F. "Shaping Life in the Lab." *Time*, March 9, 1981, pp. 50–59.

Haines, R. W., and A. Mohiuddin. *Handbook of Human Embryology*. 5th ed. New York: Longman, 1972.

Hall, M. H. "A Conversation with Masters and Johnson." *Psychology Today*, July 1969, pp. 50–58.

Hatcher, R. A., et al., *Contraceptive Technology, 1986–1987*. 13th rev. ed. New York: Irvington, 1986.

"Helping Babies in the Womb." *Time*, May 25, 1981, p. 76.

Linde, S. M. "Common Problems of Pregnancy . . . and What to Do about Them." *Today's Health*, 46 (April 1968), 50–51.

Masters, W. H., and V. E. Johnson. *Human Sexual Inadequacy*. Boston: Little, Brown, 1970.

——. *Human Sexual Response*. Boston: Little, Brown, 1966.

Morrison, M. "When the Baby's Life Is So Much Your Own. . . ." *FDA Consumer*, May 1979. Reprinted as HEW publication no. (FDA) 79-1057. Washington, D.C.: U.S. Government Printing Office, 1979.

Mosher, W. D., and C. F. Westoff. *Trends in Contraceptive Practice, United States*, 1965–76. DHHS publication no. (PHS) 82-1986. Washington, D.C.: U.S. Government Printing Office, 1982.

Naismith, G. "Conquering Male Infertility." *Today's Health*, 46 (November 1968), 68–73.

"Rebirth for Midwifery." *Time*, August 29, 1977, p. 66.

A Self-instructional Booklet to Aid in the Understanding of Contraception. DHHS publication no. (HSA) 80-5659. Rockville, Md.: Public Health Service, 1980.

"A Son's Rite." *Time*, August 31, 1981, p. 57.

"Sponge Contraceptive Approved." *The* [Bergen County, N.J.] *Record*, April 7, 1983, p. A10.

"Still Too Many Caesareans." *Newsweek*, December 31, 1984, p. 70.

"Surgery in the Womb." *Time*, August 10, 1981, p. 59.

Tay-Sachs: The Killer Is Cornered. National Tay-Sachs and Allied Diseases Association, Inc., n.d.

Toufexis, A. "Coping with Eve's Curse." *Time*, July 27, 1981, p. 59.

Chapter 8: Sexual Behavior

Bell, A. P., and M. S. Weinberg. *Homosexualities: A Study of Diversity among Men and Women*. New York: Simon and Schuster, 1978.

Bell, A. P., et al. *Sexual Preference: Its Development in Men and Women*. Bloomington: Indiana University Press, 1981.

Boxall, B. "When Rape Makes a Man One of the Boys." *The* [Bergen County, N.J.] *Record*, May 15, 1983, pp. A-1, 28.

"The Date Who Rapes." *Newsweek*, April 9, 1984, pp. 91–92.

Ellis, A., and A. Abarbanel, eds. *The Encyclopedia of Sexual Behavior*. Rev. ed. New York: Jason Aronson, 1973.

Hall, M. H. "A Conversation with Masters and Johnson." *Psychology Today*, July 1969, pp. 50–58.

How to Protect Yourself Against Sexual Assault. Washington, D.C.: U.S. Government Printing Office, 1980.

Johnson, W. R. *Masturbation*. SIECUS study guide no. 3. New

York: Sex Information and Education Council of the United States, 1974.
———, and E. G. Belzer. *Human Sexual Behavior and Sex Education*. 3rd ed. Philadelphia: Lea and Febiger, 1973.
Kinsey, A. C., et al. *Sexual Behavior in the Human Female*. Philadelphia: Saunders, 1953.
———. *Sexual Behavior in the Human Male*. Philadelphia: Saunders, 1948.
Kirkendall, L. A. *Sex Education*. SIECUS study guide no 1. New York: Sex Information and Education Council of the United States, 1974.
———, and I. Rubin. *Sexuality and the Life Cycle*. SIECUS study guide no. 8. New York: Sex Information and Education Council of the United States, 1974.
McCary, J. L., and S. P. McCary. *Human Sexuality*. 4th ed. Belmont, Calif.: Wadsworth, 1981.
Maccoby, E., and C. Jacklin. "What We Know and Don't Know about Sex Differences." *Psychology Today*, December 1974, pp. 109–12.
Masters, W. H., and V. E. Johnson. *Human Sexual Inadequacy*. Boston: Little, Brown, 1970.
———. *Human Sexual Response*. Boston: Little, Brown, 1966.
Money, J., ed. *Sex Research: New Developments*. New York: Holt, 1965.
Peterson, E., and W. D'Antonio. *Female and Male: Dimensions of Human Sexuality*. Philadelphia: Lippincott, 1974.
Pomeroy, W. B., and C. V. Christenson. *Characteristics of Male and Female Sexual Responses*. SIECUS study guide no. 4. New York: Sex Information and Education Council of the United States, 1974.
"Rape and Culture." *Time*, September 12, 1977, p. 41.
"Rape and the Law." *Newsweek*, May 20, 1985, pp. 60–64.
Riddle, D. I. "Relating to Children: Gays as Role Models." *Journal of Social Issues*, 34 (November 3, 1978).
Rubin, I. *Homosexuality*. SIECUS study guide no. 2. New York: Sex Information and Education Council of the United States, 1974.
———. *Sexual Life in the Later Years*. SIECUS study guide no. 12. New York: Sex Information and Education Council of the United States, 1970.
Schultz, D. A. *Human Sexuality*. 2nd ed. Englewood Cliffs, N.J.: Prentice-Hall, Inc., 1984.
Tripp, C. A. *The Homosexual Matrix*. New York: New American Library, 1976.

Chapter 9: Life Styles

Atwater, E. *Psychology of Adjustment*. 2nd ed. Englewood Cliffs, N.J.: Prentice-Hall, Inc., 1983.
Bell, A. P., and M. S. Weinberg. *Homosexualities*. New York: Simon and Schuster, 1978.
Blades, J. *Family Mediation: Cooperative Divorce Settlement*. Englewood Cliffs, N.J.: Prentice-Hall, Inc., 1985.
Bowker, R. *Solving Problems in Marriage*. Grand Rapids, Mich.: Eerdmans, 1972.
Brooks, A. "Corporate Ambivalence on Day Care." *The New York Times*, July 21, 1983, pp. C1, 10.
Burgess, E. W., et al. *The Family: From Traditional to Companionship*. 4th ed. New York: Van Nostrand, 1971.
"Children Having Children." *Time*, December 9, 1985, pp. 78–90.
Crawley, L., et al. *Reproduction, Sex, and Preparation for Marriage*. 2nd ed. Englewood Cliffs, N.J.: Prentice-Hall, Inc., 1973.
"Day Care on the Job." *Newsweek*, September 2, 1985, pp. 59–62.
"Growing Up Gay." *Newsweek*, January 13, 1986, pp. 50–52.
Havermann, E., and M. Lehtinen. *Marriages and Families: New Problems, New Opportunities*. Englewood Cliffs, N.J.: Prentice-Hall, Inc., 1986.
Jarmulowski, V. "The Blended Family: Who Are They?," *MS.*, February 1985, pp. 33–34.
Julian, J., and W. Kornblum. *Social Psychology*, 5th ed. Englewood Cliffs, N.J.: Prentice-Hall, Inc., 1986.
Leo, J. "Single Parent, Double Trouble," *Time*, January 4, 1982, p. 81.
Levinger, G. "Sources of Marital Dissatisfaction among Applicants for Divorce." *American Journal of Orthopsychiatry*, 36 (1966), 803–7.
Orden, S. R., and N. M. Bradburn. "Working Wives and Marital Happiness." *American Journal of Sociology*, 74 (1969), 392–407.
"Playing both Mother and Father." *Newsweek*, July 15, 1985, pp. 42–43.
Ramey, J. W. "The Sexual Bond." *Society*, 14 (1977), 161.
"The Revolution Is Over." *Time*, April 9, 1984, pp. 74–83.
Rossi, A. S. "Transition to Parenthood." *Journal of Marriage and the Family*, 30 (February 1968), 20–39.
Schulz, D. A. *Human Sexuality, 2nd ed*. Englewood Cliffs, N.J.: Prentice-Hall, Inc., 1984.
Schulz, D. A., and S. F. Rodgers. *Marriage, the Family, and Personal Fulfillment*, 3rd ed. Englewood Cliffs, N.J.: Prentice-Hall, Inc., 1985.
Sears, D. O., et al. *Social Psychology*, 5th ed. Englewood Cliffs, N.J.: Prentice-Hall, Inc., 1985.
Skolnick, A. *The Intimate Environment*. 3rd ed. Boston: Little, Brown, 1983.
Sussman, M. B., ed. *Marriage and the Family: Current Critical Issues*. Binghamton, N.Y.: Haworth Press, 1979.
"A Teen-Pregnancy Epidemic." *Newsweek*, March 25, 1985, p. 90.
Trippett, F. "The Young: Adult Penchants—and Problems." *Time*, April 6, 1981, p. 84.
Ventura, S. J. "Trends in First Births to Older Mothers, 1970–79." *Monthly Vital Statistics Report*, 31:2, Supplement 2 (May 27, 1982).
"Waiting to Wed." *Time*, July 16, 1979, p. 59.
Wallis C. "The New Baby Boom." *Time*, February 22, 1982, pp. 52–59.
"The Ways 'Singles' Are Changing U.S." *The U.S. News and World Report*, January 31, 1977.
"What Price Day Care?" *Newsweek*, September 10, 1984, pp. 14–21.

Chapter 10: Aging, Dying, and Death

Birren, J. E., and J. Livingston. *Cognition, Stress, and Aging*. Englewood Cliffs, N.J.: Prentice-Hall, Inc., 1985.

Birren, J. E., et al. *Age, Health and Employment*. Englewood Cliffs, N.J.: Prentice-Hall, Inc., 1986.
Burdman, G. M. *Healthful Aging*. Englewood Cliffs, N.J.: Prentice-Hall, Inc., 1986.
Doyle, N. *The Dying Person and the Family*. Public Affairs Pamphlet no. 485. New York: The Public Affairs Committee, 1972.
Estes, C. L. *The Aging Enterprise*. San Francisco: Jossey-Bass, 1979.
The Fitness Challenge in the Later Years. Washington, D.C.: U.S. Government Printing Office, 1980.
Foner, A. *Aging and Old Age: New Perspectives*. Englewood Cliffs, N.J.: Prentice-Hall, Inc., 1986.
Geyman, J. P. "Death and Dying of a Family Member," *The Journal of Family Practice*, 17:1 (July 1983), 125–34.
Greer, D. S., and V. Mor. *Hastings Center Report*, October 1985, pp. 5–10.
Gross, R., et al., eds. *The New Old: The Struggle for Decent Aging*. Garden City, N.Y.: Anchor, 1978.
"Happy Old Age Tied to Spouses' Health." *The New York Times*, June 12, 1980, p. C3.
Hobman, D., ed. *The Impact of Aging*. New York: St. Martin's, 1981.
"Hospices: Not to Cure but to Help." *Consumer Reports*, January 1986, pp. 24–26.
"Hospital Care for the Dying: Each Day, Some Painful Choices." *The New York Times*, January 14, 1985, pp. 1f.
How Old Is "Old"? The Effects of Aging on Learning and Working. Hearing before the Special Committee on Aging, United States Senate, 96th Congress, 2nd session, April 30, 1980. Washington, D.C.: U.S. Government Printing Office, 1980.
Hudson, R. B., ed. *The Aging in Politics: Process and Policy*. Springfield, Ill.: Charles C Thomas, 1981.
Income and Resources of the Aged. SSA publication no. 13–11727. Washington, D.C.: U.S. Government Printing Office, January 1980.
Johnson, E. S., and J. B. Williamson. *Growing Old: The Social Problems of Aging*. New York: Holt, 1980.
Jones, R. *The Other Generation: The New Power of Older People*. Englewood Cliffs, N.J.: Prentice-Hall, Inc., 1977.
Julian, J., and W. Kornblum. *Social Problems*. 5th ed. Englewood Cliffs, N.J.: Prentice-Hall, Inc., 1986.
Kiev, A. *The Courage to Live*. New York: Bantam, 1982.
Kübler-Ross, E. *Questions and Answers on Death and Dying*. New York: Macmillan, 1974.
——. *Death: The Final Stage of Growth*. Englewood Cliffs, N.J.: Prentice-Hall, Inc., 1975.
Loether, H. J. *Problems of Aging*. Belmont, Calif.: Dickenson, 1975.
Lofland, L. H. *The Craft of Dying: The Modern Face of Death*. Beverly Hills, Calif.: Sage, 1979.
McCary, J. L., and S. P. McCary. *Human Sexuality*. 4th ed. Belmont, Calif.: Wadsworth, 1981.
Ogg, E. *A Death in the Family*. Public Affairs Pamphlet no. 542. New York: The Public Affairs Committee, 1976.
Rogers, D. *The Adult Years: An Introduction to Aging, 3rd ed*. Englewood Cliffs, N.J.: Prentice-Hall, Inc., 1986.
Shneidman, E. S., and N. L. Farberow. Eds. *Clues to Suicide*. New York: McGraw-Hill, 1957.
Stein, K. "Some of Us May Never Die." In *Health 81/82*. Guilford, Conn.: Dushkin, 1981, pp. 36–39.
Stoddard, S. *The Hospice Movement: A Better Way to Care for the Dying*. New York: Vintage, 1978.
Talking to Children about Death. Washington, D.C.: U.S. Government Printing Office, 1979.
Uris, A. *Over 50*. New York: Bantam, 1979.
Ward, R. A. *The Aging Experience: An Introduction to Social Gerontology*. 2nd ed. New York: Harper, 1984.

Chapter 11: Alcohol

Abel, E. L. *Drugs and Behavior: A Primer in Neuropsychopharmacology*. New York: Wiley, 1974.
Al-Anon Faces Alcoholism. 2nd ed. New York: Al-Anon, 1984.
"Alcohol, Youth, Money, and Cancer." *Science News*, 106:3 (July 20, 1974), 39.
"Beer or Skittles?" *Harvard Medical School Health Letter*, January 1986, pp. 1–2.
Bourne, P. G., and R. Fox, eds. *Alcoholism: Progress in Research and Treatment*. New York: Academic Press, 1973.
Carroll, C. R. *Alcohol: Use, Nonuse, and Abuse*. 2nd ed. Dubuque, IA.: William C. Brown, 1975.
Chafetz, M., and H. Demone. *Alcoholism and Society*. New York: Oxford University Press, 1972.
Facts about Alcohol and Alcoholism. DHHS publication no. (ADM) 80–31. Washington, D.C.: Public Health Service, 1980.
First Statistical Compendium on Alcohol and Health. Washington, D.C.: U.S. Government Printing Office, 1981.
Israel, Y., and J. Mardones, eds. *Biological Basis of Alcoholism*. New York: Wiley, 1971.
Jones, K., et al. *Drugs and Alcohol*. 3rd ed. New York: Harper, 1978.
Kissin, B., and H. Biegleiter, eds. *The Biology of Alcoholism. Vol. 2: Physiology and Behavior*. New York: Plenum, 1972.
Lundstrom, M. "A Popular College 'Major': Drinking." *The* [Bergen County, N.J.] *Record*, October 10, 1982, p. D10.
Mirin, S. M., et al. "Alcohol Abuse in Patients Dependent on Other Drugs." *Psychiatric Annals*. 12:4 (April 1982), 430–33.
"Nightcap." *Time*, January 3, 1983, p. 51.
"Prison Study Poses Alcohol-Crime Link." *The* [Bergen County, N.J.] *Record*, January 31, 1983.
Robinson, D., ed. *Alcohol Problems: Reviews, Research, and Recommendations*. New York: Holmes and Meier, 1980.
Stone, M. "Recognizing and Treating the Alcoholic." *Behavioral Medicine*, January 1980, pp. 14–17.

Chapter 12: Tobacco

Borgatta, E. F., and R. R. Evans, eds. *Smoking, Health, and Behavior*, Chicago: Aldine, 1969.
Brody, J. E. "Personal Health: Making the Great Leap to Being a Nonsmoker." *The New York Times*, February 23, 1977.
Calling It Quits: The Latest Advice on How to Give Up Cigarettes. DHEW publication no. (NIH) 78–1824. Bethesda, Md.: Public Health Service, 1978.

Cancer Facts and Figures 1986. New York: American Cancer Society, 1985.
Cancer 1982: The Health Consequences of Smoking: A Report of the Surgeon General. DHHS publication no. (PHS) 82–50179. Washington, D.C.: U.S. Government Printing Office, 1982.
Changes in Cigarette Smoking Habits Between 1955 and 1966. DHEW publication no. (PHS) 70–1000, series 10, no. 59. Washington, D.C.: U.S. Government Printing Office, 1970.
Changing Cigarette: The Health Consequences of Smoking: A Report of the Surgeon General. DHHS publication no. (PHS) 81–50156. Washington, D.C.: U.S. Government Printing Office, 1982.
Chronic Obstructive Lung Disease: A Report of the Surgeon General. Washington, D.C.: U.S. Department of Health and Human Services, 1984.
"A Cloudy Forecast for Smokers." *Time*, April 7, 1986, p. 45.
Everyone Can Do Something about Smoking: You Too. DHEW publication no. (NIH) 79–1820. Bethesda, Md.: Public Health Service, 1979.
Gallup, G. (The Gallup Organization, Inc.). "Teens Have Few Illusions about Smoking." *The* [Bergen County, N.J.] *Record*, September 19, 1977.
The Health Consequences of Smoking for Women: A Report of the Surgeon General. Rockville, Md.: Public Health Service, 1980.
Kline, J., et al. "Smoking: A Risk Factor for Spontaneous Abortion." *New England Journal of Medicine*, 297 (October 13, 1977), 793–96.
"Passive Smoking Linked to Lung Cancer." *The* [Bergen County, N.J.] *Record*, March 13, 1983, p. A16.
"Smokeless Tobacco." *Backgrounder*, July 1985, pp. 1–6.
Smoking and Health: A Report of the Surgeon General. DHEW publication no. (PHS) 79–50066. Washington, D.C.: U.S. Government Printing Office, 1979.
Smoking, Tobacco, and Health: A Fact Book DHHS publication no. (PHS) 80–50150. Washington, D.C.: U.S. Government Printing Office, 1981.
Stewart, M. S. *Cigarettes—America's No. 1 Public Health Problem*. New York: The Public Affairs Committee, 1972.
Toufexis, A. "Report from the Surgeon General." *Time*, March 8, 1982, pp. 72f.
Williams, T. *Summary and Implications of Review of Literature Related to Adolescent Smoking*. Bethesda, Md.: Health Services and Mental Health Administration, 1972.

Chapter 13: Drugs

Altman, L. K. "Aspirin's Use in Preventing Heart Attacks Reported." *The New York Times*, November 16, 1982.
"Another Sort of Smoke." *Time*, March 8, 1982, p. 73.
Aspirin. Washington, D.C.: U.S. Government Printing Office, 1981.
Brecher, E. M. *Licit and Illicit Drugs*. Boston: Little, Brown, 1972.
Cooper, J. R., ed. *Sedative-Hypnotic Drugs: Risks and Benefits*. Washington, D.C.: National Institute on Drug Abuse, August 1977.
Darvon. Washington, D.C.: U.S. Government Printing Office, 1979.
Drug Abuse Prevention, Treatment, and Rehabilitation in Fiscal Year 1980. Washington, D.C.: U.S. Government Printing Office, 1981.
Drug Use in America: Problem in Perspective. Second Report of the National Commission on Marijuana and Drug Abuse. Washington, D.C.: U.S. Government Printing Office, March 1973.
Einstein, S. *The Drug User*. New York: Plenum, 1983.
——. *Drugs in Relation to the Drug User*. New York: Pergamon, 1980.
Fort, J. *The Addicted Society: Pleasure-Seeking and Punishment Revisited*. New York: Grove, 1981.
Generic Drugs: How Good Are They? Washington, D.C.: U.S. Government Printing Office, 1981.
Girdano, D. *Drugs: A Factual Account*. 3rd ed. New York: Random, 1980.
Grinspoon, L. *Marijuana Reconsidered*. Rev. ed. Cambridge, Mass.: Harvard University Press, 1977.
——. *Psychedelic Drugs Reconsidered*. New York: Basic, 1979.
Highlights from the National Survey on Drug Abuse: 1979. Washington, D.C.: U.S. Government Printing Office, 1980.
Hughes, R., and R. Brewin. *The Tranquilizing of America*. New York: Warner, 1980.
Hyde, M. O. *Mind Drugs*. 4th ed. New York: McGraw-Hill, 1981.
Jaffee, J. H. "Drug Addiction and Drug Abuse." In L. S. Goodman and A. Gilman, eds. *The Pharmacological Basis of Therapeutics*. 4th ed. New York: Macmillan, 1970.
Johnston, L. D. et al. *Drugs and the Class of '78*. Washington, D.C.: U.S. Government Printing Office, 1979.
——, et al. *Highlights from Student Drug Use in America: 1975–1980*. Washington, D.C.: U.S. Government Printing Office, 1981.
Lingeman, R. R. *Drugs from A to Z: A Dictionary*. 2nd ed. New York: McGraw-Hill, 1974.
Masters, R. E., and J. Houston. *The Varieties of Psychedelic Experience*. New York: Dell, 1967.
Methadone: The Drug and Its Therapeutic Uses in the Treatment of Addiction. National Clearinghouse for Drug Abuse Information, Report series 31, no. 1. Washington, D.C.: Public Health Service, July 1976.
Morganthau, T. "Guns, Grass—and Money." *Newsweek*, October 25, 1982, pp. 36–43.
"Overcoping With Valium." *FDA Consumer*, January 1980. Reprinted as HHS publication no. (FDA) 80–3100. Washington, D.C.: U.S. Government Printing Office, 1980.
"PCP: A Terror of a Drug." *Time*, July 17, 1978, p. 16.
Scarpitti, F. R., and S. K. Datesman, eds. *Drugs and the Youth Culture*, Beverly Hills, Calif.: Sage, 1980.
Schlaadt, R. G., and P. T. Shannon. *Drugs of Choice: Current Perspectives on Drug Use*. Englewood Cliffs, N.J.: Prentice-Hall, Inc., 1986.
Schmeck, H. M., Jr. "Addict's Brain: Chemistry Holds Hope for Answers." *The New York Times*, January 25, 1983, pp. C1, 6.
——. "Research on Marijuana Finds Many Risks, Some Benefits." *The New York Times*, October 9, 1979, C1.

Use of Licit and Illicit Drugs by America's High School Students, 1975–1984. Rockville, Md.: National Institute on Drug Abuse, 1985.

Valium. Washington, D.C.: U.S. Government Printing Office, 1980.

"Women Who Nurse Babies Should Skip Pot, Study Says." *The* [Bergen County, N.J.] *Record*, October 10, 1982, p. E18.

Chapter 14: *Cardiovascular Diseases and Cancer*

Arteriosclerosis, 1981. Report of the Working Group on Arteriosclerosis of the National Heart, Lung, and Blood Institute. DHHS publication no. (NIH) 81–2034. Bethesda, Md.: Public Health Service, 1981.

"The Big If in Cancer." *Time*, March 31, 1980, pp. 60–66.

Cancer Facts and Figures 1986. New York: American Cancer Society, 1985.

Cancer Treatment. NIH publication no. 80–1807. Washington, D.C.: Public Health Service, May 1980.

Cancer: *What Is It?* DHHS publication no. (NIH) 80–1806. Bethesda, Md.: Public Health Service, 1980.

Cancer: *What to Know*, *What to Do about It*. Rev. ed. DHHS publication no. (NIH) 81–211. Bethesda, Md.: Public Health Service, 1981.

"Caring for Cancer." *Harvard Medical School Health Letter*, May 1986, pp. 5–7.

"Colon Cancer: The Facts." *Newsweek*, July 22, 1985, pp. 20–21.

"A Critical Review of Adult Health Maintenance: Part 1. Prevention of Atherosclerotic Diseases." *The Journal of Family Practice*, April 1986, pp. 341–346.

"A Critical Review of Adult Health Maintenance: Part 3: Prevention of Cancer." *The Journal of Family Practice*, June 1986, pp. 511–520.

"Diet Debate: Is Cholesterol the Culprit?" *Time*, August 6, 1979, p. 68.

Dulbecco, R. "The Induction of Cancer by Viruses." *Scientific American*, April 1967, pp. 28–37.

"Early Detection." *Time*, January 16, 1978.

Epstein, S. S. *The Politics of Cancer*. San Francisco: Sierra, 1978.

"Experts Give Advice on Blood Pressure." *The New York Times*, February 13, 1977.

"A Few Kind Words for Cholesterol." *Time*, June 9, 1980, p. 51.

"First Aid for Heart Attacks." *Harvard School Health Letter*, March 1986, p. 4.

" 'Good' vs. 'Bad' Cholesterol." *Time*, November 21, 1977.

Hammond, E. C. "The Effects of Smoking." *Scientific American*, July 1962, pp. 39–51.

Heart Attacks. NIH publication no. 81–1803. Washington, D.C.: Public Health Service, August 1981.

Heart Disease: *Public Health Enemy No. 1*. Washington, D.C.: U.S. Government Printing Office, 1979.

Heart Facts 1986. Dallas: American Heart Association, 1986.

Hurst, J. W., ed. *The Heart*, *Arteries*, *and Veins*. 5th ed. New York: McGraw-Hill, 1982.

Hypertension. NIH publication no. 1714. Bethesda, Md.: National Institute of Health.

Irwin, T. *Watch Your Blood Pressure*! Public Affairs Pamphlet no. 483B. New York: The Public Affairs Committee, May 1979.

McAuliffe, S., and K. McAuliffe. "The Genetic Assault on Cancer." *The New York Times Magazine*, October 24, 1982, pp. 39–54.

"A New Look at Diet and Heart Disease." *Consumer Reports*, February 1979.

"Radon in Houses." *Harvard Medical School Health Letter*, May 1986, pp. 1–3.

"Rebuke for Radical Mastectomies." *Time*, July 13, 1981, p. 63.

Richards, V. *Cancer*, *the Wayward Cell*: *Its Origins*, *Nature*, *and Treatment*. 2nd ed. Berkeley, Calif.: University of California Press, 1978.

Rowe, R. D., and A. Mehrizi. *The Framingham Heart Study*: *Detection of Factors Increasing Risk of Coronary Disease*. Washington, D.C.: National Heart Institute, 1964.

Russell, D. S., and L. J. Rubenstein. *Pathology of Tumors of the Nervous System*. 4th ed. Baltimore: Williams and Wilkins, 1977.

Sokolow, M., and M. McIlroy. "Congenital Heart Disease." In *Clinical Cardiology*. 2nd ed. Los Altos, Calif.: Lange, 1979.

Toufexis, A. "Taming the No. 1 Killer." *Time*, June 1, 1981, pp. 52–58.

Chapter 15: *Communicable Diseases*

"The AIDS Epidemic." *The Harvard Medical School Health Letter*, 8:8 (June 1983), 1–2.

"AIDS Update (Part I)." *Harvard Medical School Health Letter*, November 1985, pp. 1–4.

"AIDS Update (Part II)." *Harvard Medical School Health Letter*, December 1985, pp. 2–5.

Altman, L. K. "Infections Still a Big Threat." *The New York Times*, July 20, 1982, p. C2.

——. "Is the Alarm over Herpes Excessive?" *The New York Times*, November 2, 1982, p. C3.

Beneson, A. S., ed. *Control of Communicable Diseases in Man*. 14th ed. Washington, D.C.: American Public Health Association, 1985.

Brock, T. D. *Biology of Microorganisms*. 4th ed. Englewood Cliffs, N.J.: Prentice-Hall, Inc., 1984.

Check, W. "The Herpes Hype." *American Health*, September/October 1982, p. 90.

"Chlamydia: The Silent Epidemic." *Time*, February 4, 1985, p. 67.

Cockburn, A., ed. *Infectious Diseases*: *Their Evolution and Eradication*. Springfield, Ill.: Charles C Thomas, 1967.

"The Cold of the Future." *Harvard Medical School Health Letter*, May 1986, p. 4.

"Dealing with Fears, Friends, and the Signs of AIDS." *The New York Times*, February 19, 1986.

Food Safety for the Family. Washington, D.C.: U.S. Government Printing Office, 1981.

Genital Herpes. DHHS publication no. (NIH) 82–2005. Bethesda, Md.: Public Health Service, 1981.

"Genital Herpes Is More Common But the Alarm Is Diminishing." *The New York Times*, July 8, 1986, pp. C1, C9.

"Hepatitis B Vaccine Approved." *The* [Bergen County, N.J.] *Record*, November 17, 1981, p. A16.

"Herpes Relief." *Newsweek*, February 11, 1985, p. 79.

Johnson, G. T., and S. E. Goldfinger. *The Harvard Medical School Health Letter Book*. Cambridge, Mass.: Harvard University Press, 1981.

King, A., and C. Nicol. *Veneral Diseases*. 4th ed. Philadelphia: Davis, 1980.

Krugman, S., and R. Ward. *Infectious Diseases of Children and Adults*. 7th ed. St. Louis: Mosby, 1980.

"Of Men and Microbes." *Time*, November 22, 1976.

"A Nasty New Epidemic." *Newsweek*, February 4, 1985, pp. 72–73.

Pelczar, M. J., and R. D. Reid. *Microbiology*. 4th ed. New York: McGraw-Hill, 1977.

Porter, R. R. "The Structure of Antibodies." *Scientific American*, October 1967, pp. 81–90.

"Separating the Myths and Fears from the Facts on How AIDS Is and Isn't Transmitted." *The New York Times*, February 12, 1986.

Sexually Transmitted Disease (STD) Statistics. Atlanta, Ga.: U.S. Department of Health and Human Services, Center for Disease Control, 1985.

Sullivan, W. "W. H. O. Immunizing Plan Seeks to Avert 5 Million Deaths a Year." *The New York Times*, February 21, 1979.

"TB Is Found Still a Danger." *The New York Times*, January 18, 1983, p. C8.

"Those Overworked Miracle Drugs." *Time*, August 17, 1981, p. 63.

Top, F. H., and P. F. Wehrle, eds. *Communicable and Infectious Diseases*. 9th ed. St. Louis: Mosby, 1981.

"2 Tests of New Drug for Common Cold Termed Promising." *The New York Times*, January 9, 1986, pp. A1, B6.

VD Fact Sheet. DHEW publication no. (CDC) 77–8195. Atlanta, Ga.: Center for Disease Control, 1978.

Wallis, C. "The New Scarlet Letter." *Time*, August 2, 1982, pp. 62–69.

Chapter 16: Consumer Health

AMA Special Task Force on Professional Liability and Insurance Action Plan. Chicago: American Medical Association, February 1985.

Bristow, L. R., M. D. *Report of the Council on Medical Service*. Chicago: American Medical Association, 1984.

Cornacchia, H. J., and S. Barrett. *Consumer Health*. 2nd ed. St. Louis: Mosby, 1980.

Erikson, J. D. "Mortality in Cities with Fluoridated and Nonfluoridated Water Supplies." *New England Journal of Medicine*, 298 (May 18, 1978), 112–16.

"Fluoridation: The Cancer Scare/The Attack on Fluoridation." *Consumer Reports*, July 1978 and August 1978.

"The Friendly New Family Doctors." *Time*, July 4, 1977.

"Health Care and Cost." *Harvard Medical School Health Letter*, February 1986, p. 1–4.

"Health Costs: What Limit?" *Time*, May 28, 1978.

Health in the United States: Chartbook. Rockville, Md.: National Center for Health Statistics, 1980.

"Law Allowing Cheaper Prescriptions Takes Effect." *The* [Bergen County, N.J.] *Record*, April 23, 1979.

May, L. "Alternative Medicine Raises Questions about Insurance." *The* [Bergen County, N.J.] *Record*, February 2, 1983.

Nelson, H. E., et al. *A Guide to Consumer Action*. HEW publication no. (OE) 77–18500. Washington, D.C.: U.S. Government Printing Office, 1977.

The Program in Health Services Research. Washington, D.C.: DHEW National Center for Health Services Research, September 1976.

Promoting Health: Issues and Strategies. Regional Forums on Community Health Promotion, January 1979.

Reinhold, R. "As Physician Supply Swells, Health Care in Rural U.S. Shows Sharp Gains." *The New York Times*, July 27, 1982, pp. C1, 4.

"Second Look at Second Opinions." *Time*, January 5, 1981, p. 87.

Sheahy, N. C. "Holistic Medicine." *Forum*, March 1979.

Shubow, M., ed. *Consumer's Resource Handbook*. Pueblo, Colo: Consumer Information Center, December 1979.

Talking to Your Doctor About Diagnosis. Washington, D.C.: U.S. Government Printing Office, 1979.

"U.S. Seeks Tighter Control of Doctors." *The New York Times*, February 4, 1986, p. A21.

Wade, N. "The Hole in Holistic Medicine." *The New York Times*, April 29, 1983, p. A30.

"Weeding Out the Incompetents." *Time*, May 26, 1986, pp. 57–58.

Wolinsky, F. D. *The Sociology of Health: Principles, Professions, and Issues*. Boston: Little, Brown, 1980.

Chapter 17: Environmental Health

"America's Polluted Parks." *Newsweek*, June 3, 1985, p. 27.

Beck, M. "The Toxic-Waste Crisis." *Newsweek*, March 7, 1983, pp. 20–24.

Beranek, L. L. "Noise." *Scientific American*, December 1966, pp. 66–76.

——. *The Hungry Planet*. Rev. ed. New York: Macmillan, 1972.

Brown, M. H. *Laying Waste: The Poisoning of America by Toxic Chemicals*. New York: Pantheon, 1980.

Carson, R. *Silent Spring*, Rev. ed. Greenwich, Conn.: Fawcett, 1978.

Chanlett, E. T. *Environmental Protection*. 2nd ed. New York: McGraw-Hill, 1979.

Church, G. J. "Radiation Sickness." *Time*, October 26, 1981, pp. 18–20.

"Comeback for the Great Lakes." *Time*, December 3, 1979.

Crittenden, A. "World Hunger Is Exacting High Human Toll." *The New York Times*, August 17, 1981, pp. A1, D10.

"Deadly Meltdown." *Time*, May 12, 1986, pp. 39–52.

DeMott, J. S. "An Industry Still in Disarray." *Time*, April 11, 1983, pp. 72f.

Dowling, M. "Defining and Classifying Hazardous Wastes." *Environment*, April 1985, pp. 18–41.

Ehrlich, P. R. *The Population Bomb*. Rev. ed. New York: Ballantine, 1976.

Environmental Quality. 11th Annual Report of the Council on Environmental Quality. Washington, D.C.: U.S. Government Printing Office, 1980.

"The Environmental Quality Index." *National Wildlife*, February–March, 1986, pp. 29–36.

Environmental Trends. Washington, D.C.: U.S. Government Printing Office, 1981.

"E.P.A. Proposes Plan to Curb Asbestos." *The New York Times*, January 24, 1986, p. A12.

Freedman, R., and B. Berelson. "The Human Population." *Scientific American*, September 1974.

Golden, F. "Hideaways for Nuclear Waste." *Time*, March 16, 1981, p. 86.

Hamer, J. "Drinking Water Safety." *Editorial Research Reports*, 1 (February 15, 1974), 121–40.

——. "Environmental Policy." *Editorial Research Reports*, 2 (December 20, 1974), 945–84.

——. "Solid Waste Technology." *Editorial Research Reports*, 2 (August 23, 1974), 641–60.

"How to Track Down Toxins." *Newsweek*, May 6, 1985, p. 81.

Julian, J., and W. Kornblum, *Social Problems*. 5th ed. Englewood Cliffs, N.J.: Prentice-Hall, Inc., 1986.

LeVeen, E. P. Review of U.S. Office of Technology Assessment. *Protecting the Nation's Groundwater from Contamination*. (Washington, D.C.: U.S. Government Printing Office, 1984.) *Environment*, May 1985, pp. 25–27.

Livernash, R. "The Environmental Legislative Agenda," *Environment*, March 1986, pp. 16–39.

Magnuson, E. "The Poisoning of America." *Time*, September 22, 1980, pp. 58–69.

Manning, R. "The Future of Nuclear Power," *Environment*, May 1985, pp. 12–38.

Martin, J. B. Review of (U.S. Office of Technology Assessment. *Managing the Nation's Commercial High-Level Radioactive Waste*. Washington, D.C.: U.S. Government Printing Office, 1985.) *Environment*, July/August 1985, pp. 25–29.

"Midpoint of 'Environmental Decade': Impact of National Policy Act Assessed." *The New York Times*, February 18, 1975, p. 14.

"National Wildlife's Tenth Annual Environmental Quality Index: A Decade of Revolution." *National Wildlife*, February/March 1979, pp.17–32.

Nature Conservancy. Annual Report. Washington, D.C.: U.S. Government Printing Office, 1981.

"Noise Pollution: Irritant of Hazard." *Harvard Medical School Health Letter*, June 1986, pp. 1–4.

" 'Not in My Back Yard': Low-Level Radioactive Waste and Health." *Harvard Medical School Health Letter*, April 1986, pp. 4–6.

Payton, B. M. "Ocean Dumping in the New York Bight," *Environment*, November 1985, pp. 26–31.

"Pollution: Now the Bad News." *Newsweek*, April 8, 1985, p. 26.

"A Problem that Cannot Be Buried." *Time*, October 14, 1985, pp. 76–84.

Reese, M. "Storm Over the Environment." *Newsweek*, March 7, 1983, pp. 16–19.

Schroeder, R. "World Food Needs." *Editorial Research Reports*, 2 (1974), 825–44.

Shabecoff, P. "Lowering of PCB's in Humans Is Found." *The New York Times*, May 10, 1983, pp. A1, 22.

——. "Study of Acid Rain Blames Pollution." *The New York Times*, June 9, 1983, pp. A1, 23.

"State of the Earth, 1985." *Natural History*, April 1985.

Stobaugh, R., and D. Yergin, eds. *Energy Future: Managing and Mismanaging the Future*. Report of the Energy Project at the Harvard Business School. New York: Random House, 1979.

"U.S. Suspends Plan for Nuclear Dump in East or Midwest." *The New York Times*, May 29, 1986, pp. 1, 20.

Woodwell, G. M. "Toxic Substances and Ecological Cycles." *Scientific American*, March 1967, pp. 24–31.

"World Population: Silent Explosion." *U.S. Department of State Bulletin*, October, November, and December 1978.

Acknowledgments

PHOTOGRAPHS

Cover: The Stock Shop

Title Page: Bicycling Magazine/Sally Shenk Ullman

Introduction: 1 C.E. Pefley.

Chapter 1: 5 Ken Karp. 10 Ken Karp. 12 Ken Karp. 14 AFL-CIO News. 15 Laimute E. Druskis. 18 Laimute E. Druskis. 23 Irene Springer. 25 Ed Lettau/Photo Researchers. 31 Susan Rosenberg/Photo Researchers. 33 Ken Karp. 35 Jean-Marie Simon/Taurus Photos.

Chapter 2: 41 Ken Karp. 45 Bertina Crone/Photo Researchers. 48 Arthur Tress/Photo Researchers. 49 Laimute E. Druskis. 52 Laimute E. Druskis. 56 Nancy Hays/Monkmeyer. 59 Irene Bayer/Monkmeyer. 61 A.T. & T. Co. Photo Center.

Chapter 3: 65 George E. Jones III/Photo Researchers. 68 Laimute E. Druskis. 70 Susan Ylvisaker/Jeroboam. 71 Michael Habicht/Taurus Photos. 72 Will McIntyre/Photo Researchers. 76 U.S. Coast Guard Official Photo. 78 Jerry Howard/Stock, Boston.

Chapter 4: 83 Ken Karp. 84 Marc P. Anderson. 88 © 1987 by Sidney Harris, *Medical Opinion.* 93 Ken Karp. 97 National Park Service. 98 Laimute E. Druskis. 99 Laimute E. Druskis. 103 Nautilus Sports/Medical Industries.

Chapter 5: 105 © 1983 Will McIntyre/Photo Researchers. 109 John Isaac, United Nations. 118 Top left, top right, and bottom left are USDA photos. Bottom right is by Laimute E. Druskis. 119 Ed Lettau/Photo Researchers. 120 Laimute E. Druskis. 123 Teri Leigh Stratford. 127 © 1986; reprinted courtesy of Bill Hoest and *Parade* Magazine.

Chapter 6: 133 Barbara Rios/Photo Researchers. 138 Teri Leigh Stratford. 141 Bonnie Schiffman/Gamma-Liaison (as previously used in John Darley et al., *Psychology,* 3rd ed. [Prentice-Hall, 1986]. 143 Drawing by Booth; © 1986, The New York Magazine, Inc. 146 Teri Leigh Stratford. 152 Peter G. Aitken/Photo Researchers.

Chapter 7: 155 Erika Stone/Photo Researchers. 166 A. L. L. Doyle, Ph.D.; J. Lippes, M.D.; H. S. Winters, M.D.; A. J. Margolis, M.D./Courtesy of Department of Gynecology-Obstetrics, the State University of New York at Buffalo. B–D. Carnegie Institution of Washington. 169 Nancy Durrell McKenna/Photo Researchers. 172 E. Mandelmann, WHO photos. 175 Eric Neurath/Stock, Boston. 176 Teri Leigh Stratford. 178 Left: Catholics for a Free Choice. Right: Eugene Gordon. 186 Nancy Durrell McKenna/Photo Researchers. 189 Teri Leigh Stratford; materials courtesy of Planned Parenthood, NYC.

Chapter 8: 199 Joseph Szabo/Photo Researchers. 202 Alice Kandell/Photo Researchers. 205 Ken Karp. 206 Ken Karp. 210 Courtesy Museum of Fine Arts, Boston. 212 Laimute E. Druskis. 216 Robert Goldstein/Photo Researchers.

Chapter 9: 223 Barbara Rios/Photo Researchers. 226 Teri Leigh Stratford/Photo Researchers. 227 Alyeska Pipeline Service Company. 229 Susan Rosenberg/Photo Researchers. 231 Ken Karp.

235 Susan Rosenberg/Photo Researchers. 238 Suzanne Szasz/Photo Researchers. 241 Drawing by Stan Hunt. © 1983 by The New Yorker Magazine, Inc. 245 Ken Karp. 247 Children's Defense Fund.

Chapter 10: 251 Ken Karp, Sirovich Senior Center. 254 Colonial Penn Group, Inc. 260 Ken Karp, Sirovich Senior Center. 261 Ken Karp. 263 Charles Gatewood. 266 RSVP/Action/Vetter. 270 Ken Karp. 271 Ann Hagen Griffiths, Omni-Photo Communications. 274 Thomas S. England/ Photo Researchers.

Chapter 11: 279 Laimute E. Druskis. 281 Wine Institute. 283 Laimute E. Druskis. 288 Ken Karp. 289 Charles Gatewood. 290 Alice Kandell/Photo Researchers. 293 Marc P. Anderson.

Chapter 12: 307 Sherry Suris/Photo Researchers. 312 WHO photo. 316 Monique Manceau/Photo Researchers. 321 American Cancer Society. 325 Eric Kroll/Taurus Photos. 326 Getsug/Anderson/ Photo Researchers.

Chapter 13: 329 Michael Kagan/Monkmeyer. 334 Bob Englehart, The Hartford Courant, © 1986 Copley News Service. 342 Drug Enforcement Administration. 343 Charles Gatewood. 349 Marc P. Anderson. 351 Ken Karp. 356 Eric Kroll/Taurus Photos. 358 Laimute E. Druskis.

Chapter 14: 363 Nancy J. Pierce/Photo Researchers. 367 New York Blood Center. 369 American Heart Association. 370 Courtesy of the National Institute of Health. 371 Ken Karp. 376 American Dairy Association. 387 American Cancer Society. 392 American Cancer Society.

Chapter 15: 399 Fred Lombardi/Photo Researchers. 402 Ray Ellis/Photo Researchers. 405 Carmine L. Galasso. 413 Courtesy National Library of Medicine. 416 Courtesy of the Department of Health, New York. 422 Bob Mahoney. 425 Jim Wilson, Woodfin Camp.

Chapter 16: 429 Ken Karp. 434 Laimute E. Druskis. 436 Ken Karp. 439 Ellen Pines Sheffield/ Woodfin Camp 1980. 442 Jim Harrison/Stock, Boston. 444 Ken Karp. 449 Laimute E. Druskis. 455 Owen Franken/Stock, Boston.

Chapter 17: 465 WHO photo by J. Mohr. 470 Marc P. Anderson. 474 Laimute C. Druskis. 476 Charles Gatewood. 478 Meryl Joseph. 479 Drawing by Stevenson; © 1970 The New Yorker Magazine, Inc. 481 USDA. 482 Georg Gerster, Rapho/Photo Researchers. 486 Eric Kroll/Taurus Photo. 490 Charles Gatewood. 496 A.T. & T. Co. Photo Center. 499 Reprinted with special permission of King Features Syndicate, Inc. 500 New York State Energy Research and Development Authority. 502 United Nations/ILO.

Appendix: 505 From Harvey Grant et al., Emergency Care, 4th ed. (Prentice-Hall, 1986). 508 American Red Cross.

Index